Clinical Anesth...
Procedures of t...
Massachusetts ...

Morgan—
Hoping for a speedy
recovery.

David J Stone MD

3/8/88

Clinical Anesthesia Procedures of the Massachusetts General Hospital

Third Edition

**Department of Anesthesia
Massachusetts General Hospital
Harvard Medical School**

**Edited by
Leonard L. Firestone, M.D.**

**Philip W. Lebowitz, M.D.
Charles E. Cook, M.D.**

**Little, Brown and Company
Boston/Toronto**

To

Richard J. Kitz, M.D.,
Henry Isaiah Dorr Professor and Chairman,
Department of Anesthesia, Massachusetts
General Hospital, for his devoted interest
in resident education and continued support
for the contributors to this manual.

Contents

Preface

The third edition of the *Clinical Anesthesia Procedures of the Massachusetts General Hospital* was undertaken by the house staff of the Department of Anaesthesia to reflect the most current practices at the Massachusetts General Hospital, the Massachusetts Eye and Ear Infirmary, the Shriners Burns Institute, the Cambridge Hospital, and the Brigham and Women's Hospital. The emphasis is still on the practical "fundamentals" involved in administering anesthesia, which, judging by the success of the previous editions, are often best conveyed by those who most recently experienced the learning process.

Like its predecessors, this Third Edition was written with the assumption that the reader has some prior knowledge of anesthesia equipment, airway management, and intubation techniques. Given this starting point, the manual is intended to be an easily accessible source of accurate, practical knowledge for anesthesiologists, anesthesia residents or nurse anesthetists in training programs, and medical students, as well as nurses, respiratory therapists, and other health professionals who provide patient care in an ICU or recovery room setting. This manual is not meant to be used as a surrogate for an experienced, knowledgeable, clinical supervisor, nor can it substitute for the exhaustive tomes that are referenced later on in the Suggested Reading sections.

Although anesthesia procedures receive the most attention, the section dealing with Preanesthetic Evaluation of patients has been expanded in the third edition. For this section, which includes three new chapters addressing the specific preanesthetic considerations that apply to patients with pulmonary, endocrine, or infectious diseases, the authors are greatly indebted to the following faculty readers who contributed valuable critical discussion and editorial comment: Drs. Robert Schneider, Henning Pontoppidan, William Latta, Sarita Walzer, and Daniel Carr, as well as Dr. Cyrus Hopkins of the Infectious Diseases Unit, M.G.H. The Administration of Anesthesia section contains new chapters on "Safety in Anesthesia," "Ambulatory Procedures," "Trauma and Burns," and "Recovery Room"; the authors gratefully acknowledge the contributions of Drs. Carl Rosow, Hassan Ali, John Savarese, Elliott Miller, Nabil Fahmy, J. Kenneth Davison, Roger Wilson, Michael D'Ambra, Nathaniel Sims, John Donlon, Gregory Crosby, Susan Firestone, Daniel Nozik, William Latta, S. K. Szyfelbein, David Cullen, and Drs. Benjamin Covino and Sanjay Datta of the Department of Anesthesia, Brigham and Women's Hospital. The final section, Patient Care in Other Settings, owes much to the input of Drs. I. David Todres, Roger Wilson, and Donald Todd, and contains a useful, entirely new chapter entitled "Pain."

To bring the manual up to the minute, there are also sections devoted to new diagnostic studies (e.g., noninvasive cardiac radionuclide tests), recently introduced drugs (midazolam, sufentanil, etomidate, and many others), the latest monitoring devices (pulse oximeters, capnographs, mass spectrometers, evoked-potential monitors), new anesthetic and surgical techniques (e.g., epidural and intrathecal administration of narcotics, laser airway surgery), discussions of important new policy guidelines (the FDA's "Anesthesia Apparatus Checkout Recommendations"; the "Standards of Practice for Minimal Monitoring" from Harvard Medical School's Department of Anesthesia; obtaining informed consent), and recommendations for managing patients with acquired immunodeficiency syndrome, outpatients, in vitro fertilization, and nonobstetrical surgery during pregnancy, extracorporeal shock wave lithotripsy, major thoracic vascular procedures, cardiopulmonary bypass, limb reimplantation, and organ (kidney, liver, heart, pancreas) transplantation. But this manual's raison d'etre remains the essentials of clinical anesthesia practice. Toward this end, the sections on endotracheal intubation and uptake of inhalation anesthetics have been expanded and enhanced by illustrations, and there are several useful new tables summarizing the clinical pharmacology of local anesthetics, narcotics, relaxants, and vasoactive infusions.

Special thanks are in order for Marissa Seligman, Pharm. D.Ph., Coordinator of Drug Information Services, M.G.H. and Susan Firestone, M.D., for providing information used in the Drug Appendix; Sara Williamson for stoically preparing the manuscript; Paul Andriesse for the expert illustrations; and Susan Pioli and her colleagues at Little, Brown and Company for advice and counsel all through this project.

L.L.F.
P.W.L.
C.E.C.

Clinical Anesthesia Procedures of the Massachusetts General Hospital

Evaluating the Patient Before Anesthesia

1

General Preanesthetic Evaluation

Leonard L. Firestone

The **overall goal** of the preoperative visit is to reduce perioperative morbidity and mortality. Its **specific objectives** include (1) becoming familiar with the present surgical illness and coexisting medical conditions, (2) establishing a doctor-patient relationship, (3) developing a management strategy for pre-, intra-, and postanesthetic care, (4) obtaining informed consent for the anesthesia plan, and (5) communicating the results of the preanesthetic evaluation in the permanent hospital record.

I. Chart review
A. History
  1. The in-hospital course usually reveals the most pertinent aspects of the **present surgical illness;** for example, has the illness led to serious intravascular volume depletion? What is the working diagnosis? What organ systems are affected?
  2. **Past medical illnesses.** Prior discharge summaries are especially useful for an overview of coexisting medical problems. Medical illnesses may complicate the surgical course and impair compensatory mechanisms.
     a. Specific preanesthetic considerations with coexisting cardiac, respiratory, hepatic, renal, endocrine, or infectious diseases are found in Chaps. 2–7.
     b. It may be appropriate to **request a consultation** from another service; consultants are most valuable when answering specific questions concerning interpretation of special laboratory studies, unfamiliar drug or other therapies, or changes from the baseline in a patient's status. Consultants should not be asked for a general "clearance" for anesthesia; this is the specific responsibility of the anesthesiologist.
     c. **Medications** may be used to treat the present or coexisting illnesses; the doses and schedules must be ascertained. When feasible, substitutions with shorter-acting preparations should be made in the perianesthetic period, to simplify interpretation of the clinical responses to anesthesia.
        (1) Whether to continue **chronic medications** preoperatively depends on the particular illness and the consequences of discontinuing the drug, the half-life of drug effects, and the importance of interactions with anesthetic agents. Specific medications used to treat diabetes melli-

tus, hypertension, angina pectoris, and other common diseases are discussed in Chaps. 2–7.

(2) Certain rare but important **drug interactions** must be anticipated because of their life-threatening nature; for example, thiopental may precipitate a fatal episode of acute intermittent porphyria, and meperidine may produce a hypertensive crisis when administered to patients treated with monoamine oxidase inhibitors.

3. **Prior surgical procedures.** Old anesthesia records should be checked for
   a. Responses to sedating premedications and anesthetic agents.
   b. Ease of laryngoscopy, and the size and type of blade and endotracheal tube used.
   c. Location of prior vascular cannulations.
   d. Prior blood transfusions.
   e. Intraanesthetic complications including allergies, dental trauma, and even surgical difficulties.

4. **Allergies.** Dysphoric responses to **morphine** are common but usually are not a manifestation of allergy; however, other opioids are available, and it is prudent to make a substitution. Many drugs besides anesthetics are administered intraoperatively, some of which (e.g., **antibiotics**) have substantial incidences of true allergy or other significant side effects. Even **food allergies** may be important; for example, allergy to **fish** may be associated with deleterious responses to protamine, a fish-derived protein preparation.

B. **Laboratory studies.** Batteries of "routine" laboratory screening tests rarely uncover abnormalities not already apparent from the history and physical examination and do little to improve patient care or even provide medicolegal protection.

1. A recent hemoglobin or hematocrit determination is evaluated in all patients.

2. For healthy adults over 40 years old, an **electrocardiogram (ECG)** is obtained prior to anesthesia.

3. A **chest x-ray** is obtained only when clinically indicated; for example, from heavy smokers, the elderly, and patients with major organ system disease, cardiac or respiratory symptoms, or occupational exposures.

4. Electrolytes, BUN, glucose, liver function and pregnancy tests, and coagulation profiles (prothrombin time for patients receiving warfarin, partial thromboplastin time for heparin, bleeding time for aspirin and other nonsteroidal anti-inflammatory compounds) are added to the screening regimen only when specifically indicated by the history and physical examination.

5. An **abnormal preoperative test result** may be associated with a significant risk of perioperative morbidity and is thus one of the most common reasons that elective surgery is unexpectedly postponed.

   a. There is no universally accepted **minimum hematocrit prior to anesthesia.** Hematocrits in the 25–30% range are usually well tolerated by otherwise healthy people but may result in ischemia in patients with coronary or cerebral vascular disease. Each case must be evaluated individually for the etiology and duration of anemia. With certain chronic illnesses (e.g., a hemoglobinopathy or chronic renal failure), transfusion may be unnecessary because other mechanisms that maximize tissue oxygen delivery compensate for reduced red cell mass.

   b. **Hypokalemia** is frequently found during treatment with thiazide diuretics. Preoperative therapy should be aimed toward repleting potassium stores, but efforts to normalize the serum potassium completely by rapid or excessive KCl administration may lead to arrhythmias and even cardiac standstill.

   c. An **abnormal ECG** should be evaluated by comparing it to previous tracings, carefully correlating cardiac signs and symptoms, and often, consulting with a cardiologist. The new onset of ECG abnormalities that are likely to alter anesthetic management include atrial fibrillation or flutter; second- or third-degree atrioventricular block; ST- or T-wave changes indicating myocardial ischemia; premature ventricular contractions (PVCs), particularly if multifocal, coupled, or in runs; or frequent premature atrial contractions (PACs).

II. **The anesthesiologist-patient relationship**

   A. Certain obstacles are inherent in the anesthesiologist's rapport with a patient. Patients may feel that the anesthesiologist spends less time caring for them than do other doctors, since patients are unconscious during the period when the anesthesiologist contributes most to treatment. Also, pre- and postoperative interviews may be conducted by staff members other than those who administer the anesthetic, and overall, the perioperative period is an emotionally stressful time for many patients and their families. Fortunately, a thorough, unhurried, and well-organized preoperative interview can overcome these intrinsic difficulties and elevate the anesthesiologist to the position of trusted and respected physician.

   B. Ideally, the individual who is to administer anesthesia should perform the preoperative evaluation. This helps to establish rapport and provides many patients with an extra measure of confidence. If the interviewer will not administer the anesthetic, the patient should be so informed but then reassured that the anesthesiologist will be of equal competence and fully aware of the results of the interview.

C. A patient's permission for, and cooperation during, special procedures (e.g., placement of invasive monitoring catheters, regional or local nerve blocks) often hinge on the relationship achieved during the preoperative visit.

III. Patient interview
A. History

1. Certain relatively common conditions contribute disproportionately to perianesthetic morbidity and mortality, and consequently should be elicited as **pertinent negatives.**

   a. **Asthma** may produce acute severe bronchospasm following induction of anesthesia or endotracheal intubation or be accompanied by cor pulmonale and/or susceptibility to pneumonia.

   b. Untreated **hypertension** (particularly a diastolic blood pressure of greater than 110 mm Hg) is associated with blood pressure lability during anesthesia and a greater incidence of postoperative cardiovascular complications; for this reason, postponement of elective surgery may be warranted until effective treatment is implemented. Diuretic therapy often leads to hypovolemia and electrolyte imbalances.

   c. **Hiatal hernia** with esophageal reflux symptoms increases the risk of pulmonary aspiration.

   d. Patients with **angina pectoris** may respond to intubation and painful surgical stimuli with myocardial ischemia, ventricular dysfunction, or frank myocardial infarction.

   e. **Other conditions** in specific patient populations (e.g., sickle cell anemia, glucose-6-phosphate dehydrogenase deficiency).

2. **Previous anesthetics,** including those administered for dental or obstetrical procedures, are detailed along with the patient's perception of these experiences.

3. A **review of systems** should explore the practical implications of any problems elucidated earlier.

   a. Orthopnea or arthritis may be too severe for the patient to tolerate lying flat on the operating room (OR) table either before induction or during regional anesthesia; a highly productive morning cough may indicate the need for pre- and postoperative chest physiotherapy.

   b. Since dental and peripheral nerve traumas are two of the most common anesthesia-related injuries, the condition of the teeth and relevant neurological evaluation should be assiduously explored for preexisting injury or disease. Similarly, a patient with chronic headaches is a likely candidate to have postspinal anesthesia

headache, independent of the dural puncture.
4. **Allergy**
   a. Patients reporting an "allergy" to **halothane** or **succinylcholine** may actually mean that either they or a close family member has malignant hyperthermia (see Chap. 28); similarly those "allergic" to **droperidol** may have the malignant neuroleptic syndrome.
   b. True allergy to **amide-type local anesthetics** is exceedingly rare, although a syncopal episode in the dentist's chair or intravascular injection during anesthesia for any procedure may erroneously lead to such a diagnosis. Allergy to **ester-type agents** does occur with slightly greater frequency and can produce anaphylaxis (see Chap. 12).
   c. Allergy to Pentothal may be indicative of true allergy, or represent a wide variety of nonallergic reactions to anesthesia, including vomiting, malaise, and slow awakening.
5. **Social histories** may reveal **tobacco, drug, or alcohol abuse.**
   a. Eliminating cigarettes for 2–4 weeks preoperatively may reduce the incidence of pulmonary complications postoperatively; excessive consumption accompanied by exercise intolerance suggests the need for preoperative pulmonary function testing.
   b. Chronic alcoholism may be accompanied by (1) functional tolerance to anesthetics (i.e., more anesthesia is needed to produce loss of consciousness than in other patients); (2) dispositional tolerance to anesthetics (i.e., hepatic metabolism of drugs is enhanced); (3) abnormal liver function tests; (4) portal hypertension; or (5) delirium tremens or seizures in the perianesthetic period.
   c. Aspects of the **employment history** may be relevant as well; it is inadvisable to use spinal anesthesia in patients who have been disabled from back ailments.
6. **Family histories** may be positive for malignant hyperthermia, which is a potentially fatal genetic disease. Moreover, any time an operation has led to the loss of a family member, whether from incurable disease or iatrogenic mishap, the experience may lead to an understandable antipathy toward anesthesia.
B. **Physical examination** for every patient should consist of
   1. All **vital signs.**
      a. **Height** and **weight** are necessary to estimate therapeutic and toxic drug dosages (in mg/kg) and to calculate the cardiac index (in $L/min/m^2$) and urine output (in ml/kg/min).

    b. Blood pressures are obtained in both arms if a reason for asymmetry exists (e.g., prior cutdowns or congenital, atherosclerotic, and other disease of the aorta or its major branches).

2. Head and neck. Evaluation should include

    a. The size of the **oral aperture** and the size of the **tongue** relative to the mouth.

    b. Dentition, especially for chipped, loose, false, capped, or missing teeth. Loose teeth may be disrupted during laryngoscopy; caps may not endure the stresses of biting against an oral airway during emergence from inhalation anesthesia. False teeth should be removed prior to arrival in the OR unless special arrangements have been made at the patient's request.

    c. Ranges-of-motion of the temporomandibular joints and cervical spine (in three planes). Limitation may help to anticipate a difficult intubation (see Chap. 10).

    d. The distance between the thyroid cartilage and the chin, which should be 3 fingerbreadths with the head in neutral position. This distance may be only 2 fingerbreadths or less in an individual with a receding jaw and may help predict difficulty with intubation.

    e. The length of the neck.

    f. The position of the trachea, whether midline or deviated, and its mobility.

    g. The patency of both nasal passages (when nasal intubation is contemplated).

    h. The carotid arteries in elderly patients, for evidence of bruits; a newly discovered bruit may indicate the need for further workup, particularly when accompanied by symptoms.

3. Heart and **lungs** should be auscultated in all patients; further details may be found in Chaps. 2 and 3.

4. Extremities. The presence of pulses, acrocyanosis, previous peripheral catheterizations, and areas of phlebitis should be noted. Needle insertion sites for regional anesthesia or invasive monitoring devices should also be inspected for local infection, cellulitis, evidence of prior trauma, or deformity.

C. Counseling the patient

1. The anesthesiologist informs the patient of the following:

    a. The time after which the patient must have nothing to eat or drink.

    b. The estimated time of surgery.

    c. That premedication will be given, including the route and time of administration, or that no premedication will be given.

    d. That after transport to the OR, the anesthesiologist in the OR will place an IV catheter; apply a blood pressure cuff, electrodes for the ECG, and a sensor for the pulse oximeter; and insert additional monitoring catheters (if appropriate).

 e. That following surgery, the patient will be brought to the recovery room.

 f. That the anesthesiologist, or another member of the anesthesia care team, will visit again following surgery.

 2. Counseling should be restricted to the endeavors specific to anesthesiologists; the surgeon is responsible for conveying opinions regarding the diagnosis, prognosis, and postoperative treatment plans.

D. Obtaining informed consent involves discussing the anesthesia management plan, alternatives, and potential complications in terms understandable to the lay person.

 1. Management may involve sophisticated regional anesthesia techniques, intubation, or vascular cannulation while awake, transfusion of blood products other than red blood cells, postoperative mechanical ventilation, or transfer to an intensive care unit. Such clinical plans are usually outside the realm of experience for lay people and therefore must be explicitly defined and discussed to obtain informed consent.

 2. The alternatives to the suggested management plan must be presented, even those that may be more dangerous than the one recommended. An alternative approach may become necessary if the planned anesthesia procedure fails or if there is a sudden change in clinical circumstances or the patient's ability to cooperate.

 3. It is also the anesthesiologist's duty to disclose the **risks** associated with the anesthesia procedure that a reasonable person in the patient's position would find material in making a decision. In general, disclosure applies to complications that occur with a relatively **high frequency** or produce **severe sequelae** rather than to all remotely possible risks.

  a. The anesthesiologist should become familiar with the incidences of the most frequent and severe complications associated with commonly employed anesthesia procedures, including (but not limited to) (1) **spinal anesthesia** (headache, neurotrauma, meningitis, arachnoiditis, respiratory arrest); (2) **lumbar epidural anesthesia** (inadvertent dural puncture, massive subarachnoid injection, intravascular injection, broken catheters, epidural hematoma or infection, and headache); (3) **general anesthesia** (aspiration pneumonitis, brain damage, cardiovascular collapse, neural and dental trauma, halothane-associated hepatitis); (4) **blood transfusion** (infection, febrile or hemolytic reaction); and (5) **vascular cannulations** (arterial or venous compromise, pneumothorax). Further detail may be found in the reference by Orkin and Cooperman in **Suggested Readings.**

  b. In cases where these risks have not been objectively defined, the patient should be so informed.

  4. Under certain extenuating circumstances, anesthesia procedures may proceed without informed consent (e.g., in dire emergency) or with limited consent (e.g., transfusion consent withheld by patients of the Jehovah's Witness faith). In such cases, it is prudent to notify the Chief of Anesthesia or his designate and the hospital administration at once.

IV. The note in the hospital record

  A. The preoperative note in the permanent hospital record is a medicolegal document containing the anesthesiologist's preoperative evaluation.

  B. Given this status, the note should contain

   1. A concise statement of the date and time of the interview and the proposed procedure, and a description of any extraordinary circumstances (e.g., an anesthetizing location outside of the OR suite).

   2. The most relevant positive and negative findings from the history, physical examination, and laboratory studies.

   3. A **problem list** that clearly delineates all disease processes and treatments and any abnormal physical or laboratory findings and allergies.

   4. An overall impression of the complexity of the patient's medical condition, which is derived from the problem list and often summarized by assignment of one of the **American Society of Anesthesiologists (ASA) Physical Status Classes:**

    a. Class 1: healthy patient.

    b. Class 2: patient with a mild systemic disease.

    c. Class 3: patient with a severe systemic disease that limits activity but is not incapacitating.

    d. Class 4: patient with an incapacitating systemic disease that is a constant threat to life.

    e. Class 5: a moribund patient not expected to survive 24 hours with or without operation.

    f. If the procedure is performed as an emergency, an *E* is added to the appropriate ASA Physical Status.

   5. **The anesthesia plan,** which is used to convey suggestions for additional preoperative studies or management strategies to make the patient ready for the procedure and to communicate the anesthesiologist's opinions regarding special needs for preoperative medications, intraoperative monitoring, transfusion or drugs, and postoperative care.

V. Premedication

  A. The **goals** of administering sedatives and analgesics prior to surgery are to allay the patient's anxiety; prevent pain during vascular cannulation, regional anesthesia procedures, or positioning; and facilitate a smooth induction of anesthesia. It has been shown that the requirement for these drugs is reduced after a good preoperative visit by an anesthesiologist.

1. Dosages of premedicants are reduced in elderly, debilitated, and acutely intoxicated patients, as well as those with Down's syndrome, upper airway obstruction, or severe pulmonary, central nervous system, or valvular heart disease.

2. Patients addicted to narcotics or barbiturates should be premedicated with enough of the relevant drug to prevent withdrawal from occurring during, or shortly after, anesthesia.

3. Premedication regimens developed for patients with specific illnesses are discussed in Chaps. 2–7.

4. Premedication administration for outpatient surgery is considered in Chaps. 10 and 24.

B. Sedatives

1. **Barbiturates. Pentobarbital** (Nembutal) and **secobarbital** (Seconal) are intermediate-acting barbiturates that are sedative and hypnotic but not analgesic; in dosages of 1–4 mg/kg (up to 200 mg) IM, they depress respiratory drive but have little effect on cardiovascular function. They may be used alone or in combination with narcotics or other sedatives or anticholinergics. The onset of effects is within 30 minutes; duration is 2–3 hours. These agents should not be used in suspected cases of acute intermittent porphyria.

2. **Benzodiazepines. Diazepam** (Valium) and **lorazepam** (Ativan) are effective tranquilizers that rarely produce significant cardiovascular or respiratory depression when used at the recommended dosages in healthy patients. Diazepam (5–15 mg PO) and lorazepam (1–4 mg IM or PO) may be used alone or in combination with other classes of premedication. Diazepam should not be given IM because injection is painful and absorption by this route is unpredictable. However, **midazolam** (Versed) is a newer, water-soluble benzodiazepine that may be administered IM (1–5 mg). Lorazepam and midazolam seem to have greater sedative and amnestic properties than diazepam without increased respiratory depression.

3. **Droperidol** (Inapsine) is a butyrophenone that produces long-acting sedation (peak is at 30–60 minutes after IM injection) in dosages of 0.03–0.14 mg/kg IM, alone or in combination with a narcotic. Droperidol has potent antiemetic activity, and low doses (1.25–2.5 mg IV in adults) seem to prevent postoperative nausea and vomiting caused by narcotics. Droperidol produces mild systemic vasodilatation from alpha-adrenergic blockade and, occasionally, extrapyramidal symptoms from its an-

tidopaminergic effects. Particularly when used alone, droperidol may also cause an unpleasant dissociative reaction, which is sometimes reversible with physostigmine (Antilirium), 1–2 mg IV, a centrally active cholinesterase inhibitor.

4. The phenothiazine **promethazine** (Phenergan) and the piperazine **hydroxyzine** (Vistaril), in doses of 25–75 mg IM, are mild tranquilizers, antiemetics, and H_1 blockers; they also potentiate the sedating and analgesic properties of narcotics. Lower doses (25 mg IM) are selected when given in combination with narcotics.

C. **Narcotics**

1. **Morphine** has both analgesic and sedative properties. It causes little cardiac depression, although it may produce hypotension through histamine-mediated vasodilatation. Morphine depresses the medullary response to carbon dioxide and causes respiration to be slow and deep. Other effects include pupillary constriction and sometimes nausea and vomiting. Occasionally, morphine may cause spasm of the sphincter of Oddi, so it is prudent to avoid its use in the presence of biliary tract disease. The typical dosage range is 0.1–0.2 mg/kg IM, often in combination with an antisialagogue or antiemetic. Patients with valvular heart disease are frequently premedicated with morphine, 0.05–0.07 mg/kg IM, in combination with scopolamine, 0.3–0.4 mg IM. Peak effects after IM doses are reached in 30–60 minutes, with analgesia lasting 4–5 hours; effects from IV doses begin almost immediately.

2. **Meperidine** (Demerol) is an analgesic that is one-tenth as potent as morphine (1.0–1.5 mg/kg IM is used for premedication). It is less sedating than morphine, so it is often combined with promethazine or hydroxyzine. Meperidine is vagolytic and may increase the heart rate; compared to morphine it seems to produce less hypotension, nausea, vomiting, and sphincter of Oddi spasm.

D. **Anticholinergics**

1. As premedication **atropine** is given primarily for its antisialagogue properties, in dosages of 0.4–0.6 mg IM for full-sized adults. Decreasing oral secretions may reduce the likelihood of laryngospasm during ketamine anesthesia or when using an irritating inhalation agent like diethyl ether. Most patients find the dry mouth sensation unpleasant, and atropine use in patients with chronic bronchitis or cystic fibrosis may lead to inspissation of mucus with plugging of small airways. Atropine premedication is sometimes employed in children to prevent the bradycardia associated with laryngoscopy and succinylcholine use; however, such protection is more reliably achieved when atropine is adminis-

tered IV immediately prior to induction. In young children, atropine may also produce flushing and exacerbation of fever.

2. **Glycopyrrolate** (Robinul) acts as an antisialagogue and inhibits the cardiac vagal reflexes during induction and intubation when used at doses of 0.2–0.3 mg IM or IV. It is also efficacious in reducing the volume and acidity of gastric fluid, and thus it provides some protection against pulmonary aspiration (see sec. **E**). Glycopyrrolate's structure contains a quaternary ammonium (i.e., charged ion), which hinders crossing the blood-brain barrier; thus there are essentially no central nervous system side effects.

3. **Scopolamine** (0.3–0.4 mg IM in adults) is a centrally active anticholinergic with potent sedative, antisialagogue, and antiemetic properties, particularly when used in combination with morphine. Scopolamine can occasionally produce delirium, hallucinations, and prolonged somnolence due to the "central anticholinergic syndrome"; such manifestations are usually reversible with physostigmine (1–2 mg IV).

E. **Prophylaxis for pulmonary aspiration** may be beneficial for patients at high risk for aspiration pneumonitis, including the parturient, and those with a hiatal hernia and reflux symptoms, "difficult" airways, ileus, obesity, or central nervous system depression.

1. **Histamine H_2 antagonists** produce a dose-related decrease in basal, nocturnal, and stimulated gastric acid production. Cimetidine (Tagamet), 200–400 mg PO/IM/IV, and ranitidine (Zantac), 150–300 mg PO or 50–100 mg IM/IV, significantly reduce both the volume of gastric juice secreted and its hydrogen ion concentration. Multidose regimens (i.e., the night before and morning of anesthesia) are most effective, although parenteral administration may be used to achieve a rapid (1 hour) onset. Cimetidine has been shown to prolong the elimination of diazepam, theophylline, propranolol, and lidocaine; ranitidine has not been associated with such side effects and is just as effective and longer acting than cimetidine.

2. **Nonparticulate antacids.** Colloidal antacid suspensions are the most effective neutralizers of stomach acid but can produce serious pneumonias if aspirated. Nonsuspension antacids, such as citric acid solutions, may be somewhat less effective in raising gastric pH, but their aspiration is less harmful.

3. **Metoclopramide** (Reglan) is a cholinergic stimulant, which in doses of 10 mg IV can improve gastric emptying in parturients requiring elective or emergency cesarean delivery. The role of this "gastrokinetic" in other populations at high risk, either

alone or in combination with an oral antacid or an H_2-receptor antagonist, is currently under investigation.

F. Preoperative administration of **chronic medications** (e.g., insulin, beta blockers, nitrates, antihypertensives, digitalis) is discussed in Chaps. 2–7.

Suggested Reading

Egbert, L. D. et al. The value of the preoperative visit by an anesthetist. *J.A.M.A.* 185:553, 1963.

New classification of physical status. *Anesthesiology* 24:111, 1963.

Orkin, F. K., and Cooperman, L. H. (eds.). *Complications in Anesthesiology*. Philadelphia: Lippincott, 1983.

Vandam, L. D. *To Make the Patient Ready for Anesthesia: Medical Care of the Surgical Patient*. Menlo Park, Calif.: Addison Wesley, 1980.

White, P. F. Pharmacologic and clinical aspects of preoperative medication. *Anesth. Analg.* 65:963, 1986.

2

Specific Considerations with Cardiac Disease

John Pawlowski

I. **Coronary artery disease.** Since the heart is an aerobic organ, the balance between myocardial oxygen supply and demand becomes critical in the presence of coronary artery disease (CAD). When myocardial oxygen demand outweighs supply, ischemia results. Both prevention and treatment involve improvement of this balance.

  A. **Determinants of myocardial oxygen demand**

   1. **Myocardial wall tension,** by the law of Laplace, is directly proportional to the chamber's distending pressure and internal radius and is inversely proportional to the wall thickness.

      a. **Preload** refers to the ventricular end-diastolic volume (EDV), which determines the end-diastolic fiber length. This in turn profoundly affects myocardial performance.

      b. **Afterload** is the force distributed in the ventricular wall during ejection; it is usually equated with the ventricular pressure during ejection and varies with time. However, it is more precisely defined by wall tension and is therefore dependent on radius as well. Lowering the EDV decreases wall tension, decreasing myocardial oxygen consumption ($M\dot{V}O_2$). Nitroglycerin, morphine, and sodium nitroprusside can accomplish this goal.

   2. **Contractility** is the ability of the myocardium to develop force and is independent of the load on the heart.

      a. **In the normal heart,** sympathetic stimulation and inotropes increase myocardial contractility and $M\dot{V}O_2$. If wall tension is constant, decreasing contractility will decrease $M\dot{V}O_2$. Calcium antagonists, beta blockers, and inhalational anesthetics decrease $M\dot{V}O_2$ in this fashion.

      b. **In the distended and failing ventricle,** increased contractility may improve emptying and reduce ventricular size and wall tension. $M\dot{V}O_2$ may then actually fall; catecholamines can work in this manner.

   3. **Heart rate** increases $M\dot{V}O_2$ by increasing the number of contractions per minute, even though myocardial oxygen demand per beat decreases. Beta blockers can effectively lower heart rate.

  B. **Determinants of myocardial oxygen supply**

   1. **Coronary blood flow** is determined by the perfusion pressure across the coronary vascular bed divided by the total coronary resistance.

      a. **Coronary perfusion pressure** (CPP) is the difference between aortic diastolic pressure and left ventricular end-diastolic pressure (LVEDP). The actual pressure usually is lower distal to a coronary stenosis.

   b. Total coronary artery **resistance** consists in the autoregulatory resistance, which is influenced by sympathetic tone and autoregulatory factors (tissue pH, PO_2, PCO_2), the basal resistance during diastole, and the compressive resistance during systole.

   c. The <u>subendocardium</u> is especially vulnerable to ischemia because it has the greatest metabolic demands, the poorest blood flow, and the greatest compressive resistance in the heart.

2. Heart rate. Coronary filling time decreases when the heart rate increases; this effect is especially important at slow rates. For example, an increase in heart rate from 60–70 beats/min can severely reduce coronary filling in an ischemic heart.

3. The **arterial oxygen content** of blood is the product of the oxyhemoglobin saturation and the hemoglobin concentration, plus a small contribution from dissolved oxygen. Anemia lowers the tissue oxygen supply and can cause ischemia.

C. Therapeutic maneuvers to improve myocardial oxygen supply-demand balance

1. Decrease MVO_2.

   a. <u>Reduce ventricular wall tension</u> by decreasing chamber size with venous and arterial vasodilators.

   b. <u>Reduce contractility</u> with calcium channel antagonists, beta blockers, or inhalational anesthetics. These agents should be used judiciously in the presence of compromised left ventricular function.

   c. <u>Slow heart rate</u> with beta blockers and anesthetics.

2. Increase myocardial oxygen supply.

   a. <u>Decrease heart rate</u> to 50–60 beats/min to maximize coronary filling time during diastole.

   b. <u>Increase CPP</u> by increasing aortic diastolic pressure and decreasing LVEDP. Often, a combination of phenylephrine and nitroglycerin will achieve these goals.

   c. **Maximize oxygen-carrying capacity** with supplemental oxygen therapy and red blood cell (RBC) transfusions to correct anemia.

D. Preoperative risk factors in CAD

1. <u>The mortality</u> from a perioperative myocardial infarction (MI) approaches 50%.

2. Factors associated with perioperative cardiac complications seem to be (in descending order of importance)

   a. Third heart sound or jugular venous distention.

   b. MI less than 6 months ago.

   c. Rhythm other than sinus.

    d. Premature ventricular contractions greater than 5/min.

    e. Age over 70 years.

    f. Emergency operation.

    g. Severe valvular or subvalvular aortic stenosis.

    h. Poor general medical condition.

    i. Vascular, intrathoracic, or upper abdominal surgery.

E. Preoperative evaluation

  1. History. Establish exercise limits, patterns and precipitants of angina, dyspnea (including paroxysmal nocturnal dyspnea), syncope, and palpitations. The medical record may reveal other relevant conditions, such as pulmonary, renal, or central nervous system disease. Doses and schedules of cardiac medications should be ascertained.

  2. The physical examination should include a record of the patient's blood pressure (both arms), heart rate, body weight and habitus, PMI, gallops, murmurs, pulses, capillary filling, cyanosis, rales, jugular venous distention, and edema. Carotid pulses, neck anatomy, radial pulses, and Allen's test should be checked in case invasive monitoring becomes necessary.

  3. Laboratory tests

    a. The electrocardiogram (ECG) should be examined for rate, rhythm, presence, and location of ischemia and/or infarction.

    b. Exercise electrocardiography or exercise tolerance testing (ETT) is the initial means to evaluate patients suspected of having CAD. This procedure can localize areas of myocardial ischemia, quantify exercise limits, and reveal ischemia-caused arrhythmias.

    c. Radionuclide studies. At present, the two most widespread and useful tests are the thallium 201 scan and the gated blood pool scan (GBPS).

      (1) Exercise-thallium scans use a potassium analog that distributes in proportion to regional myocardial blood flow and can thus identify areas underperfused from ischemia or infarction.

        (a) It does not indicate the age of an MI.

        (b) Dipyridamole (Persantine) can mimic the effect of exercise by causing coronary vasodilation. Fifty percent of patients with positive Persantine-thallium scans develop significant cardiac complications in the perioperative period following major vascular surgery.

      (2) Gated blood pool scans involve the injection of technetium (^{99m}Tc)–labeled autologous RBCs.

(a) **First-pass technique** yields high-quality images of individual chambers and intracardiac shunts and can define valvular regurgitation. In combination with exercise, this test is more sensitive for CAD than ETT or exercise-thallium scans.

(b) **Equilibrium technique** is more accurate than first-pass in the presence of arrhythmias or pulmonary hypertension.

(c) **Uses**
   (i) The GBPS **ejection fraction,** when less than 35%, correlates with a fourfold increase in postoperative cardiac complications.
   (ii) Follow-up is facilitated after congenital heart disease repair.
   (iii) GBPS can be used to demonstrate therapeutic and toxic effects of various medications on ventricular function and can thus be a guide to therapy.

(3) **Others**
   (a) ^{99m}**Tc-stannous pyrophosphate** specifically binds to calcium accumulated in mitochondria during ischemia and is particularly useful in evaluating acute transmural MIs.
   (b) **Indium 111–labeled platelets or white blood cells** (WBCs) have imaged endocarditis, mural and coronary thrombus, or rejection of cardiac allografts.
   (c) **Gallium 67** collects in lysosomes and can reveal pericarditis and congestive cardiomyopathy.
   (d) Equilibrium blood pool imaging with ^{99m}Tc-labeled RBCs has been modified for continuous beat-to-beat monitoring of left ventricular (LV) function (specifically, ejection fraction) during induction of anesthesia. This **nuclear probe technique** promises to be a useful, noninvasive method in the future.

d. **Echocardiography** uses incident sound waves to detect wall motion abnormalities, wall thickness, congenital and valvular lesions, and pericardial effusions.

(1) **M-mode,** which uses ultrasound transmitted and received along a single line at a sampling rate of 1000 Hz, provides high temporal resolution and is superior for assessing motion.

(2) **2-D,** which images cross sections in real

time, yields superior anatomic resolution.

    (3) **A combination of Doppler** (the frequency change seen when ultrasound waves strike moving RBCs) **and M-mode** can be used to identify valvular regurgitation or intracardiac shunts because of the abnormal velocity and turbulence of blood flow in these conditions.

    (4) With recent developments in imaging technology, echocardiography may even be able to define coronary anatomy and to distinguish relevant types of tissue (e.g., healthy muscle, fibrous scar, edematous muscle).

  e. Cardiac catheterization remains the "gold standard" for assessment of hemodynamics and anatomy in patients with heart disease (see Chap. 20).

4. In summary, patients suspected of having CAD should receive an ECG, exercise-thallium scan (to detect ischemia), and a GBPS (to detect ventricular dysfunction). **Consultation with a cardiologist** is specifically indicated to assist in interpreting these studies, and if time permits, to optimize drug therapy. The results of these tests will help to determine the type of monitoring and drug regimens that will be required both intra- and postoperatively.

F. Preoperative preparation

  1. The preoperative visit should provide the patient with information and realistic assurances regarding the monitoring and anesthetic procedures.

  2. Preoperative medication is ordered to reduce the stress, anxiety, awareness, and the recollection of the preoperative period. Heavy sedation is usually desirable in patients with CAD to avoid precipitating angina. For major surgery, a combination of **morphine,** 0.1 mg/kg IM; **scopolamine,** 0.3–0.4 mg IM 1 hour prior to surgery; and **lorazepam,** 1.0–2.0 mg PO 2 hours prior to surgery, will accomplish the objectives. For short or relatively nonstimulating procedures, premedication with short-acting benzodiazepines and narcotics (the narcotic given IV in the holding area) is usually sufficient. Rarely, hypotension, hypercarbia, or hypoxia is seen after heavy premedication.

  3. Medications such as nitrates, beta blockers, calcium channel blockers, and antiarrhythmics are usually continued until the operation. However, due to its slow elimination, digoxin is withheld unless needed for heart rate control. <u>Diuretics are held unless there are obvious signs of congestive heart failure (CHF).</u>

  4. Monitoring

    a. Myocardial ischemia, whether regional or global, remains difficult to detect.

        (1) **ECG changes,** most often in the form of regional S–T depression, take 30–60 seconds to appear after acute ischemic injury.

        (2) **Ventricular wall motion changes** appear after several seconds of ischemia but do not result in elevated filling pressures or decreased cardiac output until at least 20% of the ventricle is involved.

   b. Besides the equipment needed to conform to the minimal monitoring standards for general anesthesia (see Chap. 9), further monitoring for cardiac patients might include the following:

        (1) **An arterial catheter,** to provide beat-to-beat systemic blood pressures, pulse contour, and access to arterial blood for sampling.

        (2) **A central venous pressure (CVP) catheter,** which is useful for volume assessment and central access for drug administration. In patients with good LV function, the CVP changes in parallel with the LVEDP. In the presence of $(EF > 50\%)$ chronic obstructive pulmonary disease, pulmonary hypertension, or LV dysfunction, CVP correlates poorly with left-sided filling pressures.

        (3) **A Foley urinary catheter** to monitor urine output, which usually reflects the perfusion to the kidney and other vital organs.

        (4) **A thermodilution pulmonary artery (PA) catheter** with a cardiac output computer, especially in patients with the risk factors discussed in sec. **I.D.2.**

G. Anesthetic considerations of patients with CAD

   1. No adequately controlled study has shown an advantage of regional over general anesthesia. **Monitored IV anesthesia and regional anesthesia** do not impose the stress of endotracheal intubation but may require excessive sedation. **General anesthesia** allows optimal airway control but generally requires multiple drugs, many of which have deleterious effects on the cardiovascular system.

   2. Myocardial oxygen supply must equal, or exceed, demand.

   3. Whether from anesthesia or surgery, **hemodynamic perturbations** should be anticipated and prevented; at minimum, they should be recognized and treated promptly.

II. Valvular heart disease

   A. Subacute bacterial endocarditis (SBE) prophylaxis. All valvular lesions require prophylaxis against bacterial endocarditis. The mortality from endocarditis of a prosthetic valve, for example, is 50–60%. In addition, patients with congenital heart disease, asymmetric septal hypertrophy, a history of endocarditis or of rheumatic heart disease, transvenous cardiac pacemakers, mitral valve prolapse, arteriovenous shunts, or ventriculoatrial cerebrospinal fluid shunts should receive prophylactic antibiotics.

Prophylactic antibiotics are also indicated in these patients whenever they undergo dental procedures including cleaning, respiratory tract surgery including bronchoscopy, cardiac operation requiring bypass, urologic or obstetric surgery, or any operation involving infected or contaminated tissues. The incidence of bacteremia during dental surgery, for instance, approaches 90%.

1. The doses for adult patients undergoing **dental or respiratory tract** surgery include the following:
   a. **For minor surgery:** penicillin V (2 gm PO 1 hour before the procedure and 1 gm 6 hours later) or penicillin G (2 million units IM or IV 30–60 minutes before the procedure and repeat 8 hours later).
   b. **Parenteral prophylaxis before major surgery:** ampicillin (1 gm IM or IV) plus gentamicin (1.5 mg/kg IM or IV 30–60 minutes before the procedure and repeat 8 hours later).
   c. **With penicillin allergy:** erythromycin (1 gm 1 hour before the procedure and 500 mg 6 hours later) or vancomycin (1 gm IV slowly over 1 hour, beginning 1 hour before the procedure, and repeat 8 hours later).
2. For patients undergoing **urologic or GI surgery** use the following:
   a. **Oral prophylaxis:** amoxicillin (3 gm 1 hour before the procedure and 1.5 gm 6 hours later).
   b. **Parenteral prophylaxis:** ampicillin plus gentamicin (as in **1.b**).
   c. **Penicillin allergy:** vancomycin plus gentamicin (as in **1.c**).
   Note: These recommendations may require modification, depending on the particular surgical procedure, cardiac defect, and patterns of nosocomial infection. Cardiology or infectious disease consultation may be indicated in many cases. Recommendations for children may be found in the *Medical Letter* article, "Prevention of bacterial endocarditis" (see Suggested Reading).

B. **Specific lesions**
   1. **Aortic stenosis**
      a. Symptoms usually appear after a long latent phase. Life expectancy is usually 5 years after the onset of angina, 3 years after syncope, and 2 years after CHF.
      b. LV systolic pressures increase to maintain cardiac output, and LV hypertrophy follows.
      c. Aortic stenosis is severe when the aortic valve area is less than 0.6 cm²/m² and the gradient is

greater than 70 mm Hg.
  d. Myocardial ischemia is possible in the absence
      of CAD.
  e. Anesthetic considerations
      (1) Moderate premedication will avoid tachy-
          cardia from anxiety; usually morphine,
          0.05 mg/kg IM; scopolamine, 0.3 mg IM;
          and lorazepam, 1.0 mg PO, are sufficient.
      (2) A PA catheter is essential to monitor poor
          LV function or associated mitral regurgi-
          tation (MR).
      (3) Adequate preload, sinus rhythm at a rea-
          sonable rate, and maintenance of contrac-
          tility and systemic vascular resistance are
          the hemodynamic goals. Tachycardia and
          peripheral vasodilatation are poorly tol-
          erated.
      (4) A narcotic (usually fentanyl)-relaxant ox-
          ygen technique is used to control the heart
          rate while preventing a fall in systemic
          vascular resistance.
      (5) Cardiopulmonary resuscitation is noto-
          riously ineffective in patients with aortic
          stenosis; ventricular tachycardia and ven-
          tricular fibrillation are almost uniformly
          fatal.
  2. Aortic regurgitation
      a. Life expectancy is generally 4 years after the
          onset of angina and 2 years after CHF.
      b. In chronic aortic regurgitation, volume over-
          load increases LV wall tension and results in ec-
          centric hypertrophy.
      c. As EDV increases, stroke volume increases, so
          that ejection fraction is maintained until LV
          failure occurs. When cardiac output falls, the
          pulmonary capillary wedge pressure rises.
      d. Myocardial ischemia can occur in the absence
          of CAD due to increased MVO_2 from ventricular
          hypertrophy or decreased oxygen supply from
          diminished CPP.
      e. Anesthetic considerations
          (1) A light premedication should be given.
          (2) PA catheters are needed to guide the use
              of inotropes and vasodilators.
          (3) A normal or elevated heart rate main-
              tains aortic diastolic and CPP and de-
              creases left ventricular end-diastolic
              volume (LVEDV). Systemic vascular resis-
              tance should be maintained to preserve
              CPP but should not be allowed to rise high
              enough to impede forward flow.
          (4) Narcotic (usually morphine)-relaxant ox-
              ygen is the anesthetic technique of choice.
              Improved LV function from vasodilatation
              may necessitate adding an inhalational

anesthetic to control blood pressure.

(5) Vasodilators, such as sodium nitroprusside, can be used to increase forward stroke volume and to decrease LVEDP and myocardial wall tension. Care must be taken, however, to sustain CPP.

3. Mitral stenosis

a. A long latent period usually precedes symptoms of CHF, which are often manifest at the onset of atrial fibrillation (AF).

b. Left atrial pressure rises in direct proportion to flow and inversely with both diastolic filling time and mitral valve area. Severe mitral stenosis occurs when the mitral valve area is less than 1.0 cm^2 and the gradient is greater than 25 mm Hg.

c. Atrial contraction can increase LVEDV by 40%, so the development of acute AF can decrease cardiac output markedly. Therefore, sinus rhythm should be maintained. Generally, patients with chronic AF do not benefit from converting to sinus rhythm.

d. **Anesthetic considerations**

(1) A light premedication is used in patients with low cardiac output. Otherwise, premedications should be adequate to prevent anxiety, which can raise pulmonary vascular resistance.

(2) The ventricular response to AF should be well controlled with digitalis. If the heart rate is greater than 80/min, administer the usual dose of digitalis on the morning of surgery.

(3) Although often difficult to position with AF, tricuspid regurgitation, and right ventricular (RV) enlargement, PA catheters are essential for optimal management.

(4) Anesthetic agents that suppress the heart rate and maintain sinus rhythm are best. Pancuronium may produce tachycardia or nodal rhythms and thus should be avoided.

(5) Increases in PA pressures are associated with hypoxia, nitrous oxide, alpha-adrenergic agonists, calcium chloride, and Trendelenburg position and should be avoided. Judicious use of nitroglycerin can lower PA pressures without significantly affecting heart rate.

(6) For RV failure resulting from elevated pulmonary vascular resistance, a beta-adrenergic inotrope such as isoproterenol, dopamine, or dobutamine is best. In severe cases, PGE$_1$ (0.5–2.0 µg/min) has been used with some success, but

simultaneous infusion of norepinephrine through a left atrial catheter may be needed to support systemic blood pressure.

4. **Mitral regurgitation (MR)**

   a. Acute MR results in biventricular failure; chronic MR leads to fatigue, dyspnea, and CHF.

   b. MR allows blood to be ejected into the left atrium during systole. The amount of regurgitant flow depends on the ventricular-atrial pressure gradient, the size of the mitral orifice, and the duration of ejection.

   c. Compensatory mechanisms in **acute MR** result in increased heart rate, LVEDV, and contractility. Elevated PA pressures with large V waves develop, due to low left atrial compliance.

   d. Compensatory mechanisms in **chronic MR** consist of LV dilatation, low LVEDP, and eccentric hypertrophy. A compliant left atrium is the hallmark of chronic MR, so PA pressures and V waves remain low until end-stage disease.

   e. **Anesthetic considerations**

      (1) A light premedication is recommended.

      (2) PA catheters are useful for demonstrating the height of regurgitant V waves and for assessing systemic vascular resistance. Pacing, or Paceport, PA catheters may be used to prevent life-threatening bradycardias.

      (3) The goals are to maintain contractility and prevent elevation of the systemic vascular resistance. Neither narcotics nor inhalation anesthetics completely satisfy these objectives.

      (4) Vasodilators reduce impedance to forward flow, LVEDV, and possibly the size of the mitral annulus, all of which increase forward stroke volume.

5. **Mitral valve prolapse (MVP)**

   a. MVP has a prevalence of 5–10%, occurs most commonly in young women, and is associated with **von Willebrand's syndrome;** signs of easy bruisability or history of epistaxis or menorrhagia should be evaluated with a PTT, platelet count, and platelet function studies. There is also an association of MVP with skeletal and connective tissue disorders such as arched palate, thoracic deformities, and Marfan's syndrome.

   b. Most patients are asymptomatic, but some may experience atypical chest pain, palpitations, syncope, or dyspnea. **A midsystolic click** is found in only 10% of cases. The **ECG** is usually normal, but may also show inferior S–T and T-wave abnormalities. **Echocardiography** confirms the diagnosis.

    c. Supraventricular and ventricular dysrhythmias
    and bradydysrhythmias occur in a large propor-
    tion of MVP patients. Other complications in-
    clude transient cerebral ischemia, bacterial en-
    docarditis, and sudden death.

    d. Anesthetic considerations

      (1) Prophylaxis for bacterial endocarditis is
      indicated when a diagnosis of MVP has
      been established (see sec. **II.A**).

      (2) **Monitoring** should include an inferiorly
      placed ECG lead; invasive monitoring is
      usually unnecessary. Medications such as
      anticoagulants and beta blockers should
      be continued, and heavy sedative premed-
      ication is recommended.

      (3) Increasing LV volume can improve the
      prolapse; thus preload and SVR should be
      maintained. Hyperdynamic states should
      be avoided.

      (4) In general, no specific anesthetic tech-
      nique is contraindicated. However, anti-
      coagulants used to prevent transient ce-
      rebral ischemia may preclude regional
      anesthesia.

      (5) The alpha-agonist phenylephrine is the
      pressor of choice because it has little effect
      on contractility and promotes slowing of
      the heart rate.

**III. Asymmetric septal hypertrophy (or idiopathic hyper-
trophic subaortic stenosis)**

  A. A hypertrophied interventricular septum involving the
  anterior mitral leaflet causes dynamic obstruction to LV
  outflow. Typically, LV compliance is decreased, but
  ejection fraction is preserved. Although one-third of patients show some MR and one-fifth have some RV outflow obstruction, these accompanying lesions are seldom of hemodynamic importance.

  B. Conditions that worsen LV outflow obstruction

    1. Decreased LV volume
    2. Increased contractility
    3. Decreased aortic diastolic pressure

  C. Anesthetic considerations

    1. The **goals** are to reduce contractility while increas-
    ing preload and afterload. Sinus rhythm should be
    maintained; other rhythms are poorly tolerated. Al-
    though halothane has been shown to reduce the
    outflow tract gradient, other inhalational agents
    can probably be safely used as well.

    2. A heavy premedication is employed to prevent anx-
    iety, which increases myocardial contractility.

    3. Beta-adrenergic or calcium channel blockers should
    be continued until surgery.

    4. Beta blockers are indicated to treat tachycardia.

    5. Hypotension should be treated with volume admin-
    istration and phenylephrine infusion; inotropes
    may exacerbate outflow obstruction.

IV. Congenital heart disease (CHD) in adults

  A. Unrepaired congenital heart defects may lead to more severe hemodynamic derangements in adulthood than in childhood. **Atrial septal defect** is the most common congenital lesion that is diagnosed in adults.

   1. Left-to-right shunting of blood leads to RV overload, increased pulmonary blood flow, and pulmonary hypertension.

   2. Patients often present in CHF and AF. Although these findings usually resolve after surgery, Eisenmenger's physiology (irreversibly elevated pulmonary vascular resistance) may persist postoperatively. Other problems following repair include MR and conduction defects associated with supraventricular and ventricular arrhythmias.

  B. Repaired congenital lesions may still be complicated by residual pathology.

   1. Ventricular septal defects, even after repair, may leave residual RV and PA hypertension and CHF.

     a. Residual ventricular septal defects, tricuspid regurgitation, elevated pulmonary vascular resistance, and respiratory insufficiency may all occur in the early postoperative period.

     b. His bundle injury can lead to complete heart block, especially in patients with right bundle branch block and left atrial distention.

   2. Patent ductus arteriosus (PDA), once ligated, rarely has any long-term sequelae. PA hypertension is almost never irreversible; exercise tolerance is seldom impaired.

   3. Coarctation of the aorta, even after successful repair, can still involve unpredictable or labile blood pressures.

     a. Residual coarctation occurs in 10% of patients.

     b. Other cardiovascular anomalies, commonly aortic stenosis or a PDA, are present in 68% of patients with coarctation.

     c. Coarctation causes LV pressure overload, resulting in LV hypertrophy and noncompliance.

     d. If a subclavian flap is used to repair the coarctation, blood pressures obtained from the left arm may not be equal to those from the right.

   4. Tetralogy of Fallot, after correction, usually shows normalization of the RV/PA systolic gradient.

     a. Most patients have residual RV dysfunction and right bundle branch block but can still respond to exercise with an increase in cardiac output. Some show residual RV outflow obstruction or peripheral pulmonic stenosis, which can lead to RV failure and ventricular arrhythmias.

     b. Persistent pulmonary vascular hyperreactivity can result in an increased pulmonary capillary wedge pressure (PCWP) with exercise. Shunting can occur, which usually is mild, and does not alter the oxygen saturation.

   c. Pulmonic regurgitation is common but usually does not affect cardiac output.

   d. A few patients have residual ventricular septal defects or LV dysfunction with reduced ejection fractions.

5. Transposition of the great arteries

   a. Transposition of the great arteries is usually corrected by means of an intraatrial baffle that reroutes the venous return to the appropriate ventricle (e.g., Mustard or Senning procedures). Long-term postoperative problems include residual atrial septal defect, RV dysfunction, conduction disturbances, caval or pulmonary venous obstruction, and tricuspid regurgitation.

   b. Occasionally, an arterial switch procedure is employed; postoperative sequelae include LV dysfunction, biventricular outflow tract obstruction, aortic regurgitation, and coronary insufficiency.

V. Pacemakers

A. Pacemaker nomenclature. By convention, a three-letter code describes the (1) chamber(s) paced, (2) chamber(s) sensed, and (3) mode of pacing. For example, a "DVI" pacemaker paces both the atria and the ventricles, senses the ventricle, and is inhibited by the sensing circuit.

B. Interference. In general, electrocautery interferes with the **sensing mode** of the pacemaker. Usually, electrocautery will affect only one cardiac cycle, after which the pacemaker reverts to the VOO mode. A **magnet** can be used to deliberately convert a VVI pacemaker to a VOO. This maneuver should be considered in patients with adverse responses to electrocautery or with tachyarrhythmias. For patients with programmable pacemakers, discussion with a cardiologist before the operation might be useful to clarify the sensitivity of the pacemaker to electrical interference and the possible usefulness of either a magnet, a reprogramming device, or temporary pacing.

   1. **Myopotentials** can also inhibit pacemakers. If this problem is known preoperatively, fasciculations should be avoided by using only nondepolarizing muscle relaxants or else pretreating with a nondepolarizer prior to administration of succinylcholine. Shivering from hypothermia should also be avoided.

   2. With programmable pacemakers, electrocautery can actually **reprogram** the pacemaker. Although this phenomenon is rare, it is more likely in the case when a magnet is applied during electrocautery. Reprogramming can alter both the "set" rates and mode.

   3. **Complications**

     a. Improper placement of the electrocautery grounding pad can lead to myocardial burns or trigger VF. The pad should be placed away from both the heart and the pacing generator. <u>The heart or pacemaker should never be between the grounding pad and the area being cauterized.</u>

b. Central lines can dislodge or knot with pacing wires. <u>After 3 weeks</u> of implantation, a permanent pacing wire should be sufficiently covered with fibrin to <u>resist dislodgment.</u>

4. Temporary pacing can be accomplished with transvenous or epicardial wires, through appropriately designed PA catheter ports, or through pacing PA catheters. Relative indications for temporary pacing include severe conduction disturbances, sinus rhythm–dependent lesions (e.g., marginally compensated mitral or aortic stenosis), regurgitant valvular lesions, anticipated electrical interference with permanent pacing or with intraaortic balloon pumping, and heart transplantation.

Suggested Reading

Berger, H. J., and Zaret, B. L. Nuclear cardiology. *N. Engl. J. Med.* 305:799, 1981.

Braunwald, E. *Heart Disease.* Philadelphia: Saunders, 1984.

Giles, R. W., et al. Continuous monitoring of left ventricular performance with the computerized nuclear probe during laryngoscopy and intubation before coronary artery bypass surgery. *Am. J. Cardiol.* 50(4):735, 1982.

Jeffery, C. C., et al. A prospective evaluation of cardiac risk index. *Anesthesiology* 58:462, 1983.

Kaplan, J. A. *Cardiac Anesthesia.* New York: Grune & Stratton, 1979.

Kaye, D. Prophylaxis for infective endocarditis: An update. *Ann. Intern. Med.* 104:419, 1986.

Popp, R. L., et al. Echocardiography: M-mode and two-dimensional methods. *Ann. Intern. Med.* 93:844, 1980.

Prevention of bacterial endocarditis. *Med. Lett.* 26:3, 1984.

Zaidan, J. R. Pacemakers. *Anesthesiology* 60:319, 1984.

3

Specific Considerations with Pulmonary Disease

William E. Hurford

I. **General considerations.** The incidence of postoperative pulmonary complications is second only to cardiovascular complications as a cause of perioperative mortality.

  A. Patients with significant chronic pulmonary disease are at greater risk for postoperative respiratory failure than the general population, since anesthesia and surgery more easily produce hypoventilation, hypoxemia, and retention of secretions in patients with limited respiratory reserve.

  B. Approximately 7% of patients with moderate to severe chronic lung disease die within 9 weeks following general anesthesia and surgery. The death rate following thoracic and upper abdominal operations is twice that of other procedures.

  C. Postoperative morbidity and mortality can be reduced by identifying patients at risk for perioperative respiratory complications, optimizing their medical therapy, and instituting a program of chest physiotherapy prior to surgery.

II. **Effects of anesthesia and surgery on pulmonary function.** General anesthesia decreases lung volumes and promotes mismatching of pulmonary ventilation and perfusion. Many anesthetic drugs blunt the ventilatory response to carbon dioxide and hypoxia. Postoperatively, atelectasis and hypoxemia commonly result, especially in patients with preexisting pulmonary disease. Pulmonary function is further compromised by postoperative pain, which can limit coughing and lung expansion.

  A. **Respiratory mechanics and gas exchange**

   1. **General anesthesia and the supine position** decrease functional residual capacity (FRC). Atelectasis results as lung volume during tidal breathing falls below the volume at which airway closure occurs (closing capacity). Positive-pressure ventilation with large tidal volumes of positive end-expiratory pressure can minimize this effect.

   2. **Positive-pressure ventilation,** however, compared to spontaneous breathing, impairs ventilation/perfusion matching. During positive-pressure ventilation, nondependent portions of the lung receive a greater proportion of ventilation than do dependent portions. The distribution of pulmonary blood flow, however, is determined by gravity; blood flow tends to be increased in dependent portions of the lung. The end result is a variable increase in both physiologic dead space and shunt compared to spontaneous ventilation.

   3. **Diaphragmatic changes** also occur. In the supine

position, the diaphragm is displaced cephalad by abdominal contents. The addition of general anesthesia, muscle paralysis, and positive-pressure ventilation alters diaphragmatic motion: Nondependent portions of the diaphragm move more than dependent portions, the opposite of the case during spontaneous ventilation. These changes may further alter the distribution of ventilation and perfusion within the lungs.

B. Regulation of breathing

1. The ventilatory response to carbon dioxide is reduced by general anesthetics, barbiturates, and opioids. Carbon dioxide tensions are elevated during spontaneous ventilation with general anesthesia, as in the apneic threshold (the $PaCO_2$ at which patients hyperventilated to apnea resume spontaneous ventilation).

2. $PaCO_2$ may also be increased as a response to metabolic alkalosis, which commonly results from nasogastric suctioning or diuretic therapy. $PaCO_2$ normally increases about 0.6 mm Hg for every 1 mEq/L increase in base excess. Hypoventilation induced by this effect may complicate weaning.

3. The ventilatory response to hypoxia may also be blunted by general anesthetics, barbiturates, and opioids. This effect may be especially important in patients with severe chronic lung disease, who normally retain carbon dioxide and depend on a hypoxic drive for ventilation.

C. Effect of surgery. Postoperative pulmonary function is affected by the site of surgery. The ability to cough is reduced after abdominal operations compared to peripheral procedures and appears related to the pain produced by coughing. Vital capacity falls about 75% after upper abdominal procedures and approximately 50% after lower abdominal or thoracic operations. Recovery of normal pulmonary function may take several weeks. Peripheral procedures have little impact on vital capacity or the ability to clear secretions.

D. Effect on ciliary function. The upper respiratory tract normally warms and humidifies inspired air, providing an ideal environment for normal function of respiratory tract cilia and mucus. General anesthesia, often conducted with unhumidified gases at high flow rates, dries respiratory mucus and can easily damage respiratory epithelium. Endotracheal intubation exacerbates this problem by bypassing the nasopharynx. Secretions become thickened, ciliary function is reduced, and the patient's resistance to pulmonary infections is decreased. These problems may be partially prevented by lowering fresh gas flows and including a heated humidifier in the anesthesia circuit.

III. Identification of the patient at risk

A. Classification of pulmonary disease. Pulmonary disease is divided into obstructive and restrictive components.

1. The hallmark of **obstructive disease** is an increase in airway resistance.
   a. Obstructive disease may be acute, as in bronchial asthma, or chronic, as in patients with chronic obstructive pulmonary disease (COPD) or bronchitis.
   b. Pulmonary emphysema may occur as one component of chronic obstructive pulmonary disease. In this disease, alveolar air spaces are destroyed, and the elastic recoil of the lungs is lost. The airways may then collapse with exhalation, leading to increased airway resistance, air trapping, and bullae formation. Cysts and bullae may be expanded by positive-pressure ventilation or the use of nitrous oxide, resulting in rupture of the cyst or reduced venous return from mediastinal compression.
   c. Obstructive disease is characterized by regional mismatching of ventilation and perfusion as evidenced by hypoxemia while breathing room air. Dyspnea, secondary to increased work of breathing, is caused by elevated airway resistance.
   d. Increased airway irritability, air trapping, and copious airway secretions may pose serious challenges to the perioperative care of patients with severe obstructive disease. Endotracheal intubation may exacerbate bronchospasm, while positive-pressure ventilation may worsen air trapping by not allowing sufficient time for expiration. Mismatching of ventilation and perfusion slows the uptake and elimination of inhaled anesthetics. Patients may require frequent suctioning and chest physiotherapy to clear secretions and relieve mucous plugging.
2. **Restrictive pulmonary disease** is characterized by decreased compliance of the lungs or chest wall. Lung volumes are reduced while airway resistance remains normal. Restrictive disease is classified as intrinsic or extrinsic.
   a. **Intrinsic** restrictive lung disease is characterized by reduced lung compliance and is often accompanied by pulmonary fibrosis. Acute causes of intrinsic restriction include pneumonia, pulmonary edema, and the adult respiratory distress syndrome. Chronic causes include pulmonary fibrosis from hypersensitivity pneumonitis and sarcoidosis. High airway pressures may be required during positive-pressure ventilation in these patients and may increase the risk of pneumothorax.
   b. **Extrinsic** restrictive disease is caused by reduced compliance of the chest wall. Extrinsic causes of restrictive disease include defects of the pleura (such as fibrosis or effusion), de-

creased compliance of the chest wall (kyphoscoliosis, pectus excavatum, and chest wall
burns), and elevation and limitation of diaphragmatic motion (obesity, pregnancy, and
m

Normal compliance
200 cc / 1 cm H₂O

    c. Cl   dyspnea
       se   hing. Hy-
       pe   in a de-
       cr

  3. Often   ulmonary
     dysfu   estrictive
     defect   reful his-
     tory a   function
     testin   bstructive
     from   assess a
     patien

B. Medical history

  1. While a complete history should be elicited, several
risk factors deserve special emphasis, such as a
prior history of congestive heart failure, chronic
lung disease, or asthma. A prior history of treatment for pulmonary disease, occupational exposures, and the use of medications such as bronchodilators and steroids should be outlined.

  2. **Dyspnea** is the unpleasant awareness of an abnormal relation between ventilatory output and the
work of breathing. Dyspnea may arise from increased work of breathing, a reduced functional residual capacity, or increased sensory input from
pulmonary or chest wall stretch receptors. As it is
a subjective sensation, its presence may not be a
specific indicator of pulmonary disease. Occurrence
of dyspnea at rest or with minimal exertion, however, usually implies severe pulmonary dysfunction.

  3. **Tobacco.** A history of cigarette smoking is a sensitive predictor of pulmonary disease and postoperative pulmonary complications. Compared to non-
smokers, heavy smokers have a fourfold greater incidence of chronic bronchitis and three times as
many postoperative pulmonary complications.

C. Physical examination.
The physical examination is
directed toward assessing the presence and severity of
pulmonary disease.

  1. **Body habitus and general appearance.** Altered
body habitus often produces pulmonary dysfunction.

    a. **Obesity, pregnancy, and kyphoscoliosis,**
for example, reduce total lung volume and functional residual capacity, predisposing the patient to atelectasis and hypoxemia.

    b. **Cachectic,** malnourished patients have blunt-
ed respiratory drives and decreased muscle
strength and are predisposed to pneumonias.

    c. Several general signs, however, are unreliable.
Cyanosis is not a sensitive sign of hypoxemia

and may be difficult to assess. Its presence requires a capillary concentration of greater than 5 grams of reduced hemoglobin/dl. Hence, the appearance of cyanosis depends on many factors, including arterial oxygen uptake, tissue blood flow and blood volume, oxygen uptake of the tissue, and hemoglobin concentration.

    d. Clubbing also is not a reliable sign of chronic pulmonary disease; its presence may suggest interstitial fibrosis, inflammation, or malignancy.

  2. Respiratory signs. Respiratory rate, pattern, diaphragmatic coordination, and the use of accessory muscles should be assessed.

    a. Respiratory rate. Tachypnea (respiratory rate greater than 25 breaths/minute) may be the most sensitive sign of respiratory distress or underlying pulmonary pathology but may not be noticed unless the rate is carefully counted.

    b. Respiratory pattern

      (1) Prolonged expiratory time relative to inspiratory time and a total forced expiratory time greater than 5 seconds indicate airway obstruction.

      (2) Inspiratory paradox. Normally the abdominal wall should move outward with the chest wall during inspiration. Inspiratory paradox occurs when the abdomen collapses as the chest wall expands during inspiration and suggests paralysis or severe fatigue of the diaphragm.

      (3) Use of accessory muscles, such as the sternocleidomastoids, during inspiration results from decreased chest wall or diaphragmatic power and/or decreased lung compliance.

      (4) Symmetry of respiration. Tracheal deviation suggests mediastinal disease. Diminished or delayed motion of one hemithorax may be observed with pleural disease or consolidation of the lung.

    c. Auscultation of the chest. Diminished breath sounds may be due to emphysema or, when accompanied by percussive dullness, bronchial obstruction or consolidation. Inspiratory crackles may be due to atelectasis, congestive heart failure, or interstitial fibrosis. Wheezing suggests airflow obstruction. Stridor indicates upper airway obstruction or an endobronchial lesion.

  3. Cardiovascular signs

    a. Pulsus paradoxus is defined as a fall in blood pressure of greater than 10 mm Hg during inspiration. A paradoxical pulse reflects increased afterloading of the left ventricle secondary to a large decrease in intrapleural pressure and generally correlates with the degree of airway obstruction.

b. **Pulmonary hypertension and right ventricular failure.** Signs of pulmonary hypertension include a widened or fixed splitting of the S_2 with an accentuated pulmonic component, an S_4 gallop that is accentuated by inspiration, a right ventricular heave or palpable pulmonary artery (PA) pulsation, and peripheral edema with jugular venous distention and hepatojugular reflux.

c. **Coronary artery or valvular heart disease** often coexists with pulmonary disease and increases perioperative morbidity. Significant mitral disease may produce severe pulmonary hypertension.

D. **Electrocardiogram.** Electrocardiographic signs of significant pulmonary dysfunction include

1. Low voltage, a vertical axis, and poor R-wave progression due to hyperinflation.

2. **Signs of pulmonary hypertension** and cor pulmonale, including

   a. Right-axis deviation.

   b. P pulmonale (P waves greater than 2.5 mm in height).

   c. Right ventricular hypertrophy.

   d. Right bundle branch block.

E. **Chest x-ray, tomograms, and computed tomography**

1. **Abnormal PA and lateral chest x-rays** are highly specific for pulmonary disease. Signs of hyperinflation, congestive heart failure, vascular changes, consolidation, bullae, and masses must be sought, as these conditions often mandate modification of the anesthetic technique:

   a. In the presence of pneumothorax, large blebs, and cysts, nitrous oxide should be avoided, since it can rapidly increase the volume and pressure within enclosed cavities.

   b. Consolidation, abscesses, pleural effusions, and atelectasis can produce hypoxemia through mismatching of ventilation and perfusion.

   c. Mediastinal and tracheal masses may distort normal anatomy and require altered approaches to induction and intubation.

2. **Tomograms and computed tomography** are especially helpful when assessing a tracheal or bronchial stenosis, since the precise location and degree of obstruction can be identified.

F. **Arterial blood gases**

1. Preoperative measurement of arterial partial pressures of oxygen (PaO_2), carbon dioxide ($PaCO_2$), and pH serves several purposes, including

   a. Providing quantification of the severity of pulmonary dysfunction. Patients with severe hypoxemia ($PaO_2 < 60$ mm Hg) while breathing room air) or carbon dioxide retention ($PaCO_2 > 50$ mm Hg) are more likely to have postoperative pulmonary complications.

    b. Assessing the efficacy of preoperative medical and respiratory therapy.

    c. Providing a baseline to which postoperative respiratory function can be compared.

  2. The **$PaCO_2$** may be falsely depressed because of hyperventilation from apprehension and the pain of the arterial puncture.

    a. Accurate results require an experienced, unhurried approach and a relaxed patient. Prior infiltration of the puncture site with 1% lidocaine is recommended.

    b. If the measured serum bicarbonate concentration is significantly higher than that predicted by the arterial blood gas, acute hyperventilation should be suspected.

G. Pulmonary function tests

  1. Pulmonary function tests are objective measures of pulmonary mechanical function and reserve. Although there are no clear-cut guidelines for their use in the preoperative evaluation, pulmonary function tests

    a. Complement the findings of the history and physical examination, permitting a quantitative comparison of pulmonary function over time.

    b. Are useful in evaluating the effects of therapy such as pulmonary physiotherapy or bronchodilator use.

    c. Estimate remaining lung volume and function following a proposed pulmonary resection.

    d. May be of predictive value in estimating perioperative morbidity and mortality from pulmonary complications and determining the likelihood that ventilatory assistance will be required postoperatively.

  2. Spirometry measures the volume of air inhaled or exhaled over time. The data can be displayed as flow versus time or volume. Expiratory air flow is determined by airway resistance and the elastic recoil of the lung and chest wall. Lung volumes are determined by the compliance of the lung and chest wall and the power of inhalation and exhalation.

    a. The most useful tests appear to be the **vital capacity** (VC) and the **forced expiratory volume** in the first second of exhalation (FEV_1).

      (1) Vital capacity is smaller in females, decreases with age, and increases with height. Normal values ($\pm$ 20%) are 25 ml/cm for males and 20 ml/cm for females.

      (2) The FEV_1 is usually 85–90% of the vital

capacity and decreases with age. A FEV_1/VC ratio of less than 75% is considered abnormal.

(3) A reduced vital capacity in the presence of a normal FEV_1/VC suggests a restrictive defect with decreased lung volumes. A reduced FEV_1/VC implies obstructive airway disease.

b. **Additional spirometric tests of pulmonary function**

Less dependent on effort

(1) **Maximum mid-expiratory flow rate** (MMFR) is the average flow rate occurring between 25 and 75% of a vital capacity maneuver. A reduced MMFR suggests obstruction of small airways.

(2) **Maximum voluntary ventilation** (MVV) is the maximum amount of ventilation that a patient can generate by voluntary effort over 1 minute. MVV may be reduced by obstructive or restrictive disease and by poor voluntary effort.

(3) **Flow-volume loops** are useful in pinpointing the location of an airway obstruction. They are constructed by simultaneously plotting air flow and volume during a forced vital capacity maneuver that is followed immediately by an inspiration back to vital capacity. As transmural airway pressure changes during the respiratory cycle, the airway diameter at the level of an obstruction may also change. Air flow may become limited as the airway narrows maximally, producing a "plateau" on the flow-volume loop. Depending on the nature and location of the lesion, several patterns may be seen.

(a) **A fixed obstruction,** such as a goiter, is unaffected by changes in transmural pressure and limits flow during both inspiration and expiration, producing characteristic plateaus during both inspiratory and expiratory limbs of the flow-volume loop.

(b) **A variable extrathoracic obstruction,** such as that created by a paralyzed vocal cord, is worsened by forced inspiration, since the negative transmural pressure tends to collapse the airway. Forced expiration, on the other hand, increases airway caliber at the level of the lesion and minimizes its effect. Airflow therefore plateaus only during inspiration.

      (c) The opposite pattern is seen with a **variable intrathoracic obstruction.** Forced expiration decreases airway diameter at the level of the lesion and increases its obstructing effect. The plateau is produced during the expiratory phase of the loop.

3. Lung volumes may be measured by body plethysmography or gas dilution. Total lung capacity may be increased in bronchial asthma and chronic obstructive pulmonary disease. The ratio of residual volume to total lung capacity is a measure of air trapping.

4. Generally, patients with poorer spirometric performance have a greater likelihood of postoperative pulmonary complications. While cutoff values are imprecise predictors, generally a vital capacity, FEV_1/FVC, or MVV of less than 50% of predicted value is associated with increased perioperative morbidity from pulmonary complications.

5. FEV_1 of less than 800 ml following pulmonary resection correlates with an increased likelihood of early and late respiratory complications. Preoperatively, the FEV_1 following pulmonary resection may be predicted by multiplying the preoperative FEV_1 by the percentage of functioning lung to remain after resection. When significant ventilation/perfusion abnormalities exist, or when a major resection such as pneumonectomy is contemplated, the percentage of functioning lung remaining may be estimated by quantitative ventilation/perfusion lung scanning using inhaled xenon 133 and injected macroaggregated albumin labeled with technetium 99m, respectively. The proportion of functional lung remaining after resection is estimated by dividing the activity over the segments that will not be resected by the activity over all lung fields. A predicted postoperative FEV_1 of less than 800 ml is a contraindication to pulmonary resection.

H. Pulmonary artery catheterization

    1. The pulmonary circulation is normally a low-pressure, highly compliant circuit that handles increased blood flow by recruitment of underperfused vessels. Patients with chronic lung disease may have reduced pulmonary vascularity, pulmonary hypertension, and cor pulmonale. Pulmonary resection in these patients may produce considerable increases in pulmonary artery pressure, culminating in right ventricular failure.

    2. In these patients, preoperative assessment of pulmonary artery pressure during exercise or unilateral pulmonary artery occlusion may aid in assessing their pulmonary vascular reserve. While strict criteria do not exist, large elevations in pulmonary artery pressure with exercise or unilateral pulmonary artery occlusion are a relative contraindication to pulmonary resection.

IV. **Preoperative treatment of the pulmonary patient**
Preoperative therapy is directed toward reversing bronchospasm, clearing secretions, treating infection, and reducing the frequency and severity of acute exacerbations.

    A. **Reduction of smoking and environmental irritants**

        1. **Tobacco smoking** increases the amount of bronchial secretions, reduces ciliary clearance of secretions, and decreases oxygen transport by increasing carboxyhemoglobin levels in the blood. Cessation of smoking for 8 weeks or more prior to surgery reduces pulmonary secretions and may improve ciliary function. Stopping for as little as 24 hours prior to surgery lowers carboxyhemoglobin levels and increases the release of oxygen to tissues by shifting the oxyhemoglobin dissociation curve to the right.

        2. **Environmental allergens** and irritants may cause direct bronchoconstriction. Preoperative exposure to known irritants should be minimized. Elective surgery should be postponed during acute exacerbations.

    B. **Preoperative hydration, humidification, and warming of inspired gases**

        1. Asthmatics and patients with chronic obstructive pulmonary disease often have trouble clearing secretions postoperatively. Adequate perioperative hydration and humidification of inspired gases reduce drying of the airway and improve mobilization of secretions.

        2. **Cold inspired gases** may directly cause bronchoconstriction. Warming inspired gases is indicated in patients with reactive airways and especially in patients with exercise-induced asthma who may be especially sensitive to the effects of cold air.

    C. **Treatment of acute infections**

        1. Eradication of acute pulmonary infections prior to surgery may reduce the likelihood of postoperative pulmonary complications. Elective surgery should be postponed until acute infections are cleared.

        2. **Prophylactic antibiotics,** however, are not indicated, as they may merely result in the overgrowth of resistant organisms. Instead, antibiotic therapy should be directed at infections documented by sputum Gram's stain and culture.

    D. **Preoperative chest physiotherapy**

        1. A variety of preoperative chest physiotherapy protocols have been shown to decrease the incidence and severity of postoperative pulmonary complications. All are based on teaching the patient to mobilize secretions more effectively and participate in maneuvers designed to increase lung volume.

        2. Effective methods include voluntary deep breathing, coughing, and early ambulation, incentive spirometry, and chest percussion and vibration com-

[handwritten margin note: P_{50} a→26 in 12°]

bined with postural drainage.

3. **Forced expiratory maneuvers,** such as using blow-bottles, are not recommended, as they cause the patient to exhale below functional residual capacity and can lead to airway closure and alveolar collapse.

E. **Medical therapy**

1. **Theophylline**

   a. Theophylline causes bronchodilation by increasing the intracellular concentration of cyclic adenosine monophosphate (AMP) through inhibition of the enzyme phosphodiesterase.

   b. Theophylline is indicated in reversing the bronchospasm of acute bronchial asthma and may also be effective in patients with chronic obstructive pulmonary disease.

   c. The oral dose of theophylline varies from 300–1500 mg/day, aiming for plasma levels of 10–20 μg/ml. Oral theophylline may be continued until the time of surgery. If bronchospasm is well controlled, the anticipated surgery brief, and oral feedings resumed soon after surgery, no adjustments to the regimen are necessary.

   d. If the patient is bronchospastic prior to surgery, or if he will not be able to resume oral feedings soon after surgery, aminophylline should be given intravenously. Aminophylline is a 2 : 1 complex of theophylline and ethylenediamine. For those patients already taking oral theophylline, an initial infusion rate (mg theophylline/hr) may be estimated by dividing their total daily oral dose by 24. For patients not currently receiving theophylline, a loading dose of 5.6 mg/kg lean body weight should be given over at least 15 minutes. Approximate maintenance dosages are 0.9 mg/kg/hr in young patients and 0.5 mg/kg/hr in adults. Smokers generally require an increased dosage of 0.8 mg/kg/hr. Elderly patients and patients with liver disease or congestive heart failure should receive reduced dosages of approximately 0.3 mg/kg/hr.

   e. In all cases, plasma theophylline concentrations should be followed and dosage regimens modified to avoid drug toxicity. High plasma levels of theophylline are associated with nervousness, hyperexcitability, headache, nausea, vomiting, tachycardia, arrhythmias, and seizures.

2. **Beta-adrenergic agonists**

   a. Beta-adrenergic agonists, acting through beta-2 receptors to stimulate adenylate cyclase, increase intracellular levels of cyclic AMP to produce relaxation of bronchial smooth muscle.

   b. Classically, epinephrine and isoproterenol have been used, but their lack of beta-2 selectivity leads to undesirable tachycardia and arrhyth-

Table 3-1. Inhaled beta-adrenergic agonists

Generic name	Trade name	Beta-2 selectivity	Peak effect (minutes)	Duration of action (hours)
Isopro-terenol	Isuprel	0	5–15	1–3
Isoetharine	Bronkosol	+	15–60	1–4
Metapro-terenol	Alupent, Metaprel	+ +	30–60	1–5
Albuterol	Proventil, Ventolin	+ + +	30–60	4–6
Terbutaline	Brethaire	+ + +	30–120	3–6

mias in all but very low doses. Subcutaneous epinephrine (usual dose 0.3 mg SQ), however, remains useful in treating acute exacerbations of bronchial asthma.

  c. Inhalation of beta-adrenergic agonists reduces their cardiovascular side effects. Several agents are available and are summarized in Table 3-1.

3. Corticosteroids

  a. Glucocorticoids are useful in patients with asthma and COPD who have not responded adequately to theophylline and beta-adrenergic agonists. While the reason for the efficacy of steroids is unclear, possible mechanisms of action include reduction of inflammation and histamine release and inhibition of arachidonic acid metabolism.

  b. For acute exacerbations, large doses of prednisone (40–60 mg/day) are given initially and then tapered rapidly. For chronic administration, alternate-day dosage schedules or inhaled steroids may be effective and reduce the incidence and severity of side effects.

  c. Patients who have received steroids within the last 6 months are assumed to have suppressed adrenal cortical function and should receive glucocorticoid coverage (the equivalent of 100 mg hydrocortisone every 8 hours) on the day of surgery. Postoperatively, the dosage should be quickly tapered.

4. Cromolyn

  a. Cromolyn sodium prevents the degranulation of mast cells, thereby inhibiting the release of histamine and leukotrienes. It is effective as prophylaxis against acute attacks in patients with bronchial asthma. It has no value in the management of acute bronchoconstriction and has no bronchodilating effects of its own. Since cromolyn is poorly absorbed orally, it is given by inhalation.

       b. Cromolyn may be continued throughout the perioperative period.

    5. Anticholinergic drugs

       a. Anticholinergic drugs such as atropine and glycopyrrolate decrease airway resistance in normal patients and may produce bronchodilation is asthmatics.

       b. Excessive drying of airway secretions, tachycardia, and central nervous system toxicity limit the use of these agents. In the usual preanesthetic doses (atropine 0.4 mg IM or glycopyrrolate 0.2 mg IM), these drugs do not produce significant bronchodilation or protection against reflex bronchoconstriction. Their routine use is not recommended.

    6. Acetylcysteine (Mucomyst) reduces the viscosity of mucus by disrupting the disulfide bonds of mucoproteins. It may be administered by nebulizer or directly instilled through a bronchoscope. Nebulized acetylcysteine may cause bronchospasm, however, and its use should be preceded by an inhaled beta-adrenergic agonist.

  F. Nutritional support. Patients with severe pulmonary disease or carcinoma often suffer from malnutrition. Protein wasting leads to decreased muscle strength and further deterioration of pulmonary function. Concomitant hypokalemia or hypophosphatemia also may decrease respiratory muscle power. Parenteral nutrition and intravenous repletion of electrolytes may improve pulmonary function in these patients.

V. Premedication. Preanesthetic medication should reduce anxiety and reduce the discomfort of transport, line placement, and so on.

  A. Diazepam, 0.1 to 0.15 mg/kg given orally 1 hour prior to the procedure, is effective in allaying anxiety in most patients.

  B. Narcotics may be used to provide preoperative analgesia, if necessary, but the dosage should be titrated carefully in the patient with pulmonary disease. Narcotics are best avoided entirely in patients with significant airway obstruction or carbon dioxide retention. While narcotics can cause systemic histamine release, there is no evidence to suggest that narcotics, in the doses used for premedication, cause bronchoconstriction.

  C. Anticholinergic drugs are usually not indicated, as they may cause excessive drying of airway secretions and do not produce significant bronchodilation in the doses used for premedication.

  D. Oxygen therapy, if administered preoperatively, should be continued while the patient is being transported or waiting in the induction room.

VI. Choice of anesthetic technique

  A. While it seems reasonable that regional anesthesia should avert many of the pulmonary complications of general anesthesia and reduce the incidence of postoperative pulmonary complications, this hypothesis has been difficult to prove.

B. **Local or regional anesthesia** for surgery on the extremities, eye operations, and other peripheral procedures appears, in general, to be the best choice for patients with pulmonary disease.

C. **Spinal or epidural anesthesia** with levels of sensory anesthesia higher than T6, however, decreases functional residual capacity, expiratory reserve volume, and the patient's ability to cough. In patients with significant pulmonary dysfunction, retained secretions may lead to hypoxemia and respiratory failure. If a high spinal or epidural anesthetic is chosen for a patient with severe pulmonary disease, it may be combined with endotracheal intubation and a light general anesthetic. In this way, control of the airway and lung expansion can be assured.

D. **General anesthesia** is indicated for thoracic and upper abdominal procedures and prolonged peripheral operations in patients with severe pulmonary disease.

1. **Induction** may be performed intravenously or by inhalation, remembering that patients with obstructive disease have increased functional residual capacities and prolonged induction and emergence times.

    a. **Thiobarbiturates** may release histamine and worsen bronchospasm in the asthmatic. Induction with methohexital, an oxybarbiturate, has been associated with less histamine release and may be preferable. Alternatively, ketamine or an inhalational agent may be used for induction.

    b. **Intravenous lidocaine,** 0.5–1.0 mg/kg, decreases airway reflexes and is a helpful adjunct to general anesthesia in bronchospastic patients.

2. **Controlled ventilation** using large tidal volumes and slow rates is recommended to maintain lung volume.

3. **Inhalational anesthetics** depress airway reflexes, cause bronchodilation, and are recommended for maintenance of general anesthesia in patients with pulmonary disease. Of the volatile anesthetics currently used, halothane appears least irritating to the airway and causes the least respiratory depression. In patients with significant pulmonary disease, these advantages may outweigh its potential for hepatotoxicity.

4. Bronchospastic patients may be extubated while still under deep anesthesia if they do not require airway protection or postoperative ventilatory support. This practice may reduce reflex bronchoconstriction during emergence, since the continued presence of the endotracheal tube during light planes of anesthesia can increase airway reactivity.

5. **Respiratory support** should be continued post-

operatively if the patient's pulmonary status is at all in doubt.

E. **Intravenous sedation.** Barbiturates and opioids should be used sparingly in patients with pulmonary disease, since, as discussed above, these patients may be especially prone to respiratory depression from these drugs.

F. **Epidural narcotics** may be used to supplement a general anesthetic and provide postoperative analgesia as well. A lumbar epidural catheter is used routinely. Parenteral narcotic requirements are reduced by this technique. Respiratory depression, especially in patients who normally retain carbon dioxide, pruritus, and urinary retention, however, complicate the use of epidural narcotics.

VII. **Summary.** No one parameter or set of tests can identify with certainty patients who will have postoperative pulmonary complications. At best, a careful preoperative evaluation will identify patients with pulmonary dysfunction and an increased likelihood of postoperative respiratory failure. These patients may benefit from preoperative pulmonary physiotherapy and optimization of their medical regimen. Even with the best preparation, however, postoperative pulmonary complications may occur. The increased risk of surgery in patients with pulmonary disease needs to be carefully weighed against the potential benefits of the proposed procedure.

Suggested Reading

Bendixen, H. H., et al. *Respiratory Care*. St. Louis: Mosby, 1965.

Egbert, L. D., Laver, M. B., and Bendixen, H. H. The effect of site of operation and type of anesthesia upon the ability to cough in the postoperative period. *Surg. Gynecol. Obstet.* 115:295, 1962.

Harman, E., and Lillington, G. Pulmonary risk factors in surgery. *Med. Clin. North Am.* 63:1289, 1979.

Hensley, M. J., and Fencl, V. Lungs and Respiration. In L. D. Vandam (ed.), *To Make the Patient Ready for Anesthesia* (2nd ed.). Menlo Park, Calif.: Addison Wesley, 1984. Pp. 21–46.

Kaplan, J. A. *Thoracic Anesthesia*. New York: Churchill Livingstone, 1983.

LoSasso, A. M., Gibbs, P. S., and Moorthy, S. S. Obstructive Pulmonary Disease. In R. K. Stoelting and S. F. Dierdorf (eds.), *Anesthesia and Co-existing Disease*. New York: Churchill Livingstone, 1983. Pp. 171–200.

LoSasso, A. M., Gibbs, P. S., and Moorthy, S. S. Restrictive Pulmonary Disease. In R. K. Stoelting and S. F. Dierdorf (eds.), *Anesthesia and Co-existing Disease*. New York: Churchill Livingstone, 1983. Pp. 201–207.

Rehder, K., Sessler, A. D., and Marsh, H. M. General anesthesia and the lung. *Am. Rev. Respir. Dis.* 112:541, 1975.

Stein, M., and Cassara, E. L. Preoperative pulmonary evaluation and therapy for surgery patients. *J.A.M.A.* 211:787, 1970.

Tarhan, S., et al. Risk of anesthesia and surgery in patients with chronic bronchitis and chronic obstructive pulmonary disease. *Surgery* 74:720, 1973.

Tisi, G. M. Preoperative evaluation of pulmonary function. *Am. Rev. Respir. Dis.* 119:293, 1979.

4

Specific Considerations with Renal Disease

Thomas L. Higgins

I. Overview of the renal system

A. **Introduction.** Significant renal failure from a variety of etiologies is present in about 5% of patients. The presence of renal impairment will necessitate changes in anesthetic management. Optimal care requires preoperative evaluation of renal function, a knowledge of effects of anesthetics on renal function, selection of appropriate drugs, adjustment of dosages and intervals, and management of oliguria.

B. **Normal renal physiology**
1. In general, the kidneys maintain the volume, composition, and distribution of body fluids; excrete nonessential materials; and have extrarenal regulatory and endocrine functions. Specific renal functions include concentrating urine, regulating sodium (Na^+), and actively secreting wastes and other charged molecules into the urine. About 20% of cardiac output constitutes **renal blood flow** (RBF). From the 1 liter/min RBF, about 1 ml/min of urine is formed.
2. **Autoregulation** maintains blood flow to the kidneys over a wide range of mean arterial blood pressures (50–100 mm Hg). Major factors controlling salt and water excretion include volume status, Starling forces, the renin-angiotensin-aldosterone system, antidiuretic hormone (ADH), prostaglandins, catecholamines, and atrial natriuretic peptides.

II. Renal failure

A. **Acute renal failure** (ARF). Sudden loss of renal function is termed ARF and may be manifest in anuric, oliguric, or nonoliguric forms. Etiology may be *prerenal* (dehydration, low cardiac output), *intrarenal* (drug- or chemical-induced, hepatorenal syndrome, bilateral renal cortical necrosis, occluded renal artery or vein, glomerulitis), or *postrenal* (obstructive). The following problems can be expected:
1. Hypervolemia due to impaired ability to excrete water and Na^+; consequently hypertension and edema develop.
2. Lack of concentrating ability, which may lead to hypovolemia due to obligatory losses.
3. Potassium (K^+) retention.
4. Impaired excretion of drugs and toxins.
5. The possibility of progression to chronic renal failure.

B. **Chronic renal failure** (CRF)
1. A permanent decrease in glomerular filtration rate

(GFR) with a rise in serum creatinine and azotemia characterizes CRF. Patients may be well compensated until late in the course of CRF. CRF may be underdiagnosed; a serum creatinine of 1.2 mg/dl in a frail, elderly patient reflects renal compromise.

2. Common causes of CRF are glomerulonephritis, interstitial disease, cystic kidney disease, renovascular disease, end-stage diabetes or hypertension, and drug-induced renal failure.

3. The following can be expected:

    a. **Anemia.** Coagulation and platelet adhesiveness abnormalities are also seen.

    b. **Blood volume abnormalities.** Hypovolemia is common in early CRF due to obligatory loss. Volume overload occurs late in the disease, and the increased extracellular fluid may be manifest as hypertension and edema.

    c. **Electrolyte abnormalities.** Potassium retention is a late sequela and may be modified by diuretics.

    d. **Chronic metabolic acidosis,** which will interfere with the action of pressor drugs and increase the likelihood of myocardial irritability and hyperkalemia.

    e. **Hypocalcemia and hyperphosphatemia.** Bone disease is common due to elevated parathyroid hormone (PTH), and special care should be taken in positioning. Magnesium retention is seen early, and hypermagnesemia may act synergistically with relaxants. Dialysis may produce hypomagnesemia, which prevents adequate calcium (Ca^+) repletion in hypocalcemia.

    f. **Altered pharmacodynamics** of most drugs, due to changes in the volume of compartments, electrolyte and pH shifts, and rate of excretion.

    g. **Endocrinologic abnormalities** such as carbohydrate intolerance, type IV hyperlipidemia, and hyperparathyroidism.

    h. **Hypertension and accelerated atherosclerosis,** both of which predispose to myocardial ischemia.

    i. **Altered immunity** even in the absence of corticosteroid or immunosuppressive therapy. Patients may have received multiple transfusions and can harbor hepatitis B and other blood-borne pathogens.

    j. **Nausea and vomiting** are more likely; prophylactic treatment with an antiemetic is helpful. These patients have an increased incidence of gastric ulceration and should be pretreated with an H_2 blocker. A perforated ulcer may be masked by steroid therapy.

    k. **Peripheral neuropathy,** myopathy, and abnormal sympathetic responses that may contribute to hypotension under anesthesia.

III. Anesthetic implications of the causes of renal failure

A. Acute glomerulonephritis

1. Acute glomerulonephritis is characterized by abrupt onset of albuminuria, hematuria, hypertension, and edema; it is often preceded by upper respiratory infection. Serious complications are <u>hypertensive encephalopathy and heart failure.</u>

2. If the diagnosis is already established and past the point of spontaneous recovery, there is no advantage in delaying anesthesia.

3. Anesthesia in the acute stage is complicated by heart failure, volume overload, and presence of antihypertensive medication, digitalis, and corticosteroids. When possible, elective surgery should be postponed for 30 days for medical workup, by which time most patients will have recovered.

B. Pyelonephritis

1. The acute form is characterized by sudden onset of chills, fever, flank pain, and symptoms of cystitis, which may mimic an acute abdomen. Renal impairment is rarely present acutely. Elevated temperature and cardiac output may slow induction with inhaled agents.

2. The chronic form can be confused with renal ischemia, chronic interstitial nephritis, radiation injury, and obstruction. There is early impairment of urinary concentrating ability with K^+ wasting.

3. Deranged fluid balance and hypovolemia are seen in both forms. Volume should be repleted prior to induction.

C. Nephrotic syndrome

1. The nephrotic syndrome is characterized by sustained and <u>heavy proteinuria</u> (> 3.5 gm/day), resulting in hypoalbuminemia and edema. Plasma oncotic pressure is decreased, leading to decreased plasma volume, and salt and water retention. As the disease progresses, hypertension also occurs.

2. While total body water is increased, intravascular volume may be depleted. In addition, patients usually take diuretics as well as steroids and antihypertensive medications. Serum K^+ is usually low.

D. Diabetes mellitus

1. Renal involvement is common, particularly in type I (insulin-dependent; juvenile-onset) diabetes of greater than 10 years' duration. <u>Proteinuria becomes progressively more massive</u>, culminating in the nephrotic syndrome.

2. Preoperative assessment to determine presence and extent of renal dysfunction is important. In addition, there is a high correlation between renal dysfunction and diabetic neuropathy, which can involve the autonomic system. Renal papillary necrosis (destruction of the vascular supply of the papilla due to thrombosis or infection) may present with fever and uncontrolled infection.

E. **Connective tissue diseases.** Progressive renal involvement leading to uremia is common in rheumatoid arthritis, systemic lupus erythematosus, and periarteritis nodosa. Presence of any of these conditions should prompt examination of the renal system and appropriate management of fluid status and drug dosage. Elective surgery should be done during quiescent periods of activity in systemic lupus.

F. **Other systemic diseases** that produce glomerular, tubular, or vascular lesions of the kidney include subacute bacterial endocarditis, amyloidosis, gout, myelomatosis, Marfan's syndrome, Henoch-Schönlein purpura, hepatic cirrhosis, leukemia, macroglobulinemia, and sickle cell disease.

IV. **Fluid and electrolyte considerations**

A. **Perioperative fluid management in adults**

   1. **Fluid compartments in adults**

      a. **Total body water** (TBW) = 60% of body weight.

      b. **Blood volume** = 7% of body weight.

      c. **Plasma volume** = 4% of body weight.

      d. Amount of body water is proportional to lean body mass, and there will be proportionately less water in females than males and in obese patients than thin.

   2. **Normal fluid balance**

      a. **Daily water intake** is approximately 2500 ml (1350 in liquid, 800 in solid food, and 350 from metabolism).

      b. **Daily water loss** is normally the same (1500 in urine output, 400 from respiratory loss, 500 in skin evaporation, 100 in stool).

      c. There is high variability from patient to patient. Losses will be increased by fever (500 ml/°C/day), sweating, low humidity, diarrhea, solute diuresis with elevated glucose and contrast dyes, and drug therapy.

   3. **Fluid requirements**

      a. **Repletion of deficit.** Patients will be volume depleted if NPO without a maintenance IV. This deficit (in milliliters) can be estimated by adding 40 to the patient's weight in kilograms and then multiplying by the number of hours since last oral intake. Half the deficit should be replaced in the first hour and the remainder over the course of the operation. Maintenance needs increase if any of the conditions in **2.c** apply.

      b. **Intraoperative maintenance** varies by procedure.

         (1) Noninvasive or closed procedures: 1.5 ml/kg/hr.

         (2) Open procedures: 4–6 ml/kg/hr.

         (3) Major operations where retroperitoneal dissection or intestinal manipulation oc-

curs: 8–10 ml/kg/hr; up to 20 ml/hr may be needed with repair of abdominal aneurysms.

   c. **Initial blood loss** can be replaced with three times the estimated blood loss in crystalloid solution or a combination of fluids and blood products. The indications for transfusion are discussed in Chap. 27.

   d. All of the above estimates are guidelines, not rules; careful clinical observation is critical. Narrowing of the pulse pressure, exaggerated blood pressure response to anesthesia or position change, mottling of the skin, tachycardia, low urine output, and respiratory variation of the blood pressure are all signs of hypovolemia. When in doubt, central venous or pulmonary artery catheterization may be necessary.

B. **Electrolyte disorders**

  1. **Hyponatremia**

    a. Results from the alteration of the renal diluting mechanism.

    b. May be associated with high, normal, or low total body water. Hyponatremia results in a reduced serum osmolality. The relationship between electrolyte concentrations and osmolality is calculated as follows:

$$\text{Osmolality (mOsm)} = 2\,[Na^+\,(mEq/L)\,+\,K^+\,(mEq/L)]$$
$$+\,\left[\frac{\text{urea (mg\%)}}{2.8}\right]\,+\,\left[\frac{\text{glucose (mg\%)}}{18}\right]$$

    c. If larger concentrations of osmotically active substances (glucose, urea, mannitol, methyl alcohol) are present, measured osmolality will be high despite low serum Na^+.

    d. Management relies on determining the volume status of the patient. Dehydrated patients should have their intravascular stores repleted with isotonic crystalloid solutions. Volume-overloaded patients should have their free water intake restricted and undergo gentle diuresis. Hypertonic saline is relatively contraindicated.

    e. Hyponatremia associated with normovolemia occurs with the syndrome of inappropriate ADH secretion, with hypothyroidism, or in the presence of drugs that impair renal water excretion. Stress (including surgery under light anesthesia) can also induce ADH release despite normal volume status. Therapy includes free water restriction and diuresis with replacement of urinary Na^+ and K^+ losses. Although 3% NaCl or mannitol is useful in the emergency management of water intoxication with cerebral edema by promoting fluid shifts to the extracellular fluid, both must be used cautiously to prevent circulatory overload. It is not necessary to normalize serum Na^+ acutely, as most symptoms are relieved by raising the Na^+ concentration to 125–130 mEq/L.

2. **Hypernatremia**
   a. Hypernatremia may also be associated with low, normal, or excessive total body water.
   b. Diarrhea, vomiting, sweating, or osmotic diuresis may precipitate sodium and water excretion, with water loss exceeding that of salt. Therapy consists of administration of free water (5% D/W) until serum Na^+ falls and then administration of 0.45% sodium chloride (NaCl). If hemodynamic instability or evidence of hypoperfusion is present, initial therapy with 0.45% or even 0.9% NaCl is appropriate.
   c. Isolated water loss may occur with diabetes insipidus or excessive insensible loss and is treated with free water.
   d. Hypernatremia with Na^+ overload is normally prevented by thirst mechanisms but is seen with mineralocorticoid excess, dialysis treatment with hypertonic solutions, inappropriate use of 3% NaCl or sodium bicarbonate ($NaHCO_3$), and patients denied free access to water. Symptoms include lethargy, confusion, and coma. The volume of free water needed to restore sodium concentration to normal may be estimated as follows:

   $$\text{Normal TBW (liters)} = 0.6 \times \text{body weight (kg)}$$

   $$\frac{\text{Normal serum } Na^+}{\text{Current serum } Na^+} \times \text{TBW} = \text{current TBW}$$

   $$H_2O \text{ deficit} = \text{normal TBW} - \text{current TBW}$$

   The deficit should be restored slowly to avoid cerebral edema, which may accompany rapid correction.

3. **Hypokalemia**
   a. Hypokalemia may result from K^+ deficits or from shifts in the distribution of body stores. Total body K^+ correlates best with lean body mass, and serum K^+ concentration is a poor index of body stores. In a 70-kg male with normal pH, a fall in serum K^+ from 4 to 3 mEq/L reflects a deficit of 100–200 mEq. Below 3 mEq/L, each fall of 1 mEq/L reflects an additional deficit of 200–400 mEq.
   b. Losses of K^+ occur from the gastrointestinal tract (vomiting, diarrhea, ureterosigmoidostomy, and obstructed ileal loops) and from the kidney (mineralocorticoid and glucocorticoid excess, renal tubular acidosis, diuretic therapy,

and use of terbutaline to suppress premature labor). Changes in K^+ distribution occur with alkalosis as cellular H^+ shifts to the extracellular fluid and K^+ moves intracellularly. Thus, rapid overcorrection of respiratory acidosis by artificial ventilation may result in fatal hypokalemia. Vigorous correction of metabolic acidosis with $NaHCO_3$ or treatment of diabetic ketoacidosis without K^+ repletion may also produce fatal hypokalemia.

   c. **Manifestations** of K^+ deficiency rarely appear until the serum K^+ is less than 3 mEq/L unless the rate of fall is rapid. These effects include neuromuscular weakness, augmentation of nondepolarizing block, ileus, and disturbances of cardiac conduction. ECG changes of K^+ depletion include flattened T waves, U waves, S–T segment depression, and atrial and ventricular arrhythmias. Ventricular ectopy is more likely in patients taking digitalis. Serum K^+ less than 2.0 mEq/L is associated with vasoconstriction and rhabdomyolysis.

   d. In the past, elective procedures have been delayed until K^+ is greater than 2.8; and **slow** repletion accomplished with intravenous KCl (10 mEq of K^+ diluted in at least 50 ml of fluid given over 1 hour). Recent publications have questioned the necessity of repleting K^+ in the asymptomatic, chronically depleted patient. We have seen more problems due to rapid K^+ repletion than hypokalemia itself.

4. **Hyperkalemia**

   a. **Etiologies** may be decreased excretion; release from cells following surgery, hemolysis, or trauma; or iatrogenic. In renal failure patients, salt substitutes, banked blood, and potassium penicillin are all sources of exogenous K^+. Artifactual elevation is seen with thrombocytosis, hemolysis, and improper handling of the sample.

   b. **Manifestations** include neuromuscular weakness and paresthesias and cardiac abnormalities, which are increasingly dangerous as the serum K^+ rises above 7 mEq/L. Bradycardia, hypotension, ventricular fibrillation, and cardiac arrest may result. The ECG findings include high-peaked T waves progressing to depressed S–T segments, diminished R-wave amplitude, prolonged P–R interval, and ultimately widening of the QRS complex and prolonged Q–T interval.

   c. **Management** depends on the degree of urgency as assessed by ECG changes or serum K^+ level. Presence of ECG abnormalities is an indication for slow IV administration of 500–1000 mg of calcium chloride ($CaCl_2$) or calcium gluconate. The dose may be repeated in 5 minutes if ECG changes persist. $NaHCO_3$ (50 ml) moves K^+ into cells and may be given IV over 5 minutes and repeated in 10–15 minutes. A "K^+ cocktail" consisting of 150 ml of 50% D/W plus 100 ml of $NaHCO_3$ with 10–30 units of regular insulin administered at 25–50 ml/hr will reduce serum K^+ levels. Cation-exchange resins such as Kayexalate, 50 gm, with sorbitol as a retention enema will slowly remove K^+ from the body. Serum K^+ concentration can also be lowered by dialysis.

V. Assessment of renal function

A. History

1. Symptoms: polyuria, polydipsia, fatigue, dysuria, edema.
2. Medications of particular note: diuretics, K^+ supplement, carbonic anhydrase inhibitors, osmotic agents.
3. In dialyzed patients, determine dialysis schedule, wet and dry weights, and patient's symptomatic responses to fluid overload.

B. Physical examination

1. Findings usually minimal until CRF is far advanced.
2. Hypertension is common; look for evidence of cardiovascular problems (i.e., valvular murmurs, rales, edema, orthopnea, paroxysmal nocturnal dyspnea, orthostatic hypotension).
3. Hypovolemia results in oliguria, low pulse pressure, orthostatic hypotension, and tachycardia. The record of daily weights should be examined, particularly in dialyzed patients.
4. Skin turgor estimates extracellular fluid volume but is an unreliable estimate of the intravascular volume, particularly in elderly and edematous patients.

C. Laboratory data

1. Disease may be present despite normal laboratory values, but problems significant for the anesthesiologist are generally manifested by laboratory abnormalities. Trends over time are more helpful than single determinations. For example, a "normal" serum creatinine of 1.1 becomes ominous when the value 6 months previously was 0.8.
2. **Urinalysis**
   a. Presence of protein, blood, white blood cells, and casts alone or in combination may or may not be indicative of disease. Many such abnormalities are of a transient nature or of no clinical significance. Management strategy should be referral for medical workup after the procedure if there are no other contraindications to anesthesia.

    b. Ability to acidify urine suggests renal competence.

    c. Ability to concentrate urine is lost before other changes become apparent and is indicative of compromised fluid homeostasis. A specific gravity of 1.018 or more following an overnight fast suggests concentrating ability is intact. Urine specific gravity is useful to evaluate fluid status; however, intravenous pyelogram and angiography dye and osmotic agents such as mannitol will elevate specific gravity (to ≥ 1.040).

    d. Massive proteinuria indicates severe glomerular damage.

    e. Glycosuria may herald diabetes but can also indicate spillage in a patient receiving intravenous dextrose.

3. Electrolytes. Plasma Na^+, K^+, Cl^-, and HCO_3^- will usually be normal until renal failure is advanced. Careful consideration of the risks and benefits of proceeding with elective surgery should be made if Na^+ is less than 131 or greater than 150 mEq/L or if K^+ is less than 2.8 or greater than 5.7 mEq/L, because these abnormalities may exacerbate arrhythmias and seriously compromise the outcome of resuscitations.

4. Serum Ca^{2+}, PO_4^{2-}, and Mg^{2+}. Renal failure results in hypocalcemia, phosphate retention, and mild hypermagnesemia.

5. Blood urea nitrogen (BUN) reflects GFR, but is influenced by fluid status, diet, body habitus, and cardiac output. The ratio of BUN to creatinine is normally 10 to 20 : 1; disproportionate elevation of the BUN may represent hypovolemia, low cardiac output, or occult gastrointestinal bleeding.

6. Serum creatinine is normally 0.6–1.2 mg/dl, but interpretation should be tempered by knowledge of the patient's muscle mass and activity level. **Creatinine clearance** (C_{Cr}, normally 80–140 ml/min) provides the best estimate of renal reserve. A value below 25 ml/min indicates severe renal failure. Creatinine clearance can be estimated from the serum creatinine using the following formula:

$$\text{Creatinine clearance} = \frac{(140 - \text{age}) \times \text{weight (kg)}}{72 \times \text{serum creatinine}}$$

This formula overestimates creatinine clearance in females by 10–15% and is invalid in the presence of gross renal insufficiency or changing renal function. Mild renal dysfunction is present with clearance values between 50 and 80 ml/min.

7. Complete blood count (CBC). An anephric patient typically has a hemoglobin level of 6–8 gm/dl due to absence of erythropoietin. In patients with renal transplants, red blood cell, white blood cell,

and platelet counts will be depressed by immunosuppressive therapy. General debilitation, inadequate bone marrow production, and drug therapy
may predispose to coagulation abnormalities.

8. **Electrocardiogram** (ECG) may reveal pericarditis, silent myocardial infarction, or ischemia and is
a sensitive indicator of toxic effects of K^+.
   a. **Hyperkalemia.** Flattened P waves, widening
      of the QRS complex, tall peaked T waves, de-
      pressed S–T segments, ventricular arrhyth-
      mias, and ultimately sinusoidal complexes that
      become ventricular tachycardia or fibrillation.
   b. **Hypokalemia.** The T wave may be flat or in-
      verted, and a U wave may be present.
   c. **Hypercalcemia.** Shortened Q–T interval.
   d. **Hypocalcemia.** Lengthened Q–T interval.
   e. **Digitalis toxicity** is common due to decreased
      renal elimination; it manifests as shortened Q–
      T, S–T scooping, and T-wave changes.

9. **Chest x-ray.** Fluid overload, infection, pericardial
   effusion, uremic pneumonitis, or hypotensive cardiovascular disease may be revealed.

10. **Arterial blood gases** and **pH** can delineate the ex-
    tent of acid-base abnormality. Compensated meta-
    bolic acidosis is common in renal failure.

11. **Total protein** is normally 6–8 gm/dl; less than 5
    gm/dl will result in peripheral edema and changes
    in drug availability.

VI. **Anesthetic effects on the kidney**
   A. Depression of RBF, to a lesser extent GFR, accompanies
      the administration of general anesthesia. Spinal and
      epidural **anesthesia** produce decrements in RBF, GFR,
      and urine flow, with the magnitude of change tending
      to parallel the degree of sympathetic blockade. Gen-
      erally the changes are one-third to one-half those
      seen with general anesthesia if severe hypotension is
      avoided.
      1. **Indirect effects.** Myocardial depression, hypoten-
         sion, and renal vasoconstriction accompany general
         anesthesia. Halothane, enflurane, isoflurane, and
         thiopental all cause mild to moderate increases
         in renal vascular resistance to compensate for
         decreased blood pressure. Catecholamine release
         causes redistribution of renal cortical blood flow.
         Alpha-adrenergic blockers (e.g., droperidol) prevent
         redistribution of intrarenal blood flow due to cate-
         cholamine release; thus neuroleptanesthesia may
         cause the smallest change in renal function. Even
         well-hydrated volunteers with normal renal func-
         tion experience transient postanesthetic altera-
         tions in renal function. These alterations may occur
         despite insignificant changes in blood pressure and
         cardiac output, suggesting that changes in intra-
         renal distribution or regional blood flow are respon-
         sible. ADH levels do not change during halothane
         or morphine anesthesia but increase with the onset

of surgical stimulation. Hydration before the induction of anesthesia attenuates the rise in ADH produced by painful stimuli.

2. **Direct effects** are usually obscured by the marked indirect effects. The direct toxicity of fluorinated ethers is of concern since fluoride (F^-) inhibits metabolic processes, affects urinary concentration and dilution, and can cause proximal tubular swelling and necrosis. The magnitude of serum F^- elevation is concentration and duration dependent. Levels above 50 μM are associated with detectable renal dysfunction.

   a. **Methoxyflurane** (MOF) undergoes hepatic biotransformation to inorganic F^- and oxalic acid; these substances are nephrotoxins and F^- has been associated with polyuric renal failure and nephrogenic diabetes insipidus. The occurrence of renal failure is dose related; recommended maximum concentrations of MOF are 0.35% for 1 hour, 0.19% for 2 hours, and 0.09% for 3 hours, but it is contraindicated in the presence of renal dysfunction. MOF is not currently in use at Massachusetts General Hospital.

   b. **Enflurane** is metabolized to F^- more slowly than MOF and is associated with lower levels of F^- (typically < 15 μM). Since F^- clearance is about 50% of creatinine clearance, there is theoretic concern that use of enflurane in patients with renal dysfunction may lead to F^- accumulation and additional nephrotoxicity. Some authors recommend avoiding enflurane in renal failure patients, especially in high concentrations or for prolonged procedures, since it is possible that patients with preexisting disease are at risk in the presence of F^- concentrations usually considered nontoxic.

   c. **Isoflurane** is not associated with significant increases in F^-, because of much slower metabolism.

   d. **Halothane** has a different structure and metabolism and results in the lowest F^- level.

B. With short cases, changes in renal function are reversible (RBF and GFR return to normal within a few hours). With extensive surgery and prolonged anesthesia, impaired ability to excrete a water load or concentrate urine is seen and may last for several days.

VII. **Renal failure and drugs used in anesthesia.** Alterations in drug action are seen in severe renal disease due to anemia, serum protein and electrolyte abnormalities, changes in the volume of distribution, impaired biotransformation, and markedly decreased renal elimination. Uremia may be associated with central nervous system (CNS) depression, reducing the requirement for sedation by up to 50%.

A. **Lipid-soluble drugs.** In general, lipid-soluble agents are poorly ionized and metabolized by the liver to water-soluble forms before elimination by the kidney. With a few exceptions, the metabolites have little biologic activity.

1. **Atropine** and **glycopyrrolate** are eliminated largely by the kidney, and reduced dosages must be used with severe renal failure. **Scopolamine** is preferable as a drying agent but may be unnecessary, since anuric patients often have dry mucous membranes.

2. **Benzodiazepines, phenothiazines,** and **butyrophenones** are metabolized in the liver to both active and inactive compounds, which are then eliminated by the kidney. Benzodiazepines are 90–95% protein-bound. **Lorazepam,** in particular, is not recommended in patients with severe renal failure due to its potential for accumulation. **Diazepam** may be used with careful consideration of its long half-life and active metabolites. The alpha-adrenergic blockade of phenothiazine derivatives may accentuate cardiovascular instability, particularly in recently dialyzed patients.

3. **Narcotics** are metabolized in the liver to inactive forms but may have a more intense and prolonged effect in patients with renal failure, particularly in hypoalbuminemic patients where protein binding will be reduced. **Fentanyl** is less protein-bound than **meperidine** or **morphine.** All three drugs may be used in renal failure, but their duration of action may be prolonged.

4. **Halothane** may combine with hyperkalemia, hypocalcemia, and acidosis to exacerbate myocardial irritability.

5. **Thiopental** is 65–75% protein-bound, and in hypoalbuminemic patients a much greater proportion is available to reach receptor sites. Acidosis and changes in the blood-brain barrier further reduce the thiopental requirement. Intravascular volume depletion may precipitate hypotension following induction.

B. **Ionized drugs.** Drugs that are highly ionized at a physiologic pH tend to be eliminated unchanged by the kidney, and their duration of action may be prolonged by renal dysfunction.

1. **Relaxants**

   a. **d-Tubocurarine** (dTc) is normally 70–80% excreted by the kidney, but alternative biliary excretion is enhanced fourfold in the presence of CRF. Thus, it can be used in renal failure and anephric patients with appropriate reduction in dosage and frequency of administration. The functioning newly transplanted kidney can excrete dTc at a nearly normal rate.

   b. **Metocurine** relies almost exclusively on renal clearance for elimination. It is best avoided in renal failure due to the absence of significant biliary excretion.

c. **Gallamine** is eliminated entirely by the kidney and should not be used in renal failure.

d. **Pancuronium,** like dTc, is primarily eliminated by the kidney, and duration of neuromuscular blockade may be increased 80% in patients with renal failure. Presence of alternative metabolic and biliary elimination allows use of this drug in reduced dosage with proper monitoring.

e. **Atracurium** is eliminated by nonenzymatic degradation and ester hydrolysis in plasma. Initial dosage in renal patients does not differ, but a longer interval between doses may be appropriate. Laudanosine, a CNS stimulant in a variety of animal species, may accumulate in the presence of renal failure, but its clinical significance is still controversial.

f. **Vecuronium** depends on hepatic elimination, does not release histamine, and has a relative lack of cardiovascular effects, making it an ideal drug for renal failure patients. Repeated doses have a longer duration of action than in normal patients.

g. **Succinylcholine** in single doses can be used without difficulty in patients with decreased or absent renal function. Succinylmonocholine, the breakdown product that is excreted by the kidney, can produce a nondepolarizing block if large amounts accumulate. Pseudocholinesterase levels may be reduced following hemodialysis. Following succinylcholine administration, serum K^+ normally rises 0.5–1.0 mEq/L. This rise may be dangerous in the uremic patient with preexisting hyperkalemia, hypocalcemia, and acidosis.

Not c̄ neuromusc.

2. **Cholinesterase inhibitors**

a. **Neostigmine** is 50% renally eliminated, and its serum half-life is prolonged similar to that of dTc in the absence of renal function.

b. **Edrophonium** is primarily eliminated by the kidney, but nonrenal metabolism accounts for 30% of its clearance in the absence of renal function.

c. **Pyridostigmine** is 75% renally eliminated, but hepatic conversion to inactive 3-hydroxy-*N*-methylpyridinium also occurs.

d. With impaired renal function, the elimination of the reversal drugs is decreased and their half-lives prolonged. Prolongation is greater than that for pancuronium or dTc, thus the return of muscle relaxation after adequate reversal (**recurarization**) is rarely seen, and if it occurs, is probably due to abnormalities in pH or electrolytes. Recurarization has not been reported after pharmacologic reversal of vecuronium.

3. **Vasoactive agents**
    a. **Catecholamines** with alpha-adrenergic effects (norepinephrine, epinephrine, phenylephrine, ephedrine) constrict the renal vasculature and reduce RBF. **Isoproterenol** also reduces RBF, but to a lesser extent. **Dopamine** at low doses (0.5–3 μg/kg/min) stimulates dopaminergic receptors and increases RBF. However, at doses of 10 μg/kg/min or more, alpha-adrenergic effects predominate.
    b. **Sodium nitroprusside** contains cyanide and is metabolized to renally excreted thiocyanate. Toxicity (primarily neurologic) from excessive accumulation of thiocyanate is thus more likely in the renal failure patient.
    c. **Trimethaphan** (Arfonad) is a ganglionic blocker useful in control of hypertensive crisis. Trimethaphan liberates histamine, and its hypotensive effect is more pronounced in the presence of diuretic agents.
4. **Digitalis** preparations are excreted in the urine. Blood levels should be determined, and initial digitalization or changes in therapy should be avoided prior to surgery.

VIII. **General principles of management**
  A. **Assess degree of renal involvement.**
    1. If function is greater than 50% of normal ($C_{Cr} > 60$ ml/min), patients can be managed as usual.
    2. Patients with mild azotemia, nocturia, decreased concentrating ability, and slight anemia require special attention to RBF to avoid further renal compromise. Drug dosages need to be adjusted.
    3. Overt renal failure (serum creatinine ≥ 3.0, creatinine clearance 20–25 ml/min) will be accompanied by anemia, decreased oxygen-carrying capacity, blood volume and electrolyte abnormalities, coagulopathies, and susceptibility to infection.
  B. **Anticipate hypotension.** Renal failure patients often respond to induction as if they were hypovolemic, regardless of volume status. Sympathetic blockade from antihypertensive medications or chronic uremia can augment this tendency. Direct alpha-adrenergic agents such as phenylephrine are effective but decrease renal circulation. Isoproterenol will exacerbate myocardial irritability.
  C. **Anticipate hypoxia.** Decreased O_2-carrying capacity due to anemia is usually well tolerated at rest by a compensatory rightward shift in the oxygen-hemoglobin dissociation curve via 2, 3-DPG and acidosis. Thus, preoperative transfusions are not routinely indicated. Supplemental O_2 should be used preinduction. Because general anesthesia will increase intrapulmonary shunting and decrease cardiac output, nitrous oxide (N_2O) should be limited to an inspired concentration of 50% intraoperatively unless the PaO_2 or O_2 saturation is mea-

sured continuously. Increased cardiac output due to anemia will prolong induction with volatile agents.

D. Modify drug dosages, intervals, and choices to take into account altered elimination.

E. Expect coagulopathies, which are often related to abnormal platelet function.

F. Minimize susceptibility to infection with careful attention to placement of monitoring lines, Foley catheters, and endotracheal tubes. Patients receiving immunosuppressive drugs or corticosteroids are particularly at risk.

G. Expect diminished duration (up to 50%) **of regional blocks,** particularly with brachial plexus anesthesia. The mechanism is thought to be increased cardiac output with increased tissue blood flow, leading to more rapid clearance of the anesthetic agent.

H. Anticipate ARF, particularly following dye studies and after major abdominal procedures. Patients with renal stones should be maintained on intravenous fluids while NPO to avoid dehydration.

IX. Specific management problems

A. Diagnosis and treatment of intraoperative oliguria

1. **Oliguria** is defined as daily urine output of less than 400–500 ml or hourly output of less than 0.5 ml/kg.

2. **Causes of oliguria**

   a. **Prerenal.** Due to low intravascular volume, cardiac output, or RBF. Under these conditions, normal kidneys will attempt to conserve Na^+; therefore, urine osmolality should be above 400 with a urine Na^+ less than 20 mEq/L.

   b. **Intrarenal.** Due to acute tubular necrosis (ATN) secondary to ischemia or drugs. In the absence of diuretics, a urinary sodium above 30 mEq/L combined with a low urine osmolality is suggestive of ATN.

   c. **Postrenal.** Ureteral obstruction, recognized by the absence of urine output.

3. **Treatment**

   a. **Prerenal azotemia** requires volume repletion with crystalloid or, when indicated, blood products or colloid. Rapid infusion of 500 ml of saline or lactated Ringer's solution serves as both a diagnostic and therapeutic maneuver in most patients. Monitoring of the central venous or pulmonary arterial pressure is indicated if the patient fails to respond or where fluid challenge poses the risk of congestive heart failure and fluid overload. Low-dose dopamine or other inotropic drugs may improve cardiac output and RBF once adequate intravascular volume is attained.

   b. Management of **ATN** should begin with reversal of the cause, if possible. Monitoring of intravascular volume is essential to rule out coexisting prerenal causes. The use of diuretics (e.g., mannitol, furosemide) to maintain urine output is controversial. Nonoliguric renal failure carries a lesser mortality than oliguric renal failure, but it is unclear whether diuretics change the ultimate outcome. However, diuretics may produce prerenal azotemia and stimulate the renin-angiotensin system and confound the diagnostic picture for 6–12 hours after administration.

B. Patients undergoing dialysis

   1. Hemodialysis patients may have a surgically created arteriovenous fistula or synthetic cannula implanted in the forearm or lower leg. These limbs should not be used for IV lines or blood pressure monitoring by cuff. The amount of blood shunted (150–300 ml/min) may contribute to delay in induction. Hemodialysis is typically performed two or three times weekly, and serum electrolyte and volume abnormalities are corrected by adjusting the dialysis bath fluid. <u>Blood samples taken immediately after dialysis will be inaccurate</u>; redistribution of fluid and electrolytes <u>takes about 6 hours following</u> therapy. <u>We try to schedule surgery in the afternoon</u> following morning dialysis. If the dialysis team is notified, the procedure can be modified to minimize systemic heparinization.

   2. Peritoneal dialysis is accomplished using the patient's peritoneum as the exchange membrane, and these patients are at risk for peritonitis. The technique is useful after fluid overload or in the patient where hemodialysis access cannot immediately be established.

Suggested Reading

Cousins, M. J., Skowronski, G., and Plummer, J. L. Anaesthesia and the kidney. *Anaesth. Intensive Care* 11:292, 1983.

Cronnelly, R., et al. Renal function and the pharmacokinetics of neostigmine in anesthetized man. *Anesthesiology* 51:222, 1979.

Cronnelly, R. Pharmacology of muscle relaxant reversal. *1985 Annual Refresher Course Lectures.* American Society of Anesthesiologists, 1985.

Frazier, H. S., and Yager, H. Clinical use of diuretics. *N. Engl. J. Med.* 288:246, 1973.

Freitag, J. J., and Miller, L. W. (eds.). *Manual of Medical Therapeutics* (23rd ed.). Boston: Little, Brown, 1980.

Klein, L. A. Evaluation of function in the preoperative kidney. *Urol. Clin. North Am.* 3:293, 1976.

Laragh, J. H. Atrial natriuretic hormone. *N. Engl. J. Med.* 313:1330, 1985.

Levinsky, N. G. Pathophysiology of acute renal failure. *N. Engl. J. Med.* 296:1453, 1977.

Maddern, P. J. Anaesthesia for the patient with impaired renal function. *Anaesth. Intensive Care* 11:321, 1983.

Mazze, R. I., Sievenpiper, T. S., and Stephenson, J. Renal effects of enflurane and halothane in patients with abnormal renal function. *Anesthesiology* 60:161, 1984.

Mazze, R. I., and Cousins, M. J. Renal Diseases. In J. Katz, J. Benumof, and L. B. Kadis (eds.), *Anesthesia and Uncommon Diseases* (2nd ed.). Philadelphia: Saunders, 1981.

Nancarrow, C., and Mather, L. E. Pharmacokinetics in renal failure. *Anaesth. Intensive Care* 11:350, 1983.

Schrier, R. W. *Renal and Electrolyte Disorders* (3rd ed.). Boston: Little, Brown, 1986.

Textor, S. C., et al. Critical perfusion pressure for patients with bilateral atherosclerotic renovascular disease. *Ann. Intern. Med.* 102:308, 1985.

5

Specific Considerations with Liver Disease

Charles E. Cook

The liver performs a multitude of crucial biosynthetic, detoxifying, and digestive functions. Consequently, liver disease adversely affects almost all other vital organs. Anesthesia for patients with liver disease depends on knowledge of the relevant pathophysiology, but since the drugs and procedures used during surgery may affect even healthy livers, salient features of normal liver function will be reviewed as well.

I. **Energy sources for the liver**
   A. **Hepatic blood flow and oxygenation**
      1. The **hepatic artery** supplies one-half of the blood supply, but because of its higher oxygen content, it provides about one-third of the oxygen. The **portal vein** carries venous blood from the abdominal viscera to the liver and supplies the remaining two-thirds of the blood supply and one-half of the oxygen. Portal blood is rich in nutrients (and medications) absorbed from the intestine and in hormones from the pancreas (insulin, glucagon, gastrin) and intestine (vasoactive intestinal peptide, cholecystokinin). The **total hepatic blood flow** is usually about 25% of the resting cardiac output.
      2. A healthy liver can survive interruption of either blood supply, although some degree of hepatic dysfunction usually occurs. The hepatic artery may be ligated to control surgical bleeding or the portal vein may be thrombosed from trauma, parasitic infections, or sepsis. However, diseased livers have much less reserve, and infarction may follow reduction in either source of hepatic blood flow.
   B. **Substrates.** Nutrients are absorbed by the gastrointestinal tract and delivered through the portal circulation. Carbohydrates are converted to glycogen, lipids are combined with carrier proteins for transport to adipose tissue, and amino acids are used directly for protein synthesis or gluconeogenesis.

II. **Functions of the liver**
   A. **Synthetic functions**
      1. **Protein synthesis**
         a. **Albumin** is synthesized exclusively by the liver. It is the major oncotic source in the plasma and a carrier protein for many lipophilic and acidic drugs (including barbiturates, benzodiazepines, and lipophilic narcotics). **Hypoalbuminemia** results in diminished protein binding, higher free drug levels, and thus more rapid and pronounced drug effects (especially when drugs are given as a bolus). Higher free

drug levels also enhance clearance from the plasma and thus shorten half-lives. If present, elevated bilirubin levels will further enhance drug displacement and magnify these effects. Hypoalbuminemia also causes an expansion of the extracellular fluid volume (in the form of ascites and edema), increasing the volume of distribution (V$_D$) for water-soluble drugs, diluting out their effects. Even if their renal or hepatic clearance remains unchanged, the expanded V$_D$ will lengthen the half-life.

In summary, hypoalbuminemia will *enhance* the effects and clearance of lipophilic or highly protein-bound drugs and *reduce* the effects and clearance of other drugs. However, because the magnitude of these effects cannot be predicted in a given clinical setting, all drugs should be titrated to specific end points in each patient.

b. **Alpha-1 acid glycoprotein** is synthesized in the liver, secreted into the blood, and is increased with chronic inflammation, malignancy, or stress (e.g., myocardial infarction, burns, trauma, or surgery). It binds basic drugs; for example, muscle relaxants, local anesthetics, beta blockers, and some narcotics. Elevation of this **"acute phase reactant"** can cause more of a drug to be protein-bound, reducing the clinical effects and clearance.

c. **Clotting factors** are synthesized predominantly in the liver. The major exception is factor VIII, which comes from vascular endothelial cells. When levels fall below 30–50% of normal, a clinically significant coagulopathy will be evident. Vitamin K–dependent factors (II, VII, IX, and X) require carboxylation of certain of their glutamic acid residues for activity. This carboxylation step depends on vitamin K as a coenzyme. Vitamin K is synthesized by colonic flora and absorbed with the aid of bile salts secreted by the liver. Vitamin K deficiency can be caused by hepatic dysfunction, biliary obstruction, or therapies designed to reduce the colonic flora (e.g., lactulose or neomycin). Deficiency of the vitamin K–dependent factors causes a prolongation of the prothrombin time (PT) and can be treated with parenteral vitamin K (Aqua-MEPHYTON, 10 mg/day IM for 3 days) or, acutely, with transfusion of fresh-frozen plasma (FFP).

d. **Plasma cholinesterase** is synthesized by the liver, usually in such excess that even patients with severe hepatic dysfunction manifest only mild prolongation in the action of succinylcholine. However, continuous infusions of succinylcholine should be titrated with the aid of a blockade monitor (see Chap. 11). Similarly, toxic doses of ester-type local anesthetics and other drugs that are metabolized by pseudocholinesterase are easier to reach.

2. **Bile production.** Bile contains primary bile salts (synthesized by the liver), secondary bile salts (synthesized by colonic flora from primary bile salts), cholesterol, fatty acids, proteins, carbohydrates, electrolytes, bilirubin and other metabolic waste products, and many of the drug metabolites produced by the liver. Failure to produce and excrete bile results in jaundice, steatorrhea, and fat-soluble vitamin (A, D, and K) deficiencies.

3. <u>**Gluconeogenesis.**</u> <u>Normal livers can store enough glycogen to maintain the blood glucose level for about 12 hours.</u> Beyond this time, glucose is derived from hepatocellular gluconeogenesis. Adult elective patients usually fast for 8–12 hours preoperatively and therefore are <u>dependent on gluconeogenesis during surgery.</u> Although the stress hormones released at surgery (epinephrine, glucocorticoids, and glucagon) generally promote <u>glycogenolysis</u> and hyperglycemia, patients with impaired hepatic function may develop hypoglycemia.

B. **Metabolism and detoxification**

1. **Bilirubin** is the final metabolite of heme. Excess bilirubin may be caused by increased production (e.g., massive transfusion, absorption of large hematomas, or hemolysis) or decreased metabolism (e.g., hereditary abnormalities). Bilirubin is very lipophilic and is transported to the liver bound to albumin, where it is conjugated with glucuronic acid and then secreted in the bile. **Unconjugated hyperbilirubinemia** is usually due to excess production or congenital syndromes of faulty bile transport (e.g., Gilbert's syndrome). <u>**Conjugated hyperbilirubinemia** occurs with hepatocellular disease (e.g., alcoholic or viral hepatitis, cirrhosis),</u> diseases of the small bile ducts (e.g., primary biliary cirrhosis), congenital syndromes (e.g., Dubin-Johnson syndrome), or obstruction of the extrahepatic biliary ducts.

2. **Ammonia** is a product of the deamination of amino acids and other organic amines and is converted to urea by the liver. Thus, the blood urea nitrogen (BUN) may be low in acute hepatic failure. Serum ammonia levels are often monitored to assess the degree of liver impairment and sometimes, but not always, correlate with the level of hepatic encephalopathy. Another factor that could be involved in the etiology of hepatic encephalopathy is the presence of unmetabolized amines, acting as false neurotransmitters or antagonists.

3. **Steroid hormones.** Since the liver metabolizes steroid hormones, <u>hepatic failure results in signs of</u>

steroid excess. Excess aldosterone causes sodium and fluid retention (aggravating ascites and edema) and loss of potassium in the urine. Relative estrogen excess from diminished conversion to androgen may be the source of the peripheral stigmata of liver disease, including palmar erythema, spider angiomata, and gynecomastia.

4. **Drugs.** The liver is a major site of drug metabolism and elimination. Considering the large reserve of liver parenchyma, only severe hepatitis and end-stage liver disease will affect drug metabolism in a clinically significant manner. Even in illnesses that destroy hepatocytes, compensatory mechanisms increase the enzyme content of remaining cells.

   a. **Mechanisms.** Some drugs are metabolized by specific cytoplasmic enzymes such as alcohol dehydrogenase (ethanol and methanol to acetic and formic acids, respectively) and rhodanase (cyanide to thiocyanate). However, most compounds are initially metabolized by a family of **mixed-function oxidases,** the cytochrome P-450 enzymes. In a **second phase of metabolism,** many drugs are conjugated with glucuronic acid, glycine, or sulfate to enhance their water solubility for excretion in bile or urine. In some cases, metabolites are more active (e.g., prednisolone produced from prednisone), longer lasting (e.g., the desmethyl metabolite of diazepam), or more toxic (e.g., formaldehyde and formic acid produced from methanol) than the original drug.

   b. **Induction of enzymes.** The hepatic cytoplasmic enzymes (especially the cytochrome P-450 family) can be induced to increase in activity by exposure to the drugs that they metabolize. This is true for barbiturates, benzodiazepines, corticosteroids, antihistamines, ethanol, phenytoin, and chloral hydrate. In patients, enzyme induction may result in **dispositional tolerance** where increasing drug dosages are required due to accelerated metabolism. Induction is nonspecific, as cross-tolerance among some of these agents has also been reported; cross-tolerance has important implications for the toxicity of anesthetics (see sec. II.B.4.c.(1)).

   c. **Halogenated inhalational agents**
      (1) **Methoxyflurane (MOF), enflurane, and isoflurane** are degraded in the liver to produce inorganic fluoride ion (F^-), which is nephrotoxic.
         (a) Because of its very high lipid solubility, about 50% of the absorbed **MOF** is metabolized, with F^- concentration peaking 2–3 days later. The de-

fluoridation (and toxicity) of MOF can be increased by enzyme induction with barbiturates.

(b) Only 2% of absorbed **enflurane** is metabolized to produce F^-. Thus renal toxicity is unlikely with this agent, whether or not enzymes are induced with barbiturates. However, patients taking isoniazid may induce the cytochrome P-451 variant, which greatly increases the production of F^- from enflurane to potentially nephrotoxic levels. In addition, anecdotal cases of hepatic damage from enflurane have been reported.

(c) Only 0.2% of absorbed **isoflurane** is metabolized. Although this can be increased by barbiturate induction of enzymes, F^- levels are still well below the nephrotoxic range. Because of the relative inertness of isoflurane, it is probably less likely to cause hepatic damage.

(2) **Halothane.** About 20% of absorbed halothane is oxidized in the liver to form trifluoroacetic acid, chloride, and bromide. Only trace amounts of F^- are produced. Alternatively, halothane may be reduced by cytochrome P-450 in the absence of oxygen to produce [1-chloro-2,2,2-trifluoroethyl] free radicals, which can interact with fatty acids. It has been hypothesized that this reductive pathway is involved in the idiosyncratic hepatocellular injury associated with halothane, either by directly damaging hepatocellular membranes or by serving as haptens to trigger an autoimmune hepatitis.

d. **Barbiturates.** Long- and intermediate-acting barbiturates (phenobarbital, pentobarbital, secobarbital, and amobarbital), whose durations of action are determined by metabolism, will have prolonged effects in liver failure. But even the short-acting barbiturates (thiopental, thiamylal, and methohexital), whose durations (in the usual induction doses) are limited by redistribution, must still be used cautiously because hypoalbuminemia decreases the protein binding of barbiturates and thus increases the active unbound fraction (see sec. **II.A.1**).

e. **Neuromuscular blocking agents** are typically very polar and may be excreted unchanged in the urine. Their clinical durations can be prolonged in hepatic failure due to an expanded V_D. Ordinarily a small proportion of **curare** and **pancuronium** are excreted in the bile. **Vecuronium** has a significantly shorter half-life than pancuronium because of its increased uptake and metabolism by the liver. **Atracurium** is metabolized primarily by nonenzymatic Hofmann elimination, but also by nonspecific plasma esterases synthesized in the liver. However, since only very severe hepatic dysfunction reduces these enzymes, the clinical duration of atracurium is generally not significantly changed.

    f. Vasoactive amines are either metabolized by monoamine oxidase and catechol-O-methyltransferase throughout the body or are taken up into nerve terminals. Thus, hepatic dysfunction does not usually elevate the intrinsic levels of catecholamines; metabolism of parenterally administered agents may be moderately decreased. However, for many orally administered drugs (e.g., propranolol), significant clearance occurs in the liver following their absorption into the portal blood (the "first-pass" effect). With hepatocellular dysfunction or portosystemic shunting of blood, toxic doses of these drugs can reach the systemic circulation.

    g. Narcotics, benzodiazepines, and amide local anesthetics are metabolized primarily in the liver and have significantly prolonged half-lives with liver failure.

III. Anesthetic considerations with liver dysfunction

    A. Acute hepatitis. Common etiologies of acute hepatitis include viruses (hepatitis A, B; non-A, non-B; and D) and toxins (alcohol, acetaminophen, phenytoin, isoniazid, and alpha methyldopa). Generally, serum transaminase values will be elevated out of proportion to the bilirubin and alkaline phosphatase. If severe, BUN will fall while ammonia rises, and encephalopathy or coma will ensue.

    B. Cholestatic liver disease. In cholestasis, alkaline phosphatase will rise out of proportion to transaminase values. Cholestasis without an anatomic obstruction can occur in infancy, during pregnancy, and after anesthesia. Other causes include bacterial sepsis, viral hepatitis, and drugs such as alcohol, oral contraceptives, oral hypoglycemics, phenothiazines, thiazide diuretics, sulfonamides, and erythromycin estolate.

    C. Chronic liver disease and cirrhosis may result from chronic active hepatitis, alcoholism, hemochromatosis, primary biliary cirrhosis, or congenital metabolic disorders such as Wilson's disease, alpha-1-antitrypsin deficiency, glycogen storage diseases, or hereditary tyrosinemia.

        1. The end stage of chronic liver disease is **cirrhosis,** resulting in a scarred, shrunken liver, accompanied by portal hypertension, esophageal varices, hypoalbuminemia, ascites, encephalopathy, and coagulopathy. These patients may present for a portosystemic shunt procedure (portocaval, mesocaval, or splenorenal), control of bleeding varices, LeVeen peritoneovenous shunts for alleviation of ascites, or orthotopic liver transplantation.

2. The operative risks for these patients have been classified by Child: the lowest risk patients (class A) have a bilirubin less than 2.0 mg/dl, albumin greater than 3.5 gm/dl, and no ascites or encephalopathy; the highest risk patients (class C) have a bilirubin above 3.0 mg/dl, albumin below 3.0 gm/dl, and advanced ascites or encephalopathy.

IV. Anesthetic considerations in end-stage liver disease. Regardless of its cause, end-stage hepatic disease will affect most other organ systems. Since these patients are often on the verge of multiple system failure, meticulous regard to volume, acid-base status, and vital organ perfusion is needed to prevent upsetting the tenuous balance.

A. Central nervous system. The severity of hepatic encephalopathy ranges from mild confusion to deep coma. With advanced encephalopathy, patients will be unable to prevent aspiration, and the increased intraabdominal pressure from ascites makes regurgitation more likely. Thus, awake or rapid sequence inductions are indicated. Encephalopathic patients may become deeply depressed by sedatives, due to both pharmacokinetic and pharmacodynamic factors (see sec. **II.A**). Thus, premedications should be used sparingly, if at all.

B. Cardiovascular system. Alcoholic liver disease may be accompanied by alcoholic cardiomyopathy, as well as coronary artery disease from tobacco abuse. Patients are often treated with diuretics to reduce total body fluid overload, but such therapy may leave them intravascularly volume depleted. Diuretics may also cause hypokalemia (furosemide) or hyperkalemia (spironolactone). Portal hypertension and coagulopathy often combine to produce massive gastrointestinal hemorrhages from esophageal varices, diffuse gastritis, or peptic ulcers, which may require surgical control. Thrombocytopenia may be dilutional or secondary to sequestration in an enlarged spleen. Fresh whole blood, when available, is a good choice for transfusion because it also contains functionally intact platelets.

C. Respiratory system
1. **Airway protection** is often vital, for the reasons mentioned in sec. **IV.A** and because the stomach may be filled with blood. Rapid sequence induction and intubation is dealt with in Chap. 10.
2. **Gas exchange** is often abnormal. Encephalopathy seems to cause an inappropriate hyperventilation, resulting in hypocarbia and respiratory alkalosis. Hypoxemia may be present because of basilar atelectasis from abdominal distention and because of intrapulmonary arteriovenous shunting related to the liver failure.

D. Renal system
1. Intravascular depletion from hypoalbuminemia and

diuretic therapy may result in prerenal azotemia. BUN may be deceptively low because of the liver's failure to synthesize urea from ammonia.

  2. Renal failure may result from hepatorenal syndrome, the etiology of which is unknown but may be related to circulating factors that alter intrarenal hemodynamics. Since the renal parenchyma is not irreversibly damaged, normal renal function may return if the hepatic failure resolves.

  E. **Coagulopathy** occurs from clotting factor deficiencies and thrombocytopenia (from dilution or hypersplenism). In addition, portal-to-systemic circulation shunts in the abdominal wall, esophageal veins, rectal veins, and retroperitoneum will make surgery in these areas exceedingly bloody. Elective patients with prolonged PTs should be treated with vitamin K. Emergencies will require FFP to correct prolonged PTs. Platelet counts below 50,000/mm^3 or intraoperative bleeding unresponsive to FFP should be treated with platelet transfusions. An uncorrected coagulopathy (bleeding time prolonged by > 10%) is a contraindication to spinal or epidural techniques because of the potential for subarachnoid or epidural hemorrhage.

  F. **Carbohydrate support.** Since diminished reserves of glycogen will tend to decrease blood glucose levels, patients with hepatic failure should be given continuous glucose infusions, and their blood glucose levels should be intermittently measured.

V. **Effects of anesthesia on the liver.** Many of the medications and physiologic alterations that accompany anesthesia and surgery will affect hepatic physiology and blood flow.

  A. **Premedication** with morphine, scopolamine, atropine, or a barbiturate will usually not change hepatic blood flow. Chronic treatment with barbiturates will increase hepatic blood flow as well as induce hepatic enzymes.

  B. **Spinal or epidural anesthesia** to a midthoracic level will result in a 20–25% decrease in hepatic blood flow, due predominantly to lower systemic blood pressure.

  C. **General anesthesia** with a barbiturate, narcotic, nitrous oxide, and relaxant seems to have little or no effect on hepatic blood flow, as long as anesthesia is sufficiently deep and patients are normocarbic. Sympathetic discharge from light anesthesia or hypercarbia will cause vasoconstriction and decrease hepatic blood flow. MOF produces the most marked decrease in hepatic blood flow among the volatile agents, followed (in descending order) by halothane, enflurane, and isoflurane. Halothane has been documented angiographically to cause hepatic artery spasm in some patients. Because **isoflurane** markedly vasodilates the hepatic artery, it produces only a mild decrease in total flow and may actually increase oxygen delivery.

  D. **Other factors** causing decreased hepatic blood flow include alpha-adrenergic agonist, beta blocker, or vasopressin administration; hypocarbia; positive-pressure ventilation; positive end-expiratory pressure; and surgical manipulation within the abdomen (both by direct compression of vessels and stimulation of splanchnic nerves).

E. **Narcotics.** Morphine, codeine, and their synthetic derivatives can cause spasm of the **sphincter of Oddi** and the bile ducts, which aggravates biliary colic and complicates interpretation of cholangiograms. When sphincter spasm occurs, the onset is within 15 minutes, and the duration is 2–24 hours. Mixed agonist-antagonists, and possibly meperidine, seem to be less potent effectors. Narcotic antagonists will reverse the spasm but need to be given repeatedly. Atropine will provide partial relief.

F. **Histamine (H_2) receptor antagonists.** Cimetidine inhibits cytochrome P-450, thus prolonging the duration of many hepatically cleared drugs such as warfarin-type anticoagulants, phenytoin, propranolol, diazepam, lidocaine, theophylline, and metronidazole. Ranitidine binds cytochrome P-450 with lower affinity and is thus less complicated in its effects. Both drugs decrease hepatic blood flow, probably by lowering acid production, metabolic needs, and blood flow to the stomach, which in turn lowers portal blood flow from the stomach to the liver.

VI. **Postoperative hepatic dysfunction.** Liver dysfunction may follow anesthesia and surgery and ranges from mild enzyme elevations to fulminant hepatic failure. Anesthesiologists must be aware of the many causes of postoperative hepatic dysfunction.

A. **Surgical interventions** that impair hepatic blood flow or obstruct the biliary system are obvious causes of damage to the liver. Postoperative serum elevations in hepatocellular enzymes or bilirubin can also be caused by increased bilirubin loads from massive transfusion, resorption of a hematoma, or hemolysis induced by a prosthetic heart valve, sepsis, or glucose-6-phosphate dehydrogenase deficiency. A picture of "benign postoperative intrahepatic cholestasis" is usually a marker of a systemic process (e.g., sepsis) rather than intrinsic hepatic dysfunction. Overt hepatic failure can result from shock of any etiology, especially with the prolonged use of vasopressors.

B. **Nonsurgical causes.** Hepatic dysfunction from common entities like viral hepatitis, alcoholism, and cholelithiasis can exist preoperatively but may not be detected (especially in apparently healthy patients who receive only minimal laboratory evaluation) or can occur postoperatively as mere coincidence. The stresses of surgery can convert a nonicteric illness to one with frank jaundice. Drug therapy in the postoperative period must also be evaluated as a cause of jaundice.

C. **Halothane-associated hepatitis.** Following administration of halothane, hepatic dysfunction may develop that is clinically indistinguishable from viral hepatitis.

The presentation covers a broad clinical spectrum; it may occur as an asymptomatic elevation in serum transaminases, fever of otherwise unknown origin, clinical jaundice, or, very rarely, massive hepatic necrosis and death. Theoretical predisposing factors include previous exposure to halothane (especially when associated previously with mild hepatic dysfunction or fever of unknown origin), other drug allergies, obesity, advancing age, and female gender. The problem is virtually unknown in pediatric patients. **Currently, the diagnosis of halothane hepatitis can be made only by exclusion;** there is no distinctive hepatic pathology or (at the present time) pathognomonic laboratory test.

1. **The United States National Halothane Study** found that otherwise unexplained massive hepatic necrosis following halothane exposure was an exceedingly rare complication and occurred in only 1 : 35,000 cases. Risks were highest in adult patients who received multiple exposures and in those who underwent procedures that carried a higher intrinsic risk of death. Seven cases of unexplained massive hepatic necrosis occurred in 250,000 exposures to halothane; four of the seven had received an earlier halothane anesthetic in the previous 6 weeks.

2. **Possible mechanisms.** It has been hypothesized that reductive metabolites of halothane bind to hepatocytes and damage them either directly or indirectly by creating haptens that trigger an autoimmune response. Possible chemical reactions mediating this process include peroxidation of unsaturated fatty acids, depletion of antioxidants, or covalent bonding to lipids or proteins.

3. **Recommendations concerning the use of halothane.** Halothane possesses special attributes which, in certain circumstances, may make it more useful than other potent inhalational anesthetics. For example, it selectively suppresses airway reflexes, relieves bronchospasm, and is tolerated best for mask inductions. At the Massachusetts General Hospital, halothane is the agent of choice for operations on the airway (e.g., tracheal or bronchial resections and reconstructions), for asthmatics, and for pediatric patients.

    Clearly, halothane should be avoided in patients with previous histories of unexplained hepatic dysfunction after halothane anesthesia. Even in patients who have tolerated previous halothane anesthetics, the decision to repeat the exposure must be made by weighing the specific benefits of halothane for each patient. There is no clear-cut evidence elucidating the safest interval between halothane exposures.

    As elsewhere in medicine, the lower cost of halothane is relevant but is not sufficient justification for choosing halothane over other, equally appropriate agents. Because of the controversy surrounding halothane, some institutions do not use halothane in patients with liver disease or who are undergoing hepatic or biliary operations; others have abandoned the use of halothane altogether.

Suggested Reading

Brown, R. (ed.). *Anesthesia and the Patient with Liver Disease.* Philadelphia: Davis, 1981.

Bunker, J. P. (ed.). *The National Halothane Study.* Bethesda, Md.: NIGMS, National Institutes of Health, 1965.

Dykes, M. H. M., et al. Halothane and the liver: A review of the epidemiologic, immunologic and metabolic aspects of the relationship. *Can. J. Surg.* 15:4, 1972.

Mazze, R. I. Metabolism of the inhaled anesthetics: Implications of enzyme induction. *Br. J. Anaesth.* 56:27s, 1984.

Strunin, L., and Davies, J. M. The liver and anaesthesia. *Can. Anaesth. Soc. J.* 30:2, 1983.

6

Specific Considerations with Endocrine Disease

Timothy J. Herbst

Operation has long been the definitive therapy for many hormonal derangements. Anesthesiologists can also expect to see endocrine patients requiring surgery for complications of their disorders as well as for other unrelated problems. Endocrinopathy will at times profoundly affect response to anesthetic techniques; conversely, anesthesia and surgery can easily disrupt tenuous metabolic compensation. For each of the major endocrine systems, this chapter will briefly discuss the normal physiology, then cover the changes in perioperative management required by abnormal function.

I. Thyroid

A. **Physiology.** The thyroid gland, in response to thyroid-stimulating hormone (**TSH,** released by the pituitary in response to hypothalamic thyrotropin-releasing hormone, **TRH**), produces about 90 μg of tetraiodothyronine (T_4, or thyroxine) and 10 μg of triiodothyronine (T_3) each day. The disappearance half-life of T_4 from blood is about 6 days and that of T_3 is closer to a day, due in part to the significantly greater protein binding of the former substance. Peripheral tissues convert T_4 to T_3. The latter substance is more potent in the general metabolic stimulation characteristic of thyroid effect and is therefore considered by some as the true tissue thyroid hormone, while T_4 is considered a plasma prohormone reservoir. Negative feedback exists at the hypothalamus and pituitary for the control of T_3 and T_4 in physiologic range, and assay of serum levels of thyroid hormones is often supplemented by assay of TSH. Routine preoperative thyroid assessment can be accomplished by measuring T_4 and T_3RU (resin uptake, to permit correction for plasma protein binding) and multiplying the two values to obtain a "free T_4 index."

B. **Hypofunction.** Presentation can vary from the asymptomatic patient with nearly normal thyroid function tests to myxedema coma. Patients who are euthyroid on replacement therapy should present little problem and should receive their supplement on the operative day only if their regimen consists of T_3, which has a shorter half-life. The anesthesiologist confronted with a patient not adequately replaced but requiring emergency operation should anticipate cardiac depression (often refractory to catecholamines), impaired free water clearance with diffuse edema (in extreme cases manifesting as cardiomegaly, ascites, and pleural and pericardial effusions), anemia, blunted ventilatory response to hypoxia and hypercarbia, decreased carbon dioxide production (with risk of hypocarbia when normal ventilator set-

tings are used), <u>slow gastric emptying</u>, <u>hypothermia,</u>
and increased sensitivity (and slowed redistribution) for
many anesthetic agents. Occult sepsis must be suspected in severe cases. <u>Intravenous T_3 (10–25 μg every</u>
<u>8 hours)</u> or T_4 (200–500 μg acutely, followed by 100–300
μg the next day) can be given in addition to general supportive therapy but must be used cautiously in the presence of ischemic heart disease. When hypothyroidism is
associated with amyloidosis, protein deposits may cause
renal and cardiac compromise as well as an enlarged
tongue. When hypothyroidism results from autoimmune disease, there may be concurrent autoimmune adrenal insufficiency (Schmidt's syndrome). Also, cortisol
clearance in hypothyroid but otherwise normal patients
increases on replacement of thyroid hormones. For
these reasons, <u>cortisol replacement</u> (see sec. **IV.C**) is
<u>often provided</u> when initiating thyroid replacement in
severely ill patients.

C. **Hyperfunction.** The manifestations of hyperthyroidism that are of most concern involve the heart and include tachycardia, <u>dysrhythmias (especially atrial fi-</u>
<u>brillation),</u> and, rarely, papillary muscle dysfunction,
mitral regurgitation, and congestive heart failure. Hypovolemia can result from diarrhea (which, together
with abdominal pain, may be mistaken for evidence of
a surgical problem) or polyuria. Muscle wasting can be
severe. Exophthalmos associated with Graves' disease
can predispose to keratitis. The catastrophic hyperki-
nesis, tachycardia, and hypovolemia from hyperpyrexia
and vomiting, with ultimate shock and coma of **thyroid
storm** can be precipitated by surgical stress and respond imperfectly to support and beta-adrenergic blockade; the best therapy is thus preventive and only a true
life-threatening emergency justifies operation in the
thyrotoxic patient.

1. Prognosis is much improved with 1–2 weeks of
   preparation:
   a. **Beta blockade** (most easily done with pro-
      pranolol, 40–640 mg/day in divided doses as
      needed) curbs the cardiac aberrations but must
      be used judiciously in the presence of heart fail-
      ure.
   b. **Iodide** (in emergencies, as 1–2 gm of the so-
      dium salt IV; less acutely, as 2–10 gtt of SSKI
      or 10–20 gtt of Lugol's solution per day) inhibits
      synthesis and release of thyroid hormones and
      improves the surgical field by reducing vascu-
      larity. In toxic multinodular goiter, however,
      hyperthyroidism may be exacerbated by iodine
      therapy.
   c. The traditional antithyroid medications, **meth-
      imazole** (30–60 mg/day) and **propylthioura-
      cil** (150 mg every 6–8 hours), inhibit hormone
      synthesis and the latter inhibits peripheral
      conversion of T_4 to T_3, but either one will re-

quire several weeks to optimize a preoperative regimen.

  d. Generous **sedation** is often helpful.

 2. Anesthetic technique

  a. Once a euthyroid state has been achieved, and provided vital organs have not been damaged, choice of anesthetics is influenced minimally by the history of endocrine pathology. The possibility of somewhat increased drug metabolism may relatively contraindicate halothane.

  b. Operations for goiter may involve airway problems such as mass effect or tracheomalacia. After any deep neck dissection, the airway may also be compromised by hematoma, edema, or recurrent laryngeal nerve injury, and it is usual to observe such patients for at least 4 hours before transfer to regular nursing floors.

  c. Total thyroidectomy also rarely results in parathyroidectomy with severe postoperative hypocalcemia (see sec. **II.B**).

II. Parathyroid

 A. Physiology. Parathyroid hormone (PTH) acts to elevate serum calcium level; this is effected initially by increased bone resorption, followed by improved renal resorption and intestinal uptake (the last mediated by PTH-stimulated synthesis of 1,25-dihydroxyvitamin D). Release of PTH is inhibited by rising calcium, resulting in negative feedback autoregulation. Magnesium is necessary for PTH release and for its bone effect.

 B. Hypofunction. Total parathyroidectomy can result in acute, dramatic hypocalcemia. Acute presentations of idiopathic or autoimmune hypoparathyroidism are also well recognized. In the presence of vitamin D deficiency (including that caused by microsomal enzyme-inducing anticonvulsant therapy), pancreatitis, gastrointestinal malabsorption, hyperphosphatemia (from renal failure, hemolysis, trauma, or cytotoxic drug therapy), or hypomagnesemia, PTH secretion may be insufficient to maintain normal serum calcium. Transient ionized hypocalcemia can also be seen with massive citrate loads in resuscitation with fresh-frozen plasma. Symptoms can range from mild lethargy to neuromuscular irritability and tetany (of special concern when laryngeal muscles are involved). Cardiac repolarization abnormalities may be noted, but hemodynamics are rarely compromised. Coexisting hyperkalemia or hypomagnesemia will aggravate the symptoms of hypocalcemia and vice versa. Bedside elicitation of facial nerve irritability to percussion (Chvostek's sign) or carpal spasm with tourniquet ischemia (Trousseau's sign) indicates the need for supplementation (acutely, as 1–4 gm of calcium chloride or gluconate IV; chronically, as 1–8 gm/day of calcium carbonate, often with vitamin D supplementation as well).

 C. Hyperfunction. Hypercalcemia can result in severe

muscle weakness, somnolence (or psychosis), peripheral neuropathy, abdominal pain (from peptic ulcer disease, from pancreatitis, or idiopathic), hypertension, polyuria with dehydration and polydipsia, and ectopic or renal calcification. Prolonged excess of PTH results in osteopenia, with vulnerability to pathologic fractures. Other notable causes of hypercalcemia include bony involvement of malignancy (especially multiple myeloma, breast or prostate carcinomas), sarcoidosis, and, in younger patients, prolonged immobilization. Diuresis with large quantities of IV saline (6–10 L/day) and furosemide will help reduce serum calcium, but **mithramycin** (25 µg/kg) will often be necessary. When parathyroidectomy is used for definitive therapy of hyperparathyroidism, the resulting PTH deficiency can be compounded by a "hungry bone syndrome," characterized by acute postoperative decreases in serum calcium and phosphate.

III. Pancreas

A. Physiology.
The first hormone identified in the islets of Langerhans was **insulin.** Secreted in response to a meal, insulin has a disappearance half-life of 3–10 minutes in persons with normal renal function. It is the prototype hormone of anabolism and stimulates uptake of basic nutrients (glucose, amino acids, and chylomicrons) and their use in the synthesis of structural and storage molecules (glycogen, protein, fatty acids, and triglycerides). During a fast, insulin levels fall and catabolism begins with glycogenolysis, proteolysis to support liver gluconeogenesis, and lipolysis producing fatty acids and (via the liver) ketones used by various tissues as an alternative source of energy.

B. Hypofunction

1. **Diabetes mellitus** is the most common of the endrocrine diseases. Cardiovascular complications are responsible for about 80% of diabetic deaths and frequently bring diabetics to the OR (e.g., amputation is 20 times more likely in the diabetic population). It is useful to consider diabetes as being of two distinct types, though the usual blood sugar levels and prevalence of retinopathy, nephropathy, and neuropathy are no different between the two groups.

   a. **Type I.** Typically but not always juvenile onset, this disease is characterized by low or absent insulin activity with a tendency to ketosis if exogenous hormone is not furnished (insulin dependence). The disease is associated with particular HLA types, and patients often have antibodies to pancreatic islet cells.

   b. **Type II.** Usually older at onset, these patients may have low, normal, or elevated plasma insulin levels, and the majority are obese. The pancreas will secrete insulin normally in response to arginine but not to glucose. Though they often require exogenous hormone to con-

Table 6-1. Hypoglycemic agents

Agent	Typical time to onset (hours)	Typical duration of action (hours)
Insulins (SQ administration)		
Regular	1	8
Semilente	1	14
NPH	2	24
Lente	2	24
Protamine zinc	4	36
Ultralente	4	36
Sulfonylureas		
Tolbutamide (Orinase or Oramide)	1	8–12
Glipizide (Glucotrol)	1	8–24
Acetohexamide (Dymelor)	1	12–24
Tolazamide (Tolinase)	4–6	12–16
Glyburide (Micronase or Diabeta)	1–4	18–24
Chlorpropamide (Diabinese)	1–4	24–72

trol symptoms of hyperglycemia, patients are not ketosis prone and therefore not strictly insulin dependent. Major arterial vasculopathy is more common in type II diabetics, perhaps due to their greater age.

2. **Goals of management.** The first priority must be to prevent the major metabolic derangements of **hyperosmolar coma** (typically in type II patients) and **ketoacidosis** (much more common in type I but seen with sufficient stress in type II as well) without inducing the catastrophe of severe **hypoglycemia.** It is also desirable to prevent swings in blood sugar sufficient to cause increased catecholamine tone (low sugar) or fluid and electrolyte problems (from osmotic diuresis). Some animal studies suggest that tight control of blood sugar in the normal range may prevent infection and improve wound healing.

3. **Agents.** See Table 6-1.

4. **Management**

   a. All the major goals can usually be achieved with the traditional practice of administering one-half to two-thirds of the patient's usual total daily dose of insulin in the form of an intermediate- or long-acting SQ dose, followed by a glucose-containing infusion at 100–150 ml/hr. Increased rates of infusion or supplemental doses of short-acting insulin may be indicated by frequent (every 2–4 hours intraoperatively) monitoring of blood sugar; adequate estimates of glucose level can be rapidly made with capillary or venous blood and commercially available reagent strips if more formal laboratory measurement is difficult.

b. Tighter control can be achieved with constant infusion of 25–100 ml/hr of 5–10% D/W and a separate piggyback of regular insulin solution (allow an extra 10 units for absorption by plastic IV tubing when making the solution) at 1–5 units/hr, with more frequent (at least every 2 hours) blood samples to guide infusion rates.

c. Insulin and glucose infusions can induce hypokalemia; addition of 20–40 mEq of potassium chloride to each liter of dextrose solution is reasonable if renal function is satisfactory.

d. When insulin is administered exclusively by the IV route, the access must be *reliable,* since ketoacidosis can develop within 30 minutes if infusion were suddenly to stop. This can be avoided by providing a baseline low level of insulin with a SQ dose.

e. Patients on split-dose insulin regimens preoperatively should receive reduced doses of any long- or intermediate-acting insulin the night before operation. Those who usually eat after midnight should have glucose infusions overnight. Those who are on oral hypoglycemic medications should have such medications held (as long as possible before the operative day in the case of chlorpropamide) and receive insulin coverage (typically 10 units of NPH for fasting blood sugar > 180 mg/dl).

f. Diabetics should receive priority for early times on the operative schedule.

5. Other considerations

a. Diabetic neuropathy

    (1) Patients with **peripheral** neuropathy are vulnerable to positioning injury. They are less able to detect pressure points from poor positioning, and diabetic tissues are probably less able to tolerate reduced perfusion.

    (2) Patients with **autonomic** neuropathy may be less able to compensate for positional changes, or the sympathectomy of regional anesthesia, and may therefore respond with more hypotension than expected.

    (3) **Impaired gastric emptying** should be anticipated.

b. The absence of a clear history of angina should not be assumed to rule out coronary artery disease, for the incidence of **silent myocardial ischemia** is significant in diabetics.

c. Some degree of **renal insufficiency** is common.

C. **Hyperfunction**
  1. **Reactive hypoglycemia.** Some effort should be
     made to avoid large boluses of glucose, which, by
     causing delayed hypersecretion of insulin, can pre-
     cipitate rebound hypoglycemia. Rare patients will
     need overnight infusion of glucose; they can be
     identified by a history of morning hypoglycemic
     symptoms.
  2. **Insulinoma.** Rare insulin-secreting tumors re-
     quire constant dextrose infusion to avoid hypogly-
     cemia in the fasting state. **Diazoxide,** a nondi-
     uretic thiazide, may have been used to control
     symptoms preoperatively but should be discontin-
     ued at least 2 days before operation since a sudden
     (within 30 minutes) rise in serum glucose is often
     used as a criterion of successful removal of these
     difficult to locate tumors. Patients may also have
     received large doses of **corticosteroids** as part of
     their medical management.
  3. Other tumors of the endocrine or exocrine pan-
     creas, such as glucagon-secreting tumors, gastrin-
     omas (Zollinger-Ellison syndrome), or the WDHA
     (watery diarrhea, hypokalemia, achlorhydria) syn-
     drome will rarely be encountered. In such cases,
     optimum supportive medical management should
     simplify the anesthetic course.

IV. **Adrenal cortex**
  A. **Physiology.** The anterior pituitary gland, when stim-
     ulated by hypothalamic corticotropin-releasing factor
     (**CRF**), releases adrenocorticotropic hormone (**ACTH**).
     This release follows a diurnal pattern, with blood levels
     greatest in the early morning. In response to ACTH, the
     zona fasciculata and zona reticularis of the adrenal cor-
     tex produce about 20 mg of hydrocortisone (**cortisol**)
     each day; serum steroids exert negative feedback on
     CRF and ACTH release. Cortisol has anti-inflammatory
     effects but is perhaps more important for its pivotal role
     in the response to stress. It stimulates the N-methyla-
     tion of norepinephrine to epinephrine in the adrenal
     medulla and has a permissive effect for the peripheral
     actions of catecholamines. It also helps support blood
     sugar by reducing tissue uptake and stimulating glu-
     coneogenesis. **Aldosterone,** the principal mineralocor-
     ticoid, is produced by the zona glomerulosa in response
     to hyperkalemia, hypovolemia (via the renin-angioten-
     sin system), and, to a lesser extent, ACTH. It acts at the
     kidney to increase potassium wasting and sodium re-
     tention; this effect is countered by cardiac atrial natri-
     uretic peptides. The sex steroids produced in the adre-
     nal cortex are of concern to the anesthetist when
     abnormal sexual development may indicate deficiencies
     in the biosynthesis of multiple steroids, including cor-
     tisol.
  B. **Pharmacology.** A variety of synthetic steroids are
     available with varying potencies and ratios of glucocor-

Table 6-2. Steroid relative potencies and doses

| | Relative potency | | |
Steroid	Gluco-corticoid	Mineralo-corticoid	Equivalent dose (mg)
Short-acting (8- to 12-hour duration)			
Cortisol (hydrocortisone)	1.0	1.0	20
Cortisone	0.8	0.8	25
Aldosterone	0.3	3000	—
Intermediate (12- to 36-hour duration)			
Prednisone	4	0.8	5
Prednisolone	4	0.8	5
Methylprednis-olone (Solumedrol)	5	0.5	4
Fludrocor-tisone	10	125	—
Long-acting (> 48-hour duration)			
Dexametha-sone (Decadron)	25–40	0	0.5

ticoid to mineralocorticoid effects (Table 6-2). It should be noted that cortisone and prednisone are not active drugs until converted to cortisol and prednisolone, respectively, by the liver. Also, acetate salts of cortisone and cortisol, while effective orally, depend on "first-pass" liver transformation and are probably ineffective as IM agents.

C. **Hypofunction**
   1. **Hypothalamic-pituitary-adrenal axis suppression.** Though small "physiologic" doses of exogenous steroids given once each morning, and even larger doses given on alternate days, seem not to depress the endogenous response to stress, prolonged "pharmacologic" therapy often does with the potential for perioperative cardiovascular collapse. The central portion of the axis can recover within 6 months of steroid discontinuation, but the adrenal may still be unable to respond maximally for up to a year. When doubt exists whether a given patient's axis is fully intact, a stimulation test with exogenous ACTH (25 units IV or IM) can be used: A serum cortisol rise to greater than 18 μg/dl in 30 minutes indicates a normal gland. A primate study has indicated that serious complications can be avoided with only baseline replacement doses of steroids in the perioperative period, but until these findings are confirmed in humans it remains usual practice to provide "stress-dose" coverage:
      a. The equivalent of 300 mg of hydrocortisone is given the day of operation.
      b. An "on-call" IM dose of 100 mg of hydrocortisone provides an assured depot to cover mini-

mum requirements; the remainder can be given in IV divided doses through the first 24 hours.

   c. The daily steroid replacement can be rapidly tapered over 3–5 days to whatever dose kept the patient stable preoperatively.

   d. High doses can be expected to induce glucose intolerance and, with some agents, excess mineralocorticoid effect (Table 6-2).

   2. Addison's disease. The abdominal distress, hypotension, and fever of Addisonian crisis should not be mistaken for any process requiring laparotomy. Stress-dose steroid coverage for elective or other emergency procedures must include agents with mineralocorticoid effect because, in addition to their cortisol deficiency, these patients lack aldosterone, with consequent dehydration, hyponatremia, and hyperkalemia.

   3. Other considerations
   a. Significant muscle weakness can reduce relaxant requirements.
   b. Greater sensitivity to cardiovascular depressant medications and possible resistance to pressors should be anticipated.

D. Hyperfunction. Definitive operative therapy for **Cushing's disease** (an ACTH-producing pituitary tumor) or **Cushing's syndrome** (resulting from an adrenal adenoma) will induce an Addisonian state, and therefore replacement begins the day of operation with stress coverage as described in sec. **C.1.** Glucocorticoid excess, however, usually leads to glucose intolerance (see sec. **III.B** for management). Excess mineralocorticoid effect is usually present and manifests as hypertension (from hypervolemia), polycythemia, and hypokalemia; **spironolactone** is the specific antidote. Osteoporosis and thin, atrophic skin make these patients vulnerable to injury from minor trauma.

V. Adrenal Medulla

A. Physiology. Preganglionic fibers of the sympathetic nervous system end in the medullary portions of both adrenal glands and stimulate release of catecholamines, principally epinephrine, with disappearance half-lives of about 1 minute. Peripheral effects include chronotropic and inotropic stimulation of the heart, vasomotor changes, enhanced hepatic glycogenolysis, and inhibition of insulin release. These effects largely parallel the more specific effects achieved by stimulation of the sympathetic nerves to a given end organ.

B. Hyperfunction. The diagnosis of **pheochromocytoma** (usually a norepinephrine-secreting tumor) is classically made by a history of paroxysmal hypertension, tachycardic arrhythmias, sweating, and tremulousness. Patients are usually hypovolemic and may vary between fixed, baseline hypertension and orthostatic hypotension, exacerbated by possible cardiomyopathy. Hyperglycemia is common.

1. The first priority in **preoperative preparation** is to establish adequate alpha-adrenergic blockade (usually with oral **phenoxybenzamine,** starting with 20–30 mg/day and increasing to 60–250 mg/day until blood pressure is controlled). This allows adequate volume repletion, typically reflected by a fall in hematocrit. If tachycardia persists, beta blockade can then be considered. During the preoperative period, an anesthetist should be in attendance for any particularly stressful procedures, especially for angiography or embolization of the tumor (such procedures should be attempted only after adequate pharmacologic treatment).

2. **Anesthetic technique** seeks to avoid the usual sympathetic outflow occurring with induction, laryngoscopy, and incision. Generous sedation is therefore in order prior to any invasive line placement (pulmonary artery pressure monitoring is usually indicated intraoperatively, but often not for induction). Anesthesia should be well established before any stimulation; unopposed parasympathetic response to intubation can result in catastrophic bradycardia. The use of a subarachnoid catheter to produce total spinal block prior to induction of "light" general anesthesia with supplemental continuous spinal offers the advantages of ablation of sympathetic reflexes and profound muscle relaxation but eliminates endogenous support of blood pressure when the tumor is removed. Tumor manipulation often precipitates catecholamine surges, and beta blockers (propranolol or labetalol), sodium nitroprusside, hydralazine, and/or phentolamine are usually needed. In the absence of perfect preoperative alpha blockade, large fluid requirements appear with tumor removal. Hypoglycemia must also be anticipated.

VI. Other problems
A. Pituitary disorders

1. **Panhypopituitary states** can be induced by trauma (surgical or accidental), infarction (known as Sheehan's syndrome when due to postpartum hemorrhagic hypotension), tumor encroachment, or infiltrative disorders such as sarcoidosis. Symptoms of hypoadrenocorticism appear within 4–14 days, while hypothyroidism will not manifest for several weeks. Management of these problems is as outlined for the individual disorders above. **Diabetes insipidus** can be diagnosed by hypoosmotic polyuria with rising serum osmolality. Management must include adequate free water replacement until control is obtained with titrated doses of exogenous antidiuretic hormone. The preferred long-term agent is the synthetic analogue desmopressin (DDAVP, 2.5–25 μg two times a day SQ or by nasal spray), but for brief acute management Pi-

tressin tannate in oil is often useful (10 units SQ every 6 hours).

2. The syndrome of **inappropriate antidiuretic hormone secretion** (SIADH) occurs as a complication of intracranial tumors, certain other malignancies (especially small-cell lung tumors), and hypothyroidism. Intravascular volume contraction and stress also promote antidiuretic hormone release. Free water restriction is usually preferred to diuretic or hypertonic saline therapy, as too rapid restoration of normal serum sodium has been reported to cause pontine myelinolysis resulting in coma or death.

3. **Acromegaly** is caused by hypersecretion of growth hormone. Hypertrophy of the mandible (prognathism), tongue, lips, and epiglottis can complicate management of an airway already narrowed by vocal cord and nasal turbinate hypertrophy. Soft-tissue hypertrophy can also cause recurrent laryngeal nerve entrapment and paralysis. Entrapment of the ulnar artery in a narrowed carpal tunnel can result in inadequate collateral blood flow to the hand after radial artery catheterization. Sodium and potassium retention may aggravate cardiac compromise. Finally, osteoporosis, muscle weakness, and glucose intolerance, as well as possible postoperative hypopituitarism should be anticipated.

4. Patients coming to operation for pituitary problems may have had a recent **pneumoencephalogram.** Nitrous oxide is clearly contraindicated in such cases. For further operative considerations in this region, see Chap. 22.

B. **Multiple endocrine neoplasias (MEN).** The presence of certain hormonal disorders should alert the clinician to the possibility of coexisting problems.

1. **MEN type I.** Wermer's syndrome often presents with hyperparathyroidism accompanied by functioning adenomas of the pancreatic islets and pituitary. The latter range from nonsecretory to those producing growth hormone, ACTH, TSH, or prolactin. Bronchial or small intestinal carcinoid tumors, thymomas, and multiple lipomas, schwannomas and cutaneous leiomyomas have also been observed to occur with this syndrome. Though familial, this syndrome probably has multiple genetic determinants.

2. **MEN type II.** Sipple's syndrome, an autosomal dominant disease with high penetrance, consists of associated pheochromocytoma, medullary carcinoma of the thyroid, and parathyroid hyperplasia.

3. **MEN type III (or IIB).** Pheochromocytoma and medullary carcinoma of the thyroid (and, more rarely, parathyroid adenomas) also occur together in the mucosal neuroma syndrome, another auto-

somal dominant disorder characterized by multiple morphologic abnormalities. A marfanoid habitus is accompanied by soft-tissue hypertrophy of the tongue, mandible, and lips, and the airway can be further distorted by neuromas and neurofibromas of the tongue and oral and laryngeal mucosa. Diffuse lentigo or café au lait spots may signal the presence of this syndrome.

Suggested Reading

Brown, B. R. (ed.). Anesthesia and the patient with endocrine disease. *Contemp. Anesth. Pract.* 3:1, 1980.

Pender, J. W., and Basso, L. V. Diseases of the Endrocine System. In J. Katz, J. Benumof, and L. B. Kadis (eds.), *Anesthesia and Uncommon Diseases* (2nd ed.). Philadelphia: Saunders, 1981. Pp. 155–220.

Roizen, M. F. Anesthetic Implications of Concurrent Diseases. In R. D. Miller (ed.), *Anesthesia* (2nd ed.). New York: Churchill Livingstone, 1986. Pp. 255–278.

White, V. A., and Kumaga, L. F. Preoperative endocrine and metabolic considerations. *Med. Clin. North Am.* 63:1321, 1979.

7

Specific Considerations with Infectious Disease

Marie Csete Prager

All anesthetized patients are at risk of infection because of invasive procedures and impaired defenses resulting from illness, surgery, or anesthesia itself. Careful anesthetic technique should preclude direct infection from patient to patient and from patient to anesthesiologist. This chapter will focus on routine infection precautions, special considerations in caring for infected patients, and protection of the anesthesiologist from infected patients.

I. **Routine procedures.** General anesthesia undermines normal host defenses. With intubation, the protective filtering of nasal hairs is lost, and inhalation agents impair mucociliary function. Normal protective pharyngeal reflexes are bypassed. In addition, general anesthesia may impair white blood cell function. Hence, with normal defenses impaired, a clean work area and equipment are essential.

A. **Anesthesia machine.** The surface of the anesthesia machine and cart should be wiped clean with 70% isopropyl alcohol after every case. Obvious spills of blood or secretions should be cleaned as quickly as possible during the procedure. More thorough cleaning of the entire anesthesia machine with alcohol should be done about once per week and after any septic case. Fortunately, though bacteria can be easily cultured from external surfaces of anesthesia equipment, cross-contamination is rare if these basic precautions are followed.

B. **Airway and breathing circuit equipment.** Although the significance of colonized equipment in producing infection is inadequately documented, equipment in proximity to the patient's airway can become contaminated by the patient's own secretions and should be considered a potential infectious hazard to other patients. Hands are easily contaminated by dirty equipment and are an important source of pathogens.

1. Ideally all equipment that contacts the respiratory tract (oral airways, laryngoscope blades) should be decontaminated and placed on a disposable waterproof towel off to one side of the cart surface. Laryngoscope blades are often cleaned between cases with alcohol, although this method does not ensure absolute sterility. Most hospitals use completely disposable anesthesia breathing circuits and bags, endotracheal tubes, esophageal stethoscopes, and suction equipment. Reusable airway equipment such as airways and masks should be routinely sterilized with ethylene oxide in a central supply area. (This procedure requires extensive time for drying and aeration to prevent facial or laryngeal burns from residual chemical.) Reusable endotracheal tubes are steam-sterilized by autoclaving.

2. Soda lime, despite its low pH, is not an effective bacterial filter but is not routinely changed between cases unless the patient requires respiratory precautions or has AIDS. Bacterial filters on breathing circuits have not been demonstrated to reduce the incidence of postoperative pulmonary infections. Humidifiers can provide excellent conditions for growth of gram-negative rods (especially *Pseudomonas aeruginosa*) and should be cleaned, dried, and gas-sterilized between usages.

C. **Intravenous catheters.** Current practices often do not include strictly aseptic technique for the insertion of intravenous catheters and administration of intravenous drugs in the OR. However, these basic precautions are mandatory: strict handwashing, skin preparation with a germicidal agent, and securing the cannula in a clean manner. Immunosuppressed patients and those with valvular disease or indwelling prostheses should be treated aseptically. Arterial and central lines are placed with sterile technique in all patients. Multidose vials and injection ports should always be swabbed before use.

D. **Contact with secretions.** Since infected blood and secretions represent a major hazard to the anesthesiologist, gloves should always be worn during contact with blood and secretions, notably during intubation, suctioning, and extubation. Blood- or secretion-contaminated sharps should be directly discarded into puncture-proof containers, without bending or capping. Systems for disposing of these containers safely should be part of every OR routine.

II. Anesthesia for patients with infections

A. **General considerations.** Most hospitals have developed specific guidelines for identifying patients who require special precautions because of infectious disease. Anesthesiologists should be aware of these guidelines, which usually address isolation techniques on the hospital floors but can be readily adapted to the OR setting. Communication between floor personnel and anesthesia staff is necessary to maintain appropriate precautions during patient transfer.

B. **Associated conditions.** Febrile patients, in theory, require a higher MAC to achieve a given anesthetic depth. In addition, their oxygen and fluid requirements are higher. Chronically infected patients may be poorly nourished, hypoalbuminemic, and anemic. Those maintained on chronic antibiotic therapy may have limited peripheral venous access.

C. **Antibiotics.** Antibiotic schedules should be maintained as strictly as possible. Many antibiotics are known to interact with neuromuscular blocking agents to enhance and prolong paralysis (see Chap. 11). In addition, isoniazid is a potent enzyme inducer and may enhance the metabolism of enflurane, resulting in elevated serum fluoride levels.

D. Respiratory cross-contamination

1. **Droplet and contact spread.** Infected upper respiratory secretions provide a source of transient colonization of hands (and equipment) that may be transmitted to subsequent patients. Careful anesthetic technique (see Sec. **I**) and meticulous handwashing before each case should greatly decrease or eliminate this risk. Chronically intubated patients should be considered infected, as they are virtually always colonized, notably with gram-negative organisms.

2. **Airborne infection: tuberculosis.** *Mycobacterium tuberculosis* can be transmitted by aerosolized droplets but may also be a truly airborne disease, transmissible over some distance in the air through droplet nuclei.

   a. Patients with laryngeal tuberculosis or cavitary disease are particularly infectious. Anesthetic technique should be tailored to minimize aerosolization (bucking, coughing). A closed ventilation system dilutes the external concentrations of aerosolized droplets. Although the efficacy of bacterial filters in minimizing contamination of anesthesia equipment with this organism has not been tested, most anesthesiologists use filters in the circuit. If hemoptysis is a consideration, double-lumen tubes should be available. After the operation, all breathing circuitry is discarded and the soda lime changed. The same precautions apply to other respiratory infections transmitted by the airborne route and requiring respiratory precautions.

   b. Anesthesiologists themselves are at relatively high risk of tuberculosis exposure. At many institutions, anesthesiologists are encouraged to have yearly skin testing with 5 TU of PPD tuberculin. (Anesthesiologists working in a Respiratory Intensive Care Unit are considered at high risk and are tested every 6 months.) Physicians who convert on PPD testing are generally advised to accept a year of treatment with isoniazid, particularly if they are less than 35 years old.

III. Special risks to anesthesiologists

A. **Herpetic whitlow** is a herpes simplex virus (HSV) infection of the fingers. In medical personnel, the infection is most often caused by HSV type 1, but cases of HSV type 2 (the virus usually associated with genital herpes) whitlow also occur in the general population. This disorder is frequently discussed in the nursing and dental literature but represents a significant risk to anesthesiologists as well because of contact with oral secretions.

1. Classically the whitlow occurs on a previously trau-

matized area of the finger, but this trauma may be as trivial as the small skin breaks associated with frequent handwashing. Oral herpetic lesions need not be present for the disease to be transmitted. Asymptomatic patients excrete active virus as well. The use of gloves during contact with saliva should greatly decrease the risk of acquiring this disease.

2. Whitlow may be difficult to distinguish from cellulitis or abscess (paronychia or felon), but the distinction is important, since incision and drainage of whitlow significantly worsen the infection. Active lesions preclude operating room duties. The usual clinical course requires 1 month for crusting and resolution. Unfortunately, about 30% of patients experience recurrences.

B. Hepatitis. Anesthesiologists are at high risk for acquiring viral hepatitis. The three major types of viral hepatitis are hepatitis A, hepatitis B, and non-A, non-B. It should also be noted that transfusion hepatitis can result from Epstein-Barr virus and cytomegalovirus. Care of patients with impaired liver function from viral hepatitis and other forms of liver disease are discussed in Chap. 5.

1. **Hepatitis A.** This highly infectious form is acquired by the fecal-oral route, often from contaminated food. Affected patients develop lifelong immunity, and there is no progression to chronic hepatitis. An injection of pooled gamma globulin is recommended after known exposure. Anesthesiologists are not at particular risk from this, the most benign form of hepatitis.

2. **Hepatitis B.** Formerly called serum hepatitis, this form is transmitted by inoculation of blood or blood products or by sexual contact. Anesthesiologists are at greatly increased risk because of contact with blood and sharps. Since the antigen is found in saliva and other body fluids (e.g., urine), these may also be potential sources of infections. Hepatitis B has an incubation period of about 12–16 weeks.

   a. Approximately 0.1–1.0% of healthy adults are potentially infectious, as indicated by the presence of hepatitis B surface antigen (HBsAg), a viral protein marker. In-hospital patients have an estimated prevalence rate of 1.3%. Medical personnel have a rate of antibody to surface antigen (HBsAb) positivity of 2 to 4 times that of the general population. A recent study of anesthesia residents indicated that 12.7% had positive serum markers for hepatitis B. There is a direct correlation with length of hospital employment and the presence of HBsAb, and correspondingly, a 17–23% incidence of HBsAb in anesthesia faculty has been reported. The risk of acquisition of infection following a needle-stick injury from an infected patient is about 10%.

b. Hepatitis B is now rarely a posttransfusion problem, since almost all cases of acute and chronic disease will be detected with an HBsAg screen of blood donors. The presence of antibody to the surface marker, HBsAb, indicates previous exposure and immunity. In occasional patients with acute hepatitis B, the previously mentioned two markers will not be detectable, but the patient will have antibody to core antigen, anti-HBcAg. Hepatitis e antigen (HBeAg) is a marker of increased infectivity. Demonstration of hepatitis delta (D) in association with hepatitis B implies a poorer prognosis and greater likelihood of progression to chronic disease.

c. Patients with hepatitis B may be asymptomatic or have a mild form characterized by fever, fatigue, loss of appetite, nausea and vomiting, abdominal pain, and dark urine. Many patients have associated myalgia or arthralgia. Recovery is often complete in 2–4 weeks. However, some patients experience prolonged symptoms or may die of acute disease with fulminant hepatic failure. Approximately 10% progress to a chronic form; two chronic forms are distinguishable. Chronic persistent hepatitis B is milder, often asymptomatic, or associated with fatigue. Hepatic damage is usually not progressive, and immunosuppressive therapy is usually not required. The 5-year survival rate for chronic persistent hepatitis B is about 97%. Chronic active hepatitis is the more severe form but clinically can run the same spectrum as acute disease. Liver biopsy is requisite in distinguishing chronic active from chronic persistent hepatitis. The 5-year survival rate for chronic active hepatitis is about 86%. Steroids are not recommended because the drugs may actually enhance viral replication.

d. Anesthesiologists are obligated to protect themselves from this potentially fatal occupational hazard. Gloves should be worn for procedures requiring contact with blood or saliva. Needles should not be capped, bent, or otherwise manipulated before disposal. Fortunately, **a highly effective, safe hepatitis B vaccine is available and is strongly recommended for anesthesiologists.**

e. Unvaccinated anesthesiologists exposed to needlesticks from patients with known HBsAg should receive hepatitis B immune globulin (HBIG), ideally within 24 hours of exposure (but certainly within 1 week). The vaccine should also be administered at the same time. If no vaccine is given, a second HBIG dose is administered after 1 month. If vaccine was

given, the complete series should follow, and
the antibody status of the recipient retested.

3. **Non-A, non-B hepatitis** is currently the cause of
80–90% of posttransfusion hepatitis, with a mean
incubation period of 8 weeks. Only experimental
markers for non-A, non-B hepatitis are available,
and the disease is believed to be caused by one or
more retroviruses. The frequency of this type of
posttransfusion hepatitis may be related to the
level of alanine aminotransferase (ALT) in the donor, but transmission may occur when ALT and as-
partate aminotransferase (AST) are normal.

   a. The risk of transmitting clinical hepatitis with
   transfusion is ~ 1% for whole blood, packed red
   cells (regardless of preparation), fresh-frozen
   plasma, and prothrombin complex.

   b. Most cases of non-A, non-B hepatitis are anic-
   teric; however, progression to a chronic state occurs more frequently than with hepatitis B. The
   effectiveness of pooled gamma globulin after accidental percutaneous inoculation is not clear-
   cut, but this treatment is often advised.

C. **AIDS.** Acquired immunodeficiency syndrome (AIDS) is
an immune disorder caused by the retrovirus HIV (human immunodeficiency virus). The immunoincompe-
tence of full-blown AIDS results in a wide variety of op-
portunistic infections and malignancies. Patients may
present with prolonged fever, malaise, lymphadenopathy, weight loss, an infection, malignancy, or dementia.
Kaposi's sarcoma is the most frequently described malignancy. Commonly associated infections include *Pneu-
mocystis carinii, Toxoplasma gondii,* cytomegalovirus,
herpes simplex virus, candida, atypical mycobacteria,
Cryptococcus neoformans, cryptosporidium, and *Salmonella.*

1. The **immune defect** of AIDS is highly complex.
One crucial factor is depression of the T-lymphocyte
subset T4, classically designated "helper" cells,
which recognize distinct sets of antigens. In addition, there is an increased number of T8 "cytotoxic"
or "suppressor" T lymphocytes. As a result, the normal ratio of T4 to T8 cells is inverted. B-cell function is also impaired: AIDS patients have increased
levels of serum immunoglobulins but do not generate adequate responses to antigens. Lymphokine
production is diminished. Overall this malfunctioning of the immune system means that foreign antigen is not recognized and processed effectively.

2. HIV has been isolated from blood, semen, vaginal
secretions, urine, marrow, lymph nodes, spleen,
cerebrospinal fluid, brain, tears, and saliva. Blood
and semen are most important epidemiologically,
and **transmission patterns** are similar to that for
hepatitis B. In the United States high-risk groups
are homosexual or bisexual males, intravenous
drug users, hemophiliacs (or others receiving mul-

tiple blood transfusions), sexual partners of AIDS patients, and children born to mothers with AIDS.

3. It is estimated that to date more than 1 million people have been infected with HIV in the United States. Of these, an estimated 5–20% will develop the syndrome over 5 years.

   a. The greatest **epidemiologic risk,** both to the community and to health professionals, resides in this large pool of patients who are viremic but asymptomatic. Whether these people can or should be identified by screening tests remains controversial, but widespread screening is currently not recommended. Screening of blood or organ donors and certain high-risk groups, however, is desirable.

   b. Routine medical care of AIDS patients has been clearly shown to present a **low risk to medical personnel,** and this is supported by the well-documented lack of household transmission. In addition, the seroconversion rate after known needlestick exposure is low (< 1%). Nonetheless, extreme care must be taken when handling sharp instruments contaminated with blood. Needles should not be bent, capped, or manipulated prior to disposal.

4. No national **OR standards** for dealing with AIDS patients have been adopted, but the following guidelines are adapted from recommendations for care of any hospitalized AIDS patient.

   a. Sharp objects must be handled extremely carefully.

   b. Although transmission of the disease through aerosolized secretions or blood is unlikely, direct implantation of infected droplets on the eye or mucous membranes is potentially hazardous. Therefore, gloves, gown, and goggles should be used for protection if contamination is a possibility.

   c. Thorough handwashing after exposure to secretions is mandatory.

   d. Disposable breathing circuits, bags, oral airways, masks, and endotracheal tubes should be used. Laryngoscopes and other instruments can be disinfected with 70% isopropyl alcohol, although 5.25% sodium hypochlorite ("bleach") is the most effective agent, when tolerated. (The efficacy of povidone-iodine in killing HIV has not been formally tested.)

   e. All OR surfaces, including the anesthesia machine, should be disinfected with a 1 : 10 solution of bleach, and the carbon dioxide absorber changed. Contaminated disposable items should be double-bagged in plastic and clearly marked for autoclaving, or incineration, and disposal.

f. In patients with clinically significant AIDS, other anesthetic implications have been described. Renal function may be impaired. Proteinuria is common, and glomerular lesions have been demonstrated at autopsy. Episodes of acute renal failure are fairly common. Thus, it may be prudent to evaluate renal function and avoid drugs dependent on the kidney for excretion. One article has suggested that adrenal insufficiency may be common in AIDS and should be considered in the differential of unexplained hypotension during anesthesia.

5. **Blood products** for transfusion are now screened with an ELISA assay for HIV antibody titer. This method has a false-positive rate of about 15% (but this varies greatly depending on the true rate of infection in the population tested) and requires confirmation by other tests. Depending on the time of testing and the test population, the ELISA assay may have a false-negative rate of up to 5%. Since the institution of this screening assay, no national survey on the incidence of posttransfusion AIDS is yet available, but it is estimated that posttransfusion AIDS may continue to appear for up to 7 years after receiving infected blood. Unlike other viral infections, the presence of a positive antibody test does not indicate protection. To the contrary, all persons with a confirmed positive ELISA test for HIV must be considered infectious.

IV. **Risks to the patient from the anesthesiologist.** An anesthesiologist with an active infectious process may transmit his infection to a patient, and local hospital rules may preclude patient care during the most infectious stages of some diseases. These illnesses include active diarrhea due to certain pathogens (e.g., *Salmonella* or *Shigella*), childhood viral illnesses, open draining lesions on exposed areas of hands or face, and viral conjunctivitis. The common cold usually does not preclude patient care, but attention should be given to symptomatic control of secretions and careful handwashing. The carrier state of hepatitis B or HIV does not mandate cessation of most forms of employment, although these cases must be judged individually as our knowledge of these diseases increases.

Suggested Reading

Berry, A. J., et al. A multicenter study of the epidemiology of hepatitis B in anesthesia residents. *Anesth. Analg.* 64:672, 1985.

Corey, L., and Spear, P. G. Infections with herpes simplex viruses. *N. Engl. J. Med.* 314:686, 1986.

Dienstag, J. L., et al. Hepatitis B vaccine in health care personnel: Safety, immunogenicity, and indicators of efficacy. *Ann. Intern. Med.* 101:34, 1984.

DuMoulin, G. C., and Saubermann, A. J. The anesthesia machine and circle system are not likely to be sources of bacterial contamination. *Anesthesiology* 47:353, 1977.

Greene, L. W., et al. Adrenal insufficiency as a complication of the acquired immunodeficiency syndrome. *Ann. Intern. Med.* 101:497, 1984.

Hirsch, M. S., et al. Risk of nosocomial infection with human T-cell lymphotropic virus III (HTLV-III). *N. Engl. J. Med.* 312:1, 1985.

Levitz, R. E. Herpetic whitlow: A misunderstood syndrome. *Infect. Med.,* July/Aug. 1985. Pp. 205–208.

Lumley, J. Decontamination of anaesthetic equipment and ventilators. *Br. J. Anaesth.* 48:3, 1976.

McCray, E. (The Cooperative Needlestick Surveillance Group). Occupational risk of the acquired immunodeficiency syndrome among health care workers. *N. Engl. J. Med.* 314:1127, 1986.

Pardo, V., et al. Glomerular lesions in the acquired immunodeficiency syndrome. *Ann. Intern. Med.* 101:429, 1984.

Patterson, W. B., et al. Occupational hazards to hospital personnel. *Ann. Intern. Med.* 102: 658, 1985.

Administration of Anesthesia

8

Preparation for Induction

Jeffrey B. Cooper, Ronald S. Newbower, James P. Welch, Daniel F. Dedrick, and Clifford M. Gevirtz

I. **Basic requirements of anesthesia management**
   A. Regardless of the **planned** anesthetic technique, the anesthetist must **be prepared** to administer a general anesthetic. Such administration might include
      1. Establishing a patent airway.
      2. Providing supplemental oxygen.
      3. Delivering positive-pressure ventilation.
      4. Administering an inhalation anesthetic.
      5. Administering fluids and drugs intravenously.
      6. Suctioning material from the airway.
      7. Diagnosing and treating inadequate cardiac output.
      8. Diagnosing and treating cardiac arrhythmias.
      9. Performing cardiopulmonary resuscitation.
   B. Accordingly, before beginning any anesthetic procedure, the anesthetist must have available the following **equipment:**
      1. An anesthesia machine, with a verified source of oxygen and a breathing system that will allow manual administration of positive-pressure ventilation.
      2. The necessary accessories for the breathing system, including
         a. An oral airway.
         b. An airtight-fitting mask and an appropriate size or sizes of endotracheal tubes with balloon cuff seals or, for small children, uncuffed tubes.
         c. A reservoir bag.
      3. The accessories necessary for tracheal intubation, including a laryngoscope of appropriate size.
      4. A working intravenous line, preferably a plastic catheter (to minimize the chance of subcutaneous infiltration) of at least 18 gauge in adults (to allow rapid infusion of fluids in addition to medications). In infants and small children, in whom lack of cooperation is a major obstacle, the intravenous line may be placed after induction of anesthesia.
      5. A working suction system with flexible catheters and tonsil-tip suction.
      6. A blood pressure cuff and manometer or other equivalent apparatus.
      7. An ECG monitor and, if necessary, a pressure monitor.
      8. A temperature monitor and probe.
      9. A precordial or esophageal stethoscope.
      10. A readily available defibrillator and standard ECG machine.
   C. The anesthetist must also have available the following types of drugs:
      1. Muscle relaxants to facilitate intubation.

2. Rapidly acting hypnotic drugs, such as thiopental.
3. Inhalation anesthetics.
4. Resuscitative drugs.

II. Anesthesia delivery equipment and apparatus

A. The **anesthesia machine** provides a controlled flow of oxygen, nitrous oxide, and inhalation anesthetic vapors to the breathing system.

1. **Types of machines.** A wide variety of machines are in use at the Massachusetts General Hospital: Ohio Unitrol, Ohmeda Modulus II, Drager Compact, Narkomed 2A and Standard, and Foregger F500.

2. **Construction.** Figure 8-1 is a circuit diagram of a basic anesthesia machine.

   a. Oxygen (O_2) and nitrous oxide (N_2O) are usually supplied from **wall outlets**. The gauge pressure of the wall outlet should be 50–55 pounds per square inch (psi).

   b. Attached to the machine are **reserve cylinders** of O_2 (full = 2000–2200 psi, the equivalent of 660 L at atmospheric pressure and room temperature), N_2O (full = 745 psi, 1590 L), and, on some machines, compressed air (full = 1800 psi, 630 L). The N_2O pressure will not decrease until the liquid content of the tank is exhausted, at which time only about one-fourth of the contents remains.

   c. For N_2O to flow, there must be at least 25 psi of O_2 **pressure** to open the "fail-safe" valve in the machine. ("Fail-safe" is a misnomer, since it does not fail into a safe mode, i.e., it will *permit the accidental delivery of 100% N_2O if the O_2 pressure is on but the flow valve is turned off.)

      (1) The Foregger F500 and Narkomed 2A machines have an O_2/N_2O ratio alarm that monitors the ratio of flows through each control valve. It will indicate, both visually and with an audio alarm, that a mixture of less than 26% of O_2 is being delivered.

      (2) The Ohmeda Modulus II has a mechanical linkage that will not permit delivery of less than 25% O_2.

   d. Downstream from the rotameters, the mixture of O_2 and N_2O (or air) is piped to the inlet of a **temperature-compensated vaporizer** that is calibrated directly in volume percent of anesthetic. Since the calibration depends on the vapor pressure of the liquid, a separate vaporizer is required for each anesthetic. All vaporizers are "key-indexed," so that they can only be filled with the correct anesthetic. The key-indexed filler caps are designed to screw onto a specific inhalation agent bottle using a collar with defined orientation notches. The spout similarly has notches that will align only with

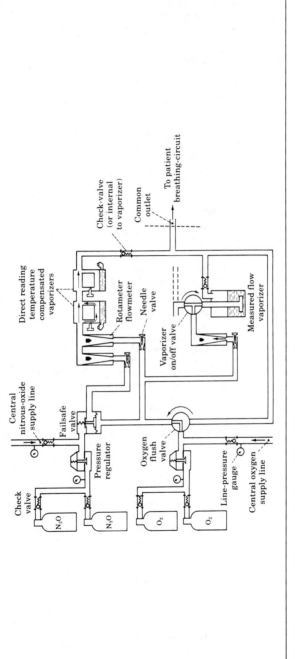

Fig. 8-1. A representative anesthesia machine. The many variations depend on vintage and manufacturer. The measured-flow vaporizer on-off valve may shunt oxygen to the common outlet or to the atmosphere in the "off" position.

the matched vaporizer. It is important to close the filler cap tightly, since failure to do so will result in a leak, which is difficult to detect in the routine inspection procedure.

e. In a machine equipped with a **measured flow vaporizer** (e.g., the Copper Kettle), O_2 is delivered from a separate rotameter to the kettle, where it is saturated with anesthetic vapor (temperature is important!). Extreme care must be taken in identifying the agent that is added to the kettle. If halothane is contained in a kettle marked "enflurane," a dangerous concentration of agent would be administered.

The concentration (C, in vol. %) of anesthetic vapor delivered to the machine common outlet is estimated as follows:

$$C = \frac{(Pv)\,(Fv)}{(Pb - Pv)\,(Fd + Fv)}$$

where Fv = O_2 flow to vaporizer (L/min)

$\quad\quad Pv$ = vapor pressure of anesthetic (at kettle temperature) (mm Hg)

$\quad\quad Pb$ = barometric pressure (mm Hg)

$\quad\quad Fd$ = diluent flow (L/min)

(1) A simplification has been used at low vapor concentrations (up to a few %), high diluent flows (more than a few L/min), and temperature close to 21°C:

   (a) For **halothane** or **isoflurane**, with a 5 L/min diluent flow, a flow of 100 ml/min through the kettle yields approximately 1% vapor; 200 ml/min yields about 2%, and so on. At 500 ml/min, the actual concentration is 4.1%.

   (b) For **enflurane**, with a 5 L/min diluent flow, a flow of 150 ml/min through the kettle yields a vapor concentration of about 1%. Again, multiples of kettle flow result in approximately multiples of vapor concentration. At a kettle flow of 600 ml/min, the actual enflurane concentration would be 3.2%, compared to the estimated 4%.

(2) The kettle control switch must be turned "on" for use. If it is not, anesthetic will not be delivered.

(3) At the end of the procedure, remember to turn the kettle control switch "off" to prevent inadvertent delivery of agent during the conclusion of the procedure.

B. The **breathing system** provides a means to deliver positive-pressure ventilation and to control alveolar

PCO_2 by minimizing rebreathing or by absorbing carbon dioxide (CO_2).

1. **Types in use.** For adults, the "circle" breathing system is used almost exclusively; T-piece configurations are usually used with children. The Bain System (modified Mapleson D) is sometimes used for adults or children. **Note:** The Bain System requires high fresh gas flows to prevent substantial rebreathing, which is a limiting factor in adult applications.

2. **Construction of the circle.** Figure 8-2 is a schematic diagram of a typical circle system. Not shown is a valve (on the side of the absorber on some machines) that is used to bypass CO_2 absorbant. Be sure to verify the absence of such a valve or its position if present. If the bypass valve is present and on, dangerous retention of CO_2 will occur.

C. The anesthesia **ventilator** is a simple version of a volume ventilator. It frees the anesthetist's hand from manual ventilation.

1. **Types in use** include the Drager AV, Ohmeda 7000, and Fraser-Harlake units, which are properly called pressure-limited, time-cycled, volume ventilators. All in use at Massachusetts General Hospital have an upright bellows, which descends during inspiration.

2. **Construction.** Figure 8-2 also includes a schematic diagram illustrating the basic function of the Ohmeda 7000 Ventilator, which is functionally similar to the Fraser-Harlake. Both are electronically controlled and must be connected to a source of **electricity** and **O_2**. The Drager AV controls are powered by O_2 or compressed air.

   a. The bellows is compressed by O_2 introduced into the surrounding chamber.

   b. The tidal volume indicated is **not** quite the same as that delivered. Fresh gas flow, compression of gas, and compliance of the breathing system affect it. Higher fresh gas flows add a little to tidal volume; higher peak airway pressures and more compliant breathing systems diminish delivered tidal volume.

   c. Instructions are provided on the chassis of each ventilator. Instructions are different for each of the units and should be reviewed prior to use.

D. The **O_2 analyzer** measures the concentration of O_2 and is usually placed in the inspiratory limb of the breathing system. If used in the expiratory limb, the sensor may need to be shaken or carefully wiped dry periodically.

1. **Types in use.** Foregger Model 450 and Ohmeda 5100.

2. **Construction.** The Foregger is based on a polarographic (Clark electrode) sensor fabricated as a replacement cartridge (approximately a 9-month

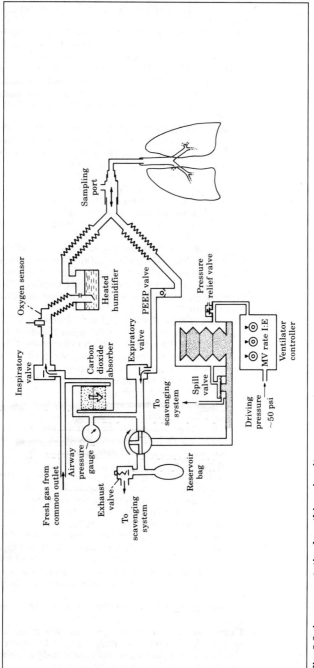

Fig. 8-2. A representative breathing circuit.

life). O_2 diffuses through a plastic membrane, where it is electrochemically reduced by a platinum cathode, which is kept negative with respect to a silver/silver chloride anode. The current produced is proportional to the concentration of O_2. The Ohmeda 5100 uses a galvanic fuel cell, which functions similarly to a polarographic cell.

   3. Operation. Instructions are printed on top of the box. A warm-up time is required.

      a. A one-point calibration at 100% O_2 and a check at 21% O_2 should be performed at the beginning of each day. A check at one point should be done before the start of each procedure.

      b. The analyzer should be left in "standby" when not in use.

E. Components of the anesthesia tray

   1. Means of maintaining an open airway

      a. An **anesthesia mask** (sizes are small to medium for women and medium to large for men), with a head strap to maintain an airtight fit.

      b. **Nasal airways** (sizes 28–30 for women and 32–34 for men) and **oral airways** (sizes 3–5 for adults), lubricated with lidocaine ointment, can be placed to keep the posterior pharynx open.

   2. Apparatus for tracheal intubation

      a. A working **laryngoscope** with a blade of appropriate size. A Macintosh #3 is the most commonly used blade, but other sizes and different blades should be available if a difficult intubation is anticipated.

      b. An **oral tracheal tube** of the appropriate size (size 30–34 Fr or 7.0–8.0 mm internal diameter [ID] for women and 36–38 Fr or 8.5–9.0 mm ID for men). Low-pressure, high-volume cuffed tubes should be used if the surgery or postoperative intubation is expected to be lengthy. The cuff should be tested for leaks with a 10-ml syringe. A clamp for a non-self-sealing pilot tube, a lubricated stylet to mold the tracheal tube, and additional oral tracheal tubes in a range of sizes should also be readily available.

   3. Commonly used drugs

      a. Atropine.

      b. Muscle relaxants to facilitate intubation and provide paralysis for surgery when necessary. Usually succinylcholine and d-tubocurarine or pancuronium are drawn up and labeled.

      c. Rapidly acting hypnotic drugs, such as thiopental.

      d. Other drugs to be used in the anesthetic, such as narcotics and tranquilizers.

      e. An anticholinesterase to reverse nondepolarizing neuromuscular blockade.

   4. A working **suction system,** including both a suction catheter and a tonsil-tip sucker.

   5. A blood pressure cuff and manometer.

6. A precordial or esophageal **stethoscope,** or both, for listening to heart tones and rhythm and breath sounds.

7. Common resuscitative drugs (on a tray or readily available): epinephrine (Adrenalin), norepinephrine (Levophed), isoproterenol (Isuprel), dopamine (Intropin), phenylephrine (Neo-Synephrine), ephedrine, calcium chloride, sodium bicarbonate, potassium chloride, atropine, lidocaine (Xylocaine), propranolol (Inderal), hydrocortisone (Solu-Cortef), mannitol, furosemide (Lasix), nitroprusside (Nipride), nitroglycerin, hydralazine (Apresoline), and naloxone (Narcan).

8. Antibiotics, ophthalmic ointment, or ocular occluders (Tegaderm) for eye protection.

III. **Monitoring apparatus, instrumentation, and techniques**

A. **Blood pressure measurement**

1. **Noninvasive.** In all the commonly used noninvasive techniques, external pressure is applied over the limb with a compression cuff. The cuff is inflated with air to a pressure above systolic, which terminates distal flow. The cuff is then slowly deflated, and arterial pressure is measured by either detecting flow (by auscultation of Korotkoff's sounds, palpation of arterial pulse, or ultrasonic flow detection) or by observing changes in the pulsations in the cuff pressure that are caused by the arterial pulse (simple or automated oscillometry). Two **sources of error** are common to all these techniques: inappropriate cuff size and rapid deflation rate. A too-narrow cuff will produce falsely high measurements, and an overly wide cuff will produce falsely low measurements. The cuff should cover about two-thirds of the upper arm or thigh; that is, the width of the cuff should be 20% greater than the diameter of the limb. If the deflation rate is too rapid, the measurement may be falsely low, especially at low heart rates. The recommended rate of deflation is 3–5 mm Hg/sec.

Typical Cuff Widths (cm)

Newborn infant	2.5
1–4 years	6.0
4–8 years	9.0
Adult (arm)	12.0
Adult (leg)	15.0

a. **Auscultation of Korotkoff's sounds** is the most common technique. As the cuff pressure deflates just below arterial systolic pressure, blood is ejected with turbulent flow. This turbulence creates sounds that can usually be detected by a stethoscope. The sounds continue as the cuff pressure is gradually decreased until the diastolic pressure is reached. At that point, Korotkoff's sounds will change or disappear, because the artery is no longer occluded at any point in the pulse cycle. Perceived **muffling of the sounds** is the standard criteria for the diastolic measurement.

b. Palpation. Blood pressures may be monitored by palpating an arterial pulse distal to the cuff. The cuff is inflated until a pulse can no longer be detected. As the cuff is slowly deflated, the point at which the pulse is first felt is recorded as systolic pressure. This value will be lower than systolic pressure determined by direct intraarterial measurements.

c. An **ultrasonic flow detector** can be used in place of the stethoscope when Korotkoff's sounds are weak or inaudible. This technique is particularly useful for infants or for low flow states in adults. An ultrasonic crystal beams a high frequency signal to the vessel wall. The motion of the vessel wall during ejection causes a shift in the frequency of the reflected wave (Doppler principle). The Parks Ultrasonic Doppler Flow Detector detects, amplifies, and converts this frequency shift into an audible sound.

d. Simple oscillotonometry is useful for monitoring blood pressure trends in infants and small children, since attaching a stethoscope to a tiny extremity is often difficult. A properly sized cuff is placed around the extremity, inflated above the estimated systolic pressure, and then slowly deflated. As the cuff pressure is reduced, oscillations will appear on the manometer. The pressure at which a sudden increase in the amplitude of oscillation occurs can be used as an **estimate** of systolic pressure.

e. Automated devices, such as the Dinamap pressure monitor, use the principle of oscillometry with automated, periodic inflation and deflation of the cuff to measure systolic, diastolic, and mean arterial pressures. The cuff pressure is monitored internally in the Dinamap by a semiconductor pressure transducer. The cuff is inflated automatically to 40 mm Hg above the previous systolic measurement (170 mm Hg, initially) and then deflated in increments of 3 mm Hg. A microprocessor in the instrument analyzes the pressure oscillations in the cuff and determines mean pressure to be the average pressure in the cuff at which the maximal oscillation occurs. The diastolic and systolic readings are not always well correlated with invasive measurements and should be interpreted cautiously, especially the extremes of measurement. (Algorithms for determining systolic and diastolic pressures are not published.) The cycling time and pressure alarm limits are set on the front panel. Motion artifact is rejected by the instrument, but will increase the inflation cycle time. The size of the cuff must be chosen correctly. Venous congestion may occur if the instrument is set to cycle the measurement too frequently; **cycle times less than 2 minutes apart should be avoided for routine monitoring.**

2. **Invasive techniques** for directly measuring blood pressure require coupling of the intravascular space to an external transducer (usually electronic) through a catheter. Blood pressures measured this way will depend, among other things, on the position of the catheter in the cardiovascular system and may be slightly different from those measured noninvasively. The accuracy of the direct measurement depends on the characteristics of the cannula and connecting tubing, assembly of the system, and calibration of the instrument.

   a. Before beginning to insert a cannula, be sure that a properly calibrated blood pressure monitor–transducer set and a fluid-filled length of connecting tubing are ready for connection to the catheter.

   b. To display an arterial or venous blood pressure waveform on an electronic monitor, a cannula must be placed and then connected to the electronic transducer through a length of fluid-filled tubing. The transducer converts the arterial pressure signal to an electronic signal, which is then amplified and displayed by the monitor. To ensure that the waveform is not distorted, the tubing must be rigid and as short as possible, preferably less than 4 feet (to prevent harmonic amplification). The number of stopcocks must be minimized and the entire system purged of air bubbles. The fluid-filled system must be assembled **aseptically.** A continuous flush device (3–5 ml/hr at 300 mm Hg infusion bag pressure) or intermittent manual flush is required to prevent clot formation at the tip of the cannula.

   c. To obtain a true zero, the transducer must be on the same horizontal plane as is the zero point in the cardiovascular system (approximately at the level of the right atrium). This is particularly important in direct measurement of venous pressures.

   d. The calibration procedure varies with each type of monitor. Refer to the manufacturer's instructions for a detailed calibration procedure. The monitor should be calibrated prior to any important pressure measurement.

B. **Cannulation**
   1. **Arterial pressure measurement**
      a. Candidates for arterial cannulation include the following: critically ill patients requiring

multiple arterial blood gas sampling, blood chemistry determinations, and/or arterial blood pressure monitoring; patients with valvular heart disease, severe coronary artery disease, or congestive heart failure; patients with significant pulmonary disease; most patients undergoing elective controlled circulation (induced hypotension); patients undergoing cardiac surgery, major thoracic or vascular surgery, and intracranial procedures; patients undergoing prolonged procedures in which massive fluid replacement or transfusion is required.

b. Although the radial artery is most commonly used, the superficial temporal and the dorsalis pedis arteries share the advantage of collateral flow. Femoral and axillary arteries, though end-arteries, may also be used because of their large diameter.

c. If the radial artery is selected, perform a modified Allen's test to ascertain whether the ulnar artery supplies the main flow to the deep palmar arch. Manually occlude both arteries at the wrist, elevate the arm to drain off venous blood, then release one artery and observe the pattern of flush. Repeat, releasing the other artery. The radial artery may be safely cannulated if, when the radial artery alone is occluded, the ulnar artery can give a flush to all parts of the hand. If it does not, another vessel must be used.

d. Mix 250 units of heparin in 250 ml of normal saline solution, and label the mixture. Fill a 10-ml syringe with this mixture and attach first a stop-cock and then a T connector (Abbott Laboratories, item 4612). Fill the T connector from the syringe. Draw up 1% lidocaine into a 3-ml syringe with a 25-gauge needle, and label it. If a wrist vessel is to be used, immobilize the forearm and hand with the wrist hyperextended over a stack of sponges. Keep the thumb abducted (Fig. 8-3A).

e. With an alcohol or iodine solution, clean the area to be punctured. Using 1% lidocaine, raise a skin wheal over the vessel, distal to the planned point of entry. Puncture the skin in the center of the wheal very superficially with a 15-gauge needle.

f. Fill the plastic catheter and its metal needle (22-gauge for infants, 20-gauge for larger children, and 18- or 20-gauge for adults) with some heparinized saline solution. Pass the catheter through the puncture site into the subcutaneous tissue. With the fingers of the opposite hand gently palpating the artery to establish its course, quickly advance the catheter completely through the vessel, impaling it. The an-

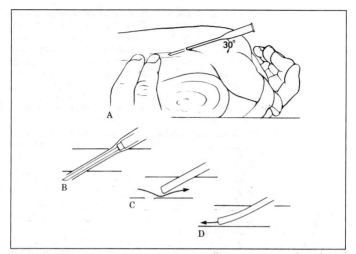

Fig. 8-3. Percutaneous radial artery cannulation. A. Direct threading method. B–D. Transfixing method. The positioning of the hand and forearm is the same for both methods.

gle between the needle and the skin should be less than 30 degrees (Fig. 8-3B). Blood will often show in the hub of the metal needle if the pass is successful (this may not be true of the 22-gauge needle).

g. Remove the metal needle from the cannula, keeping it sterile for possible reuse. Then slowly slide the cannula back until either blood is flowing freely or the tip is clearly in the subcutaneous tissue once again (Fig. 8-3C). If free flow is obtained, reduce the angle between the needle and skin to 10 degrees, and advance the cannula forward to thread it up the vessel (Fig. 8-3D). If free flow is not obtained, replace the metal needle and make another pass. After the cannula has been fully threaded with continuous free backflow, apply pressure over the proximal tip with the opposite hand to stop the bleeding. Firmly attach the T connector, stopcock, and syringe assembly, and flush the cannula free of blood; then turn the stopcock off toward the patient and remove the syringe. If a vessel is difficult to thread, insert an arterial stylet or wire through the cannula during free flow, thread it up the vessel, and then advance the cannula over it.

h. The direct threading procedure is similar to the transfixing described above, except that the catheter is advanced slowly while the anesthetist feels for pulsation until the vessel is entered (see Fig. 8-3A). When free flow of blood is observed, rigidly fix the position of the metal needle with one hand, and advance the cannula over it into the vessel with the other. Apply pressure proximally to stop the bleeding, and remove the needle carefully without dislodging the cannula; attach the T connector, stopcock, and syringe assembly as in **g.**

i. If a cutdown becomes necessary, extend the skin wheal proximally and laterally. Make a 1- to 2-cm transverse incision proximal to the puncture site and over the planned site of entry to the vessel, cutting the full thickness of the skin. With a small hemostat, spread the tissue until the vessel itself is found. Push the tip of the instrument transversely under the vessel to trap it; then open the instrument to stabilize the position. Placing silk ties under (but not tying them around) the artery will keep it within sight. Advance the catheter into the lumen of the artery under direct observation, and then remove the metal needle. Apply proximal pressure with the opposite hand to prevent further bleeding, and attach the T connector, stopcock, and syringe assembly as in **g.** Close the wound with interrupted silk sutures on a cutting needle, using the stitch closest to the vessel itself to tie the cannula and T connector in place.

j. Paint tincture of benzoin around the puncture site and onto the cannula itself, and apply antibiotic ointment over the puncture site or any skin incision. When the benzoin is completely dry, securely tape the cannula and the tip of the T connector to the skin. Tape down the other end of the T connector with its stopcock, and attach the stopcock to the fluid-filled tubing of the previously prepared pressure-transducer system.

k. Never flush the line with more than 3 ml of solution, to avoid sending a clot or air bubble to the cerebral circulation or to other end-arteries.

l. Triple check connections for tightness. Arterial exsanguination is very rapid.

m. When taking samples, first remove enough fluid to empty the volume of the T connector into a separate syringe (about 2 ml). Otherwise, the heparinized saline will dilute the arterial blood obtained.

2. **Central venous pressure measurement**

a. A central venous catheter may be employed to measure right heart filling pressures, assess tricuspid valve competence, sample central venous blood, assess the patient's blood volume to aid in intravenous fluid management, administer drugs into the central circulation, provide long-term parenteral nutrition, inject dye for cardiac output studies, or remove air emboli.

b. The right internal jugular and right subclavian veins follow an almost straight path to the right side of the heart; the left internal jugular and left subclavian veins are alternative routes. The cephalic veins bend at right angles where they pass the clavipectoral fascia to enter the axillary or subclavian veins; similarly, the external jugular veins bend at right angles where they join the subclavian veins. Consequently, it is more difficult to thread a central catheter through the external jugular or the cephalic veins. The basilic veins run deeper and more medially and offer greater success in reaching the superior vena cava from the antecubital fossa. The femoral veins are less commonly used because of the high incidence of thrombophlebitis associated with their cannulation.

c. Mix 250 units of heparin in 250 ml of normal saline solution, and label the mixture. Attach the catheter either to a transducer through a three-way stopcock or to central venous pressure (CVP) manometry for the measurement of CVP.

d. Cannulation of the right internal jugular vein (Seldinger technique)

   (1) Turn the patient's head far toward the left.

   (2) Make sure the neck is not flexed or extended.

   (3) Place the patient in the Trendelenburg position, unless the patient has pulmonary hypertension or congestive heart failure.

   (4) Palpate the mastoid process and the sternal attachment of the sternocleidomastoid muscle.

   (5) Divide the distance in two, and confirm proper position by finding the point where the external jugular vein crosses the sternocleidomastoid muscle.

   (6) Put on sterile gloves.

   (7) Clean the skin with a sterile solution.

   (8) Drape the patient so that the suprasternal notch and the clavicle are exposed.

   (9) Infiltrate the skin with 1% lidocaine between the external jugular vein and the angle formed by the sternal head and clavicular heads of the sternocleidomastoid muscle (see Fig. 8-4A).

   (10) Palpate the carotid artery medially.

   (11) Aim the 22-gauge needle and syringe so that it makes about a 30-degree angle with the skin and points toward the insertion of the clavicular head of the sternocleidomastoid muscle.

   (12) Slowly insert the needle until the vein is

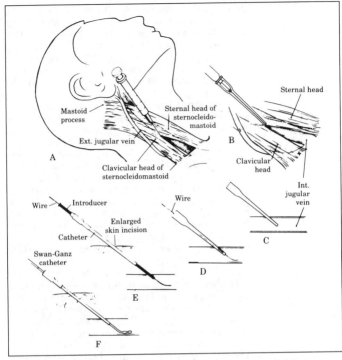

Fig. 8-4. Cannulation of the right internal jugular vein (Seldinger technique). See text for details.

punctured and free flow of blood is obtained. Never move the needle laterally when it is deep in the neck.

(13) Compare the color of the blood obtained with arterial blood to be sure that the carotid artery has not been punctured (if it has been punctured, withdraw the needle and apply pressure for 5–10 minutes).

(14) Keeping the angle and depth of the needle in view, withdraw the 22-gauge needle.

(15) Insert the 18-gauge catheter (with its needle) in the exact path of the 22-gauge needle placed above (never averting attention from the field) (Fig. 8-4B).

(16) When the vein has been punctured, advance the catheter slowly, and confirm successful cannulation by withdrawing the needle and seeing blood return (Fig. 8-4C).

(17) Pick up the guide wire and hold it next to the catheter.

(18) Remove the needle and syringe from the catheter, and insert the "soft" end of the guide wire through the catheter until the wire is about three-quarters inserted. Do not force; the wire must slide easily (Fig. 8-4D). If inserted too far, the guide wire may cause atrial or ventricular arrhythmias.

e. The **external jugular vein** runs superficially and laterally from the edge of the sternocleidomastoid muscle toward the clavicle. The skin adjacent to the vein should first be punctured superficially with a 15-gauge needle. The 14-gauge needle is then placed superficially at this site and directed along the course of the vein until free flow is encountered in an attached syringe or attached catheter–plastic shield assembly. The catheter is then advanced and treated as described in **d.** Gentle skin traction rostrally and finger occlusion of the vein at the clavicle will make the vein a larger, less mobile target.

A modified Seldinger technique can be used with this approach also. A J wire is introduced through an 18- or 16-gauge short catheter and rotated under the clavicle into the central circulation. A larger CVP catheter can then be placed over the wire after making a nick in the skin and platysma with a #11 scalpel blade.

f. The **subclavian vein** should be located with a 22-gauge needle placed under the clavicle just medial to the midclavicular line and directed toward the sternal notch. Once free flow is obtained, the procedure is duplicated with a 14-gauge needle, and the catheter is introduced and treated as in **d.** During needle insertion, always remain close to the inferior edge of the clavicle, and do not penetrate directly posteriorly (to avoid causing a pneumothorax).

g. To enter the **cephalic or basilic vein,** position the arm in moderate abduction with the elbow in the neutral position. A proximal tourniquet or blood pressure cuff may be used to distend the vein. Enter the vessel through a lidocaine skin wheal with a 14-gauge needle, watching for blood return in the catheter–plastic sheath assembly or syringe. Advance the catheter freely, and release the tourniquet. Remove the plastic sheath, and treat the catheter as described in **d.** If the catheter is difficult to thread, try removing the end of the plastic sheath, attaching a stopcock and the prefilled CVP manometry tubing, and allowing free flow of the solution to distend the vein while advancing the catheter. If a problem is encountered while advancing the catheter to the shoulder, try positioning the arm in more extreme abduction, that is, <u>raise the arm to 90 degrees from the trunk. Turning the head of the patient toward the arm of insertion</u> with placement of the <u>chin on the shoulder</u> will decrease the incidence of catheter passage into the jugular vein. The most recalcitrant veins, particularly the cephalic vein, may require insertion of a guide wire and threading of the catheter over it. If a cutdown is necessary, the deep brachial veins are also available and may be located easily by dissecting over the brachial pulse.

h. To find the **femoral vein,** palpate the femoral artery at the inguinal crease, and, using 1% lidocaine, raise a skin wheal 1 cm inferiorly and 1 cm medially to the palpated artery. Advance the 14-gauge needle through the skin wheal until blood return is seen; then, using the plastic sheath, advance the catheter into the vessel and treat it as described in **d.** The procedure may be made easier by raising the patient's buttocks on towels or a pillow.

i. The yellow Intracath set includes a 16-gauge catheter with a 14-gauge needle and is commonly used for adults; 24 inches in length for femoral, basilic, and cephalic veins; 8 or 12 inches in length for subclavian and external and internal jugular veins. In children, the green Intracath with a 19-gauge catheter and 17-gauge needle; in infants, the blue Intracath with a 22-gauge catheter and 19-gauge needle is appropriate.

j. To ensure the catheter's placement in the **central circulation,** perform one of the following:

   (1) Attach an electrically conductive stopcock to the end of a CVP line, fill the latter with normal saline, and connect an ECG to it. As the catheter is advanced, examine P waves until a cavitary pattern is observed, signifying entry into the right atrium.

   (2) Connect the CVP line to a transducer, and observe pressure waveforms as the catheter is advanced. Once a right ventricular trace has appeared, withdraw the catheter slightly, so that the tip lies within the right atrium.

   (3) Observe the position of the radiopaque catheter on an anteroposterior or posteroanterior chest x-ray.

k. Complications of CVP catheter insertion and use include the following:

   (1) **Arrhythmias.** Ventricular arrhythmias may occur when the catheter is within the

right ventricle. Atrial arrhythmias may occur if it is within the right atrium, especially if near the tricuspid valve.

(2) Carotid or subclavian artery puncture.

(3) Pneumothorax, hydrothorax, chylothorax, and air embolism.

3. Pulmonary artery pressure measurement

a. The flow-directed, or Swan-Ganz, catheter may be used to monitor pulmonary artery (PA) pressure, to assess left heart filling (via PA-occluded or pulmonary capillary wedge [PCW] pressures), to sample true mixed venous blood, and to inject dye or iced saline solution for cardiac output determination.

Indications for PA catheterization include those patients whose history or physical examination suggest poor cardiac function, recent myocardial infarction, known valvular disease, episodes of congestive heart failure, or frequent or uncontrolled angina. It is commonly used in coronary artery revascularization or valve replacements; patients in cardiogenic, hemorrhagic, or septic shock requiring inotropes or vasodilators; patients in respiratory failure; and patients with massive trauma. Any of the veins that have been mentioned may be used, although the right internal jugular is preferred because of the lower incidence of pneumothorax associated with this approach.

b. The following items should be made ready: iodine and alcohol solutions; several sterile sponges; 1% lidocaine in a 3-ml syringe with a 25-gauge needle; a 3-ml syringe with a 22-gauge needle; a 16-gauge over-the-needle catheter; a #11 scalpel blade; an 8 Fr introducer set; sterile gloves; a pack of sterile towels; a 7 Fr Swan-Ganz catheter; a flush solution with 250 units of heparin in 250 ml of normal saline; and one tuberculin syringe. If a 5 Fr Swan-Ganz catheter is used, a 7 Fr introducer set is appropriate.

c. Swan-Ganz line insertion

(1) Remove the Swan-Ganz catheter from its package, and keep it sterile.

(2) Have an assistant flush the PA and CVP (and right atrium, if present) lumens with heparinized saline solution. Pass the catheter through the protective sheath (Arrow Cath-Gard or equivalent), then check the balloon integrity with 1 ml of air. Remove the air from the balloon. Attach both PA and CVP lumens to calibrated pressure transducers through three-way stopcocks. Shake the distal end of the Swan-Ganz catheter to confirm measurement by the transducer. Contin-

uous monitoring of pressure through the PA lumen should be made during insertion of the catheter.

(3) Use the Seldinger technique to place a wire into the internal jugular vein as described in section **2.d.** The skin is incised using a #11 scalpel blade edge pointed away from the wire. The introducer and overlying catheter are then threaded over the wire and through the incision with a twisting motion. If resistance is encountered, use the scalpel blade to deepen or enlarge the opening in the platysma muscle (Fig. 8-4E).

(4) Ask the patient to exhale and hold his breath, then remove the wire and introducer from the large catheter and immediately insert the PA line to 20 cm, measured from the skin (Fig. 8-4F).

(5) Insert 1.0–1.5 ml of air into the balloon to cover the tip of the catheter and thus reduce the incidence of ventricular arrhythmias. The line should now be in the right atrium, confirmed by observing central venous pressure waves (Fig. 8-5).

(6) Continue to insert the PA line to 35–45 cm, which should place the tip in the right ventricle. Confirm this by observing the ventricular pressure wave (Fig. 8-5).

(7) Failure to see the expected waveforms despite the continued advancing of the catheter may be handled by flushing the catheter lumen with heparinized saline; by examining the transducer and noncompliant tubing for air in the line causing a dampened trace; by checking the monitor for function and proper scale selection; and by withdrawing the catheter (with the balloon deflated) to the 20- to 30-cm mark, reinflating the balloon, rotating the catheter slightly, and advancing it once again. Large inspirations may augment stroke volume to help float the catheter into the pulmonary artery.

(8) Continue to insert the line until the PA tracing is obtained at 40–50 cm (Fig. 8-5).

(9) Continue to insert the PA line with the balloon inflated until the wedge tracing is obtained at about 50–55 cm (Fig. 8-5). Do not insert the line any further than 65 cm.

(10) Let the air out of the balloon. The PA tracing should reappear. If it does not, flush the line; if it still does not appear, pull back the line until the PA tracing does reappear.

(11) Reinflate the balloon to confirm wedge po-

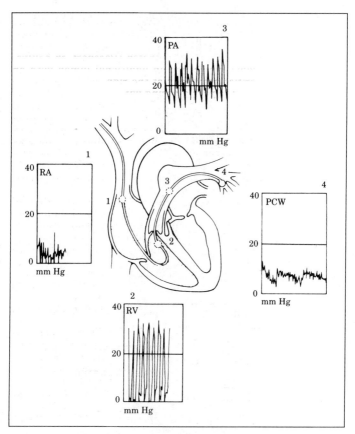

Fig. 8-5. Characteristic pressure waves seen during insertion of a Swan-Ganz catheter.

sition; deflate to confirm the PA position. Adjust as necessary.

(12) Tape the catheter securely to the patient's forehead and to the distal end of the large introducing catheter.

(13) If the CVP port is in the right ventricle rather than the right atrium, the right ventricular end-diastolic pressure can be transduced directly.

d. Always be ready to treat **arrhythmias** while the catheter is passing through the ventricle. If the patient has a history of premature ventricular contractions, consider giving a bolus of lidocaine (1 mg/kg) and starting a lidocaine infusion (2 mg/min) before inserting the line.

e. Insertion of the Swan-Ganz catheter may cause

transient **right bundle branch block,** and additional precautions are required in the presence of left bundle branch block. A right ventricular pacing catheter (Paceport or equivalent), which has an additional lumen with an orifice positioned at the right ventricle, can be used to pass a pacing wire quickly should complete heart block with bradycardia develop. If the patient has first-degree block and left bundle branch block, then an atrioventricular pacing Swan-Ganz catheter is indicated. This special catheter is also used in "redo" cardiac surgery where epicardial pacing may be problematic or in aortic regurgitation where bradycardia is extremely poorly tolerated.

f. Never keep the balloon inflated for an extended period because of the possibility of pulmonary infarction. When the wedge pressure tracing is desired, inflate the balloon slowly, and stop when the tracing is obtained. Do not inflate the balloon further.

g. A Swan-Ganz catheter may also be inserted in other large veins. Many people prefer to use the basilic or brachial veins with a cutdown, although the Seldinger technique may sometimes work.

h. The catheter is placed using fluoroscopic visualization when a pacemaker has been placed within the past 3 months or when selective PA placement is necessary as in pneumonectomy. If a PA catheter is required in the presence of significant structural abnormalities, such as the Eisenmenger complex or atrial septal defect, then fluoroscopy will be of great assistance in proper placement.

i. A three-port catheter (Edwards VIP or equivalent; an additional port is positioned in the right atrium) is commonly used to minimize the number of central catheters required for fluid and drug administration.

j. A protective sheath (Arrow Cath-Gard catheter contamination shield) should be placed over the Swan-Ganz catheter prior to insertion. Once the catheter is properly placed, this sheath will keep the catheter sterile while allowing additional manipulation, if needed. A Velcro locking device is placed over the contamination shield to maintain catheter position. The introducer is sutured in two places to the skin using 2–0 silk on a straight cutting needle. This will minimize the to-and-fro motion of the introducer and reduce bacterial contamination. A sterile dressing is then applied over the entry site.

C. Electrocardiographic monitoring

1. The ECG is monitored in all patients undergoing surgery. It is used for the detection of arrhythmias, myocardial ischemia, electrolyte imbalance, heart block, and pacemaker function.

2. Electrocardiographic monitoring requires the proper placement of two sensing electrodes and a third reference electrode. In practice, four electrodes are usually used, so that any one of three different lead configurations can be selected. Since the ECG is a small electrical signal (about 1 mV), its measurement is very susceptible to electrical interference from other sources, especially power cords, electrosurgical instruments, and motion. Modern ECG monitors deal effectively with these problems. A noisy or drifting ECG display is usually due to an inappropriately applied, dry, or loosened electrode or to loose or dirty connections.

3. To apply electrodes:
   a. Clean and gently rub skin areas with gauze.
   b. Inspect each electrode to ensure that the gel is present and wet.
   c. Connect lead wires (before applying the electrodes).
   d. Apply the electrodes to the skin.

4. Lead II is most commonly monitored because the P wave is easily seen, allowing ready detection of junctional and ventricular arrhythmias. The reported incidence of arrhythmias during induction, intubation, and surgery is 60%.

5. Lead V5 is monitored for the detection of myocardial ischemia, since the bulk of the left ventricular myocardium lies beneath it. If only a three-electrode system is available, a modified V5 lead can be followed by placing the right-arm lead under the clavicle, the left-arm lead in the V5 position, and the left-leg lead as usual, while monitoring lead I.

6. A five-lead system should be used with simultaneous monitoring of leads II and V5 during cardiac surgery, major vascular surgery, or any surgery on patients with significant cardiac disease.

D. **Temperature monitoring**

1. The ever-present danger of the syndrome of malignant hyperthermia is not the sole indication for temperature monitoring. Infants and small children (with a high ratio of surface area to mass) have poor thermal stability, as do adults subjected to low room temperatures, large evaporative losses from burns or exposed peritoneum, cold fluids, or extensive irrigations. Cardiopulmonary bypass with deliberate hypothermia also requires monitoring, particularly during rewarming, to assess temperature gradients between the core and periphery.

2. Several routes may be used for temperature monitoring by means of a thermistor probe and telethermometer, including the skin, axillae, rectum, esophagus, nasopharynx, and tympanic membranes. The following facts about these routes should be noted:
   a. The **skin** may not reflect core temperature.

b. The **axilla** can be used for temperature determination if the probe is secured over the artery and the arm fully adducted to the patient's side. The measured temperature will usually be about 1°C lower than core temperature after equilibration.

c. **Rectal** temperatures do not accurately reflect the early departures from normal body temperature during anesthesia and should only be employed when alternatives are not available. Rectal perforation can occur as a rare complication.

d. **Esophageal** measurements are acceptable if the probe is placed in the lower third of the esophagus, a position that is difficult to determine. Taping the probe to an esophageal stethoscope and inserting the assembly so that the heart sounds are maximal will probably achieve the proper position, though radiography is the only reliable test. A probe in this position will indicate the temperature of the heart and blood. The probe is very stiff and can perforate the esophagus.

e. The **nasopharynx** gives a good indication of the temperature of the blood coming to the brain, since it is in close proximity to the carotid artery. The probe can be correctly placed by measuring the distance between the external meatus of the ear and external nares and very slowly inserting the probe exactly that distance. The probe should be taped over the bridge of the nose and cotton inserted into the external nares to prevent skin necrosis during long procedures. Nasopharyngeal probes should not be used if the patient has had head trauma or has cerebrospinal fluid rhinorrhea. Epistaxis is a common occurrence.

E. Neuromuscular blockade monitoring

1. The extent of muscle relaxation (see Chap. 11) can be assessed by external stimulation of selected nerves (usually the ulnar) and by simultaneous observation of the corresponding muscular contraction (thumb adduction). The train-of-four technique is employed using a suitable constant-current output stimulator. The same instrument can also be used for other methods of neuromuscular monitoring (single twitch or tetanus).

2. In the train-of-four mode, the stimulator generates four short-duration electrical pulses 0.5 second apart (2 hertz). Supramaximal stimulation of the nerve and proper positioning of the electrodes over the ulnar nerve are important for accurate interpretation.

3. To use the instrument:

   a. Clean and gently rub the skin area over the ulnar nerve at the wrist.

   b. Connect lead wires to two gel-coated electrodes.
   c. Apply the negative lead directly over the nerve.
   d. Adjust the output control to its lowest setting.
   Turn the stimulator on. Increase the output
   control until maximal thumb adductor response
   is obtained. If supramaximal stimulation cannot be achieved at an output of 50 milliam-
   peres, replace or reposition the electrodes, or
   both. Needle electrodes should be avoided, since
   direct trauma to the nerve has been reported as
   well as local burns.
F. Pulse oximetry. Nellcor pulse oximeters (Model C) are
   available for every anesthetizing location.
   1. Principle. Blood O_2 content (CaO_2) is the equivalent volume of O_2 contained in 100 ml of blood.
   Since O_2 is both dissolved in the plasma and bound
   to hemoglobin, the calculation of the O_2 content has
   two terms:

$$CaO_2 = [(1.37)(Hgb)(SaO_2)] + [(0.003)(PaO_2)]$$

   where 1.37 is the number of milliliters of O_2 bound
   to 1 gm of fully saturated hemoglobin, Hgb is the
   hemoglobin concentration in gm/dl, SaO_2 is the oxygen saturation, 0.003 is the solubility of O_2 in
   plasma, and PaO_2 is the arterial O_2 tension.
   Pulse oximetry uses spectrophotometry and Beer's
   law to measure changes in light absorption in
   blood. Beer's law is as follows:

$$I_{transmitted} = [I_{incident}][e^{-(D)(C)(\alpha)}]$$

   where $I_{transmitted}$ is the intensity of transmitted light,
   $I_{incident}$ the intensity of the incident light, D is the
   distance light transmitted through the liquid, C is
   the concentration of the solute (in this case, oxyhemoglobin), and α is the extinction coefficient of
   the solute (which is a constant for the solute at a
   specific wavelength of light).
   Two different wavelengths of light are used; one
   an infrared frequency and the other a visible red
   frequency. At each frequency, oxyhemoglobin and
   reduced hemoglobin absorb light differently. The
   light comes from light-emitting diodes (LED), which
   are housed in a sensor that is placed around a vascular bed (usually the finger). The amount of light
   reaching the detector (a light-sensitive resistor) on
   the other side of the sensor changes as blood pulses
   through the vasculature because the relative
   amounts of hemoglobin and oxyhemoglobin change
   with the added volume of arterial blood. At each
   wavelength, the difference in absorption caused by
   the arterial pulse is measured, canceling the effects
   of other tissues, venous blood, and background
   light. The differences are used to solve the equations relating absorption to saturation.

The light source and detector must be aligned properly. A sufficient peripheral pulse is required. Alternate probes for other placements are available (nasal, foot) for special situations.

2. **Limitations** of pulse oximeters are
   a. Abnormal hemoglobins (e.g., methemoglobin, carboxyhemoglobin, sulfhemoglobin) and cardiac and vital dyes (e.g., indocyanine green and methylene blue) cause lower saturation readings.
   b. Venous congestion, secondary to frequent tourniquet use, will lower the saturation.
   c. Overhead infrared lights will cause falsely elevated values. Covering the area with an opaque cloth will correct the problem.
   d. Intrinsic tremors or vibrations from the bed may alter the pulse rate reading.
   e. The absence of a peripheral pulse, as from hypothermia, hypotension, or nonpulsatile flow on cardiopulmonary bypass, will result in no reading and the instrument will indicate that it is "searching" for a pulse.

G. **Capnometry.** A Puritan Bennett (PB) capnometer is used routinely on the pediatric and neurosurgical anesthetic services and often in other circumstances.
   1. **Principle.** The PB capnometer also uses spectrophotometry and Beer's law, but to measure the concentration of a species in a gas mixture. Some gas is withdrawn from the breathing system at a steady rate (150 ml/min for adults) and passed into a small measurement chamber (about 1 ml volume) in the instrument. Pulses of infrared light of a frequency that is most absorbing for CO_2 are beamed through the gas. Every other pulse from the same light source is beamed instead through a "reference" gas of known CO_2 concentration. The difference in the amount of light absorbed between the sample and reference chambers is used to determine the concentration in the sample. This referencing technique is required to keep the instrument stable, because the amounts of light absorbed are so small. The instrument measures the instantaneous concentration during each breath. The accuracy will depend on the rate of withdrawal from the breathing system, the length and size of the sample tubing, and the pressure at which calibration was made.

   The end-tidal CO_2 value is typically several mm Hg below arterial PCO_2 and follows changes fairly well under most conditions. But, changes in ventilation/perfusion matching, dead space, and so on, can change the end-tidal–arterial difference, so that end-tidal changes may not accurately reflect the change in arterial. Also, the end-tidal value itself may be misleading, since a plateau in concentration at the end of expiration is necessary to represent alveolar gas accurately. For this reason, the *waveform* should be displayed whenever practical (capnograph). Careful observation of the movement of the pointer of an analog meter may substitute when necessary.

The end-tidal measurement and waveform together can identify many equipment problems and physiologic events, such as airway or breathing system obstruction, disconnection, excessive rebreathing, malignant hyperthermia, hypoventilation, or air embolism.

2. **Limitations and problems**

   a. High respiratory rates, as are typical in infants and children, may result in substantially lower readings. A lower sample flow rate (about 50 ml/min) is required, but an end-tidal plateau still may not be reached, and readings should be interpreted cautiously.

   b. Nitrous oxide interferes with the measurement. In the PB instrument, electronic compensation (activated from the front panel switch) is necessary above 30% N_2O.

   c. Anything that changes the pressure in the measurement chamber will alter the calibration; positive end-expiratory pressure (PEEP) and continuous positive airway pressure (CPAP) cause higher readings, and lower sample flow rate or longer or smaller diameter sample tubing result in lower readings. For an accurate measurement, calibration should be repeated under the actual conditions of use.

H. **Transcutaneous oxygen monitoring ($P_{tc}O_2$).** These monitors are used in the neonatal and pediatric intensive care units and may be brought to the operating rooms for continuous monitoring of infants at risk for the development of hypoxia. $P_{tc}O_2$ monitoring offers an alternative to the episodic removal and analysis of arterial blood samples, since it is comparatively noninvasive and allows for continuous as opposed to periodic determination of PaO_2.

   1. **Principle.** Oxygen in the blood diffuses through tissues and skin. The PO_2 measured on the skin surface correlates well with arterial PO_2. The skin must be heated (to approximately 43°C) to arterialize the capillaries. The sensor is a Clark-type electrode and integral heater. The current required to maintain the heater at constant temperature is an indicator of perfusion; for example, increasing current implies increasing perfusion.

   $P_{tc}O_2$ is substantially affected by O_2 delivery, so cardiac output is a major factor. Skin perfusion decreases early in a low-flow state, resulting in lower $P_{tc}O_2$. But the difference between PaO_2 and $P_{tc}O_2$ increases, and the $P_{tc}O_2$ is more an indicator of low flow than decreased PaO_2.

2. **Limitations and problems**

   a. Calibration is required with each use. An equilibration period of approximately 10 minutes is necessary.

   b. To prevent burns, monitor the skin sensor temperature. It should not be permitted to rise above 44°C. Change the electrode position every 2 hours in neonates and every 4 hours in adults.

   c. Falsely high values may result from an air bubble in the electrolyte solution or contamination of the electrode. If the monitor seems fixed at 155 mm Hg (room air O_2), check the skin contact. If the reading remains constant despite changing the FIO_2, then additional contact gel may be needed.

   d. Falsely low readings can result from improper calibration, direct pressure applied to the electrode (e.g., from leaning on it), or a burn at the electrode site.

   e. $P_{tc}O_2$ varies with skin location (truncal values tend to be higher than the extremities). The practice at the Massachusetts General Hospital is to place the electrode on the chest or abdomen.

I. **Mass spectrometry.** Mass spectrometers are in use at several hospitals in the Harvard system.

   1. **Principle.** A sample of gas is withdrawn through a side port in the breathing system near the Y-piece and is carried through a long nylon catheter to a central mass spectrometer. The sample is ionized in an electron beam. The resulting fragments are accelerated through a high-voltage field and then subjected to a deflecting magnetic field. The specific fragments are detected on collectors, and the relative concentration of each species is determined. Calibration is performed automatically at the central system. The instrument measures the concentration of O_2, CO_2, N_2, and N_2O, and the three major potent inhalation anesthetics.

   By a switching system, the mass spectrometer samples from as many as 32 locations. The time between measurements in each room may be one or several minutes depending on the number of rooms "on line." A "stat" sample may be requested. The composition of the last sample is displayed on a cathode-ray tube. One system also provides a breath-to-breath qualitative CO_2 waveform.

   The mass spectrometer provides the ability to identify equipment problems and to monitor respiratory status in the same way as an infrared capnometer (see sec. **III.G**). It provides additional information about anesthetic concentrations that can warn of vaporizer malfunction and can track the process of

uptake and distribution.
2. **Limitations and problems**
   a. The sampling interval is short enough to provide sufficient early warning of most untoward events and physiologic changes, but detection of some events, such as esophageal intubation, may not be sufficiently rapid if long measurement delays are being encountered.
   b. Overlap of fragments on some detectors can cause small erroneous readings of some inhalation anesthetics. An aerosol of isoproterenol will result in a false high measurement.

IV. **Anesthesia apparatus checkout recommendations** This checkout, or a reasonable equivalent, should be conducted before administering anesthesia. Users of this guideline are encouraged to modify to accommodate differences in equipment design and variations in local clinical practice. Such local modifications should have appropriate peer review. Users should refer to the operators manual for special procedures or precautions.
   A. The following guidelines are promulgated by the U.S. Food and Drug Administration (August 1986).
      1. **Inspect anesthesia machine for:***

         machine identification number
         valid inspection sticker
         undamaged flowmeters, vaporizers, gauges, supply hoses
         complete, undamaged breathing system with adequate CO_2 absorbent
         correct mounting of cylinders in yokes
         presence of cylinder wrench

      2. **Inspect and turn on:***

         electrical equipment requiring warm up (ECG/pressure monitor, oxygen monitor, etc.)

      3. **Connect waste gas scavenging system:***

         adjust vacuum as required

      4. **Check that:***

         flow-control valves are off
         vaporizers are off
         vaporizers are filled (not overfilled)
         filler caps are sealed tightly
         CO_2 absorber by-pass (if any) is off

      5. **Check oxygen (O_2) cylinder supplies:***
         a. Disconnect pipeline supply (if connected) and return cylinder and pipeline pressure gauges to zero with O_2 flush valve.

If an anesthetist uses the same machine in successive cases, the steps marked with an asterisk (*) need not be repeated or may be abbreviated after the initial checkout.

    b. Open O_2 cylinder; check pressure; close cylinder and observe gauge for evidence of high pressure leak.

    c. With the O_2 flush valve, flush to empty piping.

    d. Repeat as in **b.** and **c.** above for second O_2 cylinder, if present.

    e. Replace any cylinder less than about 600 psig. At least one should be nearly full.

    f. Open less full cylinder.

6. **Turn on master switch (if present):***

7. **Check nitrous oxide (N_2O) and other gas cylinder supplies:***

    Use same procedure as described in **5.a** and **b** above, but open and **CLOSE** flow-control valve to empty piping.
    Note: N_2O pressure below 745 psig. indicates that the cylinder is less than ¼ full.

8. **Test flowmeters:***

    a. Check that float is at bottom of tube with flow-control valves closed (or at min. O_2 flow if so equipped).

    b. Adjust flow of all gases through their full range and check for erratic movements of floats.

9. **Test ratio protection/warning system (if present):***

    Attempt to create hypoxic O_2/N_2O mixture, and verify correct change in gas flows and/or alarm.

10. **Test O_2 pressure failure system:***

    a. Set O_2 and other gas flows to mid-range.

    b. Close O_2 cylinder and flush to release O_2 pressure.

    c. Verify that all flows fall to zero. Open O_2 cylinder.

    d. Close all other cylinders and bleed piping pressures.

    e. Close O_2 cylinder and bleed piping pressure.

    f. CLOSE FLOW CONTROL VALVES.

11. **Test central pipeline gas supplies:***

    a. Inspect supply hoses (should not be cracked or worn).

    b. Connect supply hoses, verifying correct color coding.

    c. Adjust all flows to at least mid-range.

    d. Verify that supply pressures hold (45–55 psig).

    e. Shut off flow control valves.

12. **Add any accessory equipment to the breathing system:***

    Add PEEP valve, humidifier, etc., if they might be used (if necessary remove after step 18 until needed).

13. **Calibrate O₂ monitor:**

   a. Calibrate O_2 monitor to read 21% in room air.*
   b. Test low alarm.*
   c. Occlude breathing system at patient end; fill and empty system several times with 100% O_2.
   d. Check that monitor reading is nearly 100%.

14. **Sniff inspiratory gas:**

   There should be no odor.

15. **Check unidirectional valves:***

   a. Inhale and exhale through a surgical mask into the breathing system (each limb individually, if possible).
   b. Verify unidirectional flow in each limb.
   c. Reconnect tubing firmly.

16. **Test for leaks in machine and breathing system:†**

   a. Close APL (pop-off) valve and occlude system at patient end.
   b. Fill system via O_2 flush until bag just full, but negligible pressure in system. Set O_2 flow to 5 L/min.
   c. Slowly decrease O_2 flow until pressure **no longer rises** above about 20 cm H_2O. This approximates total leak rate, which should be no greater than a few hundred ml/min (less for closed circuit techniques).
   Caution: Check valves in some machines make it imperative to measure flow in step **c** above when pressure **just stops rising.**
   d. Squeeze bag to pressure of about 50 cm H_2O and verify that system is tight.

17. **Exhaust valve and scavenger system:**

   a. Open APL valve and observe release of pressure.
   b. Occlude breathing system at patient end and verify that negligible positive or negative pressure appears with either zero or 5 L/min flow and exhaust relief valve (if present) opens with flush flow.

18. **Test ventilator:**

   a. If switching valve is present, test function in both bag and ventilator mode.
   b. Close APL valve if necessary and occlude system at patient end.
   c. Test for leaks and pressure relief by appropriate cycling (exact procedure will vary with type of ventilator).
   d. Attach reservoir bag at mask fitting, fill system and cycle ventilator. Assure filling and emptying of the bag.

---

†A vaporizer leak can only be detected if the vaporizer is turned on during this test. Even then, a relatively small but clinically significant leak may still be obscured.

19. **Check for appropriate level of patient suction.**

20. **Check, connect, and calibrate other electronic monitors.**

21. **Check final position of all controls.**

22. **Turn on and set other appropriate alarms** for equipment to be used.

    (Perform next two steps as soon as is practical.)

23. **Set O_2 monitor alarm limits.**
24. **Set airway pressure and/or volume monitor alarm limits** (if adjustable).

B. **Review of Safety Procedures.** Having prepared the anesthesia machine and monitoring equipment, it is appropriate to pause for a few moments and consider the philosophy and mechanisms for the safe conduct of anesthesia. In the next chapter, some of the safety procedures used at the Massachusetts General Hospital and other Harvard-affiliated institutions are reviewed.

Suggested Reading

Bruner, J. M. R. *Handbook of Blood Pressure Monitoring.* Littleton, Mass.: PSG, 1978.

Cooper, J. B. Anesthesia Delivery Apparatus Hazards. In F. Orkin and L. Cooperman (eds.), *Complications in Anesthesia* (2nd ed). Philadelphia: Lippincott. In press.

Dorsch, J. A., and Dorsch, S. E. *Understanding Anesthesia Equipment: Construction, Care and Complications* (2nd ed.). Baltimore: Williams & Wilkins, 1984.

Gravenstein, J. S., and Paulus, D. A. *Monitoring Practice in Clinical Anesthesia.* (2nd ed.). Philadelphia: Lippincott, 1987.

Kaplan, J. A. Hemodynamic Monitoring. In J. A. Kaplan (ed.), *Cardiac Anesthesia.* New York: Grune & Stratton, 1979. Pp. 71–115.

9

Safety in Anesthesia

Jeffrey B. Cooper and Clifford M. Gevirtz

Assuring that no harm befalls the patient is the most fundamental consideration of anesthesia management. Although the risk of injury from anesthesia is relatively low, serious injuries and death are not unknown. Data are sparse, but it has been estimated that, on average, an anesthesiologist will be involved in a preventable fatality or serious injury to a patient at least once during his or her professional career. Other instances of lesser morbidity occur with some regularity. Although vigilance remains the most important principle for prevention of injuries, it is not by itself sufficient. Several different strategies must be used to maintain the lowest risk exposure possible, with the ultimate objective that every anesthetic administration be complication-free. We describe here some specific suggestions to help achieve this goal, as well as some of the safety systems that have been implemented at the Massachusetts General Hospital.

I. **The risk of anesthesia**
   A. The overall risk of death related to anesthesia is about 1 per 10,000 anesthetic administrations. The risk to a relatively healthy patient presenting for elective surgery is far less, perhaps 1 per 50,000 administrations. Potentially injurious, life-threatening incidents or complications occur at a much higher rate, on the order of 1 per 10 administrations for non-ICU-bound patients.
   B. Serious mishaps are typically the result of a combination of errors, lapses in vigilance, environmental influences, and human-factor deficiencies, all of which can combine to obscure the prompt detection or correction of a problem. Some of the most frequent errors identified in studies of critical incidents and some suggested preventive tactics are listed in Table 9-1.
   C. Some of the factors frequently associated with critical anesthesia incidents and mishaps are
      1. Failure to prepare adequately for anesthesia, including a complete patient history and thorough inspection of equipment and apparatus.
      2. Inadequate familiarity with instrumentation or equipment, the surgical procedure, or the anesthetic technique.
      3. Poor communication within the surgical team.
      4. Haste.
      5. Obstruction of the visual field.
      6. Fatigue.
      7. Inattention and carelessness.

II. **Standardized protocols**
   A. The Harvard Medical School Department of Anaesthesia has adopted **Standards of Practice for Minimal Monitoring** and, for pre-use, **Inspection of Anesthesia Apparatus.** These standards apply for

Table 9-1. Frequent errors and prevention strategies in anesthesia critical incidents

Incident description	Prevention strategies
Breathing system disconnection	Airway pressure alarm Capnography
Syringe or drug ampule swap	Distinct label Organized system
Gas flow control error	Oxygen analyzer
Loss of gas supply	Oxygen analyzer
Intravenous line disconnection	Keep IV in view
Vaporizer on/off unintentionally	Anesthetic analyzer Vaporizer interlock
Drug overdose (judgment error)	Review of appropriate dosage Adequate supervision
Breathing system leak	Pre-use leak test Capnography
Unintentional extubation	Secure tube well
Misplaced tracheal tube	Capnography
Breathing system misconnection	Patency test Airway pressure alarm
Inadequate fluid replacement	Preanesthetic history review Lower threshold for invasive monitoring
Laryngoscope malfunction	Pre-use check Spare scope
Hypoxemia	Pulse oximetry

any administration of anesthesia involving Department of Anaesthesia personnel and are specifically referable to preplanned anesthetics administered in a designated anesthetizing location (specific exclusions: administration of epidural analgesia for labor or pain management). In emergency circumstances in any location, immediate life-support measures of whatever appropriate nature come first with attention turning to the measures described in these standards as soon as possible and practical. These are minimal standards, which may be exceeded at any time based on the judgment of the involved anesthesia personnel. These standards encourage high-quality patient care, but observing them cannot guarantee any specific patient outcome. These standards are subject to revision from time to time, as warranted by the evolution of technology and practice.

1. **Standard of practice for minimal monitoring**
   a. **Anesthesiologist's or nurse anesthetist's presence in the OR.** For all anesthetics initiated by or involving a member of the Department of Anaesthesia, an attending or resident anesthesiologist or nurse anesthetist shall be present in the room throughout the conduct of

all general anesthetics, regional anesthetics, and monitored anesthetic care. An exception is made when there is a direct known hazard (e.g., radiation) to the anesthesiologist or nurse anesthetist, in which case some provision for monitoring the patient must be made.

b. **Blood pressure and heart rate.** Every patient receiving general anesthesia, regional anesthesia, or monitored anesthetic care shall have arterial blood pressure and heart rate measured at least every 5 minutes where not clinically impractical. Under extenuating circumstances, the attending anesthesiologist may waive this requirement after so stating (including the reasons) in a note in the patient's chart.

c. **ECG.** Every patient shall have the ECG continuously displayed from the induction or institution of anesthesia until preparing to leave the anesthetizing location, where not clinically impractical. Under extenuating circumstances, the attending anesthesiologist may waive this requirement after so stating (including the reasons) in a note in the patient's chart.

d. **Continuous monitoring.** During every administration of general anesthesia, the anesthetist shall employ methods of continuously monitoring the patient's ventilation and circulation. The methods shall include, for ventilation and circulation each, at least one of the following or the equivalent:

    (1) **For ventilation.** Palpation or observation of the reservoir breathing bag, auscultation of breath sounds, monitoring of respiratory gases such as end-tidal carbon dioxide (CO_2), or monitoring expiratory gas flow. Monitoring end-tidal CO_2 is an emerging standard and is strongly preferred.

    (2) **For circulation.** Palpation of a pulse, auscultation of heart sounds, monitoring of a tracing of intraarterial pressure, pulse plethysmography, or ultrasound peripheral pulse monitoring.

It is recognized that brief interruptions of the continuous monitoring may be unavoidable.

e. **Breathing system disconnect monitoring.** When ventilation is controlled by an automatic mechanical ventilator, there shall be in continuous use a device that is capable of detecting disconnection of any component of the breathing system. The device must give an audible signal when its alarm threshold is exceeded. (It is recognized that there are certain rare or unusual circumstances in which such a device may fail to detect a disconnection.)

f. **Oxygen analyzer.** During every administration of general anesthesia using an anesthesia machine, the concentration of oxygen (O_2) in the patient breathing system will be measured by a functioning O_2 analyzer with a low concentration limit alarm in use. This device must conform to the American National Standards Institute (ANSI) Z.79.10 Standard. Under extenuating circumstances, the attending anesthesiologist may waive this requirement after so stating (including the reasons) in a note in the patient's chart.

g. **Ability to measure temperature.** During every administration of general anesthesia, there shall be readily available a means to measure the patient's temperature.

Rationale: A means of temperature measurement must be available as a potential aid in the diagnosis and treatment of suspected or actual intraoperative hypothermia and malignant hyperthermia. The measurement/monitoring of temperature during every general anesthetic is not specifically mandated because of the potential risks of such monitoring and because of the likelihood of other physical signs giving earlier indication of the development of malignant hyperthermia.

2. **Standard of practice for preanesthetic apparatus checkout**

a. **The "first-use check."** The function of the anesthesia machine shall be tested prior to its first use during any work day. The specific protocol used shall be at the discretion of the responsible anesthesiologist or anesthetist insofar as it is consistent with the policy of the individual hospital department. At minimum, the following shall be determined:

(1) There is no external damage that compromises function.

(2) Adequate main and reserve O_2 supplies are available.

(3) The following components if present have *no visible damage* and *function correctly*: flow-sensitive fresh gas ratio protection or warning system; inspired gas O_2 analyzer and its audible lower-limit alarm; breathing system; mechanical ventilator and the monitor for breathing system disconnect; and waste gas scavenging system.

(4) There are no clinically significant leaks in the anesthesia machine or the breathing system.

b. **The "case check."** Prior to the start of *each anesthetic* (including the first one of the day), the responsible anesthesiologist or anesthetist shall verify the following and after so doing, note on the anesthetic record that the case check has been performed. The specific protocol used shall be at the discretion of the responsible anesthesiologist or anesthetist insofar as it is consistent with the policy of the individual hospital department. At minimum, the following shall be verified:

(1) Function of the breathing system (patency, absence of leaks, venting through the scavenging system).

(2) Flow of O_2 through both flowmeter and flush valves.

(3) Presence of functioning suction.

(4) Presence of apparatus for airway maintenance, including tracheal intubation.

(5) Presence of apparatus for starting and maintaining an intravenous infusion.

(6) Presence of appropriate anesthetic drugs as determined by departmental policy. When a vaporizer is present, the liquid level should be confirmed and the filler cap tightened.

(7) Presence of appropriate resuscitative drugs as determined by departmental policy.

B. Relief protocol

1. It is the policy at the Massachusetts General Hospital to provide periodic breaks for the primary individual providing anesthesia. No firm rule is enforced; rather, the decision is based on the individual's needs and request. However, current practice is to afford a 20-minute break approximately every 2–3 hours.

2. Reliefs should be avoided in short cases and should be used with extra caution in cases characterized by complexity, that is, where the primary anesthetist's intuitive sense of the anesthesia management cannot be satisfactorily transferred to another person.

3. When an anesthesiologist is relieved, the replacement should sign or initial the record at the time of the change. Upon return, the original anesthesiologist should similarly make a note on the record.

4. During a relief changeover, the following information should be exchanged and actions taken before the original anesthesiologist exits:

   a. The situation

   (1) Presentation of the patient's diagnosis, operation, past medical history, allergies, abnormal laboratory values, chest x-ray, and ECG.

   (2) Description of the anesthetic technique and logic.

   b. Surgical course

   (1) Determination of anesthetic course and the status of surgical procedure.

      (2) Assessment of blood loss and fluid replacement.

      (3) Inspection of IV catheters and monitoring lines.

      (4) Present level of anesthesia (lightening or deepening); time at which the patient will need additional anesthesia.

      (5) Inspection of drug administration syringes and containers for drug names and concentrations.

      (6) Determination of current settings of gas flows and anesthetic concentration, readings on the O_2 analyzer, and the cylinder and pipeline supply pressures.

      (7) Measurement of current clinical signs and vital signs.

  c. Anticipated course

      (1) The availability of blood products.

      (2) The anesthetic plan, including fluid and drug therapies.

      (3) The plan for postoperative respiratory and drug support.

C. Standardized monitoring array. To the extent possible, monitoring apparatus has been organized in a standardized array on all anesthesia machines. Also, pulse oximeters are available for every anesthetizing location.

D. Standardization of the anesthesia system and inspection

  1. Because differences in the function and location of components of breathing systems are an important cause of errors, all anesthesia machine breathing systems are based on a single standard system (the Ohio Model 21 absorber) with identical location and types of components.

  2. All anesthesia apparatus is inspected systematically at 6-month intervals. An inspection sticker is affixed to each anesthesia machine and to each portable item. Inspection and service records are maintained.

  3. An identifying number is affixed on the front surface of each anesthesia machine. This number should be noted on the anesthesia record so that, in the event of an actual or suspected problem, the equipment used can be identified.

E. Organization of drugs and supplies. Supply carts are organized in standardized array to facilitate location of drugs or equipment in emergencies and identification of depleted stocks.

III. Specific safety suggestions

  A. Syringe identification

    1. All syringes should be identified with a label.

    2. Medication must never be administered from a syringe unless the *name* and *concentration* of the medication are clearly identified on the syringe.

3. A syringe should not be labeled by anyone other than the individual who drew up the drug.

4. When more than one IV container is used, each should be numbered consecutively.

5. When adding medications to the IV container, a label that specifies the name of the drug, the total amount added, and the resulting concentration should be affixed. The date and time of additions and the name of the person who made the dilution should also be noted.

B. Patient history. The patient's allergy history should always be checked prior to the administration of any medication. It is recommended that antibiotics be administered before induction whenever possible to avoid the development of allergic reactions during anesthesia.

C. Availability of suction. A properly functioning, dedicated suction must always be readily available during anesthesia.

D. Intravenous connections. When IV connections are obscured from view (e.g., under the drapes), they must be doubly secured.

E. Obscured breathing system connections. When these connections are obscured, frequent, periodic checks of the integrity of the connection should be made. Tube-trees will relieve stress on connections, and tape applied in a spiral or longitudinal fashion may lessen the likelihood of disconnection.

F. Visitors and observers. Particular caution is indicated during the presence of visitors and observers. Absolutely no one should tamper with or lean on anesthesia equipment.

G. Workspace arrangement. To the extent possible, all anesthesia equipment and apparatus should be arranged to be within a close visual field. Placement of the anesthesia machine behind the anesthesiologist should be avoided.

IV. Quality assurance in anesthesia. Some means for monitoring the quality of anesthesia services rendered and for documenting problems is necessary. Specifically, **recovery room impact events** that occur in the OR or the recovery room are documented on a standard form.

A. A recovery room impact event is an unanticipated, undesirable, possibly anesthesia-related effect that required intervention, is pertinent to recovery room care, and did or could cause mortality or at least moderate morbidity.

B. The **objectives** of this quality assurance system are

1. To aid the anesthesiologist in organizing information reported to the recovery room nurse.

2. To evaluate the care rendered to individual patients.

3. To monitor overall complication rates in search of trends or peculiar problems.

4. To serve as a source of identifying problem cases requiring further screening.

C. A **postoperative visit** by the anesthesiologist is a key component of quality care and is required by the Joint Commission on Accreditation of Hospitals. Adverse outcomes may be discovered by this route and discussed at departmental case conferences.

D. **Departmental case conferences** serve an important role in both quality assurance and education. By this means, both systematic and random problems in anesthesia practices may be detected.

V. **What to do after an adverse event.** No matter how experienced or skilled, there is a high probability that an anesthesiologist will be involved in a mishap during the span of a career. When such an event occurs, the foremost issues are early recognition and correction and discovery of the factors that led to the mishap to avoid a repetition.

A. **Notify** the responsible attending physicians and clinical director who should, in turn, notify the hospital risk manager.

B. **Document the event.** Describe the complication, how it happened, and what diagnostic tests and treatments have been ordered.

C. Prevent the irretrievable loss of information; **remove and sequester equipment and apparatus associated with the event.** The equipment should be secured to prevent tampering. Retain and preserve any disposable products that may have been involved, including packaging. Do not test or tamper with any equipment or apparatus.

D. **Special precautions for equipment-related incidents**

1. The manufacturer should be notified and consideration should be given regarding notification of the Food and Drug Administration through its Product Problem Reporting System (1-800-638-6725).

2. If there has been a serious injury, an independent, qualified examiner should perform an equipment inspection, under the auspice of the hospital insurance company.

Suggested Reading

American Society of Anesthesiologists. *Patient Safety Program.* Video Cassette Program, Vol. 1–6. Evanston, Ill., 1985.

Cooper, J. B., Newbower, R. S., and Kitz, R. J. An analysis of major errors and equipment in anesthesia management: Considerations for prevention and detection. *Anesthesiology* 60:34, 1984.

Pierce, E. C., and Cooper, J. B. Analysis of anesthetic mishaps. *Int. Anesthesiol. Clin.* 22(2):190, 1984.

Patient Safety Manual (2nd ed.). Chicago: American College of Surgeons, 1985.

Duberman, S. *Quality Assurance in the Practice of Anesthesiology.* Park Ridge, Ill.: American Society of Anesthesiologists, 1986.

10

Administration of General Anesthesia

Randall S. Hickle

General anesthesia consists in three essential characteristics: **amnesia (or unconsciousness), analgesia,** and **lack of movement.** Inducing, maintaining, and reversing general anesthesia may be accomplished in many, equally acceptable ways. Modifications for specific patient populations, disease states, and emergencies are described in later chapters.

I. **Preoperative preparations.** The anesthesiologist is responsible for a patient from the time the sedating preoperative medication is administered, or, for an unstable patient, from the time the patient leaves his or her nursing unit. Provision should be made to accompany patients with an unstable hemodynamic or respiratory status. Once in the OR holding area, each patient should be reassessed with respect to

  A. **Level of anxiety,** which may increase with even "routine" procedures (e.g., IV catheter placement). Apprehension may be treated effectively by both verbal and nonverbal support; a calm voice and assured manner may be as effective as a bolus of diazepam. Loud discussions about difficult airways, malfunctioning machines, missing instruments, or staff fatigue should be minimized.

  For some patients, further premedication may also be needed. For this purpose, a benzodiazepine (e.g., diazepam in increments of 1–5 mg IV for adults or midazolam in 0.5–1.0 mg IV increments) may be used.

  B. **Effect of sedating premedication.** Occasionally, excessive central nervous system (CNS), cardiovascular, and respiratory depression may result from preoperative sedation. The time of administration should also be confirmed; mis-timing may explain (an apparent) lack of response.

  C. **Preoperative problem list.** The chart should be reviewed for data not available during the preoperative interview (e.g., laboratory studies, consultant notes) and interim changes in condition (e.g., angina during the night). It should be confirmed that antacids, antibiotics, or antianginal and other chronic medications have been administered when indicated.

  D. **NPO status.** Patients should be asked explicitly when they last ate. Elective cases are usually postponed if preoperative NPO orders have been violated. In emergency cases, when the stomach may be "full," either "rapid sequence" induction or an awake intubation is indicated (see Sec. **II.D.2**).

  E. **Intravascular volume.** Most general anesthetics are systemic vasodilators, and some depress myocardial contractility. This combination of effects can lead to marked hypotension, particularly when fluid deficits have not been replaced. Common causes for preoperative hypovolemia (see also Chap. 17) include protracted NPO status, hemorrhage, fever, vomiting, diuretic use, and surgical bowel preparations. Hypovolemia should be strongly suspected if hypotension and tachycardia result from tilting the OR table to a head-up position prior to induction.

F. Personal possessions. Eyeglasses, contact lenses, and hearing aids may sometimes accompany the patient to the OR; prior to induction they should be removed and safely stored. The oral cavity should be checked to confirm that **false teeth** and other dental appliances have been removed.

II. Induction

A. Monitoring. See Chap. 8.

B. Positioning. For induction, patients are usually placed supine, with all their extremities resting on padded surfaces in neutral anatomic position. Occasionally, placement into a position appropriate for surgery may occur prior to induction; for example, a severely arthritic patient requiring surgery in lithotomy position. Positioning should be systematically reevaluated at intervals throughout the procedure since the presence of unyielding metal against body parts is one of the more frequent, and preventable, causes of patient injury.

C. Medications

1. Induction may be accomplished by the IV, IM, rectal, or respiratory routes. Induction agents all produce dose-dependent CNS depression as outlined in Table 10-1. The most commonly used induction agents are **ultrashort-acting barbiturates** (usually administered IV to adults and either IV or rectally in children). Other IV induction agents that are used in specific contexts include **ketamine, etomidate,** and **benzodiazepines. Potent inhalation agents** can be used for induction by mask: "single-breath induction," voluntary inhalation induction, and "steal" inductions are discussed in Chap. 23.

2. Certain drugs (e.g., IV narcotics or lidocaine 1.0–1.5 mg/kg IV) may be used as adjuvants to induction agents in order to attenuate reflexes following airway stimulation. Such agents also make it possible to induce unconsciousness with lower doses of IV hypnotics and may be particularly useful in hypertensive or asthmatic patients.

D. Airway management

1. **Mask ventilation.** With unconsciousness, airway reflexes (e.g., cough, gag) are obtunded, and the posterior pharyngeal muscles relax. Upper airway obstruction may be diagnosed by the presence of "paradoxical" or "rocking" chest wall motions during inspiration (i.e., the abdomen rises while the thorax moves inward); a tugging motion on the tra-

Table 10-1. The stages of general anesthesia

The "stages" or planes of anesthesia were defined by Guedel after careful observation of patient responses during induction with diethyl ether. Induction with modern anesthetic agents is sufficiently rapid that these descriptions of individual stages are often not applicable or appreciated. However, modification of these categories still provides useful terminology to describe progression from the awake to the anesthetized state.

Stage I: Amnesia	This period begins with induction of anesthesia and continues to loss of consciousness. The threshold of pain perception is not lowered during stage I.
Stage II: Delirium	This period is characterized by uninhibited excitation and potentially injurious responses to noxious stimuli, including vomiting, laryngospasm, hypertension, tachycardia, and uncontrolled movement. The pupils are often dilated, gaze may be divergent, respiration is frequently irregular, and breath holding is common. Desirable induction drugs accelerate transition through this stage.
Stage III: Surgical anesthesia	In this target depth for anesthesia, the gaze is central, pupils are constricted, and respirations are regular. Anesthesia is considered sufficient when painful stimulation does not elicit somatic reflexes or deleterious autonomic responses (e.g., hypertension, tachycardia).
Stage IV: Overdosage	Commonly referred to as "too deep," this stage is marked by shallow or absent respirations, dilated and nonreactive pupils, and hypotension that may progress to circulatory failure. Anesthesia should be lightened immediately.

chea during labored breathing also indicates obstruction. Shallow breathing or apnea may also occur.

a. Specific maneuvers to support the airway include neck extension at the atlanto-occipital joint, forward thrust on the angle of the mandible, and placement of an oral or nasal airway.

b. Unobstructed spontaneous ventilation is confirmed by appropriate movement of the reservoir bag (provided there is a tight mask fit), by the presence of breath sounds through a precordial stethoscope, and by the absence of "snoring" or other upper airway sounds associated with obstruction.

c. Positive-pressure ventilation may also be applied by mask. Care must be exercised to prevent inflating the stomach; usually <u>inspiratory pressures less than 20 cm H_2O are safe.</u>

d. Mask fit is often a problem in edentulous or bearded patients; it may be improved by the use of a rubber head strap.

e. **Laryngospasm** is airway obstruction secondary to tonic contraction of the laryngeal and pharyngeal muscles. It may be caused by respiratory efforts against a partially obstructed airway or occurrence of a noxious stimulus before a sufficiently deep plane of anesthesia has been achieved. It may be <u>treated by continuous positive airway pressure with 100% oxygen.</u> <u>Thiopental</u> or other rapidly acting IV agents may also be used to deepen the plane of anesthesia while minimizing other stimulation. <u>Small doses of succinylcholine IV (10–20 mg) may be needed</u> if the preceding measures do not work (see Chap. 28).

f. **The anesthesiologist's routine use of gloves is highly recommended during all airway manipulations.** Exposure to hepatitis, herpes, acquired immunodeficiency syndrome (AIDS), and other infectious diseases carried in saliva and blood may be minimized by this precaution (see Chap. 7).

2. **Endotracheal intubation**

a. "Mask anesthesia" (e.g., without endotracheal intubation) is often used for relatively short, uncomplicated, peripheral procedures. "Endotracheal anesthesia" is indicated when surgery involves a major body cavity or when there is a risk of aspiration. Other indications include difficult mask airway, need for intraoperative or postoperative mechanical ventilation, awkward positioning, and surgery on the head or neck.

b. **Neuromuscular blocking agents** are used to facilitate endotracheal intubation, but only after the ability to ventilate with positive pressure by mask has been unequivocally established (see **II.D.2.j** for an exception to this principle). The choice of relaxant for endotracheal intubation is discussed in Chap. 11.

   c. In lighter planes of anesthesia, airway reflexes are heightened rather than depressed. Before attempting endotracheal intubation, an adequate depth of anesthesia should be achieved.

   d. The method for **direct laryngoscopy** is illustrated in Fig. 10-1.

     (1) **Elevate the occiput** with 2–4 inches of firm padding to eliminate the angle between the pharynx and larynx (Figs. 10-1A and 10-1B).

     (2) **Extend the neck** at the atlanto-occipital joint; the head is now in the **"sniffing" position** (Fig. 10-1C). Patients with cervical rheumatoid or osteoarthritis or prior cervical trauma may be vulnerable to injury from this maneuver; however, it generally is safe to move the neck to the extent tolerated by a patient when awake. Considerations for intubating trauma victims may be found in Chap. 27.

     (3) **Open the mouth widely** to the point of temporomandibular joint subluxation. The thumb and index finger of the right hand, which separate the teeth, are placed in the right corner of the mouth, where they will not interfere with insertion of the laryngoscope blade by the left hand.

     (4) **Insert the laryngoscope blade** along the **right side** of the tongue; the lips should not be pinched between the blade and teeth. The blade is then advanced toward the midline, sweeping the tongue to the upper left corner of the mouth, until the epiglottis comes into view. The tongue and pharyngeal soft tissues are then lifted to expose the glottic opening. (If the blade is initially placed in the midline, the tongue may fall to either side, obscuring vision and obstructing the path of the endotracheal tube). The laryngoscope should be used to lift in the direction of the arrow in Fig. 10-1C, rather than as a lever (arrow in Fig. 10-1D), to prevent damaging the maxillary incisors or gingiva.

   e. There are two commonly used **laryngoscope blades,** curved and straight.

     (1) **Curved blade** (e.g., Macintosh #3 for the average adult). The tip of this blade is placed in the vallecula, so that lifting upward indirectly lifts the epiglottis and exposes the glottis (Fig. 10-1D).

     (2) **Straight blade** (e.g., Miller #2 or #3 for

the average adult). The method of insertion is the same, but the epiglottis is lifted directly with the tip of the blade (Fig. 10-1C) to expose the glottis.

f. If the vocal cords cannot be visualized by this method, application of pressure on the thyroid cartilage by an assistant may help. If only the posterior glottis is visible, the tube may be **gently** advanced anterior to the arytenoid cartilage (Fig. 10-1E) and, if there is no resistance, into the trachea.

g. Positioning of the endotracheal tube

(1) The tube is advanced through the oral cavity from the right corner of the mouth and then past the vocal cords. The tube should not be guided alongside the flange of the blade; doing so will obstruct vision and obscure the glottis.

(2) The proximal edge of the endotracheal tube cuff is placed just below the vocal cords, and the marking on the tube is noted in relation to the patient's incisors.

(3) The cuff is inflated just to the point of obtaining a seal in the presence of 20–30 cm H_2O positive pressure ventilation. Later, the cuff pressure is rechecked; overdistention from initial overinflation or nitrous oxide (N_2O) diffusion into the cuff can damage the tracheal mucosa (see Chap. 32).

(4) Tube position is confirmed by auscultation over both lung fields and the stomach. Listening for breath sounds high in each axilla will usually avoid being misled by breath sounds transmitted from the opposite lung or stomach.

Capnometry will confirm endotracheal placement by the presence of metabolic carbon dioxide (CO_2); esophageal tube placement is indicated by an end-tidal CO_2 reading of zero.

(5) The tube is taped securely in place. The position of the markings on the tube should be unchanged and an oral airway or bite block inserted to prevent occlusion of the tube should the patient "lighten" during anesthesia. Breath sounds are then rechecked after taping.

h. Patient factors that increase the difficulty of endotracheal intubation include a short neck, large tongue, small mouth, limited neck extension, receding mandible, altered airway anatomy (from burn injury or trauma), or large and protruding incisors.

(1) If a **difficult intubation** is anticipated, H_2-antagonists and possibly metoclo-

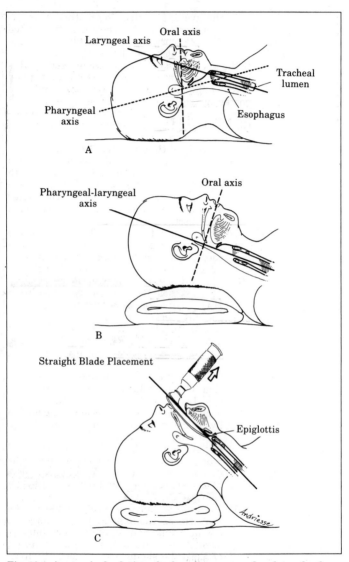

Fig. 10-1. Anatomical relations for laryngoscopy and endotracheal intubation.

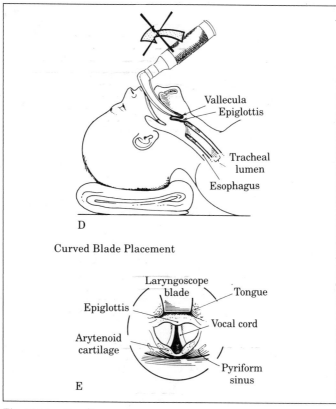

D

Curved Blade Placement

E

Fig. 10-1 (continued)

pramide should be started 12 hours before induction to decrease the acidity and volume of gastric secretions; nonparticulate antacids (e.g., sodium bicitrate) may be used 30 minutes before induction. Administration of atropine or glycopyrrolate at this time will decrease the secretions resulting from airway stimulation, but is usually not required.

(2) Extra equipment may prove helpful: a variety of smaller than predicted endotracheal tubes, an assortment of laryngoscope blades, a tube stylet, nasal airways, Magill forceps, and possibly, a fiberoptic laryngoscope.

(3) **Preoxygenation** is prudent when difficulty is anticipated, since hypoxemia can occur during prolonged laryngoscopy. Maintenance of spontaneous ventilation

may sometimes facilitate intubation, but with rare exceptions, <u>no relaxants should be administered until the ability to ventilate has been established</u>. It is helpful to have an assistant available who is familiar with airway management and equipment.

i. If intubation is not accomplished on the first try, but the patient is not at risk for aspiration, calm preparation should be made for a second attempt. Oxygenation, maintenance of adequate anesthesia and laryngeal relaxation, and hemodynamic stability must, however, be ensured before further intubation attempts are made. If regurgitation and aspiration are considered to be added risks, cricoid pressure (see Sec. **j.(2)(e)**) should, in addition, be maintained. On subsequent attempts, one or more elements of the first laryngoscopy **should be changed:**

(1) The occiput may be elevated further, or an assistant may apply pressure to the larynx, or the mouth may be opened wider.

(2) The plane of anesthesia may be deepened.

(3) The laryngoscope blade may be changed or a stylet introduced into the endotracheal tube.

(4) A more experienced laryngoscopist may be called.

(5) Fiberoptic laryngoscopy may be attempted, provided the patient is breathing spontaneously (see Sec. **k. (6)**).

(6) If all of the above fail, the patient may need to be awakened and preparations made for awake intubation; perhaps by fiberoptic laryngoscopy. Alternatively, anesthesia may be continued by mask but at the risk of having an unintubatable patient should a crisis arise.

(7) If the ability to ventilate is lost, a tracheostomy may be necessary. Fortunately, such emergency interventions are rarely necessary. A valuable temporizing move is **transtracheal oxygenation.** A 14-gauge IV catheter is inserted percutaneously through the cricothyroid membrane, the needle removed, and the catheter then connected to a 3-ml plastic syringe (without the plunger). A 15-mm universal endotracheal tube adapter pushed into the barrel of the syringe allows the breathing circuit to be connected.

j. **"Rapid sequence" induction**

(1) **Indications.** Pulmonary aspiration of as little as 20 ml of gastric fluid at pH 2, may

produce a potentially lethal chemical pneumonitis. Patients who are at risk for aspiration (e.g., history of recent meal, significant esophageal reflux, pregnancy, ileus or bowel obstruction, nausea/vomiting, extreme anxiety, or trauma) are candidates for intubation by this method.

(2) Method

(a) Nonparticulate antacids (sodium bicitrate), H_2-antagonists (cimetidine or ranitidine), or gastrokinetics (metoclopramide) may be used preoperatively to decrease the acidity and volume of gastric secretions. If the stomach is dilated, decompression with a nasogastric tube is advisable.

(b) Equipment is similar to that for any intubation but commonly includes a cuffed endotracheal tube one size smaller than usual, with stylet and cuff-inflation syringe in place. There should also be an assortment of laryngoscope blades, an extra laryngoscope handle, and a strong suction.

(c) Preoxygenation should be long enough to wash out nitrogen (N_2) and wash in oxygen (O_2) (i.e., 3 minutes, or at least seven vital capacity breaths).

(d) Induction is accomplished with thiopental (2–7 mg/kg), but a test dose is not given. Ketamine (1–3 mg/kg) may be indicated instead of thiopental (see sec. **V.A.2**).

(e) Cricoid pressure (known as the Sellick maneuver) is applied as the patient loses consciousness. When the neck is extended, firm pressure on the cricoid cartilage compresses the esophagus against the cervical vertebrae. This maneuver will prevent passive reflux of fluid into the oropharynx during intubation. The technique is *not* intended to obstruct the esophagus should active vomiting occur during induction; in this case pressure must be released and other maneuvers used to secure and protect the airway. Cricoid pressure should be maintained by an assistant until the endotracheal tube cuff is inflated and breath sounds are heard bilaterally.

(f) Paralysis is provided by succinylcholine (1 mg/kg) given *immediately* after the thiopental. *There is no attempt to ventilate the patient at any time by mask.* Intubation can usually be performed within 30–60 seconds. A "defasciculating" dose of curare (3 mg IV for adults) or pancuronium (0.5 mg) may be given just prior to induction to minimize the increase in abdominal pressure caused by succinylcholine-induced fasciculations, but may, at the same time, delay the onset of neuromuscular blockade. If "precurarization" is used, the intubating dose of succinylcholine is 1.5 mg/kg. Contraindications to the use of succinylcholine and appropriate substitutions may be found in Chaps. 11 and 27.

(g) **Intubation** should be performed as soon as succinylcholine has produced jaw relaxation. The styletted tube is used on the first attempt. The endotracheal tube cuff is inflated with 5–10 ml of air and the position confirmed by auscultation *before* cricoid pressure is released (making sure that there is no leak at 30 cm H_2O peak inspiratory pressure).

(h) If the first attempt fails, cricoid pressure should be maintained continuously during all subsequent intubation maneuvers, while mask ventilation with 100% O_2 is administered.

(i) At the end of anesthesia, **extubation** should not take place before a nasogastric tube has been passed to empty the stomach (see sec. **IV.B** for a discussion of the criteria for extubation).

(3) A rapid sequence induction involves added risk, since the patient receives a relaxant **before** the ability to ventilate has been established (see sec. **II.D.2.b**). When difficult intubation is known or suspected, an awake intubation is a safer approach.

k. "Awake" intubations

(1) **Indications**

(a) Difficult intubation anticipated in a patient at risk for aspiration.

(b) Uncertainty about the ability to intubate or ventilate after induction of general anesthesia (e.g., after trauma or for surgery on the mandible or maxilla).

      (c) Need to assess neurologic function after intubation or positioning for surgery (e.g., a patient with an unstable cervical spinal column).

(2) **IV sedation** should not cause obtundation or airway obstruction, since it is essential that patients maintain adequate spontaneous respiration.

(3) **Local anesthesia** by superior laryngeal nerve block and oral spray or transtracheal injection should also be provided to blunt gag and cough reflexes. Patients with "full stomachs," however, are usually lightly sedated, and topical anesthesia is not applied to the trachea until a cuffed endotracheal tube is in place to protect from aspiration. (These criteria are not absolutely rigid; for example, a patient with a full stomach and severe coronary artery disease may require somewhat more sedation and topical anesthesia.)

(4) **Awake intubation by direct laryngoscopy**

      (a) Awake intubation under direct vision may be oral or nasal. The nasal route is usually avoided if there has been recent nasal surgery, sinusitis, coagulopathy, anticoagulation, or basilar skull fracture.

      (b) Local anesthesia and sedation are provided as in **(2)** and **(3).** For nasal tube placement, application of swabs soaked in either 4% cocaine or 4 ml of 4% lidocaine mixed with 5 mg of phenylephrine will provide both topical anesthesia and vasoconstriction of the nasal mucosa. The larger of the two nares is chosen after patency is confirmed.

      (c) **For nasal intubations,** the endotracheal tube must pass through the bony choana of the posterior naris without producing epistaxis. A 6–7-mm tube is appropriate for most adults. Patients are initially placed in "sniffing" position, with firm padding under the occiput and full neck extension (see Fig. 10-1C). The tube is lubricated, then advanced gently but firmly through the nasal opening, directly perpendicular to the plane of the face. Oxygen may be administered by mask or by a connection to the end of the tube. The tube is then slowly advanced until resistance suddenly decreases, just past the nasal turbinates. If very firm resistance is met, a smaller tube or other nostril may be tried.

(d) Laryngoscopy is performed after coating the blade with viscous lidocaine (2%), taking care to avoid sensitive midline structures like the uvula. Additional anesthetic spray may be needed to prevent coughing and gagging. The endotracheal tube is advanced to the vocal cords under direct vision. If necessary, a Magill forceps can be used to guide the tip of the tube through the cords, taking care not to damage the tube cuff. A 180-degree rotation is sometimes needed to advance the tube into the trachea. If intubation cannot be accomplished nasally, the tube may be removed and an awake oral intubation performed.

(5) Awake "blind" nasal intubation

(a) **Indications.** This technique is particularly useful in <u>patients with severe trismus</u> or in other circumstances that preclude direct laryngoscopy. (Blind nasotracheal intubations can also be performed in the spontaneously ventilating, anesthetized patient). However, <u>blind intubations should not be attempted in patients with airway tumors or abscesses or following trauma to the nasopharynx, oropharynx, or larynx.</u>

(b) Techniques for IV sedation, topical anesthesia, patient positioning, as well as contraindications to nasal intubation, were discussed in sec. **II.D.2.k.(4).**

(c) The tube is advanced past the nasal turbinates during inspiration until the tip is just above the larynx. (Air movement through the tube can be felt during exhalation, clear plastic tubes will also show condensation, but phonation is still possible). At this point, touching the larynx may elicit a cough. Intubation is accomplished by asking the patient to take a deep breath and quickly advancing the tube 3–5 cm.

(d) During tube advancement, the patient's neck superficial to the larynx should be palpated to appreciate anterior or lateral deviation of the tube. If the tube tip is "felt" anteriorly, neck flexion may correct the problem; lateral adjustments are made by rotating the tube in the nostril. In some cases, the tube may enter a pyriform sinus (see Fig. 10-1E); gentle compression lateral to the hyoid bone will collapse this space and allow the tube to pass into the trachea.

(e) If phonation still occurs, the tube has not entered the glottis but has probably entered the esophagus. This may be prevented on subsequent attempts by exaggerating the sniffing position or applying pressure to the larynx.

(f) After successful intubation, the cuff is inflated, breath sounds are checked, and induction of anesthesia is begun.

(6) Fiberoptic laryngoscopy

(a) Endotracheal intubation, either by nasal or oral route, can be facilitated by the use of a fiberoptic laryngoscope or bronchoscope. Use of this device may be indicated in patients with cervical spine, facial, or upper airway trauma or with congenital deformities that make simpler forms of intubation difficult. When possible, fiberoptic laryngoscopy should be used prior to "blind" techniques or repeated direct laryngoscopy, since airway secretions and bleeding make glottic visualization much more difficult.

(b) After a nasotracheal tube has been inserted through a nasal opening into the pharynx, the flexible tip of the scope is advanced through the tube, beyond the epiglottis and vocal cords, and into the trachea. The endotracheal tube is then advanced over the scope into the trachea, and the scope is withdrawn.

(c) Even in experienced hands, intubation by fiberoptic laryngoscopy may proceed slowly and therefore should be used only in spontaneously breathing (awake or anesthetized) patients. For this same reason, fiberoptic laryngoscopy is not a substitute for emergency tracheostomy or cricothyroidotomy.

III. Maintenance of general anesthesia
A. General considerations
1. Surgical stimulation varies in intensity from moment to moment, so even a constant blood level of a volatile or IV agent will not necessarily produce a stable depth of anesthesia. The depth of anesthesia must be continually reassessed by gauging the patient's response to each surgical stimulus and subsequent anesthetic administration.
2. Responses to pain may be **somatic** (movement, coughing, breath-holding, grimacing) or **autonomic** (tachycardia, hypertension, mydriasis, sweating, tearing). Both somatic and autonomic responses may be influenced by factors other than pain. For example, when muscle relaxants are employed, somatic manifestations of pain are largely abolished. Autonomic responses may arise from hypoxia, hypercarbia, or hypovolemia, as well as from pain. Clearly, interpreting the level of anesthesia requires integration of many clinical observations; responding appropriately requires judgment and experience.
B. Methods. Once general anesthesia has been induced, it can be maintained by a number of alternative methods.
1. With a pure **inhalational technique,** autonomic or somatic responses are treated by adjusting the inspired concentration. A falling heart rate and blood pressure are generally reliable indicators of increasing depth under halothane or enflurane anesthesia; however, isoflurane or enflurane may increase heart rate even in surgical planes of anesthesia. The rate and depth of respirations are useful guides in spontaneously breathing patients, because rate increases and tidal volume decreases in a dose-related manner over the clinical range. Pupil size is less useful, because modern anesthetics lack the consistent pupillary responses seen with diethyl ether (see Table 10-1).
2. With **N$_2$O-narcotic-relaxant** or **"balanced"** anesthesia, specific drugs are used to provide the separate components of general anesthesia (i.e., amnesia, analgesia, lack of movement).
   a. This technique is frequently chosen for patients with depressed or uncertain cardiovascular status, although it is also a perfectly reasonable choice for healthy individuals.
   b. It is the technique of choice for patients susceptible to malignant hyperthermia.
   c. Awareness during surgery is of particular concern with N$_2$O-narcotic-relaxant technique. Unfortunately, there are no absolutely reliable clinical signs to ensure that amnesia (or unconsciousness) has been produced. Narcotic analgesics do not reliably produce unconsciousness unless administered in extremely high doses

  (2) Cardiovascular system. The barbiturates produce vasodilatation and direct myocardial depression. The magnitude of the hemodynamic alteration depends on underlying myocardial function and intravascular volume, and it may be minimized by slowing the rate of administration.

 b. Dosage. The usual IV induction dose of thiopental is between 2 and 7 mg/kg.

  (1) Low doses are appropriate for patients who have received other CNS depressants or when it is desirable to maintain spontaneous ventilation during induction (e.g., blind nasal intubation). A low dose is also appropriate when there is any question of hemodynamic instability or hypovolemia.

  (2) Higher doses are used in young, healthy patients, in patients who are tolerant of barbiturates or alcohol, during rapid sequence inductions when hypovolemia is not present, and in extremely anxious or agitated patients.

 c. Pharmacokinetics. The rapid onset and short duration of the ultrashort-acting barbiturates are a consequence of their physiochemical properties; they are extremely fat soluble and are distributed into brain and other highly perfused (blood vessel–rich) organs within 30 seconds. Redistribution into muscle and skin rapidly follows, which causes a fall in plasma and brain concentrations. The **redistribution half-life** ($t_{1/2\alpha}$), which is the time it takes for the peak blood concentration to decrease by 50%, is approximately 3 minutes for thiopental, thiamylal, and methohexital. Therefore, additional doses may be required for "prolonged" (> 5 minutes) induction periods. There is little clinically apparent difference in onset and duration of these drugs, although the **elimination half-life** ($t_{1/2\beta}$) for thiopental is greater than 10–12 hours versus 1.5–5 hours for methohexital. The barbiturates are biotransformed in the liver to inactive metabolites.

 d. Adverse effects

  (1) Allergy. Anaphylactic responses to barbiturates do occur but are rare; manifestations include bronchospasm or cardiovascular collapse and should be treated with epinephrine (0.3–1.0 mg IV). Somewhat more common are reactions ranging from local urticaria to generalized skin flushing and tachycardia; treatment for these reactions usually consists of diphenhydramine (50 mg IV for adults).

  (2) Local tissue damage may be caused by extravascular infiltration of thiopental, which is <u>strongly alkaline (pH 11)</u>; intraarterial injection can cause frank tissue necrosis. The use of relatively dilute (2.5%) solutions minimizes the potential for damage.

(3) The use of <u>methohexital</u> is associated with a <u>higher incidence of **hiccoughs**</u> and <u>**myoclonic muscle movements**</u> than thiopental or thiamylal.

e. **Absolute contraindications** to barbiturate administration include

(1) Previous history of anaphylaxis to a barbiturate.

(2) Inability to support ventilation or secure the airway.

(3) Acute intermittent porphyria (AIP), a congenital defect in hemoglobin production resulting in increased production of porphyrin. Life-threatening episodes of AIP can be triggered by barbiturates. Symptoms include onset of abdominal pain, hemoglobinuria, paralysis, and psychiatric disturbances shortly after IV barbiturate administration.

2. **Ketamine**

a. **Pharmacodynamics**

(1) **Central nervous system.** Ketamine is a phencyclidine derivative that produces a "dissociative" state characterized by mental disconnection from the environment and profound analgesia. High doses administered IV rapidly result in unconsciousness, increased muscle tone, and exaggerated, uncoordinated eye movements. Ketamine is less likely to produce apnea than thiopental, and upper airway tone is frequently maintained. However, airway reflexes are not normal, so aspiration may occur. <u>Ketamine alone is usually insufficient for visceral surgery</u>, but it is widely used for short, painful procedures such as dressing changes. Ketamine is also useful for inductions in children or uncooperative patients who do not have IVs, since it may be administered intramuscularly. Its other pharmacodynamic properties (see sec. **a. (2)**) make it useful in other specific settings as well.

(2) **Cardiovascular system.** <u>Heart rate and blood pressure</u> usually <u>increase</u> because of <u>sympathetic nervous system activation</u>. Ketamine may have **less of a hypotensive effect** than other induction agents, so it is often chosen for emergency inductions in hypovolemic patients (e.g.,

trauma cases or obstetrical emergencies) and elective inductions of children with congenital heart disease. Ketamine (and its metabolites) are direct myocardial depressants, so hypotension may still occur in patients who have exhausted all sympathetic reserves.

(3) **Respiratory system.** Because ketamine is a potent bronchodilator, it is a reasonable choice for induction of symptomatic asthmatic patients.

b. **Dosage.** Anesthesia is produced by 1–3 mg/kg IV or 5–10 mg/kg IM. The **onset** of unconsciousness is about 1 minute after an IV dose and 5–8 minutes after an IM dose.

c. **Pharmacokinetics.** Ketamine is rapidly redistributed ($t_{1/2\alpha}$ = 10 minutes), which terminates the action of a single IV dose in 5–15 minutes. The $t_{1/2\beta}$ is 3 hours, and elimination is primarily by hepatic biotransformation.

d. **Adverse effects and contraindications**

(1) Nightmares, hallucinations, and emergence delirium may occur in up to 30% of patients who receive ketamine. Concomitant use of benzodiazepines decreases this incidence, but it is prudent to avoid the use of ketamine in the presence of a psychiatric disorder.

(2) Because it increases blood pressure and myocardial O_2 consumption, ketamine should be used with caution in patients with coronary artery disease or vascular aneurysms. Ketamine increases cerebral blood flow, so its use is contraindicated in patients with intracranial hypertension.

(3) There is a marked stimulation of oral secretions with ketamine, so pretreatment with an antisialagogue is recommended when endotracheal intubation is not planned. Atropine use, however, increases the risk of emergence delirium.

(4) Ketamine is rarely used in ophthalmologic procedures because it can cause diplopia, exaggerated eye movements, blepharospasm, and nystagmus. Myoclonic movements and phonation during induction with ketamine are also relatively common.

3. **Etomidate**

a. **Pharmacodynamics.** Etomidate is an ultrashort-acting benzylimidazole that rapidly produces unconsciousness but little analgesia. It causes minimal cardiovascular depression and (like thiopental) reduces cerebral blood flow and intracranial pressure.

    b. Dosage. The usual IV induction dose is 0.3–0.4 mg/kg.

    c. Pharmacokinetics. The **onset** is rapid (30–60 seconds), and **duration** is determined by rate of redistribution to well-perfused tissues (generally 3–5 minutes). Etomidate is rapidly biotransformed in the liver.

    d. Adverse effects and contraindications.

       (1) Minor but annoying side effects, including pain on IV injection and vomiting on emergence, are relatively frequent. Myoclonic muscle movement occurs in up to 50% of patients; this effect is reduced by premedication with benzodiazepines or narcotics.

       (2) Etomidate inhibits two steps in adrenal steroid biosynthesis; inhibition of adrenocorticotropic hormone (ACTH) response is measurable after a single dose, although this has not been shown to be the cause of perioperative complications. However, adrenal insufficiency may have contributed to increased mortality following continuous IV infusions of etomidate for long-term sedation in an intensive care unit.

4. Benzodiazepines include diazepam and midazolam.

    a. Pharmacodynamics

       (1) Central nervous system. The benzodiazepines are more often used for their anxiolytic and sedative effects than to produce hypnosis. Higher doses may be used to induce anesthesia, but the onset is usually not as rapid as with barbiturates or ketamine. Other centrally mediated actions include skeletal muscle relaxation, anterograde amnesia, and anticonvulsant effects.

       (2) Cardiovascular system. The benzodiazepines produce minimal reductions in cardiac output and blood pressure. Large doses may decrease systemic vascular resistance, especially when given together with an opioid.

       (3) Respiratory system. Low doses of midazolam or diazepam may slightly reduce tidal volume and respiratory rate. However, respiratory depression, particularly after large IV doses, occurs in patients with chronic obstructive pulmonary disease, in older, debilitated individuals, and (rarely) even in healthy people.

    b. Dosage

       (1) The induction dose of **midazolam** follow-

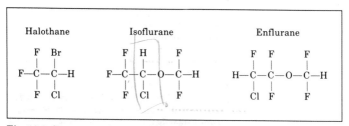

Fig. 10-2. Structure of three potent inhalation anesthetics.

dium to the arrhythmogenic effects of catecholamines, which is of particular concern when epinephrine-containing local anesthetic solutions are used for infiltration or when sympathomimetic agents (e.g., pressors or bronchodilators) are administered. With halothane, subcutaneous infiltration with epinephrine should not exceed 2 μg/kg/20 min in adults. Isoflurane is less of a myocardial depressant but a more potent vasodilator than the other potent agents. Overall, it tends not to reduce blood pressure as much, but the heart rate may increase dramatically.

(3) **Respiratory system.** Halothane, enflurane, and isoflurane cause dose-related respiratory depression, which is exacerbated by concurrent administration of narcotics and benzodiazepines. Respiratory depression stems from direct effects on the medullary respiratory centers, as well as on the thoracic respiratory muscles and diaphragm. In surgical planes of anesthesia, intercostal muscle movement is diminished, respiratory rate is increased, and tidal volume is decreased. All three agents cause marked bronchodilation and depression of airway reflexes. However, these agents are also airway irritants (isoflurane > enflurane > halothane) and during light levels of anesthesia may precipitate laryngospasm or bronchospasm, particularly in heavy smokers and asthmatics.

(4) **Hepatic effects.** Postoperative liver enzyme elevations are often attributed to "halothane hepatitis," although this is a diagnosis of exclusion and other possible causes must be ruled out (for a full discussion, see Chap. 5).

(5) **Effects on muscle.** The potent inhalational agents directly relax skeletal muscle, which reduces the doses of nondepolarizing muscle relaxants required. All inhalational anesthetics may trigger malignant hyperthermia in susceptible individuals (see Chap. 28).

(6) **Renal effects.** The volatile anesthetics reduce systemic arterial pressure and correspondingly lower renal blood flow and glomerular filtration rate (GFR). These effects are normally of little clinical consequence. Methoxyflurane (MOF), another inhalational agent, has largely been abandoned because it produced polyuric renal failure. The nephrotoxin was actually fluoride ion (F^-), a product of MOF metabolism. Enflurane is also metabolized to inorganic fluoride in small amounts, but even prolonged enflurane anesthesia has not been linked conclusively to postoperative renal dysfunction in normal patients.

b. **Pharmacokinetics.** Although mostly eliminated unchanged through the lungs, the potent inhalational agents are also metabolized to a varying extent, primarily by hepatic mixed-function oxidases. About 20% of **halothane** molecules are degraded to trifluoroacetic acid (the major metabolite, which is eliminated in the urine), and trace amounts of Br^-, Cl^-, and F^-. About 2% of **enflurane** undergoes biotransformation into F^- and nonvolatile fluorinated metabolites. **Isoflurane** is metabolized least (only 0.2%), producing F^- and trifluoroacetic acid.

C. **Narcotic (opioid) analgesics** share the ability to interact with opiate receptors and produce a characteristic set of effects. The clinically available agents range from the naturally occurring alkaloid morphine to synthetic compounds like meperidine, fentanyl, and sufentanil. Although they vary widely in potency, the opioids are equally effective for most applications. The choice of one opioid instead of another is usually based on its onset or duration.

1. **Pharmacodynamics**

a. **Central nervous system.** Opioids interfere with the rostral processing of pain information, by acting on the dorsal horn of the spinal cord and inhibitory pathways originating in the brainstem. They also act on higher centers (e.g., limbic cortex) to alter the affective responses to pain. Besides analgesia, all of these compounds produce some degree of sedation, but none reliably produces unconsciousness un-

Table 10-3. Narcotic dosages and pharmacokinetics

Narcotic	Dose A[a]	Dose B[b]	Dose C[c]	Time to peak (min)	$t_{1/2\alpha}$ (min)	$t_{1/2\beta}$ (hr)
Morphine	0.05–0.2 mg/kg	0.2–0.3 mg/kg	1–2 mg/kg	30	9–19	3.0–4.5
Meperidine	0.5–2.0 mg/kg	2–3 mg/kg		15	7–17	3–4
Fentanyl	0.5–2.0 µg/kg	2–8 µg/kg	50–150 µg/kg	5–7	13	4–7
Sufentanil		0.2–0.8 µg/kg	10–30 µg/kg	3–4	10–13	2.5
Alfentanil		10–100 µg/kg[d]		1–2	10–13	1.5

Key: $t_{1/2\alpha}$ = the half-time of redistribution; $t_{1/2\beta}$ = the half-time of elimination.
[a]Typical doses for perioperative analgesia, given in divided IV increments.
[b]Typical initial doses used in the N_2O-narcotic-relaxant technique for a patient who may be extubated within 4 hours.
[c]The dose range for induction of anesthesia (e.g., for cardiac surgery) in patients who will need prolonged postoperative mechanical ventilation.
[d]Doses of 10–20 µg/kg seem suitable for brief outpatient procedures.

less very high doses are administered (Table 10-3).

b. **Respiratory system.** All narcotics produce dose-related depression of respiration; in this regard, none of the pure agonists are safer than any other. When the medullary respiratory centers become less sensitive to $PaCO_2$, respiratory rate slows and minute ventilation decreases; such effects can linger well into the postoperative period. Ventilation may also be impaired due to narcotic-induced muscle rigidity. This centrally mediated increase in muscular tone usually occurs after rapid administration of potent narcotics like fentanyl and sufentanil. Although this effect is reversed by naloxone, rigidity that occurs during induction of anesthesia is more appropriately treated with a muscle relaxant.

c. **Cardiovascular system.** Narcotics by themselves produce little or no direct myocardial depression. Cardiac output, however, does decline with the addition of N_2O or benzodiazepines. All narcotics decrease systemic vascular resistance (SVR) by decreasing medullary sympathetic outflow. For this reason, patients with the highest sympathetic tone (e.g., those with congestive heart failure) tend to undergo the greatest reduction in SVR. Capacitance (venous) beds dilate also, and significant volume may be pooled in the splanchnic vasculature. Morphine and meperidine also decrease SVR by direct release of histamine, an effect that is not produced by fentanyl or its congeners. All narcotics, with the exception of meperidine, produce bradycardia by stimulating the central vagal nuclei; it may be treated (or prevented) with vagolytic agents (e.g., atropine or pancuronium).

d. **Other effects.** The narcotics produce stimulation of smooth muscle throughout the body and may result in constipation, urinary retention, and biliary colic. Nausea and vomiting are produced by stimulation of the medullary chemoreceptor trigger zone. Dopaminergic antagonists like droperidol greatly reduce the likelihood of this particular side effect. Narcotics also constrict the pupils by stimulating the Edinger-Westphal nucleus. Even a small dose of narcotic will cause miosis, so pupil size is not a very useful guide for titrating narcotics intraoperatively.

2. **Pharmacokinetics.** All narcotics are rapidly distributed throughout the body following IV injection, and all have large apparent volumes of distribution. Elimination is primarily by the liver, and the inactive metabolites are excreted in the urine. Ta-

ble 10-3 lists the narcotics that are most widely used during anesthesia. Alfentanil has just recently received FDA approval but has already been widely used in Europe and the U.K. The dosages and durations of narcotics vary substantially for individual patients and different procedures, so those listed should be regarded only as a starting point. Doses are administered IV incrementally, according to patient response.

D. **Narcotic antagonists** can be used to reverse hypoventilation, rigidity, biliary colic, and the other effects of narcotics. The only pure narcotic antagonist available for intravenous use is naloxone.

1. **Pharmacodynamics.** Naloxone is a competitive antagonist at all opiate receptors. It reverses the analgesia, respiratory depression, and all other receptor-mediated effects produced by narcotic agonists. (In narcotic-dependent individuals, naloxone will acutely precipitate a violent withdrawal syndrome). It may have some stimulant properties, but it is not a reliable means of reversing nonnarcotic CNS depression.

2. **Dosage.** The amount of naloxone needed for reversal depends on the total dose of narcotic administered; in most cases, partial reversal is the desired end point. Postoperatively, naloxone should be titrated to a particular effect (e.g., an increase in respiration or wakefulness) by administering incremental IV doses of 0.04 mg or less to adults.

3. **Pharmacokinetics.** The effect of an IV dose of naloxone is rapid; obvious signs of reversal of respiratory and CNS depression occur within 1–2 minutes. Naloxone undergoes secondary redistribution, so brain levels rapidly fall. The duration of reversal is typically 30–60 minutes after IV administration and somewhat longer if given IM. Naloxone crosses the placenta, so that its maternal administration before delivery is an effective way to treat neonatal narcotic-induced depression. Since many narcotics have a longer duration of action than naloxone and opioid depression may reappear, all patients require observation after narcotic reversal.

4. **Adverse effects.** Narcotic reversal following surgery may indirectly produce significant changes in heart rate and blood pressure, associated with abrupt onset of pain. On rare occasions, naloxone has been reported to produce acute pulmonary edema and arrhythmias (ventricular tachycardia, ventricular fibrillation) even in normal, healthy patients. The mechanism for this effect is unknown, but it seems clear that naloxone should be used cautiously in individuals with preexisting cardiac disease. Short-term ventilatory support may be preferable to naloxone use in this group of patients. Other undesirable effects of naloxone are nausea

and vomiting, which may pose added risk during emergence from anesthesia.

Suggested Reading

Clements, J. A., and Nimmo, W. S. Pharmacokinetics and analgesic effects of ketamine in man. *Br. J. Anaesth.* 53:27, 1981.

Eger, E. I. *Anesthetic Uptake and Action.* Baltimore: Williams & Wilkins, 1974.

Giese, J. L., et al. Etomidate versus thiopental for induction of anesthesia. *Anesth. Analg.* 64:871, 1985.

Halothane-associated liver damage. *Lancet* 1:1251, 1986.

Hudson, R. J., Stanski, D. R., and Burch, P. G. Pharmacokinetics of methohexital and thiopental in surgical patients. *Anesthesiology* 59(3):215, 1983.

Jack, M. L., and Colburn, W. A. Pharmacokinetic model for diazepam and its major metabolite desmethyldiazepam following diazepam administration. *J. Pharm. Sci.* 72:1318, 1983.

Johnston, R. R., Eger, E. I., and Wilson, C. A comparative interaction of epinephrine with enflurane, isoflurane, and halothane in man. *Anesth. Analg.* 55:709, 1976.

Roberts, J. T. *Fundamentals of Tracheal Intubation.* New York: Grune & Stratton, 1983.

Rosow, C. E. Newer Synthetic Opioid Analgesics. In G. Smith and B. Covino (eds.), *Acute Pain.* London: Butterworth's, 1985. Pp. 68–83.

Stock, J. G., and Strunin, L. Unexplained hepatitis following halothane. *Anesthesiology* 63:424, 1985.

Yukioka, H. et al. Intravenous lidocaine as a suppressant of coughing during tracheal intubation. *Anesth. Analg.* 64:1189, 1985.

11

Neuromuscular Blockade

Janice Bitetti

I. Neuromuscular transmission

A. The neuromuscular junction is a **synapse.** As a motor nerve approaches the muscle, it divides into many nonmyelinated nerve filaments, each of which innervates a muscle fiber. The motor nerve terminal and the muscle end plate face each other across a narrow synaptic cleft. This cleft divides the junction into presynaptic and postsynaptic areas (Fig. 11-1).

B. The neurotransmitter **acetylcholine** (ACh) is synthesized in the nerve ending by the enzyme choline acetyltransferase (CAT). CAT catalyzes the transfer of an acetate moiety from intracellular acetylcoenzyme A (CoA), to choline, which is derived from extracellular sources. ACh is stored in synaptic vesicles that are clustered in triangular arrays around presynaptic "active zones" (Fig. 11-1). When an action potential invades the nerve terminal, calcium (Ca^{2+}) channels open, and Ca^{2+} fluxes inward, leading to fusion of synaptic vesicles with nerve membrane and release of ACh into the synaptic cleft. ACh is released in uniform amounts, termed *quanta.* Under normal conditions, much more ACh is released than is necessary to depolarize the muscle membrane, and so there is a large safety factor for this process.

C. Fast rates of stimulation require that the nerve increase its stores of releasable ACh, a process known as **mobilization.** Mobilization includes choline transport, synthesis of acetyl CoA, and movement of vesicles to the release site. Under normal conditions, even with tetanic stimulation, nerves are able to mobilize transmitter rapidly enough to replace that which has been released. In the presence of d-tubocurarine (dTC), however, mobilization of transmitter is impaired, and during superphysiologic stimulation (> 50 Hz), ACh output cannot keep pace with demands, and hence the muscle response fades.

D. Released ACh diffuses across the synaptic cleft and interacts with receptors on the muscle end plate, which are located in high density at the crests and shoulders of the junctional folds opposite the release sites. The ACh receptor is well-characterized and contains five membrane-spanning subunits, two of which are structurally identical and are the binding sites for ACh. When both sites are occupied, the ion channel formed by the five subunits opens and allows sodium (Na^+) and Ca^{2+} ions to move inward and potassium (K^+) ions to move outward. The change in the transmembrane potential generated is called the end-plate potential. If enough channels are opened simultaneously, the muscle membrane adjacent to the end plate will become depo-

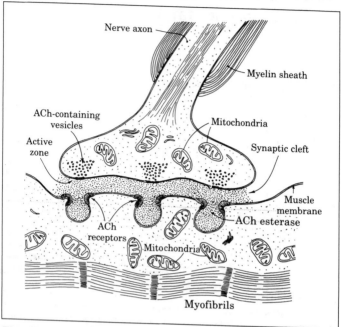

Fig. 11-1. The neuromuscular junction.

larized beyond threshold and an action potential is propagated throughout the muscle fiber. This in turn activates the excitation-contraction coupling mechanism and leads to muscle contraction. The muscle action potential is an all-or-none phenomenon, so the gradations observed in muscle contraction are the result of varying numbers of muscle fibers stimulated. There are many more receptors on the muscle end plate than are necessary to depolarize the adjacent muscle membrane (the "margin of safety"), which explains why most postsynaptic receptors must be blocked by relaxants before there is clinical evidence of neuromuscular blockade.

E. Membrane repolarization is achieved once ACh diffuses away from its receptor and is broken down by the enzyme acetylcholinesterase present in the synapse.

II. Types of neuromuscular blockade. There are classically three types of neuromuscular blockade: depolarizing, nondepolarizing, and phase II.

A. Depolarizing blockade occurs when drugs mimic the action of the neurotransmitter ACh. The archetype is succinylcholine (SCh), which, like ACh, is a quaternary amine. They bind and activate the ACh receptor, which leads to depolarization of the end plate and adjacent muscle membrane. SCh is the most commonly used drug, but since it is not degraded as rapidly as ACh, end-plate depolarization persists and leads to a state of

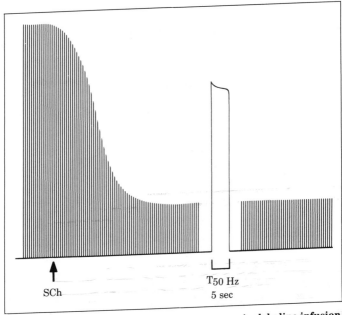

Fig. 11-2. A diagram showing the response to succinylcholine infusion at the arrow. During the beginning of the steady state block, tetanus at 50 Hz showed no fade or posttetanic potentiation.

accommodation or inexcitability of the muscle membrane adjacent to the junctional membrane.

  1. Depolarizing block is **characterized** by
      a. Muscle fasciculation followed by relaxation.
      b. Absence of fade during a tetanic or train-of-four stimulus from a blockade monitor.
      c. Absence of an enhanced twitch following tetanic stimulation ("posttetanic potentiation") (Figs. 11-2 and 11-3).
      d. Potentiation of blockade by anticholinesterases.
      e. Antagonism of blockade by nondepolarizers.
  2. Depolarizing blockade from SCh **ends** when the molecule diffuses from the receptor and is hydrolyzed by plasma cholinesterase, also called pseudocholinesterase, although some molecules may diffuse into the muscle fiber through open channels.
  3. The **clinical pharmacology** of SCh is summarized in Table 11-1.
B. **Nondepolarizing blockade** is classically attributed to a pure, reversible competition between antagonist molecules and ACh for occupancy of the ACh binding site. Thus, binding of the two ACh molecules necessary to open the channel is sterically prevented.

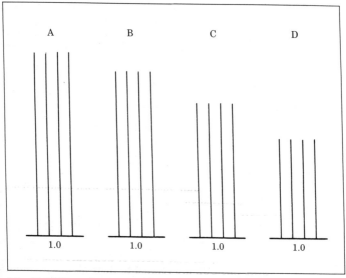

Fig. 11-3. The train-of-four response at *A* prior to the administration of a <u>depolarizing relaxant</u>. Responses *B, C,* and *D* show a decrease in the amplitude of the train-of-four response with <u>no change in the T4 ratio</u> (i.e., no fade).

1. **Other mechanisms** that may also be involved in nondepolarizing blockade include
   a. <u>Steric blockade</u> of the ion channel.
   b. <u>Blockade of the entrance to closed channels.</u>
   c. <u>Binding to another "allosteric" site</u> on the receptor that renders it unresponsive to ACh.
   d. <u>Interference with presynaptic Ca²⁺ influx or ACh mobilization.</u>
2. Nondepolarizing blockade is **characterized** by
   a. <u>Absence of fasciculation</u> prior to onset of blockade.
   b. <u>Fade</u> during tetanic stimulation and during train-of-four.
   c. <u>Posttetanic potentiation</u> (Figs. 11-4 and 11-5).
   d. <u>Antagonism of block by depolarizing agents and anticholinesterases.</u>
   e. <u>Potentiation of block by other nondepolarizing drugs.</u>
3. **Nondepolarizing relaxants** are quaternary ammonium compounds and include two major categories: <u>steroidals</u> (pancuronium and vecuronium) and <u>benzylisoquinolines</u> (dTC, metocurine, and atracurium). Combinations of pancuronium with either dTC or metocurine act synergistically, while combinations of the two related agents, dTC and metocurine, do not. The newest agents, vecu-

ronium and atracurium, were introduced for their much shorter durations and lack of "cumulative" actions (i.e., intervals between doses that maintain an ED_{95} do not get progressively longer with these relaxants).

4. The **clinical pharmacology** of the nondepolarizing relaxants is summarized in Table 11-1.

C. **Phase II block,** or desensitization block, occurs with repeated or continuous administration of a depolarizing agent over a long period, in doses of 5–6 mg/kg with halothane and enflurane, and 8–12 mg/kg with nitrous oxide–narcotic anesthesia. The mechanism is not clear but may be due to a conformational change in the receptor. Phase II block is **characterized** by

1. Fade on tetanic stimulation of train-of-four.
2. Increasing requirement for drug with prolonged use (tachyphylaxis).
3. Posttetanic potentiation.
4. Partial or complete reversal with anticholinesterases.

D. **Side effects**

1. In general, the side effects of **depolarizing relaxants** like SCh are related to their ability to mimic the action of ACh at ACh receptors (both muscarinic and nicotinic) of other tissues.

   a. **Side effects of SCh**

      (1) **Fasciculations and postoperative muscle pains** may be prevented by a small dose of a nondepolarizing relaxant (e.g., 3 mg of dTC) given 3 minutes prior to SCh or by pretreatment with 0.05 mg/kg of diazepam. If pretreating for a rapid sequence induction, the dosage of SCh is increased to 1.5 mg/kg. Pretreatment with a nondepolarizing relaxant may cause diplopia, weakness, and a decreased vital capacity; awake patients should be warned and resuscitation equipment should be made available.

      (2) **Ganglionic stimulation.** SCh may cause increased heart rate and increased blood pressure in adults or decreased heart rate in children and adults receiving a second dose of SCh. Pretreatment with atropine will prevent the bradycardia.

      (3) **Hyperkalemia.** SCh normally causes K^+ to increase 0.5–1.0 mEq/L, but K^+ may significantly rise in patients with burns, upper and lower motor neuron disease, trauma, prolonged bed rest, muscle diseases, or closed head injury. This usually occurs after the first week and may last from 3–9 months after the injury.

      (4) **Increased intraocular pressure,** due to contraction of tonic eye muscles. SCh is

Table 11-1. Comparative clinical pharmacology of relaxants[a,b]

Drugs	ED$_{95}$[c] (mg/kg IV)	Intubating Dose[d] (mg/kg IV bolus)	Onset time[e] (min)	Potency factor[f]	Time to 25% recovery[g] (min)	Elimination
Succinylcholine[h]	0.25	1 (1.5–2.0 IM)	1		5–10	0% renal; breakdown by plasma cholinesterase
Pancuronium	0.07	0.08–0.1	3–5	1	80–100	70–80% renal, 15–20% biliary excretion and liver metabolism[i]
Vecuronium	0.06	0.1–0.12	2–3	1.2	25–30	10–20% renal, 80% biliary excretion and hepatic metabolism[i]
d-Tubocurarine (dTC)	0.51	0.5–0.6	3–5	0.14	80–100	70% renal, 15–20% biliary excretion, which increases in renal failure
Metocurine	0.28	0.3–0.4	3–5	0.25	80–100	80–100% renal
Atracurium	0.25	0.4–0.5	2–3	0.28	25–30	Ester hydrolysis independent of plasma cholinesterase and Hofmann elimination (pH and temperature dependent)[j]
Gallamine	3.0	3.0–4.0	3–5	0.023	80–100	100% renal
Pancuronium and dTC	0.02 + 0.15	0.02 + 0.15	3–5	1	40–60	
Pancuronium and metocurine	0.02 + 0.07	0.02 + 0.07	3–5	1	40–60	

[a]All doses were determined under balanced (N$_2$O-narcotic) technique.
[b]There is a large variability in patient response to all relaxants, especially at the extremes of age. Therefore, patients should be monitored as described in sec. **IV.**

Table 11-2. Location and function of nicotinic and muscarinic receptors

Type of receptor	Function
Nicotinic	
Neuromuscular junction	
Presynaptic	Maintains ACh release at high-frequency stimulation
Postsynaptic	Initiates depolarization of muscle membrane
Autonomic ganglia cell bodies—both sympathetic and parasympathetic	Initiate depolarization of ganglion cell, leading to generalized sympathetic effects (increased vessel wall tone, increased sweating) and parasympathetic effects listed below
Muscarinic	
Peripheral postganglionic parasympathetic nerve endings	
Heart (via vagus nerve)	Slows sinus node, lowers atrial conduction, lowers atrioventricular node conduction
Smooth muscles at bronchi and bronchioles	Bronchoconstriction
Gastrointestinal	Raises tone
Genitourinary	Raises bladder tone, lowers sphincter tone
Eye	Miosis
Secretory glands	Stimulates salivary, tracheobronchial, lacrimal, digestive, and exocrine sweat glands

agents that inhibit the enzyme acetylcholinesterase, thereby increasing the ACh available to compete with the relaxants for their binding site. Other drugs like 4-aminopyridine increase the release of ACh presynaptically; however, only the anticholinesterases are in widespread clinical use. The latter, in addition, may act presynaptically by increasing ACh mobilization and/or release and also by direct depolarization of the postjunctional membrane.

B. Reversal of **phase II blockade** occurs spontaneously within 10–15 minutes in approximately 50% of patients. The remainder have prolonged responses. It is advisable to allow these patients to recover spontaneously for 20–25 minutes after turning off the SCh infusion. After this period, reversal with anticholinesterase agents may be attempted if a plateau in recovery

Table 11-3. Cardiovascular side effects of relaxants

Drugs	Histamine release[a]	Ganglionic effects	Vagolytic activity	Sympathetic stimulation
Succinylcholine	+	Stimulates	0	0
Pancuronium	0	0	+	+
Vecuronium	0	0	0	0
d-Tubocurarine	+ +	Blocks	0	0
Metocurine	+	Weak block	0	0
Atracurium	+[b]	0	0	0
Gallamine	0	0	+ +	+

[a]Histamine release is dose- and rate-dependent and therefore less pronounced if drugs are given slowly.
[b]At doses > 0.5 mg/kg.

(as judged by blockade monitoring) is reached. Earlier reversal could worsen the block.

C. **Anticholinesterases.** The three principal drugs are edrophonium, neostigmine, and pyridostigmine. Like ACh, all have muscarinic as well as nicotonic effects. Muscarinic stimulation leads to salivation, bradycardia, tearing, miosis, and bronchoconstriction. Administration of an anticholinergic drug (e.g., atropine or glycopyrrolate) prior to an anticholinesterase will minimize the muscarinic receptor activation. Table 11-4 summarizes the clinical pharmacology of these three relaxant antagonists.

D. **Time to reversal** is related to degree of spontaneous recovery prior to the administration of anticholinesterases; it will take longer for a deeper block. Antagonism is also more difficult in the presence of respiratory acidosis, hypothermia, electrolyte abnormalities, and other blocking drugs like antibiotics. The main offenders are streptomycin and aminoglycosides used for peritoneal lavage, the polymyxins, tetracycline, and clindamycin. Attempts to reverse blockade when no twitches are elicited by a peripheral nerve stimulator can possibly deepen blockade by promoting open-channel blocking effects of the nondepolarizing drugs. Once reversal occurs, "recurarization" is not seen.

IV. **Monitoring neuromuscular function**

A. There are several **reasons to monitor** neuromuscular blockade under anesthesia:

1. As an objective addition to clinical assessment in determining degree of relaxation during surgery and degree of recovery before extubation.

2. To help adjust dosage according to patient response.

3. To monitor for the development of phase II block.

4. For early recognition of patients with abnormal plasma cholinesterase.

5. To assess whether depression of respiratory function after anesthesia is due to residual neuromuscular blockade.

B. Most peripheral nerve stimulators (also called blockade monitors) in use today employ various patterns of stimuli: single twitch, tetanic stimulation, and train-of-four stimuli. Any muscle can be monitored; the adductor pollicis response to ulnar nerve stimulation at the wrist is used most often, since it is easily accessible and results are not complicated by direct muscle activation. Surface-stimulating electrodes are placed on the wrist over the ulnar nerve and are attached to a battery-driven pulse generator, which delivers a graded impulse of electrical current at a specified frequency. Evoked muscle tension can be estimated by feeling for thumb adduction or measured and recorded through a strain gauge attached to the thumb. Following administration of a muscle relaxant, the developed tension and twitch height decrease with the onset of neuromuscular blockade beyond the threshold of 75% receptor blockade.

Table 11-4. Clinical pharmacology of reversal drugs

Drugs	Dosage	Time to peak antagonism (min)	Duration of antagonism (min)	Excretion pattern[a]	Dosage of atropine required[b] (μg/kg)
Edrophonium	0.5–1 mg/kg	1	40–65	70% renal 30% hepatic	7–10
Neostigmine	0.03–0.06 mg/kg up to 5 mg	7	55–75	50% renal 50% hepatic	15–30
Pyridostigmine	0.25 mg/kg	10–13	80–130	75% renal 25% hepatic	15–20

[a]The increased duration during renal failure exceeds the increased durations of pancuronium and curare, and so there is no "recurarization." The onset time of atropine is much faster than that of glycopyrrolate and it peaks in a little over a minute compared to 4–5 minutes for glycopyrrolate. Therefore, glycopyrrolate is a good choice with pyridostigmine, which has a longer time to peak antagonism. However, glycopyrrolate should be given at least 3 minutes before edrophonium. There appears to be less tachycardia, fewer arrhythmias, and a greater secretory drying effect with glycopyrrolate.

[b]Dosage of glycopyrrolate = ½ dosage of atropine.

Table 11-5. Clinical assessment of blockade

Evoked response (by blockade monitor)	Clinical correlate
95% suppression of single twitch at 0.15–0.1 Hz	Adequate intubating conditions
90% suppression of single twitch; train-of-four count of 1 twitch	Surgical relaxation with N_2O-narcotic anesthesia
75% suppression of single twitch; train-of-four count of 3 twitches	Adequate relaxation with inhalational agents
25% single-twitch suppression	Decreased vital capacity
Train-of-four ratio > 0.75; sustained tetanus at 50 Hz for 5 seconds	Head lift for 5 seconds; vital capacity 15–20 ml/kg; inspiratory force − 25 cm H_2O; effective cough
Train-of-four ratio = 1.0	Normal expiratory flow rate, vital capacity, and inspiratory force

C. The **electrical response** of a muscle to nerve stimulation can also be evaluated by electromyography (EMG), and in general, results correlate with those of mechanical assessment. Its advantages are more rapid assessment of response, simplicity, and no need for transducers. Although self-contained compact EMG monitors are now available, EMG is still largely a research tool.

D. The relationship between patterns of stimuli and relevant clinical information (Table 11-5) are discussed below.

    1. Single twitch. A supramaximal stimulus each lasting 0.2 msec at a frequency of 0.1 Hz is generally used. A control height of muscle twitch is established prior to administration of the muscle relaxant, and then degree of blockade can be assessed by comparing the percentage of twitch height to that of control. A supramaximal stimulus assures recruitment of all muscle fibers, and a short duration like 0.2 msec prevents repetitive firing. Stimulus frequency affects twitch height and degree of fade, and 0.1 Hz is chosen because at that frequency, 95% twitch height depression corresponds to satisfactory intubation conditions and adequate surgical relaxation. The single twitch is useful in studying relaxants and in assessing recovery times, but careful documentation of control height is required. It is not a sensitive indicator of onset of or recovery from blockade, since 75% of receptors must be blocked before twitch height begins to decrease, and at recovery to control height, approximately 75% of receptors are still occupied.

2. **Tetanic stimulus.** This pattern of nerve stimulation detects whether the response is sustained or fades during the stimulus. The stimulus frequency ranges from 50–200 Hz. During depolarizing blockade, the peak tension is reduced but sustained. With nondepolarizing blockade and with phase II block, the peak height is reduced and fades. Tetanic fade appears to be a prejunctional phenomenon due to the effects of curare-like drugs on mobilization of ACh during high-frequency stimulation. A tetanic stimulus of 50 Hz for 5 seconds is clinically useful, since sustained tension at this frequency correlates with maximal voluntary effort. However, tetanic stimuli are painful, and frequent tetanic stimulation can induce muscle recovery.

3. **Posttetanic single twitch** is resumption of single-twitch stimulation 6–10 seconds after a tetanic stimulus. An increase in twitch height after a tetanus is known as posttetanic potentiation (PTP) and can be explained by increased mobilization and synthesis of ACh during and after tetanic stimulation during partial curarization. Both nondepolarizing blockade and phase II block will exhibit PTP; depolarizing blockade will not. A normal muscle will show no PTP by EMG but may exhibit mechanical PTP due to a change in the contractile response of the muscle induced by tetanic stimulation. During a deep nondepolarizing block, when there is no response to single twitch or to a tetanus, the appearance of a response after a 5-second 50-Hz stimulus precedes return of the train-of-four by 30–40 minutes. The presence of electromyographic PTP is indicative of residual nondepolarizing blockade.

4. **Train-of-four (T4).** Four supramaximal stimuli at a frequency of 2 Hz are repeated at intervals no less than 10 seconds apart. Responses at this frequency are well separated yet show fade during partial curarization. During nondepolarizing neuromuscular blockade, elimination of the fourth response in the train corresponds to 75% depression of the first response when compared to control. Likewise, disappearance of the third, second, and first responses correspond to 80%, 90%, and 100% depression of the first twitch respectively. The ratio of the height of the fourth twitch to that of the first (the "T4 ratio") correlates with the degree of clinical recovery. A T4 ratio of 0.75 indicates that the single twitch has returned to control, and tetanus at 50 Hz for 5 seconds is fully sustained. This level of recovery correlates with adequate clinical recovery. Train-of-four is the most useful method for clinical monitoring, since it does not require a control height, it is not as painful as tetanic stimulation, and it does not induce changes in subsequent recovery. It is a good measure of relaxation in the range of blockade required for surgical relaxation (75–

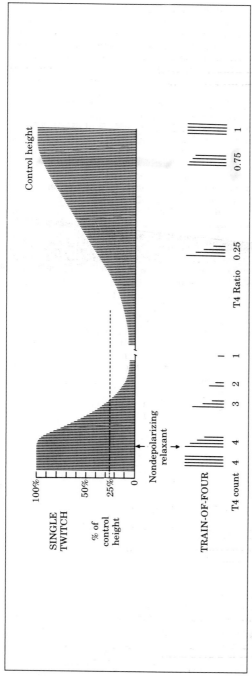

Fig. 11-6. A display of simultaneous tracings of single twitch at 0.1 Hz, and train-of-four (T4) response, during onset and recovery from a nondepolarizing relaxant. Train-of-four count: 1 = equivalent to 90% block; 2 = > 80% block; 3 = > 75% block; 4 = > 75% block. T4 ratio: 0.25 = significant block; 0.75 = minimal residual block; 1.0 = complete recovery of T4.

90% blockade) and is useful in assessing recovery from blockade (Fig. 11-6). It is not helpful in quantifying the degree of depolarizing blockade, because twitch height will decrease but no fade will be evident. However, onset of phase II block results in the appearance of fade and so train-of-four monitoring is useful for surveillance of depolarizing blockers.

Suggested Reading

Ali, H. H. Monitoring of neuromuscular function. Semin. Anesth. 3:284, 1984.

Ali, H. H. Monitoring of neuromuscular function and clinical interaction. *Clin. Anesthesiol.* 3:447, 1985.

Ali, H. H., and Savarese, J. J. Monitoring of neuromuscular function. *Anesthesiology* 45:216, 1976.

Ali, H. H., and Saverese, J. J. Neuromuscular Blockade. In R. R. Attia (ed.), *Practical Anesthetic Pharmacology.* New York: Appleton-Century-Crofts, 1978. Pp. 36–58.

Dreyer, F. Acetylcholine receptor. *Br. J. Anaesth.* 54:115, 1982.

Lebowitz, P. W., et al. Potentiation of neuromuscular blockade by combinations of pancuronium and metocurine or pancuronium and *d*-tubocurarine. *Anesth. Analg.* 59:604, 1980.

Miller, R. D. The priming principle. *Anesthesiology* 62:381, 1985.

Miller, R. D. (ed.), *Anesthesia.* New York: Churchill Livingstone, 1986. Pp. 835–943.

12

Local Anesthetics

Mark Dershwitz

I. General principles

A. Chemistry. The local anesthetics are weak bases whose structure consists of an aromatic moiety connected to a substituted amine through an ester or amide linkage. The pKa values of the local anesthetics are near physiologic pH; thus in vivo both charged and uncharged forms are present to a significant degree. The clinical differences between the ester and amide local anesthetics involve their potential for producing adverse effects and the mechanisms by which they are metabolized. *± cocaine*

1. **Esters:** procaine, chloroprocaine, and tetracaine.
2. **Amides:** lidocaine, mepivacaine, bupivacaine, and etidocaine.

B. Mechanism of action

1. Local anesthetics block conduction in nerves by **impairing propagation of the action potential** (AP) in axons. They have no effect on the resting or threshold potentials but decrease the rate of rise of the AP such that the threshold potential is not reached.

2. Local anesthetics act at a specific **receptor site** in the nerve membrane. This receptor is the sodium channel and is accessible primarily from within the nerve cell. The anesthetic molecule must traverse the cell membrane, through passive nonionic diffusion of the molecule in the uncharged state, and then bind to the sodium channel in the charged state.

3. Commercially available solutions of local anesthetics are supplied with the **pH** adjusted to the acidic side to enhance chemical stability. Plain solutions are usually adjusted near pH 6, while those containing a vasoconstrictor are adjusted near pH 4 because of the lability of catecholamine molecules at alkaline pH. Lower pH values, by decreasing the proportion of molecules in the uncharged form, result in a slower onset time of anesthesia.

4. **Differential blockade of nerve fibers** (Table 12-1)

   a. In general, thinner nerve fibers are more easily blocked than thick ones. However, myelinated fibers are more readily blocked than nonmyelinated ones because of the need to produce blockade only at the nodes of Ranvier.

   b. By careful choice of an appropriate agent and concentration, it is possible to selectively block pain and temperature sensation (A-δ and C fibers) in the absence of significant motor blockade (A-α fibers).

Table 12-1. Classification of nerve fibers

Fiber type	Myelin	Diameter (microns)	Function
A-α	+ +	6–22	Motor efferent, proprioception afferent
A-β	+ +	6–22	Motor efferent, proprioception afferent
A-γ	+ +	3–6	Muscle spindle efferent
A-δ	+ +	1–4	Pain, temperature, touch afferent
B	+	< 3	Preganglionic autonomic
C	–	0.3–1.3	Pain, temperature, touch afferent; postganglionic autonomic

5. **Sequence of clinical anesthesia.** The blockade of peripheral nerves usually progresses in the following order:
   a. Peripheral vasodilatation and skin temperature elevation.
   b. Loss of pain and temperature sensation.
   c. Loss of proprioception.
   d. Loss of touch and pressure sensation.
   e. Motor paralysis.
C. **Metabolism of local anesthetics**
   1. **Esters.** The ester linkage is readily cleaved by plasma cholinesterase. Thus, their half-lives in the circulation are very short (about 1 minute). The degradation product of ester metabolism is p-aminobenzoic acid, a compound associated with hypersensitivity reactions in some individuals.
   2. **Amides.** The amide linkage is cleaved through initial N-dealkylation followed by hydrolysis, reactions occuring primarily in the liver, and to little or no extent in the plasma. Persons with severe liver disease may be more susceptible to adverse reactions to amide local anesthetics. The elimination half-lives for the amide local anesthetics are about 2–3 hours.
II. **Characteristics of specific agents**
   A. **Esters**
      1. **Procaine** (Novocain)
         a. Short acting, low potency, low toxicity.
         b. Used for local infiltration and for spinal anesthesia when very short duration is desired.
      2. **Chloroprocaine** (Nesacaine)
         a. Short acting, low potency, very low toxicity, very rapid onset.
         b. Very rapid hydrolysis by plasma cholinesterase accounts for low toxicity and short duration.

      c. Used for local infiltration, nerve blocks, and epidural anesthesia.

      d. Subarachnoid administration must be avoided because neurologic deficits of long (or permanent) duration may result. The mechanism of this effect is believed to be due to the low pH of the solution and the bisulfite preservative.

      e. Some clinicians recommend chloroprocaine as the agent of choice when regional anesthesia is to be administered to a patient susceptible to malignant hyperthermia.

  3. Tetracaine (Pontocaine)

      a. Long acting, high potency, high toxicity.

      b. Used primarily for spinal anesthesia.

      c. Produces motor blockade of longer duration and greater intensity than sensory blockade.

B. Amides

  1. Lidocaine (Xylocaine)   "*LimBE*"

      a. Rapid onset, moderate duration, moderate potency and toxicity.

      b. Most frequently used local anesthetic for all types of local and regional anesthesia.

  2. Mepivacaine (Carbocaine)

      a. Moderate potency and toxicity, duration in excess of that of lidocaine.

      b. Used for local infiltration, nerve blocks, and epidural anesthesia.

  3. Bupivacaine (Marcaine, Sensorcaine)

      a. Slow onset, very long duration, high potency and toxicity.

      b. Frequently used for all types of local and regional anesthesia when a prolonged duration is desired.

      c. Sensory blockade is of greater intensity and duration than motor blockade.

      d. Inadvertent intravascular injection may result in cardiac arrest remarkably resistant to therapy; pregnant patients in labor may be more susceptible.

  4. Etidocaine (Duranest)

      a. Rapid onset, very long duration, high potency and toxicity.

      b. Used in nerve blocks and epidural anesthesia.

      c. Produces motor blockade in excess of the accompanying sensory blockade; the degree of sensory anesthesia with epidural anesthesia may be inadequate for intraabdominal procedures, unless the 1.5% concentration is employed.

III. Methods of regional anesthesia (See Chap. 13 for relevant anatomy and techniques.)

  A. Infiltration

    1. Local infiltration

      a. The injection of local anesthetic solutions intradermally or subcutaneously to produce anesthesia at the site of surgery.

    b. Large volumes of low concentration solutions are typically used.

    c. Epinephrine may be added to the solution at a concentration of 5 μg/ml (1 : 200,000) to double the duration of the anesthesia with some (but not all) local anesthetics.

    d. **Agents** (Table 12-2). Any of the local anesthetics may be used for local infiltration, the choice depending on the duration desired and the volume required.

2. Intravenous regional

    a. The injection of an anesthetic solution into a limb (usually arm) vein after exsanguination with an Esmarch bandage and occlusion of the vein with a tourniquet.

    b. A large volume of dilute local anesthetic is used (e.g., 40–50 ml 0.5% lidocaine without epinephrine).

    c. Anesthesia persists as long as the tourniquet is inflated; 2 hours is the maximum recommended time for tourniquet inflation.

    d. Anesthesia disappears rapidly after deflation of the tourniquet.

    e. **Agents.** Only lidocaine is approved for intravenous regional anesthesia in the United States. Bupivacaine has been used; however, cardiac toxicity from rapid systemic vascular administration due to a defective tourniquet, or a tourniquet deflated too soon after anesthetic injection, makes the choice of this agent unsafe. Since the duration of anesthesia is limited by tourniquet time, little is to be gained from using agents other than lidocaine.

B. Peripheral nerve blockade

  1. Nerve block

    a. The injection of a local anesthetic solution in proximity to a peripheral nerve (e.g., median, femoral).

    b. Onset is rapid, and a duration of up to several hours can be achieved.

    c. The block of a nerve at the elbow or wrist requires about 5 ml; the block of a larger nerve such as the femoral requires about 10–20 ml.

    d. Nerves in areas supplied by arteries lacking collaterals (e.g., finger, toe, nose, ear, penis) should not be blocked with epinephrine-containing solutions because of the possibility of gangrene.

  2. Plexus block

    a. The injection of a local anesthetic solution in proximity to a nerve plexus (e.g., brachial).

    b. Onset is slow, but a duration of many hours may be achieved.

    c. Large volumes of local anesthetic solution are required, typically 20–40 ml for the axillary approach to the brachial plexus. Epinephrine-con-

Table 12-2. Agents for infiltration anesthesia

Agent	Concentration	Duration (hr)		Dosage range*
		Without epinephrine	With epinephrine	
Procaine	0.5–1.0%	0.25–0.5	0.5–1.5	Up to 60 ml
Chloroprocaine	0.5–1.0%	0.25–0.5	0.5–1.5	Up to 100 ml
Lidocaine	0.5–1.0%	0.5–2	1–3	Up to 50 ml
Mepivacaine	0.5–1.0%	0.5–2	1–3	Up to 50 ml
Bupivacaine	0.25–0.5%	2–4	4–8	Up to 45 ml

*Maximum recommended dosage is for a 70-kg patient, using the higher concentration solution, containing epinephrine. Frequently, lower dosages are effective.

taining solutions should be used to delay systemic absorption and minimize toxicity.

3. **Agents** (Table 12-3)

   a. The agent is chosen according to the duration of anesthesia desired: chloroprocaine for short duration, lidocaine or mepivacaine for intermediate duration, and bupivacaine or etidocaine for long duration.

   b. Since commercial epinephrine-containing solutions are supplied at a much lower pH than plain solutions, a faster onset of anesthesia may be achieved by adding epinephrine to the commercial plain solution just prior to injection. Using 0.1 ml of 1 : 1000 epinephrine, added with a tuberculin syringe, for each 20 ml of local anesthetic, gives a final concentration of 5 µg/ml of epinephrine (1 : 200,000).

C. Central nerve blockade

   1. **Epidural anesthesia**

      a. The injection of a local anesthetic solution into the epidural space through a lumbar vertebral (or less commonly, caudal or thoracic vertebral) approach.

      b. The duration of anesthesia is dependent on the choice of agent, its concentration, and the presence or absence of vasoconstrictor.

      c. Most commonly, a continuous epidural anesthetic is performed by the introduction of a small catheter through the epidural needle into the epidural space. The duration of anesthesia that may be achieved by repeated injections through the catheter may be limited by the development of tachyphylaxis, particularly when shorter acting agents such as lidocaine are employed.

      d. Caudal anesthesia is a type of epidural anesthesia where the epidural space is entered through the sacral hiatus; it is used when effective anesthesia of the sacral roots is mandatory.

      e. **Agents** (Table 12-4)

         (1) Local anesthetics used in epidural and caudal anesthesia are chloroprocaine, lidocaine, mepivacaine, bupivacaine, and etidocaine.

         (2) Considerations for the choice of an agent for epidural or caudal anesthesia are the same as for plexus block (see sec. **III.B.3**).

         (3) It would appear attractive to **combine** two local anesthetics in solution to take advantage of different properties of the two drugs; for example, a combination of chloroprocaine and bupivacaine (which might be expected to have a rapid onset and prolonged duration) has been studied. The combination has a rapid onset, but a duration no longer than that of chloropro-

Table 12-3. Agents for peripheral nerve block

Agent	Concentration	Duration (hr)[a]	Dosage range[b]
Chloroprocaine[c]	2–3%	0.5–1.5	Up to 40 ml of 2% solution
Lidocaine	1–2%	2–4	Up to 50 ml of 1% solution
Mepivacaine	1–2%	3–5	Up to 50 ml of 1% solution
Bupivacaine	0.25–0.5%	6–12	Up to 45 ml of 0.5% solution
Etidocaine	1–1.5%	6–12	Up to 40 ml of 1% solution

[a]Epinephrine-containing solution.
[b]Maximum recommended dosage is for a 70-kg patient, using epinephrine-containing solution. Frequently, lower dosages are effective. Values given are for epinephrine-free solution.
[c]Epinephrine-containing solution.

Table 12-4. Agents for epidural and caudal anesthesia

Agent	Concentration	Duration (hr)[a]	Dosage range[b]
Chloroprocaine[c]	2–3%	0.5–1.0	Up to 40 ml of 2% solution
Lidocaine	1–2%	0.75–1.5	Up to 50 ml of 1% solution
Mepivacaine	1–2%	1–2	Up to 50 ml of 1% solution
Bupivacaine[d]	0.25–0.75%	2–4	Up to 45 ml of 0.5% solution
Etidocaine	0.5–1.5%	2–4	Up to 40 ml of 1% solution

[a]Epinephrine-containing solution. Time given is that between doses in continuous epidural anesthesia.
[b]Maximum recommended dosage is for a 70-kg patient, using epinephrine-containing solution. Frequently, lower dosages are effective. Values given are for epinephrine-free solution.
[c]The 0.75% solution is not recommended in obstetrical anesthesia.
[d]

caine alone. Thus, extemporaneous mixing of anesthetic solutions for epidural use is to be discouraged; **sequential** administration of the two agents may provide the characteristics desired.

2. **Spinal anesthesia**

   a. The injection of local anesthetic solution into the subarachnoid space through a lower lumbar vertebral approach.

   b. A small volume of concentrated solution is used. The duration of anesthesia is dependent on the choice of agent, the amount (in milligrams) injected, and (in the case of tetracaine) the presence or absence of vasoconstrictor.

   c. Two of the factors determining sensory level (height) are the amount (in milligrams) injected, and the baricity of the solution.

   d. **Agents** (Table 12-5)

      (1) Local anesthetics used in spinal anesthesia are procaine, lidocaine, tetracaine, and bupivacaine.

      (2) **Procaine** is supplied as a 10% solution. It is mixed with an equal volume of 10% glucose to form a *hyperbaric* solution.

      (3) **Lidocaine** for *hyperbaric* use is supplied as a 5% solution containing 7.5% glucose. A solution of 2% lidocaine without glucose has been used for *isobaric* spinal anesthesia.

      (4) **Tetracaine** is commercially supplied as a 1% isobaric solution and as tetracaine crystals, 20 mg/ampul. A *hyperbaric* solution is prepared by mixing equal volumes of the 1% solution with 10% glucose. An *isobaric* solution is prepared by mixing equal volumes of the 1% solution with cerebrospinal fluid (CSF) obtained at the time of lumbar puncture. Alternatively, 4 ml of CSF may be used to dissolve 20 mg of tetracaine crystals. A *hypobaric* solution is prepared by dissolving 20 mg of tetracaine crystals in 20 ml of sterile, preservative-free water.

      (5) **Bupivacaine** for *hyperbaric* use is supplied as a 0.75% solution containing 8.25% glucose. Solutions of 0.5% and 0.75% bupivacaine without glucose have been used for *isobaric* spinal anesthesia.

IV. **Toxicity** (Table 12-6)

   A. **Preventive measures**

      1. **Avoidance of excessive doses.** For each patient, the dose to be administered should be chosen according to the site to be anesthetized, the patient's size, and the patient's physical status.

         a. The recommended maximum dose (in mg/kg of lean body mass) should not be exceeded.

Table 12-5. Agents for spinal anesthesia

Agent	Concentration	Baricity[a]	Usual dose[b]	Duration (hr)
Hyperbaric				
Procaine[c]	5% in 5% glucose	1.018	120 mg (2.4 ml)	0.5–1.0
Lidocaine	5% in 7.5% glucose	1.028	60 mg (1.2 ml)	0.75–1.5
Bupivacaine	0.75% in 8.25% glucose	1.030	9 mg (1.2 ml)	2–4
Tetracaine[c]	0.5% in 5% glucose	1.018	12 mg (2.4 ml)	2–3
Tetracaine + epinephrine[c]	0.5% in 5% glucose + 0.2 ml epinephrine	1.016	12 mg (2.6 ml)	3–5
Isobaric				
Lidocaine[d]	2%	1.009	60 mg (3 ml)	1–2
Bupivacaine[d]	0.5%	1.008	15 mg (3 ml)	2–4
Tetracaine[c]	0.5%	1.006[e]	15 mg (3 ml)	3–5
Hypobaric				
Tetracaine[c]	0.1%	1.000	10 mg (10 ml)	3–5

[a]Baricity is defined as the ratio of the mass of 1 ml of solution at a specified temperature to the mass of 1 ml of water at 4°C. The values listed are approximate and vary according to temperature.

[b]Usual dosage suggested is for a patient of "average" height undergoing perineal, leg, or lower abdominal surgery. For surgery in the upper abdomen, the dosage of the hyperbaric solutions may be increased. For short or pregnant patients, the dosage must be reduced.

[c]Solutions prepared as described under sec. III.C.2.d.

[d]These solutions are not FDA approved in the United States for spinal anesthesia at present. However, a number of studies exist in the anesthesiology literature concerning the intrathecal use of these solutions.

[e]Baricity depends on that of the patient's CSF, because CSF is used as the diluent to prepare the solution.

Table 12-6. Relative toxicity of local anesthetics

| Agent | Approximate potency ratios[a] | | | Maximum recommended doses[b] | |
| | Anesthetic potency | | CNS toxicity | Plain solution (mg) | Epinephrine-containing (mg) |
	Spinal	Ulnar block			
Procaine	1	1	1	400	600
Chloroprocaine	1	1	1	800	1000
Lidocaine	2	2	3	300	500
Mepivacaine		2	2	300	500
Etidocaine		4	6	300	400
Bupivacaine	14	6	12	175	225
Tetracaine	10		8	100[c]	200

[a]Potency ratios and equivalent doses depend on the method of anesthesia used.
[b]Maximum dose as recommended by the manufacturer in the United States for peripheral nerve blocks in 70-kg individuals.
[c]Tetracaine is used only for spinal anesthesia, primarily because of its toxic potential. When used at the recommended doses for spinal anesthesia, CNS and cardiovascular toxicity are unlikely.

    b. When large volumes of local anesthetic solution are required for a particular block, a lower concentration (than the highest available) will almost always provide adequate sensory anesthesia without exceeding the maximum recommended dose.

    c. Older patients require a lower total dose than younger patients of comparable size.

2. Avoidance of rapid absorption

    a. Unless contraindicated due to the anatomic site to be anesthetized or the presence of peripheral vascular or cardiac disease, vasoconstrictors should be added to local anesthetic solutions used in nerve, plexus, epidural, and caudal blocks.

    b. When an intravenous regional anesthetic has been administered, the tourniquet should not be deflated less than 20 minutes after the injection of the lidocaine, even if the surgical procedure has been completed, to prevent the effects of a bolus injection of the anesthetic.

3. Avoidance of intravascular injection

    a. The syringe containing the anesthetic solution should be aspirated prior to commencing injection and after each 5 ml of the total volume has been injected. If blood is obtained after aspirating, the needle or catheter tip must be repositioned.

    b. The patient must be constantly monitored for symptoms and signs of intravascular injection. If the anesthetic solution contains epinephrine (5 µg/ml), 2 or 3 ml injected IV will produce a dramatic tachycardia. Local anesthetics injected IV may result in the patient experiencing light-headedness, dizziness, a metallic taste in the mouth, numbness of the tongue or lips, slurred speech, or tinnitus. These symptoms occur with doses lower than those required to cause unconsciousness and seizures.

B. Central nervous system toxicity

  1. Signs and symptoms

    a. The symptoms of central nervous system (CNS) toxicity that frequently precede a seizure are listed in sec. **IV.A.3.b.**

    b. If further anesthetic is injected or absorbed, grand mal seizures may result.

    c. Blood and tissue levels of local anesthetics higher than those required to cause seizures may result in unconsciousness, apnea, and cardiovascular collapse.

  2. Treatment

    a. CNS toxicity of local anesthetics is exacerbated by hypercarbia; thus hyperventilation is important in therapy.

    b. The convulsing patient should be hyperventilated with Ambu bag and mask using 100% oxygen. In the presence of a full stomach, endotracheal intubation facilitated by the administration of succinylcholine should be performed.

    c. If the seizure does not terminate spontaneously with hyperventilation, IV administration of diazepam (0.1 mg/kg) or thiopental (2 mg/kg) is indicated to end it within a minute or so.

C. Cardiovascular toxicity

1. Signs and symptoms

    a. In low doses (1 mg/kg), intravascular injection of lidocaine has an antiarrhythmic effect on the heart. The automaticity of ectopic pacemakers is decreased, and the threshold for fibrillation in ventricular muscle and Purkinje fibers is increased.

    b. Local anesthetics depress electrical and contractile activity in isolated hearts, but this effect is rarely seen in vivo. <u>Cardiac stimulation is the usual result from local anesthetic toxicity and is due to increased CNS activity</u>.

    c. The intravascular injection of bupivacaine or etidocaine, however, may result in cardiovascular collapse, often refractory to therapy, because of the large degree of tissue binding displayed by these agents.

    d. Thus, depending on the agent and the prior health of the patient's heart, cardiovascular toxicity may be manifested as hypotension, tachy- or bradyarrhythmias, ventricular fibrillation, or electrical standstill.

2. Treatment

    a. <u>Hypotension</u> is treated by the administration of fluids, a peripheral vasoconstrictor such as phenylephrine, and placement of the patient in the Trendelenburg position. In the presence of low cardiac output, an <u>inotrope</u> such as dopamine is also administered.

    b. Cardiac arrhythmias are difficult to treat but subside over time if the patient can be hemodynamically maintained. For an arrhythmia in which cardiac output is compromised, or in the case of asystole, prolonged administration of cardiopulmonary resuscitation is warranted; as the drug redistributes, the cardiotoxic effects may subside.

D. Hypersensitivity reactions

1. Signs and symptoms

    a. Local anesthetics of the <u>ester type</u> may result in allergic reactions due to the metabolite p-aminobenzoic acid. In addition, <u>these anesthetics may produce allergic reactions in persons sensitive to sulfonamides or thiazide diuretics</u>.

    b. Local anesthetics of the amide class are essentially devoid of allergic potential; only one documented true allergic reaction has been reported. However, many anesthetic solutions contain methylparaben as the preservative; this compound may produce an allergic reaction in someone sensitive to *p*-aminobenzoic acid.

    c. Local hypersensitivity reactions may be manifest as local erythema, urticaria, edema, or dermatitis.

    d. Systemic hypersensitivity reactions are much rarer and present as generalized erythema, urticaria, edema, bronchoconstriction, or hypotension.

  2. Treatment is symptomatic and supportive.

    a. Bronchoconstriction is treated by the administration of epinephrine, 0.3 mg SQ and repeated every 15 minutes as needed.

    b. Hypotension should be managed by the administration of fluids and a vasopressor such as phenylephrine and placement of the patient in the Trendelenburg position. In the presence of low cardiac output, an inotrope such as dopamine should also be administered.

    c. Cutaneous reactions may respond to antihistamines, such as diphenhydramine (Benadryl). More severe reactions may require a systemic glucocorticoid such as methylprednisolone (Solu-Medrol).

Suggested Reading

Covino, B. G., and Vassallo, H. G. *Local Anesthesia: Mechanisms of Action and Clinical Use.* New York: Grune & Stratton, 1976.

Ritchie, J. M., and Greene, N. M. Local Anesthetics. In A. G. Gilman et al. (eds.), *Goodman and Gilman's The Pharmacological Basis of Therapeutics.* New York: Macmillan, 1985.

Savarese, J. J., and Covino, B. G. Basic and Clinical Pharmacology of Local Anesthetic Drugs. In R. D. Miller (ed.), *Anesthesia.* New York: Churchill Livingston, 1986.

13

Regional Anesthesia

Ronald J. Botelho

Regional anesthesia encompasses a variety of techniques that interrupt nerve conduction by proximate administration of local anesthetic drugs. When properly performed, regional anesthesia provides excellent operative conditions along with analgesia. The benefits obtained using regional anesthesia as compared to general anesthesia include less postoperative confusion, more postoperative analgesia, and potentially less interference with cardiovascular and pulmonary function.

I. Preparation

   A. Preoperative visit. Regional anesthesia may be contraindicated in cases of anticoagulation or coagulopathy (bleeding time prolonged by 10% or more), sepsis, neurologic disease, cellulitis near or at the needle entry site, and physical or mental inability to cooperate. After the assessment is performed and the patient found to be a suitable candidate for a particular regional anesthetic technique, complete explanation of the procedure should be given, including expectations of patient cooperation and anticipated paresthesias. Reassurance that sedation or additional analgesia and anesthesia will be given, if necessary, reduces patient anxiety. Consent for general anesthesia as well as the regional anesthesia procedure should be obtained. Although unlikely, a general anesthetic may become necessary if the operation is prolonged or a complication occurs.

   B. Preoperative and intraoperative medication. The amount of patient cooperation needed during the operation must be determined before prescribing preoperative medication. More sedation can be given for procedures that require little cooperation, such as spinal or epidural anesthesia. Often it is difficult to estimate the optimal dose; it is better to err by giving too little sedation than too much, since supplemental drugs can be given in the operating room. The use of atropine or other antisialagogues is usually unnecessary and may dry the patient's mouth uncomfortably.

   C. Preinduction preparation. Oxygen should be available for immediate positive-pressure ventilation and delivery by disposable mask or nasal cannulas. Other considerations in the immediate preinduction period include the availability of equipment and drugs for administration of the block, monitoring, and resuscitation (see Chap. 8). Sterile, disposable trays that contain the necessary equipment are available for most types of blocks; sterile technique must always be applied when opening and using these trays.

II. Spinal anesthesia.
Subarachnoid administration of local anesthetic drugs is one of the simplest techniques used for blocking spinal nerves. After a single injection (or place-

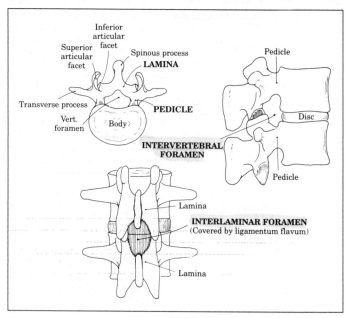

Fig. 13-1. Vertebral anatomy.

ment of a subarachnoid catheter) is performed, excellent anesthesia with muscle relaxation will result. Knowledge of the anatomy and the physiologic changes produced by sympathetic blockade is fundamental to successful and safe spinal anesthesia.

A. Anatomy

1. Spinal anesthesia is administered by inserting a needle through the lumbar interspinous space (Fig. 13-1) to the subarachnoid space. In the lumbar region, the interspinous space can be markedly enlarged by flexion of the spine.

2. Three **ligaments** bind the vertebral arches together. The **supraspinous ligament** connects the apices of the spinous processes. The **interspinous ligament** links one spinous process to another and connects posteriorly to the supraspinous ligament and anteriorly to the ligamentum flavum. The **ligamentum flavum** forms the posterior border of the spinal canal. It connects the caudal edge of the lamina below. This ligament can usually be recognized by increased resistance to needle insertion until the needle passes through it to the epidural space.

3. The **spinal cord** descends caudally in the spinal canal to the upper border of L1 in adults. At birth, the spinal cord ends at L3, but because of differen-

tial cord–vertebral growth rates, it rises to L1 by 1 year of age. The lumbar, sacral, and coccygeal nerve roots branch from the conus medullaris and form the **cauda equina.** The mobility of these nerve roots reduces danger of impalement when a needle is inserted in this region.

4. There are three **meninges** or covering membranes in the central nervous system (CNS). The **pia mater** closely invests the spinal cord as it descends to the second sacral vertebra, where it becomes the filum terminale. The **dura mater** is the tough fibrous sheath that surrounds the cord in the spinal canal. The **arachnoid** lies between the pia and dura and is loosely adherent to the dura.

5. The **blood supply** to the spinal cord involves end arteries, including the anterior spinal artery and radicular arteries. Radicular arteries enter the spinal canal through the intervertebral foramina; interruption by ligation or direct trauma can cause ischemic damage to the spinal cord.

6. The **cerebrospinal fluid** (CSF) is a clear, colorless ultrafiltrate of blood that fills the subarachnoid space. The total volume of CSF is 100–150 ml; the volume contained in the spinal subarachnoid space is 25–35 ml. The specific gravity ranges from 1.003–1.009.

B. **Determination of the anesthetic level needed.** Knowledge of the cutaneous nerve distribution (Fig. 13-2) and the autonomic afferents from organs will help determine the segmental level needed for a particular operation (the afferent autonomic nerves mediate visceral sensation and viscerosomatic reflexes). Although it is difficult to define the absolute level of anesthesia needed for a particular operation, Table 13-1 provides some minimum suggested levels for operations involving particular anatomic regions.

A **differential nerve block** (see Chap. 12) occurs in spinal anesthesia, because diffusion of local anesthetics in CSF creates concentration gradients. Thin fibers (e.g., sensory nerves carrying pain and temperature and autonomic nerves) are more sensitive to local anesthetic blockade than thicker fibers (e.g., somatic motor and sensory nerves carrying touch and pressure), leading to a more cephalad level of block for thin fibers. For example, block of sympathetic innervation usually occurs 2–4 segments higher than the cutaneous sensory level.

C. **Factors influencing the level of anesthesia.** Knowledge of the following factors will help to avoid obtaining too high or too low a level.

1. The level varies directly with the **dose of agent** used.

2. **Specific gravity of the anesthetic solution relative to patient position,** both during and after drug administration, can cause dramatic differences in the level. The three types of solutions used are **isobaric, hypobaric, and hyperbaric.** Al-

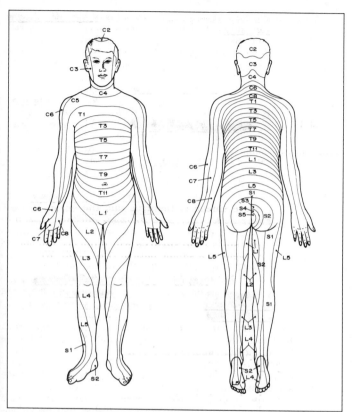

Fig. 13-2. Skin dermatomes corresponding to respective sensory innervation by spinal nerves.

though patient position is of little consequence when isobaric solutions are used, placing a patient in the Trendelenburg position (head-down tilt) will increase the level by cephalad migration of a hyperbaric solution and decrease the level by caudad movement of a hypobaric solution. Further change in the anesthetic level usually stops within 5–35 minutes after injection (referred to as "fixation"). Patient position will not influence the level after fixation.

3. The level of anesthesia obtained varies directly with the **volume** of solution injected, particularly when isobaric solutions are used. Volume also plays a significant role with hypobaric solutions when large volumes are required.

4. **Turbulence** created during or after administration of anesthetic solution (prior to fixation) will in-

Table 13-1. Suggested minimum cutaneous levels for spinal anesthesia

Operative site	Level
Lower extremities	T12
Hip	T10
Vagina/uterus	T10
Bladder/prostate	T10
Lower extremities with tourniquet	T8
Testis/ovaries	T8
Lower intraabdominal	T6
Other intraabdominal	T4

crease spread of the drug and the level obtained. Turbulence is created by rapid injection rate, barbotage, cough, and excessive patient movement.

5. The **spinal curvatures** will influence the spread of agent in a supine patient (Fig. 13-3). With a hyperbaric solution, the thoracic curvature limits cephalad spread to approximately T4. This may be overcome by increasing the dose of agent or using the Trendelenburg position.

6. The required dose to obtain a specific level is directly related to spinal subarachnoid volume, which varies directly with height, and inversely with age in adults, obesity, and pregnancy.

D. **Technique**

1. **Positioning.** Lateral decubitus and the sitting positions are the two that are used most often. With the lateral decubitus position, the affected side should be placed down with use of hyperbaric solutions and up with hypobaric solutions. The spine should be horizontal and at the edge of the bed. The knees are drawn up to the chest to obtain spinal flexion, increasing the size of the interlaminar foramina. The vertebral column should then be inspected to ensure that it is horizontal and there is no rotation.

   The sitting position is useful in obese patients and for performing a saddle block (low-level spinal anesthesia). With this position, the knees are elevated with the feet resting on a stool to obtain maximum spinal flexion.

2. Palpating the iliac crests identifies the relevant **anatomy.** A line connecting the iliac crests should either cross the spinous process of L4 or the L4–L5 interspace. The L2–L3, L3–L4, or L4–L5 interspaces are commonly used for lumbar puncture.

3. **Skin preparation.** A large area (T12–S1) is painted with an appropriate antiseptic solution (not soap). Sterile technique must be maintained, and care should be taken to avoid contamination of

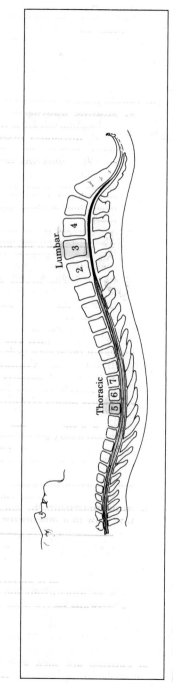

Fig. 13-3. Spinal column curvatures that influence the spread of anesthetic solutions.

the spinal kit with antiseptic solutions that can potentially cause arachnoiditis if injected.

4. A **skin wheal** is placed over the intended site of entry with a 25-gauge, ¾-inch needle using either 1% lidocaine or 1% procaine. Deeper infiltration with the same or a 22-gauge, 1-inch needle is then performed.

5. **Spinal needle approaches**
   a. **Midline approach.** A 25- or 26-gauge, 3½-inch spinal needle is frequently used with a 19-gauge introducer needle (1½-inch). The introducer needle (or the spinal needle itself) is placed into the interspinous ligament and should lie in the same plane as the spinous processes with slight (10–30 degrees) angulation cephalad. A 22-gauge spinal needle can also be used, but it does not require an introducer needle.
   b. **Paramedian approach.** The spinal needle is placed 1.5–2.0 cm lateral to the center of the selected interspace (no introducer needle is needed even when using a 25- or 26-gauge needle). The needle is directed medially and slightly cephalad. The path of the needle is lateral to the supraspinous ligament. This approach is particularly useful when this ligament is ossified.

6. **Needle placement.** The needle is advanced until increased resistance is felt as it passes into the ligamentum flavum. Continuing past the ligament, a sudden loss of resistance ("pop") is felt when the dura is punctured. The use of small-gauge needles sometimes makes identification of these sensations difficult. When the needle is at an appropriate depth (3–5 cm), periodic stylet removal to check for CSF return may prove helpful. There is usually free flow of CSF with correct placement. Aspiration may be necessary to obtain CSF flow if the needle becomes plugged with tissue or when CSF pressure is low. To avoid plugging, always have the stylet in place when advancing the needle.

7. **Administration of anesthetic.** There should be CSF flow in a 360-degree rotation of the needle to ensure that the entire bevel is within the subarachnoid space. While holding the needle firmly, the stylet is removed, and the syringe containing the predetermined dose is attached. Gentle aspiration of less than 0.1 ml is performed to ensure free flow of CSF, at which point the anesthetic drug is slowly injected (no faster than 0.5 ml/sec to avoid turbulence). Reaspiration of CSF at the end of injection confirms that the needle point is still in the subarachnoid space. The needle and introducer are then removed together.

8. Patients are then **gently repositioned** by the anesthesiologist; patients should not assist, strain,

Table 13-2. Drugs and dosages for hyperbaric spinal anesthesia

Drug	Level (mg)*			Duration (min)
	T10	T8	T6	
Tetracaine	10	12	14	90–120
Bupivacaine	7.5	9.0	10.5	90–120
Lidocaine	50	60	70	30–90

*Doses are based on a 66-inch patient. An additional 2 mg of tetracaine, 10 mg of lidocaine, or 1.5 mg of bupivacaine, should be added or subtracted for each 6 inches in height above or below 66 inches. 5'6"

or cough at this point. The level of sensory blockade is checked using pinpricks or alcohol cooling. Excessive patient movement is avoided until fixation of the block.

9. The blood pressure should be **closely monitored** (every 60–90 seconds) for 10–15 minutes so that hypotension can be treated quickly if it develops.

E. **Drugs and dosage** (see Chap. 12)

1. **Hyperbaric solutions.** See Table 13-2.

2. **Isobaric.** For tetracaine, the dosage (in milligrams) for a given level is approximately the same as when using a hyperbaric tetracaine technique.

3. **Hypobaric.** The dosage of these agents is approximately 1 ml/segment anesthetized.

4. **Vasoconstrictors.** Epinephrine (0.2 mg) or phenylephrine (2–5 mg) can be used to prolong the duration of spinal anesthesia by tetracaine (although apparently not with lidocaine or bupivacaine). If one of these agents is added to the solution immediately prior to use, it can roughly double the duration yet delay the onset of spinal anesthesia. In the elderly, vasoconstrictors may prolong the duration by a factor of 3 or more.

F. **Complications**

1. **Hypotension** is a common complication of spinal anesthesia, resulting from sudden sympathetic blockade and vasodilatation. Specifically, there is a decrease in systemic vascular resistance and an increase in venous capacitance. In addition, the sympathetic innervation to the heart arises from T1–T4, and a **high spinal** can be accompanied by bradycardia and a decrease in cardiac output. Because of differential nerve block, sympatholysis is usually 2–4 segments higher than the sensory level achieved; thus bradycardia may be noted even with a sensory level of T3. Prevention of hypotension (in euvolemic patients) can usually be accomplished by administration of 500–1000 ml of lactated Ringer's solution prior to induction. Hypotension may be treated with ephedrine (5–10 mg IV boluses) or

phenylephrine infusion. The latter may exacerbate bradycardia, which can be treated with atropine if needed.

2. **Apnea** can occur either as a result of reduced medullary blood flow from severe hypotension or from direct C3–C5 blockade, inhibiting phrenic nerve function. Ventilatory support is required immediately.

3. **Dyspnea** is a common complaint with high spinal anesthesia and is usually the result of proprioceptive block of abdominal and chest wall movement. Reassurance of the patient is usually all that is required.

4. As a consequence of continued CSF leak through the dura, low CSF pressure results in traction on pain-sensitive structures (particularly in the upright position) and manifests as **headache,** characteristically in the occiput and neck. The incidence of headache is higher in younger patients and when larger needles are used to perform the dural puncture. The incidence of postspinal headache is about 2% when a 25-gauge needle is used. The headache will usually resolve with IV fluids, bed rest, and analgesics. Rarely, an epidural blood patch is necessary for resolution of symptoms.

   Other causes of headache include arachnoiditis and meningitis. These complications are rare but should be considered with an atypical headache.

5. **Spinal cord damage** is an exceedingly rare complication, but it is the focus of the most patient concern.

6. **Nausea and vomiting** are nonspecific symptoms that can be caused by hypotension or unopposed vagal stimulation. Treatment involves normalizing the blood pressure, oxygen administration, and atropine IV.

G. **Contraindications**

   1. **Absolute**
      a. Lack of patient consent.
      b. Allergy to that specific class of local anesthetic drug.
      c. Increased intracranial pressure.
      d. Infection at the intended puncture site.

   2. **Relative**
      a. Hypovolemia.
      b. Coagulopathy or anticoagulation treatment.
      c. Systemic sepsis.
      d. Progressive neurologic diseases.
      e. Chronic back pain.

III. **Epidural anesthesia** is achieved by administration of local anesthetic solutions into the epidural space by a single injection or by catheter for repeated injections. Compared to spinal anesthesia, onset is slower and intensity of both sensory and motor block is less, even though the epidural technique requires significantly more drug. Because of the slower onset, however, cardiovascular changes are less dramatic, and, when performed correctly, headache (from dural puncture) will not occur.

A. **Anatomy.** The spinal epidural space lies between the dura anteriorly and the ligamentum flavum posteriorly. It contains areolar and lymphatic tissue, as well as epidural veins that can occupy a significant volume within the epidural space. The cephalad limit of the spinal epidural space is the foramen magnum, where the dura fuses with the periosteum of the skull. The caudad limit is the sacrococcygeal membrane.

B. **Determination of the anesthetic level is needed.** The factors that determine the level needed for epidural anesthesia are the same as for spinal anesthesia. Epidural anesthesia can be administered at any vertebral level, although the L2–L5 interspaces are most commonly used because of increased safety against spinal cord injury. The earliest and most intense block occurs at the level of injection, from which point nerve block proceeds in both caudad and cephalad directions. Thus a **segmental block** which leaves sensation intact above and below the blocked segments may be achieved. A **differential block** is also obtained with epidural anesthesia and often is more pronounced than that produced by spinal anesthesia.

C. **Factors influencing the level of anesthesia**
   1. The **volume** of anesthetic solution injected.
   2. The **concentration** of the anesthetic solution (particularly affecting the intensity of block).
   3. **Patient position.** In the lateral position, the dependent side will develop more dense anesthesia as a result of gravitational spread. Likewise, perineal anesthesia is obtained using the sitting position during injection.
   4. **Pregnancy, age, and height.** A reduction in dosage of 25–50% is required for pregnancy and extremes of age. The dosage requirement increases directly with height.

D. **Technique.** The object is to place the epidural needle carefully into the epidural space by piercing only the ligamentum flavum and not the dura. In a transverse plane, the epidural space is triangular, the base of which is the dura with the apex posterior in the midline. Although either the midline or paramedian approach may be used, the needle should be angled to enter the epidural space at its widest point.
   Palpation of landmarks, skin preparation, and draping are the same as described for subarachnoid block.
   1. **Epidural needle approaches.** A midline approach will ensure entry into the widest portion of the epidural space. The paramedian approach may be used if midline entry proves difficult. In either case, a 17-gauge Tuohy or Weiss needle with stylet is placed through the skin wheal. The needle is advanced into the interspinous ligament 1.5–3.0 cm from the skin. The stylet is then removed, and one

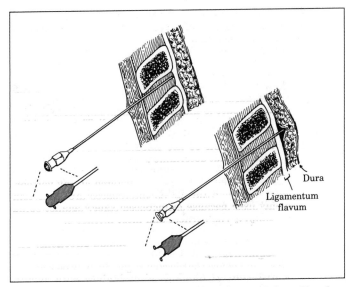

Fig. 13-4. Hanging-drop technique for identification of the epidural space. The drop retracts into the hub as the tip of the needle enters the epidural space.

or both of the procedures for identification of the epidural space (see sec. **2**) are used with needle advancement. If a "single-shot" technique is to be performed, a 22-gauge 3½-inch epidural or spinal needle is usually used.

2. **Identification of the epidural space**
   a. **Hanging-drop technique** (Fig. 13-4). A drop of local anesthetic solution is placed in the hub of the needle. The needle is then slowly advanced until the drop retracts into the hub, indicating that the bevel has entered the epidural space. At this point, the test for loss of resistance to injection of air or local anesthetic solution can be performed as described in **b**. The advantage of this technique is that both hands can be used for careful needle advancement. However, drop retraction occurs only 80% of the time.
   b. **Loss of resistance technique.** The barrel of a glass syringe is lubricated by drawing up a small amount of local anesthetic solution so that the plunger moves freely. The syringe, containing approximately 3 ml of air, is then firmly attached to the needle hub. Constant pressure is applied to the plunger as the needle is slowly advanced. When the bevel enters the epidural space, there is marked loss of resistance to

plunger displacement. Following the injection of air, no more than 1 ml should return into the syringe.

3. **Test dose.** The syringe is disconnected and evidence of CSF or blood return sought. Careful aspiration must be performed. If either CSF or blood returns, the needle must be repositioned. A test dose is administered with 3 ml of anesthetic solution, preferably containing 1 : 200,000 epinephrine, which should not result in a major anesthetic effect if the needle is in the epidural space. However, if the dura has been punctured, a block should be obtained within 3 minutes. If the local anesthetic solution containing epinephrine has been injected into an epidural vein, a 20–30% rise in heart rate will occur. Chloroprocaine should not be used for the test dose, as intrathecal injection of this agent has been reported to cause nerve damage.

4. **Administration** of local anesthetic solution should proceed in increments with 3–5 ml injected every 3–5 minutes until the total dose is given. Aspiration is performed prior to each injection to assure continued needle or catheter placement in the epidural space.

5. **Catheter placement for continuous block.** When a block is required for a prolonged period, a catheter is placed for ease of repeated injections.

   a. The needle is placed in the epidural space with the bevel pointing cephalad or caudad. Place the bevel cephalad when high levels are required and caudad when low levels are desired.

   b. An 18- to 20-gauge radiopaque plastic catheter with 1-cm graduations at the tip should be used. If a catheter with a stylet is used, the wire stylet is withdrawn to a point 2–3 cm from the tip.

   c. The catheter is then threaded into the epidural needle until increased resistance is encountered as the catheter reaches the bevel of the needle. As the catheter is advanced 2–3 cm past the bevel, the patient may abruptly experience a paresthesia. If the paresthesia is sustained, the catheter must be repositioned. At this point, the catheter must not be withdrawn into the needle because shearing of the catheter may result. If the catheter must be withdrawn, the needle and catheter are removed together.

   d. The distance from the surface of the patient's back to a mark on the catheter is measured (the graduated glass syringe is useful for this purpose).

   e. Once the catheter is in place, the needle is carefully withdrawn over the catheter. The catheter must be stabilized so that it is not inadvertently withdrawn with the needle. The distance from the patient's back to the mark on the catheter should again be measured. If necessary, the catheter should be withdrawn, leaving only 2–3 cm in the epidural space.

f. The catheter is then fitted with an adapter at the end to allow syringe attachment. Aspiration is performed, and the catheter and syringe are inspected for CSF or blood return. The catheter is then taped to the patient's back, and increments of anesthetic solution then administered.

E. Dosage (see Chap. 12)

1. A useful "rule of thumb" for the **initial dose** is to use 1.0 ml of anesthetic solution per segment and an additional 0.1 ml/segment for every 2 inches in height above 5 feet. In the elderly, the dose is reduced approximately 50%, while a reduction of 25–30% is made for pregnant women.

2. **"Top up" doses.** To maintain a constant level of anesthesia, approximately two-thirds of the initial dose should be given in anticipation of a receding block.

3. **Vasoconstrictors.** Epinephrine is usually added in a concentration of 1 : 200,000. It will diminish systemic uptake and the plasma levels of local anesthetic as well as prolong the duration of anesthesia. When added to lidocaine, the prolongation is approximately 50%; the effect is not as strong when used with bupivacaine. Commercially prepared epinephrine-containing solutions are buffered at a relatively low pH, which slows onset of block. Delaying onset can be avoided by adding the epinephrine to the solution immediately prior to use.

F. Complications

1. **Unintentional subarachnoid injection** of a large volume of anesthetic solution can result in a **total spinal block.** This complication can be prevented by aspirating before every injection and administering local anesthetics in increments. Treatment consists in controlled ventilation and correction of the hypotension accompanying a complete sympathetic block.

2. **Intravascular injection** of local anesthetics into an epidural vein usually causes CNS and cardiovascular toxicity and may result in convulsions or cardiopulmonary arrest.

3. **Wet tap.** If the dura is punctured with the 17-gauge needle, there is a 75% chance that a young patient will develop a postdural puncture headache. If the dura has been punctured, either another attempt is made as far removed as possible from the interspace of dural puncture or the method changed to subarachnoid block.

4. **Local anesthetic overdose** is possible with this technique, unlike spinal anesthesia, where small amounts of drug are used.

5. **Hypotension** resulting from epidural sympathetic

block is usually less severe than that occurring with subarachnoid block.

6. **Direct spinal cord injury** is possible if the epidural technique is performed above L1.

G. **Contraindications** are the same as for spinal anesthesia.

IV. **Caudal block** is epidural anesthesia performed by injection of local anesthetic into the caudal canal. Compared to a lumbar epidural technique, there is less chance of dural puncture or development of significant sympathetic block. It is most often used to obtain anesthesia in lumbosacral dermatomes.

A. **Anatomy.** The sacrum is a triangular bone formed by fusion of the five sacral vertebrae. The **sacral hiatus** is formed by failure of the laminae of S5 to fuse. There are several variants in the size and configuration of the sacral hiatus. The majority are congenital defects in the caudal roof, which tend to enlarge the hiatus and facilitate, rather than hinder, needle placement. In approximately 5% of cases, the hiatal deformities prevent needle insertion. The lateral margins of the sacral hiatus are formed by the **sacral cornua,** which are the inferior articulating processes of S5. The **sacrococcygeal membrane** is a thin layer of fibrous tissue that covers the sacral hiatus. The caudal canal contains the sacral venous plexus, the sacral nerves, the dural sac which usually ends at the lower border of S2, and the filum terminale. In neonates, the dural sac may extend to the lower border of S4.

B. **Technique**

1. **Position.** Patients may be placed in the prone, jackknife, lateral, or knee-chest position. Prone and jackknife allow the easiest identification of landmarks. However, the lateral position may be less objectionable and more comfortable for some patients. For pregnant women, either the lateral or the knee-chest position can be used.

For the prone position, a pillow is placed beneath the patient's hips, and the table is flexed to lift and tilt the sacrum. The gluteal muscles are relaxed by abduction and internal rotation of the legs.

2. **Palpation of landmarks.** The sacral cornua are located; if they are difficult to palpate directly, the location of the sacral hiatus can be estimated by measuring 5 cm cephalad from the tip of the coccyx in the midline. Then estimation of the S2 level can be made. The S2 foramina are located ½ inch caudally and medially to the posterior iliac spines. A line can be drawn at this level before preparing the skin.

3. **Skin preparation.** Sterile prep and drape procedures follow placement of a sponge between the gluteal folds to protect the perineum from antiseptic solution when using the prone position.

4. A **skin wheal** is raised with lidocaine between the sacral cornua. After subcutaneous infiltration, the

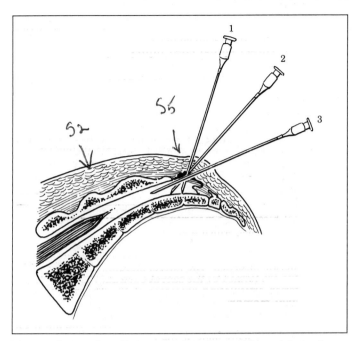

Fig. 13-5. Stages of needle insertion into the caudal canal. Lowering the hub after contact with the anterior sacral plate allows further advancement.

same needle may be used to locate the sacral hiatus.

5. **Needle placement** (Fig. 13-5). A 22-gauge spinal needle is inserted at an angle of 70–80 degrees through the skin wheal. The needle is advanced through the sacrococcygeal membrane until the point contacts the anterior sacral plate. The needle is then withdrawn slightly, the hub lowered so the needle is parallel to the plane of the sacrum, and then advanced 1½ inches into the caudal canal. If the needle contacts bone, the hub is lowered further. Lateral needle movement should be avoided, since it can result in nerve damage. The stylet is then withdrawn and used to measure the distance of the needle within the canal. The tip of the needle should not extend past the S2 level.

The needle hub is inspected for passive CSF or blood return, and the needle is aspirated. If no CSF or blood appear, 3 ml of air is injected. When the needle is correctly placed, there should be no resistance to injection of air, although patients will occasionally note a sensation of pressure during the injection. Subcutaneous crepitus indicates that the needle has been placed in soft tissue, dorsal to the sacrum, and must be withdrawn.

6. **Test dose.** After the needle has been positioned properly in the caudal canal, a test dose of 3 ml of anesthetic solution is injected. Patients are then observed for 3–5 minutes to detect development of subarachnoid block or symptoms of intravenous injection (see sec. **III.D.3**).

C. **Drugs and dosage.** The guidelines for drugs and dosage are generally the same as for lumbar epidural anesthesia. The extent of the caudal block is less predictable than other epidural techniques because of variability in the content and volume of the caudal canal, as well as the amount of local anesthetic solution that leaks out through the sacral foramina. To obtain sacrococcygeal anesthesia, a volume of 10 ml should be sufficient. For a T10 level, 15–30 ml should be administered.

The effect of epinephrine is the same as with other epidural techniques.

D. **Complications** are the same as previously described for lumbar epidural anesthesia. When caudal block is used in obstetrical anesthesia, it should not be performed if the presenting part of the fetus is below the ischial spines. Injection of anesthetic solution into the presenting part of the baby has been reported.

V. **Brachial plexus block** is accomplished by single injection into the interfascial compartment surrounding the plexus and the axillary artery. The compartment is formed from the prevertebral fascia that extends from the scalene muscles to the distal axilla, where it becomes the axillary sheath. The brachial plexus mediates all motor control and most sensation to the upper extremity. (Cutaneous sensation over the medial aspect of the upper arm and the whole shoulder area is not included in brachial plexus distribution. These are supplied by the intercostobrachial nerve and the cervical plexus, respectively.) Five techniques have been described for brachial plexus blockade; those most commonly used are described below.

A. **Anatomy** (Fig. 13-6). The brachial plexus is formed from the anterior rami of C5–8 and T1. For descriptive purposes, the brachial plexus is divided into the roots, trunks, divisions, cords, and branches, as illustrated in Fig. 13-6. The lateral, posterior, and medial cords are formed from divisions and are named according to their position around the axillary artery. The nerves that supply motor and sensory function of the arm arise from the cords as branches. The major branches continue as extensions of the cords and include the ulnar, radial, and median (formed from both lateral and medial cords) nerves. At a more proximal point, the musculocutaneous, median cutaneous, and axillary nerves branch from the lateral, medial, and posterior cords, respectively. There are two median cutaneous nerves: one to the upper arm and the other to the forearm (Fig. 13-7).

B. **The axillary approach** is the most common method of blocking the brachial plexus. It is easy to identify the

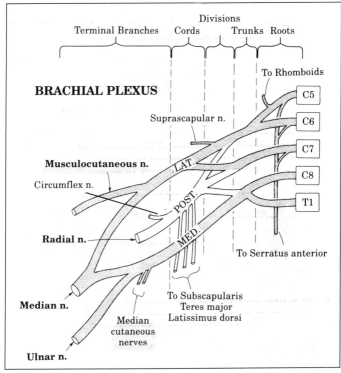

Divisions

Terminal Branches   Cords   Trunks   Roots

BRACHIAL PLEXUS

To Rhomboids

C5

C6

Suprascapular n.

C7

Musculocutaneous n.   LAT.

C8

Circumflex n.   POST.

T1

Radial n.   MED.

To Serratus anterior

Median n.   To Subscapularis
Teres major
Latissimus dorsi

Median
cutaneous
nerves

Ulnar n.

Fig. 13-6. Diagram of the brachial plexus and peripheral nerve formation.

landmarks used to determine needle placement, and there are fewer complications than with the interscalene or supraclavicular approaches. Axillary block is particularly useful for operations on the hand and forearm but is not a useful technique for operations involving the shoulder because there is no block of the cervical plexus (Fig. 13-7).

1. **Technique.** Anesthetic solution is injected into the axillary sheath at the most proximal point that the axillary artery is palpable. Blocking the branches that arise proximally from the cords is still difficult because of the relatively distal point of injection in the interfascial compartment. Applying digital pressure over the sheath, distal to the needle, both during and after injection, directs proximal spread of anesthetic solution within the sheath. Occasionally, the musculocutaneous and median cutaneous nerves will be left unblocked because of their proximal location.

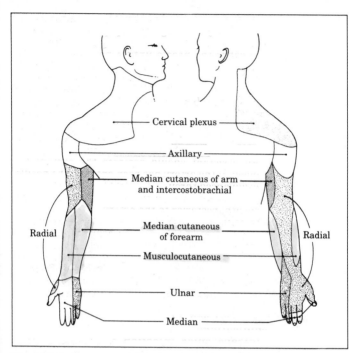

Fig. 13-7. Cutaneous peripheral nerve supply of the upper extremity.

The musculocutaneous nerve can be blocked by infiltration of 5 ml of anesthetic solution into the coracobrachial muscle, lateral and deep to the sheath (a paresthesia does not have to be elicited for blockade to be successful). Median cutaneous and intercostobrachial nerves can be blocked by subcutaneous infiltration of 10 ml of anesthetic solution in a half-ring around the medial aspect of the arm.

a. **Position.** In the supine position, the patient abducts the arm and flexes the elbow. The arm is also externally rotated, so that the hand lies alongside the patient's head.

b. The axilla is prepared and draped, but shaving is not necessary.

c. **Equipment.** A 23-gauge, 1½-inch short-bevel needle, extension tubing, and a 35-ml syringe are connected and filled with anesthetic solution.

d. The axillary artery is palpated and fixed at its most proximal point in the axilla. A skin wheal is then raised superficial to the artery.

e. The 23-gauge needle is advanced through the

wheal and aimed toward the lateral border of the artery. Feeling for a "pop" when entering the sheath, the anesthesiologist continues to advance the needle until a paresthesia in the distribution of either the median, radial, or ulnar nerves is elicited. If a paresthesia is not obtained, the needle should be withdrawn and redirected. If a paresthesia occurs in the distribution of the musculocutaneous nerve, the needle should be withdrawn and redirected because the musculocutaneous nerve may not lie within the sheath at this location. An assistant should aspirate the syringe for blood. If the artery has been entered, the needle is advanced through it until blood cannot be aspirated. The needle tip is then resting in the sheath, posterior to the artery.

    f. Once the needle tip is in the axillary sheath and blood does not return upon aspiration, the anesthetic solution is injected. A total of 30–40 ml of anesthetic solution is injected in increments with intermittent aspiration for blood. Prior to removing the needle, the musculocutaneous, median cutaneous, and the intercostobrachial nerves can be blocked.

2. Drugs. See Chap. 12.

3. Complications

    a. Intravascular injection of anesthetic solution, which can result in cardiovascular collapse or convulsions, can be prevented by intermittently checking for blood return while injecting.

    b. Nerve damage is a rare complication that can occur with all regional nerve blocks. Most nerve injuries result from pressure against unyielding metal parts of the OR table; stretch injury may also occur. Less commonly, injury may result from the needle trauma, use of inappropriately high concentrations of local anesthetics, prolonged tourniquet times, and ischemia from vasoconstrictors.

    c. Hematomas may develop from arterial puncture but usually resolve without residua.

4. Contraindications

    a. Infection over the needle entry site or in the axillary lymph nodes; cellulitis of the affected arm.

    b. Malignancy involving the axillary lymph nodes.

    c. Preexisting nerve damage (relative contraindication).

C. Interscalene block. A paravertebral approach that is useful for upper extremity, and, notably, shoulder surgery, interscalene block is achieved at the level of the cervical roots and can provide both brachial and cervical plexus blocks. Although this technique can be used for hand and forearm operations, <u>the lower cervical and T1 roots are occasionally spared, resulting in a failure of block in the ulnar distribution.</u>

1. **Technique**

   a. **Position.** In the supine position, the patient turns the head away from the side to be blocked. The arm is placed at the side with downward displacement of the shoulder to facilitate palpation of landmarks.

   b. **Landmarks.** The needle entry site is located between the <u>middle</u> and <u>anterior scalene</u> muscles <u>at the C6 level</u> (Fig. 13-8). The anterior scalene muscle lies below the posterior edge of the sternocleidomastoid. By rolling the fingers posteriorly over the anterior scalene muscle, a groove will be palpable between the anterior and middle scalene muscles, through which the roots of the brachial plexus pass in a vertical column. The intersection of this groove with a transverse plane at the <u>level of the cricoid cartilage is the point at which the needle should enter the skin (C6 level).</u>

   c. Prepare, drape, and infiltrate the skin with local anesthetic as usual.

   d. A 23-gauge, 1½-inch short-bevel needle is advanced through a wheal, <u>perpendicular to the skin in all planes</u> until a paresthesia is obtained (the direction should be 45 degrees caudal to a sagittal plane and 10–20 degrees posterior to a coronal plane). After the needle has been stabilized and aspirated to detect intravenous or subarachnoid placement, the total volume of anesthetic solution is slowly injected. If only brachial plexus block is desired, digital pressure superior to the needle can be applied to encourage caudad spread of anesthetic solution.

2. **Drugs and dosage.** The agents used are the same as for the axillary approach. Chloroprocaine should be used with caution because of possible subarachnoid injection (see sec. III.D.3).

3. **Complications**

   a. <u>**Inadvertent epidural or spinal** anesthesia</u> is a potentially serious complication resulting from incorrect needle placement.

   b. Local anesthetic drugs can be delivered directly to the cerebral circulation by **<u>vertebral artery injection.</u>** This can result in convulsions and loss of consciousness.

   c. **<u>Phrenic nerve block</u>** is frequently obtained; this complication precludes bilateral use of this technique.

   d. The <u>recurrent laryngeal</u>, <u>vagus</u>, and <u>cervical sympathetic nerves</u> are sometimes blocked.

   e. **<u>Pneumothorax</u>** is an infrequent complication

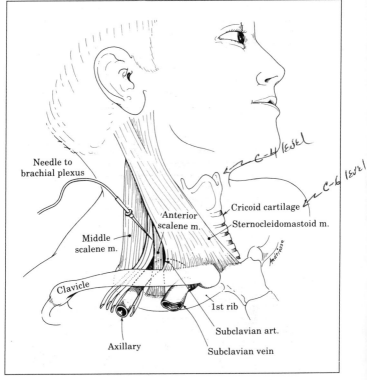

Fig. 13-8. Interscalene approach to brachial plexus block.

but can happen with inappropriately deep placement of needles.

 4. **Specific contraindications.** This technique should not be used in patients with diminished pulmonary reserve because of the possibility of causing unilateral diaphragmatic paralysis.

VI. **Ankle block** provides anesthesia for the foot by blocking five nerves at the level of the malleoli: the posterior tibial, sural, saphenous, deep peroneal, and superficial peroneal nerves. This block is useful for most operations limited to the foot.

 A. **Anatomy** (Fig. 13-9). The dorsum of the foot is innervated by the saphenous, the superficial peroneal, and the deep peroneal nerves. At the ankle, the saphenous nerve is superficial and located between the medial malleolus and the tendon of the anterior tibialis muscle. At the superior border of the malleoli, the deep peroneal nerve is located directly beneath, or beneath and medial to, the extensor hallucis longus tendon. More distally it is located lateral to the extensor hallucis longus tendon.

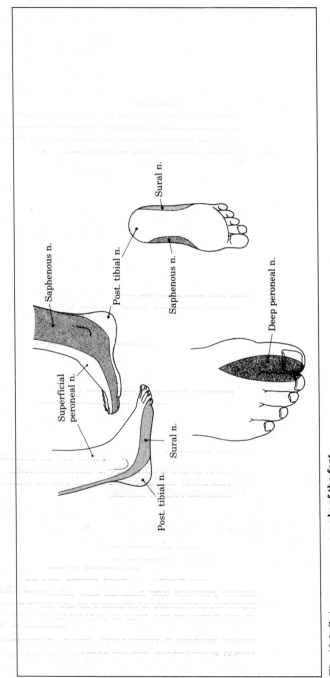

Fig. 13-9. Cutaneous nerve supply of the foot.

The superficial peroneal nerve can be found adjacent to the extensor digitorum longus. It often divides into terminal branches above the ankle. The branches descend superficially between the extensor hallucis longus tendon and the lateral malleolus. The posterior tibial nerve is located lateral to the posterior tibial artery, behind the medial malleolus. The sural nerve is located posterior to the lateral malleolus.

B. **Technique.** The deep peroneal, sural, and posterior tibial nerves are easily located by palpable landmarks. The saphenous and superficial peroneal nerves may be blocked along with the deep peroneal nerve using a single entry site. Following block of the deep peroneal nerve, anesthetic solution is infiltrated subcutaneously both medially and laterally to block the other two nerves.

Paresthesias are not mandatory for blocking these nerves. However, if obtained, they do assure correct needle placement and thereby reduce the total amount of anesthetic solution necessary.

1. **Position.** Patients may lie supine for block of the superficial peroneal, deep peroneal, and saphenous nerves. External and internal rotation of the leg with hip and knee flexion will allow access to the posterior tibial and sural nerves. If leg rotation is difficult, patients may be placed prone for these blocks.

2. The skin around the ankle and dorsum of the foot is prepared and draped as usual.

3. **Landmarks** (Fig. 13-10).

   a. The deep peroneal nerve is located between the anterior tibialis tendon and the extensor hallucis tendon on a cross section through the superior border of the malleoli. These tendons are easily palpable with dorsiflexion of the foot and extension of the great toe.

   b. The posterior tibial nerve is found behind the medial malleolus and lateral to the posterior tibial artery. The artery is usually palpable.

   c. The sural nerve is superficial and located behind the lateral malleolus, between it and the Achilles tendon.

4. A 23- or 25-gauge 1½- to 3½-inch needle is directed toward the lateral border of a palpable nerve. When the needle is at the same depth as the nerve or if a paresthesia is obtained, the needle is stabilized, and 3–5 ml of anesthetic solution is injected. To block the **deep peroneal nerve,** the needle is placed between the tendons and advanced until either a paresthesia is obtained in the distribution of the nerve or the tibia is contacted. If a paresthesia is obtained, then 3–5 ml of solution is injected; without a paresthesia, use 5–10 ml while slowly withdrawing. For the **saphenous nerve,** direct the needle medially, and infiltrate subcutaneously to the anterior surface of the medial malleo-

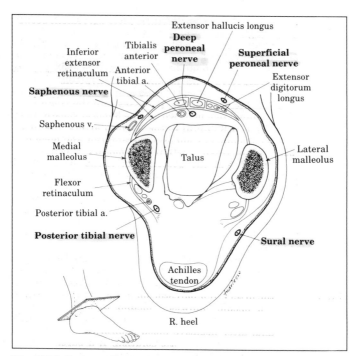

Fig. 13-10. Cross section at the level of the ankle.

lus. The **superficial peroneal nerve** is blocked by directing the needle laterally from the initial entry site and infiltrating subcutaneously to the anterior surface of the lateral malleolus. For the **posterior tibial nerve,** insert the needle posterior to the medial malleolus and direct it toward the lateral border of the posterior tibial artery. A paresthesia is usually obtained, but if not, then withdraw 1 cm from the point of bone contact and inject 5 ml.

For the **sural nerve,** the needle is placed just lateral to the Achilles tendon and directed superficially toward the posterior surface of the lateral malleolus. Without a paresthesia, slowly withdraw the needle from the point of bone contact and inject 5–8 ml.

C. **Drugs.** Any anesthetic agents suitable for peripheral nerve block can be used (see Chap. 12). However, epinephrine-containing solutions are not used because of possible end-artery vasoconstriction and subsequent tissue ischemia.

D. **Complications and contraindications.** The only specific contraindications are lack of patient consent and infection at a needle entry site. Preexisting foot ischemia, particularly in diabetics, is a relative contraindication and necessitates prior agreement between the surgeon and anesthesiologist.

VII. **Femoral and lateral femoral cutaneous nerve blocks.** These two nerves are blocked to biopsy the quadriceps muscle—for example, to obtain a diagnostic muscle biopsy from patients suspected of having malignant hyperthermia.

    A. **Anatomy.** The femoral nerve is formed from the posterior divisions of L2–L4. It passes into the thigh under the inguinal ligament within the femoral sheath. In the sheath, it lies lateral to the femoral artery. It supplies cutaneous innervation over the anterior and medial aspects of the thigh. The lateral femoral cutaneous nerve is formed from the posterior divisions of L2–L3. It passes into the thigh beneath the inguinal ligament and close to the anterior superior iliac spine. Cutaneous innervation to the lateral aspect of the thigh is provided by this nerve.

    B. **Technique**

        1. Prepare, drape, and raise a wheal at the site as usual.

        2. **Femoral nerve.** Palpate the femoral artery just below the inguinal ligament, and advance a 22-gauge, 1½-inch needle toward the lateral border of the artery. If a paresthesia is not obtained, redirect the needle "fanwise," medial to lateral, until a paresthesia is obtained. Then stabilize the needle and, after negative blood aspiration, inject 10–15 ml of local anesthetic solution. If a paresthesia is not obtained, the nerve can be blocked by injecting in a fanwise manner medial to lateral, from the lateral border of the femoral artery.

NAVL ➞ ○ (handwritten margin note)

        3. **Lateral femoral cutaneous nerve.** After the femoral nerve is blocked, withdraw the needle to the subcutaneous level and redirect it laterally along the lower border of the inguinal ligament. Inject 10 ml along the lower border of the inguinal ligament toward the anterior superior iliac spine (ASIS). A more direct approach is to place the needle 2–3 cm medial and 2–3 cm inferior to the ASIS. If a paresthesia is obtained, the needle is stabilized and 5 ml is injected. Without a paresthesia, inject 5–8 ml fanwise, medial to lateral.

    C. **Drugs.** See sec. **VI.C.**

    D. **Complications and contraindications.** See sec. **VI.D.**

VIII. **Intravenous regional anesthesia** (Bier block) is a simple way to produce analgesia and muscle relaxation in an extremity. It is performed by IV administration of local anesthetic distal to a tourniquet providing complete vascular occlusion.

    A. **Technique**

        1. **Intravenous access** is obtained by placement of a 20- to 22-gauge catheter in the distal extremity near the operative site. Attach a plastic extension tubing from the catheter to a 50-ml syringe.

2. **Place a pneumatic double tourniquet** proximal to the operative site.
3. **Exsanguinate the extremity** by application of an Esmarch bandage or by elevation when use of an Esmarch bandage is not possible. The bandage is applied, distal to proximal, and the tourniquet is inflated before removing the bandage.
4. **Inflate the proximal pneumatic tourniquet** above systolic blood pressure. If the tourniquet does not provide complete vascular occlusion, the anesthetic solution will escape from the extremity and gain access to the central circulation. Check pulses after tourniquet inflation to ensure arterial occlusion; (usually 250–300 mm Hg in the arm and 350–400 mm Hg in the legs). The local anesthetic solution is then injected and the IV catheter removed. The area anesthetized includes the distal extremity up to, but not including, the area beneath the proximal tourniquet. Once tourniquet discomfort begins, the second (distal) tourniquet can be inflated over an area already anesthetized. The proximal tourniquet is then deflated, and the patient will be better able to tolerate the tourniquet. In long operations, **tourniquet pain** is usually the limiting factor for success of this technique.
B. **Drugs and dosage.** Unlike other regional techniques, the duration of action is limited by tourniquet time rather than the agent. Patchy analgesia may remain after tourniquet release, but usually for less than 20 minutes. The amount of drug administered depends on the size of the extremity to be anesthetized. Average doses are 40–50 ml of lidocaine 0.5% for an arm and 100 ml of lidocaine 0.25% for a leg. Leg anesthesia should be undertaken only with extremely reliable tourniquets because of the large doses required. Obviously, agents should not be mixed with vasoconstrictors.
C. **Complications**
    1. **Local anesthetic drug toxicity.** Blood levels may be minimized by rapidly releasing and reinflating the tourniquet at the end of the procedure. In addition, the extremity should be kept immobile immediately after release of the tourniquet to minimize the increase in the central blood levels.
    2. **Nerve damage secondary to tourniquet application.** Tourniquet times should be as brief as possible and not exceed 2 hours. Tourniquet pressure should be continuously monitored with a manometer.
D. **Relative contraindications**
    1. Distal infection of the extremity.
    2. Ischemia of the involved extremity.
    3. Heart block.
    4. Seizure disorder.
    5. Sickle cell

Suggested Reading

Clemente, C. D. *Anatomy: A Regional Atlas of the Human Body.* Baltimore: Urban & S, 1981.

Cousins, M. J., and Bridenbaugh, P. O. *Neural Blockade in Clinical Anesthesia and Management of Pain.* Philadelphia: Lippincott, 1980.

Covino, B., and Scott, D. B. (eds.). *Handbook of Epidural Anesthesia and Analgesia.* Orlando, Fla.: Grune and Stratton, 1985.

Katz, J. *Atlas of Regional Anesthesia.* East Norwalk, Conn.: Appleton-Century-Crofts, 1985.

Lund, P. C. *Principles and Practice of Spinal Anesthesia.* Springfield, Ill.: Thomas, 1971.

Moore, D. C. *Regional Block: A Handbook for Use in the Clinical Practice of Medicine and Surgery* (4th ed.). Springfield, Ill.: Thomas, 1981.

14

Closed Circuit Anesthesia

W. Andrew Kofke and William B. Latta

This chapter presents a review of the basic concepts integral to an understanding of closed circuit anesthesia (CCA) and of various techniques of safe administration. The method described is primarily adapted from the work of Lowe and Ernst.

I. **Anesthetic circuits**
   A. **Open circuit.** The anesthetic gases are carried into the respiratory tract with atmospheric air. The respiratory tract is open to the atmosphere at all times during inspiration and expiration, and there is no rebreathing (e.g., open drop ether).
   B. **Semiopen circuit.** The anesthetic gases are carried into the respiratory tract by fresh gas inflow and may be diluted with atmospheric air. The respiratory tract is open to the atmosphere on both inspiration and expiration, except that a reservoir is placed in the circuit (e.g., Mapleson circuit). Some rebreathing of carbon dioxide can occur.
   C. **Semiclosed circuit.** The anesthetic gases are carried into the respiratory tract completely by fresh gas inflow and rebreathed gases. The respiratory tract and the reservoir are closed to the atmosphere on inspiration and are open to the atmosphere on expiration. Partial rebreathing can occur, although carbon dioxide is absorbed from the circuit.
   D. **Closed circuit.** Anesthetic gases are carried into the respiratory tract completely by the fresh gas inflow and rebreathed gases. The respiratory tract and the reservoir are closed to the atmosphere on both inspiration and expiration. Total rebreathing of exhaled gases occurs, except for carbon dioxide, which is absorbed.
II. **Anesthetic uptake.** When a gaseous anesthetic is delivered into an anesthetic circuit at a given concentration, the following factors act to alter the anesthetic concentration ultimately achieved in the brain.
   A. **Anesthetic circuit characteristics.** Several aspects of a semiclosed or closed circuit can produce an inspired anesthetic concentration different from that initially delivered into the circuit.
      1. **Circuit size** relative to fresh gas inflow rate. Equilibration of the circuit (plus the functional residual capacity) occurs more quickly at higher fresh gas flows. For example, a 10-liter circuit is 86% equilibrated after 2 minutes of a 10-L/min fresh gas flow, whereas approximately 10 minutes are required to achieve 86% equilibration of the same circuit with a 2-L/min fresh gas inflow.
      2. **Fresh gas inflow rate.** In addition to the factors described in sec. **1,** decreased fresh gas inflow rate to below the patient's minute volume produces re-

breathing. Thus, anesthetic-depleted exhaled gas is added to the inspiratory limb of the circuit, decreasing the concentration of inspired anesthetic.

3. **Solubility in circuit components.** Until anesthetic tubing and soda lime are fully equilibrated with the inflowing anesthetic, the inspired anesthetic concentration will be decreased by uptake of anesthetic by these components. In general, the more fat-soluble an anesthetic is, the more pronounced this effect will be. In addition, soda lime can absorb or release anesthetic in a fashion related to its state of hydration (see sec. **VI.B.1**).

B. **Rate of rise of anesthetic in alveoli.** In general, alveolar anesthetic concentration correlates with the concentration of anesthetic in the blood leaving the alveolus. Accordingly, factors affecting the rate of rise of the alveolar anesthetic concentration (relative to inspired concentration, F_A/F_I) can have pronounced effects on the speed of induction of anesthesia. Two opposing processes, anesthetic delivery to and uptake from alveoli determine the F_A/F_I at a given time after starting administration of a volatile anesthetic.

1. **Anesthetic delivery** is a prescribed constant in a closed system. In a nonrebreathing system, it can be altered by the following:

   a. **Alveolar ventilation.** Changes in alveolar ventilation have pronounced effects on F_A/F_I with effects being more pronounced with the more blood-soluble agents (higher $\lambda_{B/G}$; see Table 14-1). Increased ventilation, without alteration of other processes that affect anesthetic delivery or uptake, increases F_A/F_I (Fig. 14-1).

   b. **Ventilation-perfusion (V/Q) matching.** With constant $PaCO_2$ and increasing dead-space ventilation, increased ventilation of unperfused alveoli has little effect on the rate of rise of arterial anesthetic concentration. Conversely, with constant $PaCO_2$, decreased perfusion of ventilated alveoli (venous admixture) leads to a decreased rate of rise of arterial anesthetic concentration. This effect becomes more pronounced with the less soluble anesthetics (e.g., nitrous oxide).

   c. **Concentration effect.** With anesthetics requiring administration of high concentrations (e.g., nitrous oxide), uptake concentrates the remaining alveolar gas, and augments the input of additional gas (anesthetic) into alveoli to replace that lost by uptake.

   d. **The second gas effect.** When a first anesthetic, requiring high concentrations, such as nitrous oxide, is administered, uptake of large volumes of the first anesthetic increases delivery and accelerates the alveolar rate of rise of a second gas such as halothane.

Table 14-1. Properties of inhalational anesthetics

Gas	MAC (%)	$\lambda_{B/G}$*	Vapor pressure (20°C) (mm Hg)	Milliliters of vapor per milliliter of liquid (37°C)
Halothane	0.74	2.3	243 (0.32 atm)	240
Enflurane	1.68	1.8	175 (0.24 atm)	210
Isoflurane	1.15	1.4	239 (0.33 atm)	206
Methoxyflurane	0.16	10.2	23 (0.03 atm)	219
Nitrous oxide	104	0.47	39,000 (52 atm)	—

*$\lambda_{B/G}$ is the blood-gas partition coefficient.

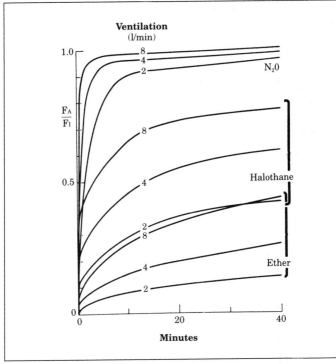

Fig. 14-1. The ratio of alveolar to inspired gas concentrations (F_A/F_I) as a function of time with varying minute ventilation. At constant cardiac output increasing minute ventilation increases the alveolar rate of rise of anesthetic concentration. This effect is more marked with anesthetics with higher blood solubility (e.g., ether), decreasing correspondingly with lower solubility (e.g., nitrous oxide). (From E. I. Eger. *Anesthetic Uptake and Action.* Baltimore: Williams & Wilkins, 1979.)

2. **Anesthetic uptake** can be altered by the following:

   a. **Cardiac output.** Increased cardiac output increases anesthetic uptake. However, in the absence of other changes in factors affecting F_A/F_I, increased cardiac output will slow the rise in alveolar concentration, with an opposite effect resulting from decreased cardiac output. These cardiac output effects occur in both rebreathing and nonrebreathing systems, although they are more pronounced in nonrebreathing circuits and early on in the course of anesthetic administration (Fig. 14-2).

   b. **Anesthetic solubility.** Increasing solubility in blood increases uptake, thereby slowing the rate of rise of F_A/F_I (see Table 14-1). Effects of changes in solubility are similar to those seen

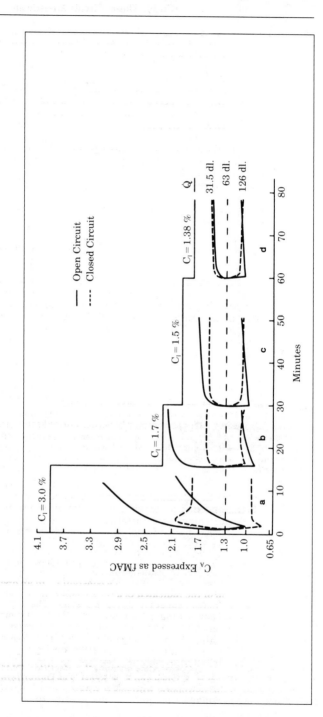

with changes in cardiac output. Solubility of halogenated volatile anesthetics in blood is increased somewhat with hypothermia and hyperlipidemia.

c. **Anesthetic loss.** Anesthetics can be lost from the body percutaneously and through visceral membranes and may be lost due to metabolism. Such percutaneous, visceral, and metabolic losses are probably negligible.

C. **Time constant for cerebral uptake of anesthetic.** The time constant for entry of an anesthetic into the brain is described by $(V \times \lambda_t)/f$, where V is brain volume, λ_t is the brain tissue–blood partition coefficient, and f is cerebral blood flow. The brain time constants (in minutes) for the commonly used volatile anesthetics are as follows:

Nitrous oxide	Halothane	Enflurane	Isoflurane
2.2	4.8	3.3	5.0

Three time constants are required for 95% equilibration of brain with blood to occur. Thus, even when the desired arterial concentration is achieved and maintained early in an anesthetic (as in the ideal closed circuit case), the desired cerebral concentration is not usually approached for 10–15 minutes (three time constants, assuming constant cerebral blood flow). Agents with higher tissue solubility will have longer time constants, as the "effective" tissue volume in which it can dissolve is greater. Conversely, increasing delivery of anesthetic agent to the brain with increased cerebral blood flow decreases the time constant.

D. **Opposing effects** commonly occur. For example, inhalation of halothane will act to decrease cardiac output ($\uparrow$ FA/FI) and decrease ventilation ($\uparrow$ FA/FI). In addition, nitrous oxide may be given concomitantly, thereby augmenting rate of rise of alveolar halothane concentration while the cerebral blood flow may have increased with halothane and hypoventilation, decreasing the time needed to achieve equilibration of brain and blood. Accordingly, the factors that can make the brain

---

Fig. 14-2. Alveolar halothane concentration as a function of time with variations in circuit type, cardiac output, and inspired halothane concentration. C_I indicates the inspired concentration initially required at each time interval to maintain a constant C_A in an open system. Continuation of the indicated C_I after a change in cardiac output produces the noted changes in C_A (open system). The horizontal line at 1.3 MAC and $\dot{Q} = 63$ dl represents the C_A that would be maintained with the proper reduction in delivered concentration with time in an open or closed system. The noted changes in C_A for a closed system presuppose reductions in delivered amounts of anesthetic vapor as required by a dosage schedule. C_A = alveolar anesthetic concentration, $\dot{Q}$ = cardiac output, dl = deciliter, fMAC = fraction of MAC. (From H. J. Lowe and E. A. Ernst. *The Quantitative Practice of Anesthesia.* Baltimore: Williams & Wilkins, 1981. Copyright 1981, The Williams & Wilkins Co.)

anesthetic concentration different from that on the vaporizer dial often oppose each other, and should be considered in an overall context.

III. **Advantages of closed circuit anesthesia**
   A. Additional monitoring of the patient is the most significant advantage.
      1. Oxygen consumption ($\dot{V}O_2$) equals inflow oxygen. Its measurement allows early detection of changes in the depth of anesthesia.
      2. Circuit volume is continually assessed and allows early detection of small circuit leaks.
      3. It facilitates assessment of lung compliance.
      4. Muscle relaxation can be assessed, because, at low flows, the reservoir bag or the ventilator bellows becomes a sensitive indicator of small diaphragmatic movements.
      5. Cardiac output changes become qualitatively apparent as changes in the uptake rate of anesthetic gas.
      6. With use of an upright bellows ventilator, the duration and rate of exhalation as well as spontaneous tidal volume (when the ventilator is turned off) may be visually determined.
   B. Circuit humidity is maintained at 92–100% (*Anaesth. Intensive Care* 1:415, 1973).
   C. The patient's body heat is conserved.
   D. Less anesthetic is used, with consequent financial saving.
   E. Operating room pollution by anesthetics is decreased.
   F. It is an excellent technique for learning uptake and distribution of anesthetics as well as the signs of anesthetic depth.
   G. Anesthetics can be precisely volatilized in the circuit without complex individual vaporizers for each agent.
   H. Nitrous oxide–free techniques using air-oxygen are easily done without air tanks and flowmeters.

IV. **Disadvantages and precautions**
   A. The CCA technique involves specific equipment requirements and cautions (see sec. **VI**).
   B. If nitrous oxide or nitrogen is used, an oxygen analyzer must be employed.
   C. Circuit contamination by nitrogen or other gases can result in delivery of less nitrous oxide than desired.
   D. If a ventilator is used and the circuit volume is not adequately monitored, the patient can conceivably be hypoventilated.
   E. Changes in the vaporizer settings take longer to be reflected in uptake from the alveolus.

V. **Basic theory of closed circuit anesthesia**
   A. **Definitions** (1 dl = 100 ml)

   C_A = alveolar concentration (ml vapor/dl)
   C_a = arterial concentration (ml vapor/dl)
   C_D = delivered gas concentration (ml vapor/dl) in fresh gas inflow
   MAC = minimal alveolar concentration (ml vapor/dl)

λ_t = tissue-blood partition coefficient

$\lambda_{B/G}$ = blood-gas partition coefficient

$\dot{Q}$ = cardiac output (dl/min)

$\dot{Q}_{AN}$ = anesthetic uptake rate (ml vapor/min)

Q_{AN} = total anesthetic uptake (ml vapor)

$\dot{V}O_2$ = minute O_2 consumption (ml/min)

$\dot{Q}_t$ = tissue blood flow (dl/min)

t = duration of anesthetic administration (min)

V_t = tissue volume (dl)

$\dot{V}_A$ = minute alveolar ventilation (dl/min)

B. At constant arterial concentration, the rate of whole body anesthetic vapor uptake, $\dot{Q}_{AN}$, at any time, t, after the start of anesthesia equals the sum of organ uptakes.

$$\dot{Q}_{AN} = Ca \sum \dot{Q}_t \exp\left(-\frac{\dot{Q}_t \times t}{V_t \times \lambda_t} \right)$$

C. It has been empirically determined that $\dot{Q}_{AN}$ can be approximated as follows:

$$\dot{Q}_{AN} = Ca \times \dot{Q} \times t^{-0.5}$$

With $Ca = CA \times \lambda_{B/G}$, integrating this equation gives the cumulative anesthetic dose, Q_{AN}, after a given period of anesthesia, t:

$$Q_{AN} = 2 \times Ca \times Q \times t^{+0.5}$$

and therefore $Q_{AN} \propto \sqrt{t}$ and $\dot{Q}_{AN} \propto 1/\sqrt{t}$. Thus, the amount of anesthetic vapor absorbed between squares of time is equal; that is, the amount absorbed between 0–1, 1–4, 4–9 . . . minutes is the same. This amount is called the **unit dose.**

1 Q_{AN} unit = 2 (Ca) ($\dot{Q}$) ($\sqrt{1}$),

2 Q_{AN} units = 2 (Ca) ($\dot{Q}$) ($\sqrt{4}$)

3 Q_{AN} units = 2 (Ca) ($\dot{Q}$) ($\sqrt{9}$), etc.

D. In a closed circuit, $\dot{Q}_{AN}$ is independent of ventilation.

VI. Equipment

A. The vaporizer (out of circuit) used for closed circuit anesthesia should be able to perform accurately at flow rates of 200 ml/min or less. There are limitations to accuracy with some vaporizers at low flows, with changes in nitrous oxide concentration, with positive-pressure ventilation, and with upstream oxygen flushing (*Anesth. Analg.* 59:359, 1980).

B. Carbon dioxide absorber

　1. Soda lime

　　a. The cannister should be large enough to accommodate the patient's breath in the intergranular space. Therefore, a minimum of 500 gm of soda lime is needed for the average size patient.

　　b. The soda lime should not be allowed to dry out. It begins to absorb carbon dioxide less effectively when it contains less than 15% water. In addition, when dry, soda lime can absorb significant amounts of volatile anesthetic, which is then released into the circuit with rehydration of the soda lime by exhaled water vapor.

    c. Halothane reacts with soda lime, producing CF_2CBrCl, which reaches a level of about 5 ppm after an hour of CCA (*Anesthesiology* 50:2, 1979). There is indirect evidence that it is a normal metabolite of halothane in humans but is toxic to mice at 250 ppm. It is rapidly cleared on opening the circuit.

   2. **Baralyme** does not absorb volatile anesthetics and does not become dehydrated with anhydrous flow (because the water of hydration is bound).

C. Circuit

   1. Rubber hoses tend to absorb significant amounts of volatile anesthetics. A relatively nonabsorptive circle with Baralyme and hoses of polyethylene, polyolefin, or polyurethane is ideal, absorbing only one-fifth as much anesthetic as rubber hoses and soda lime.

   2. The system should be airtight. Snug metal-to-metal connections tend to provide good airtight fits. Leaks can be detected by applying a wet scrub brush to joints and looking for bubbling at leaky connections.

   3. The expiratory valve should not be adjacent to the fresh gas inflow line, to ensure that all of the fresh gas reaches the patient.

D. Oxygen analyzer

   1. The oxygen analyzer should be calibrated, and its battery should be checked at the start of each anesthetic. It must be accurate at oxygen concentrations less than 30% and should be equipped with upper and lower concentration alarms.

   2. Polarographic oxygen analyzers, when erroneous, tend to register falsely low oxygen concentrations.

   3. The oxygen analyzer should be placed on the expiratory limb of the circuit, since this more closely approximates alveolar oxygen concentration.

E. Rotameters. It is preferred, but not essential, that the oxygen and nitrous oxide rotameters be accurate at low flows; if they are not, the advantage of quantifying oxygen consumption is lost. If there is no anesthetic in a Copper Kettle vaporizer, oxygen can be introduced utilizing its low-flow oxygen rotameter.

F. A T piece and syringe are required for the injection of liquid volatile anesthetic into the circuit (Fig. 14-3). A T-piece metal connector placed in the expiratory limb capped with a one-holed stopper may be used to inject liquid anesthetic. A catheter plug (PRN adapter) may be useful to insert into the hole in the stopper to make it airtight. A three-way stopcock is inserted through a needle into the catheter plug. A syringe should be attached to the stopcock horizontally to minimize the risk of accidental discharge of its entire contents into the circuit. The stopcock must be turned off to the circuit when

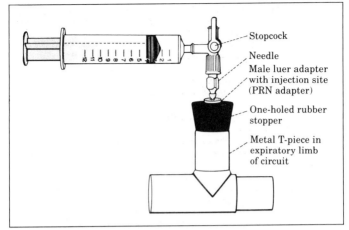

Fig. 14-3. Apparatus for injection of liquid anesthetic directly into the circuit as part of closed circuit anesthesia.

not injecting. To prevent accidental IV injection, the syringe should be labeled in unmistakable fashion and should never be left on the drug tray.

G. Timer. A stopwatch or electronic timer is useful early in the anesthesia but is not essential.

H. Ventilators. Only ventilators with upright bellows can be used. By not allowing the bellows to inflate fully and "pop off," the anesthetist can assess the breath-to-breath gas volume of the circuit.

VII. **Principles of closed circuit anesthesia administration**

A. Prior to starting, it is useful to approximate anticipated metabolic needs based on the patient's weight in kilograms (Table 14-2):

$$kg^{3/4} \times 10 = \dot{V}O_2 \text{ (ml/min)}$$

$$kg^{3/4} \times 8 = \dot{V}CO_2 \text{ (ml/min)}$$

$$kg^{3/4} \times 2 = \dot{Q} \text{ (100 ml/min) (assume}$$

$$[a - v]O_2 = 5 \text{ vol \%)}$$

$$kg^{3/4} \times 1.6 = \dot{V}A \text{ (100 ml/min)}$$

(for 5 vol % alveolar CO_2 concentration)

B. The gas volume and the F_EO_2 of the circuit are kept constant by manipulation of nitrous oxide and oxygen flow rates.

C. Unless nitrogen–oxygen is the desired gas mixture, the patient must be denitrogenated prior to closing the circuit. After the start of the anesthetic, nitrogen will be released from tissues (approximately 15 ml/kg) (*Br. J. Anaesth.* 47:350, 1975), resulting in lowering of nitrous

Table 14-2. Relationship of weight to physiologic variables

Kilograms	$\dot{V}O_2$ (ml/min)	$\dot{Q}$ (100 ml/min)	$Kg^{3/4}$
5	33	6.7	3.3
10	56	11	5.6
20	95	19	9.5
30	128	26	12.8
40	159	32	15.9
50	188	38	18.8
60	216	43	21.6
70	242	48	24.2
80	268	54	26.8
90	292	58	29.2
100	316	63	31.6

oxide concentrations. Therefore, to maintain the appropriate nitrous oxide concentration and wash out accumulated volatile metabolites, the circuit should be opened with high flows for approximately 5 minutes every 1–3 hours.

D. **Dose**

1. The anesthetic dose decreases over the course of the anesthesia in a predictable manner, so that dosage schedules can be derived, as will be shown. However, it must always be borne in mind that **the anesthetic dose ultimately must be titrated to match patient needs.**

2. As noted earlier, the cumulative anesthetic dose is directly proportional to the square root of time, so that the same dose—the unit dose—is likely to be given between each square of time after induction (1, 4, 9, 16 . . . minutes) to match predicted tissue uptake. Thus, one unit dose should be taken up by 1 minute after induction, two doses by 4 minutes, three doses by 9 minutes, and so on. This calculation, however, does not account for the amount of anesthetic needed to prime the circuit, nor does it account for uptake by the circuit tubing or carbon dioxide absorber. Consequently, in the average adult, one extra unit dose, the priming dose, is usually given in the first 9 minutes or prior to surgical incision, as tolerated or indicated by the patient's clinical condition. The priming dose may be less than the unit dose in very large patients or may be larger than the unit dose in very small patients.

3. The dosage used corresponds to approximately 1.3 MAC (i.e., approximately effective dose in 95% of patients). For each percent of nitrous oxide used, the MAC for the other volatile anesthetic used decreases by approximately 1%. At any given time af-

ter induction, volatile anesthetic uptake rate is as follows:

$$\dot{Q}_{AN} = f \times MAC \times \lambda_{B/G} \times t^{-0.5}$$

where $f = 1.3 - \% N_2O/100$.

Vapor unit dose (ml) $= 2 \times f \times MAC \times \lambda_{B/G} \times \dot{Q}$

and the unit dose of liquid anesthetic equals about $\frac{1}{200}$ of the vapor unit dose.

4. Utilizing these equations, a unit dose, and therefore a dosage schedule, can be derived for any volatile anesthetic (Tables 14-1 to 14-4).
5. The actual rate of uptake of nitrous oxide is 70% of predicted; therefore, the calculated unit dose for nitrous oxide must be multiplied by 0.70.

E. The anesthetic can enter the circuit as follows:
   1. **Via vaporizer.** This provides a rather steady concentration of anesthetic in the circuit, although there are the aforementioned limitations to accuracy with some vaporizers. In addition, it can be difficult to administer enough anesthetic during induction.
   2. **Via Copper Kettle.** This also provides a steady concentration of anesthetic, and higher concentrations can be achieved than with a vaporizer. However, it can be difficult maintaining a constant total oxygen flow, and with enflurane or methoxyflurane it is impossible to give enough anesthetic in the first few time periods without exceeding the patient's $\dot{V}O_2$.
   3. **Via injection of liquid anesthetic into the circuit.** This provides a mode of introducing any amount of anesthetic into the circuit but produces fluctuations in the concentrations of anesthetic in the circuit.

VIII. **Conduct of closed circuit anesthesia**
   A. **Checking the equipment**
      1. An oxygen analyzer is placed in the expiratory limb and calibrated. The batteries are checked, and the low oxygen alarm is set at 0.3–0.4.
      2. The carbon dioxide absorber is inspected.
      3. The circuit is examined for leaks.
      4. Circuit compression volume can be measured by occluding the patient port of the circuit, which is connected to a volume ventilator. The ventilator is turned on and adjusted through a series of small volumes, generating circuit pressures in the physiologic range, thereby developing the compliance curve for that circuit.
      5. Rotameters can be calibrated by connecting the circuit to a known volume (e.g., an upright bellows ventilator) and measuring the time to expand the bellows a known volume at a rotameter flow rate of 50–300 ml/min.
   B. The patient is denitrogenated for 3–5 minutes with ox-

Table 14-3. Unit doses of volatile anesthetics (ml)[a]

Weight (kg)[b]	Phase	Halothane	Enflurane	Isoflurane	Methoxyflurane	65% N2O
10	Vapor	50	92	55	47	475
	Liquid	0.21	0.44	0.27	0.21	
20	Vapor	86	160	95	81	813
	Liquid	0.36	0.76	0.46	0.36	
30	Vapor	116	215	128	108	1095
	Liquid	0.48	1.02	0.62	0.49	
40	Vapor	145	269	160	136	1368
	Liquid	0.61	1.28	0.78	0.62	
50	Vapor	172	319	190	161	1625
	Liquid	0.72	1.52	0.92	0.74	
60	Vapor	195	361	215	182	1839
	Liquid	0.81	1.72	1.04	0.83	
70	Vapor	218	403	240	204	2053
	Liquid	0.91	1.92	1.16	0.93	
80	Vapor	241	445	265	225	2267
	Liquid	1.00	2.12	1.29	1.03	
90	Vapor	264	487	290	246	2481
	Liquid	1.10	2.32	1.41	1.12	
100	Vapor	286	529	315	267	2694
	Liquid	1.20	2.52	1.53	1.22	

[a]Doses of anesthetic at 1.3 MAC (except N2O) given in O2 or O2—N2. All doses are halved if given in 65% N2O.
[b]Effects of absorption by the circuit are more pronounced at lower weights.

ygen at 6–10 L/min, after which time he is intravenously anesthetized. At this point, closed circuit anesthesia through a tight-fitting mask can begin, or the patient is paralyzed and intubated, after which CCA starts.

C. Over the first 9 minutes, about four unit doses of volatile anesthetic are introduced into the circuit.

  1. If nitrous oxide is to be used, it is given at 5–8 L/min, initially with the oxygen off, until the FeO_2 is approximately 0.3–0.4, at which time the oxygen is reintroduced at the $\dot{V}O_2$ rate. During this period and subsequently, the nitrous oxide rate is decreased to maintain approximately constant circuit volume and FeO_2 at approximately 0.3. Thus, FeO_2 and circuit volume are the main determinants of nitrous oxide flow. The dosage schedule for nitrous oxide is consulted secondarily.

  2. Coincident with the introduction of nitrous oxide, the four unit doses of volatile anesthetic are introduced over the first 9 minutes as tolerated, or required, by the patient's clinical status.

  3. If a vaporizer is used, it should not be turned on until the circuit is primed with nitrous oxide.

D. After the initial 9-minute induction period, closed circuit anesthesia is continued, giving approximately one unit dose per time interval, each interval being the period between the squares of time after induction (0–1, 1–4, 4–9, 9–16, 16–25 . . . minutes).

E. If controlled mechanical ventilation is utilized, the circuit volume of compression can be significant at such low flows. V_T, the tidal volume on the ventilator, is not equivalent to the tidal volume delivered to the patient but is as follows:

$$V_T = \dot{V}A/RR + V_D + V_{comp}$$

$\dot{V}A$ = desired minute ventilation (ml/min), RR = respiratory rate/min, V_D = anatomic dead space (1 ml/kg intubated), and V_{comp} = circuit volume of compression (ml).

After $\dot{V}O_2$ is determined, ventilator V_T can be adjusted to yield a desired $PaCO_2$, assuming a normal respiratory quotient and a barometric pressure of 760 mm Hg.

$$PaCO_2 = \frac{570 \times \dot{V}O_2}{RR \times (V_T - V_D - V_{comp})}$$

F. Circuit leak with spontaneous ventilation is essentially nonexistent. With controlled ventilation, after relatively steady-state conditions are obtained, circuit leak can be estimated by turning the ventilator off for 60 seconds and noting the volume through which the bellows rise, an amount that approximates the leak.

G. If the seal between the circuit and the environment is broken at any time, room air nitrogen enters the circuit, and high flows are needed for approximately 5 minutes to denitrogenate.

Table 14-4. Anesthetic dosage schedule (70-kg patient in 65% N_2O; $\dot{V}O_2 = 242$)[a]

| Unit doses | | | Halothane | | | | Enflurane | | | | Isoflurane | | | | N_2O |
| | | | 109 ml Vapor | | 0.46 ml Liquid | | 202 ml Vapor | | 0.96 ml Liquid | | 120 ml Vapor | | 0.58 ml Liquid | | 2053 ml Vapor |
t	Δt	√t	Vapor (ml/min)	Kettle O_2 (ml/min)	Vaporizer[b] (%)	Total liquid (ml)	Vapor (ml/min)	Kettle O_2 (ml/min)	Vaporizer[b] (%)	Total liquid (ml)	Vapor (ml/min)	Kettle O_2 (ml/min)	Vaporizer[b] (%)	Total liquid (ml)	Vapor (ml/min)
0		0													
	1		48	96	4.9	0.6	90	270	8.9	1.3	53	106	5.4	0.8	684
1		1													
	3		48	96	4.9	1.2	90	270	8.9	2.6	53	106	5.4	1.5	684
4		2													
	5		48	96	4.9	1.8	90	270	8.9	3.8	53	106	5.4	2.3	684
9		3													
	7		16	32	2.9	2.3	29	90	5.1	4.8	17	34	3.1	2.9	293
16		4													
	9		12	24	2.5	2.8	22	66	4.5	5.8	13	26	2.8	3.5	228
25		5													
	11		10	20	2.3	3.2	18	54	4.1	6.7	11	22	2.5	4.1	187
36		6													
	13		8	16	2.1	3.7	16	48	3.7	7.7	9	18	2.2	4.6	158
49		7													

			7	14	1.9	4.1	13	39	3.4	8.6	8	16	2.1	5.2	137
15	8	64	6	12	1.7	4.6	12	36	3.1	9.6	7	14	1.9	5.8	121
17	9	81	6	12	1.6	5.1	11	33	3.0	10.6	6	12	1.8	6.4	108
19	10	100													

[a]Schedule for first 9 minutes represents 3 unit doses plus priming dose.
[b]Vaporizer dosage schedules are valid at all patient weights.

H. The patient should be given a high-flow anesthetic for 5–10 minutes every 1–3 hours. During these periods, the volatile anesthetic should be administered through a vaporizer at a clinically indicated concentration.

I. The format can be altered in the following ways:

1. The anesthesia can be induced with a semiclosed circuit for a period of time (9 minutes or more) and then can be closed. This variation is particularly useful if adequate denitrogenation is not feasible with the patient awake or if a more prolonged induction is desired.

2. The anesthesia can be done without nitrous oxide, thereby doubling the unit dose of volatile anesthetic (over the dose given with 65% nitrous oxide). Room air can be conveniently added to the circuit as needed by connecting the bulb and tubing from a sphygmomanometer to an unused port on a stopcock on the T-piece portal in the circuit. (See Fig. 14-3.)

3. The anesthesia can be done with nitrous oxide–narcotic-hypnotic without the volatile anesthetics.

4. The patient can be allowed to breathe spontaneously or can be ventilated with either an upright bellows ventilator or by reservoir bag. If the ventilator is used, it is maintained so that the bellows never fully inflates, thereby providing the most quantitative means of assessing and maintaining constant circuit volume.

5. Closed circuit anesthesia is usually done with the patient intubated, but it can also be done with a tight-fitting mask, accepting no leak.

J. Example. A 70-kg patient receiving a halothane–nitrous oxide (65%) anesthetic has a predicted $\dot{V}O_2 = 242$ ml/min. The unit dose of halothane = 109 ml vapor, or 0.46 ml liquid (see Table 14-4).

1. Check the equipment, and set the oxygen analyzer's low oxygen alarm at 0.35.

2. Denitrogenate the patient with mask oxygen.

3. Induce with thiopental, and intubate using succinylcholine.

4. Give nitrous oxide at 5–8 L/min with the oxygen off. Decrease the nitrous oxide flow as circuit volume dictates. When FEO_2 is approximately 0.35–0.40, reintroduce oxygen at 240 ml/min. Manipulate nitrous oxide and oxygen flows as indicated by FEO_2 and circuit volume, aiming for $FEO_2 = 0.30$.

5. Introduce halothane into the circuit after the circuit has been primed with nitrous oxide.

   a. When given by vaporizer, the halothane concentration is set at approximately 5% for the first 9 minutes, then is decreased to approximately 3.0% from 9–16 minutes, then approximately 2.6% from 16–25 minutes, and so on, according to the dosage schedule, with alterations as dictated by the patient's clinical status.

   b. When halothane is given by Copper Kettle, the

kettle oxygen is set at 96 ml/min for the first 9 minutes to introduce the first four-unit doses and altered thereafter according to the dosage schedule, with further alterations as dictated by the patient's clinical status.

   c. When the halothane is given by injection of liquid into the circuit, the first 9-minute, four-unit dose requirement of 1.8 ml is given in increments of 0.2–0.4 ml. Thereafter, the patient receives about 0.46 ml of liquid halothane per time interval.

6. Ventilate the patient with a bellows-up ventilator, adjusting flows to keep FEO_2 about 0.30 and to keep the bellows about 100 ml short of completely filling and popping off gases.

7. Every 1–3 hours, run the circuit at 2 L/min of oxygen and 4 L/min of nitrous oxide with 0.5–1.0% halothane for 5 minutes.

8. Discontinue halothane approximately one to two time intervals before the anticipated end of the operation.

9. Open the circuit with 100% oxygen to speed emergence.

Suggested Reading

Aldrete, J. A., Lowe, H. J., and Virtue, R. W. (eds.). *Low Flow and Closed System Anesthesia*. New York: Grune & Stratton, 1979.

Eger, E. I. *Anesthetic Uptake and Action*. Baltimore: Williams & Wilkins, 1974.

Goldberg, I. S., et al. A pharmacokinetic model of closed circuit inhalation anesthesia. *Ann. Biomed. Eng.* 6:231, 1978.

Lowe, H. J. *Dose-Regulated Penthrane Methoxyflurane Anesthesia*. Chicago: Abbott Laboratories, 1972.

Lowe, H. J., et al. Quantitative closed circuit anesthesia. *Anesthesiol. Rev.* 1:16, 1974.

Lowe, H. J., and Ernst, E. A. *The Quantitative Practice of Anesthesia*. Baltimore: Williams & Wilkins, 1981.

Severinghaus, J. W. The rate of uptake of nitrous oxide in man. *J. Clin. Invest.* 33:1183, 1954.

Waters, D. J., and Mapleson, W. W. Exponentials and the anaesthetist. *Anaesthesia* 19:274, 1964.

15

Common Intraanesthetic Problems

Philip W. Lebowitz

I. **Airway control**
  A. **Securing and maintaining a patent airway** is essential for safe anesthesia.
    1. Selecting a **face mask** that provides an airtight seal prevents loss of the anesthetic agent and allows for the use of positive-pressure ventilation. A good fit may be difficult on edentulous patients, as well as on those with a prominent nose, receding jaw, or indwelling nasogastric tube. The application of mask straps may obviate this problem. When necessary, stuffing gauze pads into the cheeks of edentulous patients may provide an acceptable seating for a mask fit.
    2. **Once induction has occurred,** the patient's jaw may relax and the tongue may fall backward, obstructing the glottis. Lifting the jaw forward and upward into a prognathic position by exerting pressure behind the vertical ramus of the mandible and hyperextending the neck to carry the tongue farther forward and upward should solve this problem. The latter maneuver is most easily performed by applying firm, yet gentle, pressure upward against the mandibular mentum. In addition, placing a lubricated oropharyngeal or nasopharyngeal airway (provided the anesthetic level is deep enough) often relieves the obstruction. Turning the head to a lateral position is another useful technique.
    3. **Glottic obstruction,** ranging from mild to acutely life-threatening, can be caused by acute epiglottitis, laryngospasm, subglottic edema and/or stenosis, and the presence of foreign bodies (e.g., poorly chewed food, teeth, dentures, blood, mucus, and vomitus). The removal of such foreign bodies by hand, suction, or Magill forceps can be lifesaving.
    4. **Airway obstruction** may be revealed by snoring sounds, by the failure of the reservoir bag to empty and fill with the respiratory cycle, and by "rocking" movements of the chest and abdomen. Rocking is seen when the chest retracts rather than expands as the diaphragm descends with inspiration.
  B. Glottic obstruction cannot occur in the presence of a **tracheostomy appliance or an endotracheal tube.** However, airway obstruction may still be seen
    1. When foreign material occludes the lumen.
    2. When aspiration of foreign material blocks the distal bronchial tree.
    3. When the endotracheal tube kinks.
    4. When the balloon cuff herniates over the end of the

tube or compresses the endotracheal tube lumen
from without.

C. Placing the tracheostomy appliance in a false passageway or placing the endotracheal tube in the esophagus
will not secure a patent airway.

D. Do not, unless necessity dictates otherwise, paralyze a
patient in anticipation of placing an endotracheal tube
until it has been determined that the patient can be
ventilated by mask should the intubation attempt prove
unsuccessful.

II. Apnea and ventilatory inadequacy

A. Making the distinction between **central depression of
respiration** and **inadequate strength in the muscles of respiration** is important in guiding therapy.

1. The primary drive to breathe issues from the **medulla** in response to an elevated $PaCO_2$. Severe
neurologic dysfunction of this medullary center as
a result of edema, compression, or invasion can
cause irregular breathing and even apnea.

2. **Controlled ventilation** that lowers the $PaCO_2$ below normal levels will cause apnea until the $PaCO_2$
rises to restart spontaneous ventilation in normal
patients.

3. Apnea may occur in patients who **chronically retain carbon dioxide** if the $PaCO_2$ falls below their
usual level.

4. Other central causes of hypoventilation are narcotics, barbiturates and benzodiazepines, both as premedicants and as anesthetics, and narcotics that
are given epidurally or intrathecally.

   a. **Narcotics.** Intrathecal morphine is more likely
   to cause respiratory depression than is epidural
   morphine; epidural fentanyl is safer still. When
   apnea does occur after intrathecal or epidural
   morphine, it results from rostral spread and
   may be seen several hours after administration. A narcotic overdose from any route may be
   reversed specifically by naloxone (Narcan).
   Naloxone should be given slowly in increments
   of 0.01 mg to reverse the respiratory depression, avoiding the acute onset of pain or anxiety. Because of the shorter half-life of naloxone,
   it is important to observe the patient for 20–40
   minutes after giving naloxone to be certain that
   respiratory depression does not recur. If breathing becomes inadequate on the basis of prolonged narcotic effect, either another dose of
   naloxone may be administered or the patient
   may be ventilated. Nalbuphine (Nubain), a
   narcotic agonist-antagonist, may also be given
   to reverse narcotic-induced respiratory depression without complete loss of analgesia.

   b. **Barbiturates** have no comparable reversal
   agent. However, the breath holding commonly
   seen in anesthetic induction with barbiturates

is transient and can be treated with controlled ventilation.

    c. **Benzodiazepines,** such as diazepam or midazolam, may cause respiratory depression when given in high doses or in old or debilitated patients. Benzodiazepine antagonists are now experimental and are not clinically available.

  5. **Inhalational agents,** such as halothane, enflurane, and isoflurane, depress respiration and may produce hypoventilation in deeper planes of anesthesia. Additionally, in lighter planes, **noxious stimuli,** such as periosteal irritation and traction on the peritoneum or diaphragm, may reflexly stop respiration for a brief period.

  B. Peripheral causes of hypoventilation usually stem from the use of **muscle relaxants.**

    1. Prolonged block from the use of succinylcholine is caused either by its inadequate hydrolysis by plasma cholinesterase or by a phase II (nondepolarizing) block, which may occur when large amounts of the drug are used.

    2. Nondepolarizing muscle relaxation may persist because of overdose, particularly in patients with myasthenia gravis and in patients with renal and hepatic failure. Similarly, insufficient reversal by anticholinesterase agents will allow the block to continue. In addition, hypothermia, hypokalemia, respiratory alkalosis, or the use of local anesthetics, magnesium sulfate, quinidine, or absorbed antibiotics, such as aminoglycosides and polymyxin B, may potentiate the block.

    3. Monitoring evoked muscle strength with a twitch or train-of-four peripheral nerve stimulator can prevent excessive or continued neuromuscular blockade from going unrecognized.

  C. Other reasons for inadequate muscle strength include **high spinal anesthesia** and **quadriplegia.**

  D. **Surgical packing of the upper abdomen** may hinder diaphragmatic movement, and **splinting postoperatively** due to pain from thoracic or upper abdominal incisions may result in hypoventilation.

III. Hypotension

  A. Hypotension represents a significant lowering of systemic arterial blood pressure below the patient's normal range. Generally, it may derive from a combination of decreased intravascular volume, decreased venous or arterial tone (or both), and decreased cardiac output.

  B. **Decreased intravascular volume** may result from

    1. Hypovolemia due to acute hemorrhage.

    2. Volume loss from vomiting, diarrhea, enteric drains or fistulas, or cathartic bowel preparation.

    3. Polyuria secondary to diabetes mellitus, diabetes insipidus, or high-output acute tubular necrosis; or diuresis from diuretic drugs, radiographic dye, or relief of urinary obstruction.

4. Adrenal insufficiency. An Addisonian patient or one treated with steroids prior to surgery may have a marginal adrenal reserve, which may prove insufficient during the stress of surgery unless additional steroids are given. Hydrocortisone (Solu-Cortef), 300 mg daily, will cover surgical stress; 100 mg should be given IV preoperatively and a second 100 mg during surgery.

C. **Venous return may be decreased by**

1. Surgical compression of the inferior or superior vena cava.

2. Pneumothorax, which may distort the great vessels by mediastinal shift.

3. Increased airway pressure, especially with large tidal-volume mechanical ventilation, or positive end-expiratory pressure, or both. The magnitude of respiratory variation in arterial blood pressure indicates the degree of hypovolemia.

4. Increased venous capacitance, as caused by nitroprusside, nitroglycerin, or sympathetic block.

D. **Arteriolar resistance may also be lowered** by

1. Sympathetic block, as in spinal or epidural anesthesia.

2. Drugs, such as vasodilators (nitroprusside, nitroglycerin, hydralazine), alpha-adrenergic blockers (droperidol, chlorpromazine, phentolamine), histamine releasers (d-tubocurarine, morphine), and ganglionic blockers (trimethaphan).

3. Inhalation anesthetics, because they lower central catecholamine release and act as direct vasodilators.

4. Septic shock.

E. **Myocardial dysfunction**

1. Halothane, enflurane, and isoflurane cause negative inotropic effects upon the heart.

2. Propranolol, by blocking cardiac beta receptors, may decrease cardiac output and lower systemic pressure.

3. Coronary artery disease, ventricular dysfunction, valvular heart disease, acute myocardial infarction, pulmonary embolism, and rhythm or conduction disturbances may each contribute to decreased cardiac output and hypotension.

4. Vagal reflexes may decrease inotropy and will produce bradycardia, leading to hypotension.

5. Systemically absorbed local anesthetics in large doses may cause cardiac depression.

6. Barbiturates depress cardiac output.

F. **Arterial hypotension may be treated** by

1. First and foremost, using volume expansion, pressor drugs, or both to improve cardiac filling.

2. Repositioning the patient toward the Trendelenburg posture to increase venous return. Avoiding reverse Trendelenburg or sitting positions when the patient is or has been rendered hypovolemic

will head off this difficulty.

3. Choosing anesthetic agents that do not worsen the hypotension or discontinuing the anesthetic in cases of severe hypotension.

4. Correcting of mechanical causes by placing a chest tube for pneumothorax, reducing or eliminating positive end-expiratory pressure, changing from mechanical ventilation to hand ventilation, or relieving obstruction of the venae cavae. Turning a pregnant patient onto her side (usually the left) will move the gravid uterus off the inferior vena cava. Adequately supporting the chest and pelvis with the patient in the prone position will prevent compression of the inferior vena cava as well.

5. Improving cardiac output by decreasing myocardial oxygen consumption in the ischemic heart.

6. Treating cardiac rhythm disturbances.

7. Adding positive inotropic drugs to increase stroke volume.

8. Cardiac pacing or employing vagolytic drugs to increase heart rate.

IV. Hypertension

A. The most common cause of high systemic blood pressure during anesthesia is **preexisting hypertension** that is not well controlled. In addition, **increased intracranial pressure** developing during anesthesia may be signaled by hypertension.

B. **Catecholamine release** causing hypertension is seen both in patients with preexisting disease and in normal patients in response to anesthesia that is too light for a given stimulus. Pheochromocytoma in particular may become unmasked for the first time under anesthesia.

1. Catecholamine release may be due to pain or excitement, especially during induction and emergence from anesthesia.

2. Catecholamine release is notably present during tracheal intubation.

3. Two other causes for catecholamine release are a high $PaCO_2$ and a low PaO_2. Here, hypertension will be present until bradycardia and hypotension supervene from myocardial ischemia.

C. **Iatrogenic or preventable causes of hypertension** include

1. Pressors such as ephedrine and phenylephrine.

2. Vagolytic drugs, such as pancuronium and gallamine.

3. Ketamine.

4. Prolonged tourniquet application during peripheral procedures.

5. Hypervolemia from overhydration.

6. Full bladder in anesthetized patients.

D. **Significant hypertension during anesthesia may be treated** by

1. Most importantly, deepening the anesthesia in parallel with the change in surgical stimulus.

2. Anesthetizing the airway with local anesthetics prior to intubation.
3. Sedating the anxious patient.
4. Preventing hypercarbia and hypoxia through adequate ventilation.
5. Using the following kinds of drugs:
   a. Anesthetics with myocardial depressant action (halothane, thiopental).
   b. Direct vasodilators (nitroprusside, nitroglycerin, hydralazine).
   c. Narcotics and muscle relaxants that release histamine (morphine, *d*-tubocurarine).
   d. Alpha-adrenergic blockers (phentolamine, droperidol).
   e. Beta-adrenergic blockers (propranolol).
   f. Ganglionic blockers (trimethaphan).
   g. Beta- and selective alpha$_1$-adrenergic blockers (labetalol).

V. Bradycardia

A. Although occasionally seen in healthy individuals, a heart rate slower than 60 beats/min is usually caused by intrinsic disease, by vagal reflexes, or by vagotonic medications.
1. **Intrinsic cardiac diseases** include
   a. Sick sinus syndrome.
   b. Complete (third-degree) heart block.
   c. Acute myocardial infarction.
   d. A failing myocardium.
2. The following stimuli initiate **vagus-mediated slowing of the sinoatrial node:**
   a. Traction on the peritoneum or spermatic cord.
   b. Direct eye pressure or traction on an extraocular muscle.
   c. Direct pressure on the vagus or the carotid sinus during neck or intrathoracic surgery.
   d. Centrally mediated anxiety or pain responses, such as during IV catheter placement (vagal reaction).
   e. A Valsalva maneuver.
   f. Suctioning the oropharynx or laryngoscopy in neonates and infants.
3. **Medications that slow heart rate** include
   a. Succinylcholine, when given to neonates and young children, and when given to adults twice within a 2–10-minute period.
   b. Anticholinesterase agents (neostigmine, pyridostigmine, edrophonium).
   c. Propranolol.
   d. Digoxin.
   e. Narcotics (though not meperidine).
   f. Phenylephrine (reflex bradycardia).
4. **Increased intracranial pressure** may result in bradycardia along with systemic hypertension and irregular respiration.
5. **Hypoxia,** when severe in adults and moderately so

in infants, will slow the heart rate.

B. Treatment

1. In patients with sick sinus syndrome or complete heart block, a pacing wire should be inserted prior to surgery.

2. For bradycardia due to vagal reflexes, rapid discontinuation of the provocative stimulation may be sufficient, but atropine may be needed as well.

3. For bradycardia caused by vagal stimulation, atropine, 0.3–0.8 mg IV, depending on the severity of the slowing, is the treatment of choice, but 0.02 mg/kg IV is suggested for administration with anticholinesterase reversal of muscle relaxants.

4. After a myocardial infarction, the abolition of severe bradycardia is even more important than usual, since premature ventricular contractions may induce fatal ventricular tachyarrhythmias. A pacing wire or chronotropic agents, such as isoproterenol or epinephrine, may be indicated in particular cases.

5. Vagolytic drugs, such as pancuronium and gallamine, and ephedrine, as a beta stimulant, will all increase heart rate.

VI. Tachycardia

A. Sinus tachycardia, or a heart rate of 100–160 beats/min in an adult and up to 200 beats/min in an infant, may be seen in the following situations:

1. Hypotension or hypovolemia. Relative hypovolemic states, such as adrenocortical insufficiency, septic shock, or transfusion reaction can elicit the same response (an increased heart rate), which raises cardiac output.

2. Catecholamine release caused by anxiety and by noxious stimuli when anesthesia is too light.

3. Hypoxia.

4. Hypercarbia.

5. Fever.

6. Malignant hyperthermia.

7. Pheochromocytoma.

8. Thyrotoxicosis.

9. Myocardial infarction or pulmonary embolism.

B. Medications that increase heart rate include pancuronium, gallamine, isoproterenol, epinephrine, dopamine, atropine, and ephedrine.

C. Tachyarrhythmias

1. **Atrial fibrillation** (atrial rate 350–600) with rapid ventricular response may be seen with an ischemic myocardium, with mitral valvular disease, with hyperthyroidism, or with excessive sympathetic stimulation. Rapid atrial arrhythmias commonly develop following pneumonectomy or when the heart has been excessively manipulated. The ventricular rate may be slowed by the administration of digitalis; normal sinus rhythm may even be restored. Doses of 0.25 mg PO or IV of digoxin may be given up to a total of 1 mg in 24 hours,

followed by 0.125–0.25 mg daily. <u>Propranolol in increments of 0.25 mg</u> or <u>verapamil, 5–10 mg, may</u> also be used IV to slow the rate. <u>Caution, however, is advised in not giving both propranolol and verapamil together in doses high enough to cause cardiac failure.</u> If necessary, cardioversion may be employed.

 ✳
2. **Atrial flutter** (atrial rate 250–350) with 1 : 1 or 2 : 1 block will result in a rapid ventricular rate and may be treated with digitalization, if digitalis toxicity is not, in fact, its cause. <u>Propranolol,</u> <u>verapamil,</u> and <u>cardioversion</u> are alternative treatments.

3. <u>**Paroxysmal supraventricular tachycardia**</u> (atrial and ventricular rates of 150–250) may be treated with <u>carotid sinus massage</u> or <u>verapamil,</u> although <u>edrophonium,</u> <u>digoxin,</u> <u>propranolol,</u> and phenylephrine have also been proved effective.

4. **Ventricular tachycardia** (ventricular rate 150–250) should be treated with <u>lidocaine</u> and cardioversion in urgent cases, although propranolol, procainamide, and bretylium have a role in preventing recurrence.

VII. Additional arrhythmias

A. **Premature atrial contractions** are frequently detected on continuous electrocardiographic monitoring but are usually benign and require no treatment. Characteristically, the <u>P wave of a premature atrial contraction looks different from preceding P waves,</u> and the P–R interval may vary from normal; however, except in the cases of nonconduction or aberrant conduction, the QRS complex remains unchanged. When sufficiently problematic, treatment may be attempted with digoxin or with propranolol.

B. **Junctional or atrioventricular nodal rhythms** are characterized by absent or abnormal P waves and a normal QRS complex. <u>Although they may indicate underlying ischemic cardiac disease, junctional rhythms are commonly seen under primarily inhalational anesthesia in normal individuals.</u> Again, most of the time, this rhythm need not cause undue alarm. However, <u>in the patient whose cardiac output depends heavily on the contribution from atrial contraction, stroke volume and blood pressure may decline precipitously,</u> and congestive heart failure or marked hypotension may rapidly ensue. <u>Reduction of the anesthetic</u> concentration may bring about a return to sinus rhythm. <u>Atropine</u> in increments of 0.2 mg <u>may convert a slow junctional rhythm to sinus rhythm, particularly if a vagal mechanism is at the root.</u> <u>If the rate is fast,</u> <u>propranolol in increments of 0.25 mg may be used.</u> If the arrhythmia is associated with hypotension, raising the blood pressure and right atrial filling with volume or vasopressors (phenylephrine) may convert the rhythm. If necessary, atrial pacing may be instituted to restore the atrial contraction.

C. <u>**Premature ventricular contractions**</u> (PVCs) are

notable for their bizarre, widened QRS complexes. When coupled alternatively with normal beats, bigeminy is said to occur. Although PVCs are occasionally seen in normal individuals, they may signify ischemic cardiac disease or even acute myocardial infarction; also they may represent digitalis toxicity. They become more worrisome when they are multifocal, occur in runs, increase in frequency, or land on or near the preceding T wave; these situations portend the development of ventricular tachycardia, ventricular fibrillation, and cardiac arrest. Under anesthesia, PVCs are a common occurrence and are usually related to excessive sympathetic stimulation, hypercarbia, and hypoxia.

Accordingly, appropriate therapies in the otherwise normal individual include deepening the anesthesia, increasing the alveolar ventilation to lower $PaCO_2$, and supplying sufficient quantities of oxygen. For the patient with coronary artery disease who continues to have ventricular irritability in spite of these measures, lidocaine, 1 mg/kg IV, may be given, and if necessary, a lidocaine infusion at 2 mg/min may be used to maintain drug levels. If the PVCs represent left ventricular failure, adjusting volume and inotopic support may be required, using a pulmonary arterial catheter to guide therapy. For long-term suppression of ventricular irritability, procainamide, propranolol, disopyramide, quinidine, or mexiletine may be used.

VIII. Hypercarbia

A. In simplest terms, hypercarbia is due either to **increased production of carbon dioxide** or to **inadequate ventilation.**

1. Inadequate spontaneous ventilation may be central or mechanical in origin, as discussed in sec. **II.**

2. Additionally, controlled and assisted patterns of ventilation may be considered inadequate when they fail to keep the $PaCO_2$ within the normal range. The deficiency may be caused by partial or complete airway obstruction, by inadequate squeezing of the reservoir bag, or by ventilator settings too low for the patient's lung and chest wall compliance.

3. An increased $PaCO_2$ may be caused by the following:

   a. Giving the patient carbon dioxide to breathe.

   b. Bypassing the carbon dioxide absorber or using a malfunctioning absorber in a closed or semi-closed system.

   c. Intraperitoneal carbon dioxide insufflation.

   d. Allowing partial rebreathing in an open system.

4. The spontaneously breathing patient may **hyperventilate** in an attempt to blow off the increased carbon dioxide, although the drive to do so may be profoundly altered by a general anesthetic.

5. An increased ratio of dead space to tidal volume (V_D/V_T), either anatomic (as caused by using a

      large mask on an infant) or physiologic (as occurs with pulmonary embolism), will increase $PaCO_2$.

    6. Increased carbon dioxide production is seen in sepsis and is marked in malignant hyperthermia.

B. Hypercarbia is unpleasant to the awake patient, and in the anesthetized patient, it produces hypertension, tachycardia, and cardiac arrhythmias. Attention to the patient's ventilation, whether spontaneous or controlled, can avert these difficulties most of the time.

IX. Hypoxia

A. The delivery to tissues of oxygen sufficient to meet their metabolic needs requires

    1. An adequate oxygen supply.

    2. Satisfactory alveolar ventilation.

    3. A relative balancing of ventilation and perfusion in the lung.

    4. An alveolar capillary membrane that allows diffusion of oxygen.

    5. A suitable cardiac output with appropriate regional blood flow.

    6. An appropriate hemoglobin content to carry oxygen to the tissues.

B. Hypoxia during anesthesia may be due to

    1. A malfunctioning oxygen source.

    2. An oxygen supply that is empty, disconnected, or shut off.

    3. A tank containing something other than oxygen connected to the oxygen yoke.

    4. An oxygen flowmeter that is not turned to a sufficiently high flow.

    5. A leak in the oxygen flowmeter.

C. Hypoxia may further be due to poor oxygen delivery secondary to a leak in the breathing system, airway obstruction, or misdirected oxygen flow (esophageal intubation). Alveolar ventilation, whether spontaneous or controlled, must be maintained.

D. The greater the amount of arteriovenous shunting in the pulmonary circulation, the lower are the PaO_2 values for any given FIO_2. The problem arises in alveoli that receive a pulmonary capillary blood supply but are not ventilated to proportionate degrees. This ventilation/perfusion $(\dot{V}A/\dot{Q})$ imbalance is accentuated in atelectasis, pneumonia, pulmonary edema, and other parenchymal pathologic states. Some correctable reasons for increased shunting include atelectasis due to surgical compression from packs and retractors, poor compliance in the lower lung when kept in a lateral position for long periods, and endobronchial intubation.

E. A low, fixed cardiac output or intracardiac right-to-left shunting will lower PaO_2 values for any given FIO_2.

F. Interstitial pulmonary parenchymal disease may occasionally cause an alveolar capillary block syndrome, with resulting hypoxia.

G. Anemia, in the absence of full, compensatory, increased cardiac output, will diminish oxygen transport capabilities.

H. By definition, shock from any cause produces tissue hypoxia.

X. Sweating

A. Sweating, like tearing, may be observed in response to the sympathetic discharge caused by anxiety, pain, or noxious stimuli in the presence of too-light anesthesia. Sweating may be seen in conjunction with bradycardia, nausea, and hypotension as part of a generalized vagal reaction.

B. As a mechanism for heat release, sweating is seen with fever from infection, from the combination of high ambient room temperature and heavy surgical drapes, and from malignant hyperthermia.

C. Sweating, except insofar as it causes evaporative fluid loss, is not harmful in itself but may be used as a sign to gauge the depth of anesthesia. Atropine tends to suppress sweating and promote heat retention.

XI. Hiccoughs

A. These intermittent spasms of the diaphragm are thought to be reflex responses to visceral stimulation, such as gastric dilatation, and may be vagally mediated. When the patient is intubated, hiccoughs are a problem only in that diaphragmatic movement may disturb the surgical field. However, with mask ventilation, closure of the glottis accompanies the spasms and increases the risk of laryngospasm.

B. Possible avenues of **treatment** include

1. Discontinuing the offending surgical stimulation.
2. Deepening the anesthesia, particularly with a small amount of halothane.
3. Emptying the stomach with a nasogastric tube.
4. Increasing the degree of neuromuscular blockade.
5. Giving chlorpromazine (Thorazine) IV in 5-mg increments.

Suggested Reading

Brodsky, J. B. (ed.). Clinical aspects of oxygen. *Int. Anesthesiol. Clin.* 19(3):1, 1981.

Fink, B. R. The etiology and treatment of laryngeal spasm. *Anesthesiology* 17:569, 1956.

Goldman, L., and Caldera, D. L. Risks of general anesthesia and elective operation in the hypertensive patient. *Anesthesiology* 50:285, 1979.

Kaplan, J. A. Electrocardiographic Monitoring. In J. A. Kaplan (ed.), *Cardiac Anesthesia*. Orlando, Fla.: Grune & Stratton, 1979. Pp. 117–166.

McKay, R. D., et al. Internal carotid artery stump pressure and cerebral blood flow during carotid endarterectomy. *Anesthesiology* 45:390, 1976.

16

Controlling the Circulation

Blake M. Paterson

The ability to control the circulation is of fundamental importance to anesthesiologists. Valuable anesthetic techniques may have undesirable cardiovascular side effects and frequently require intervention to maintain homeostasis. Controlling the circulation may be necessary to treat ischemic, hypertensive, or hypotensive emergencies. Elective induction of hypotension may be undertaken to optimize surgical conditions. To safely achieve these benefits, an understanding of circulatory physiology is required.

The purpose of the circulation is to supply organs with oxygen and nutrients; consequently local tissue perfusion is more important than absolute blood pressure. Unfortunately, other than gross function, few indices exist to assess organ perfusion. Furthermore, anesthesia complicates the evaluation of tissue perfusion and cardiovascular function, and organ function may be altered by both anesthesia and surgery. Consequently, **systemic blood pressure** is widely regarded as the best approximation of circulatory integrity. Arterial pressure represents a complex interaction of cardiac and peripheral factors: **blood volume, cardiac output,** and **systemic vascular capacitance and resistance** (SVR). When using the blood pressure to quantify circulatory integrity, all of these factors must be considered; for example, hypotension combined with vasodilatation will compromise organ function less than hypotension accompanied by vasoconstriction.

I. **Autoregulation**
   A. Metabolic regulation controls 75% of all local blood flow in the body. Most organs have a specific blood flow regulatory system to maintain perfusion at levels sufficient to meet their metabolic needs. In general, anesthetics inhibit autoregulation, making organ perfusion pressure-dependent.
   B. **Brain.** Cerebral blood flow is kept constant over a wide range of mean arterial pressure (MAP) (60–160 mm Hg in normotensive patients) and PaO_2 (> 50 mm Hg). If MAP falls below 60 mm Hg, cerebral autoregulation is lost and perfusion becomes pressure-dependent. Since cerebral perfusion pressure equals MAP minus intracranial pressure, increased intracranial pressure limits cerebral perfusion. Hypoxia, acidosis, and hypercarbia may increase regional blood flow by vasodilatation, while hypocarbia (< 35 mm Hg) reduces cerebral blood flow by vasoconstriction.
   C. **Kidneys.** Under normal conditions, autoregulation maintains constant renal blood flow over a MAP range of 60–150 mm Hg. Glomerular filtration rate (GFR) remains relatively constant with decreasing pressures until it drops off sharply at systolic pressures near 70 mm Hg. During induced hypotension, GFR and urine output

may fall toward zero, while renal blood flow, in the absence of vascular disease, may be adequate to meet the metabolic needs of the kidney.

D. Heart. Coronary artery perfusion is affected principally by <u>diastolic blood pressure</u>. During systemic hypotension, coronary blood flow decreases, while myocardial work and oxygen consumption decrease due to reduced afterload, restoring the balance of oxygen supply and demand. <u>In normal individuals, ischemic ECG changes are absent until diastolic blood pressure drops below 30–40 mm Hg</u>. Ischemia is likely to occur at higher pressures in patients with coronary artery disease, hypertension, or cardiomyopathy.

E. Lungs. <u>V_D/V_T may rise from 0.3 to 0.6–0.8 during hypotension;</u> this may be due to a worsening of the regional balance between ventilation and perfusion. Because oxygenation may be a problem, endotracheal intubation and controlled ventilation with an increased F_{IO_2} are always indicated during induced hypotension.

II. Supporting the circulation

A. Perioperatively, hypotension may result from impaired myocardial contractility or decreased filling pressures. Reduction of preload leading to decreased cardiac output may occur with hypovolemia, displacement of blood from the thorax (positive-pressure ventilation), or cardiac compression. Alterations of afterload may result from changes in vascular tone and resistance, changing the cardiac output and blood pressure. When there is inadequate pressure to perfuse vital organs, any pharmacologic agent that augments cardiac output or increases MAP will increase, at least transiently, blood flow to all vital structures. However, increased overall flow may not reflect drug effects on a local vascular bed. To determine the most appropriate pharmacologic intervention, the etiology of a low-perfusion state must be determined and the specific pharmacology and side effects of the agent(s) understood.

B. Sympathomimetic agents. The inotropic and chronotropic state of the heart is modulated by myocardial beta-1 receptors, while beta-2 receptors are responsible for bronchial, uterine, and vascular smooth-muscle relaxation. Alpha-1 receptors mediate vascular smooth-muscle contraction throughout the body; alpha-2 receptors mediate a negative feedback control at central and peripheral nerve terminals, reducing sympathetic outflow. Before selecting a sympathomimetic agent, the underlying sympathetic tone and acid-base status should be considered, since patient responses will be modulated by these factors.

1. **Alpha agonists.** The alpha-1 agonists presently in use are synthetic derivatives of phenylethanolamine. They produce profound vasoconstriction and are particularly useful, in patients with good cardiac function, as temporizing agents while the underlying cause of hypotension is corrected. <u>Their use is contraindicated in parturients</u>; unopposed al-

pha effects will reduce uterine blood flow by increasing uterine vascular resistance. Renovascular and coronary artery resistance may also be increased by these agents, with deleterious effects on organ flow.

- a. **Phenylephrine.** A short duration of action makes it easily titratable. At its usual IV dosage (Table 16-1), phenylephrine provides relatively pure alpha stimulation, while with profound overdosage some cardiac stimulation is seen, reducing the incidence of cardiac failure from excessive afterload. The latter effects are mediated through either cardiac beta receptors or recently identified cardiac alpha-1 receptors.

- b. **Methoxamine.** A long duration of action makes methoxamine difficult to titrate. No cardiac stimulation is seen with overdosage, so increased afterload and congestive heart failure may ensue. This agent is infrequently used during operations.

2. **Beta agonists.** The clinical use of beta agonists is limited by the following side effects: positive chronotropy, which tends to exacerbate arrhythmias, and stimulation of beta-2 receptors, causing vasodilatation.

   Isoproterenol is a pure beta agonist that has powerful bronchodilating and cardiac stimulating effects, while also causing vasodilatation, hypotension, and tachycardia. Isoproterenol is indicated in the presence of pulmonary hypertension and for immediate control of hemodynamically significant, atropine-resistant bradycardia from complete heart block. The use of agents such as epinephrine and dopamine may be preferable when bradycardia is associated with hypotension.

3. **Mixed agonists.** This category includes agents that are naturally occurring catecholamines or synthetic sympathomimetics possessing varying alpha, beta, and dopamine receptor-stimulating abilities. Some may cause indirect (tyramine-like) sympathomimetic effects by triggering the release of endogenous norepinephrine stores in the body.

   $\alpha > \beta$

   - a. **Norepinephrine.** A potent alpha- and beta-receptor agonist, norepinephrine causes predominant alpha effects at low IV dosages, resulting in vasoconstriction, hypertension, and occasionally, reflex bradycardia. Increasing dosages will produce a positive inotropic effect from stimulation of beta-1 receptors, making it a useful agent in the setting of vasodilatation with mild myocardial depression. Norepinephrine reduces renal blood flow, even at low dosages. As with most pressor/inotropic agents, use of direct arterial pressure monitoring is highly recommended.

   - b. **Epinephrine.** Both alpha and beta receptors

   $\beta > \alpha$

Table 16-1. Agents used to support the circulation*

Drug (trade name)	IV dose range (duration of action)	Adrenergic effects			Comments
		Dose	Alpha	Beta	
Phenylephrine (Neo-Synephrine)	0.1–20 µg/kg/min (5–10 min)		+ + +		Increases renovascular resistance
Isoproterenol (Isuprel)	0.5–4.0 µg/min (5–10 min)			+ + + +	Marked arrhythmogenesis
Norepinephrine (Levophed)	2–30 µg/min (1–2 min)	Low	+ +	+	Reduces renal blood flow even at low doses
		High	+ + + +	+ +	Moderate arrhythmogenesis
Epinephrine (Adrenalin)	100–200 µg bolus 1–4 µg/min (1–2 min)	Low	+	+ +	Reduces renal blood flow
		High	+ +	+ + + +	Marked arrhythmogenesis
Dopamine (Intropin)	3–15 µg/kg/min (5–10 min)	Low	+	+	Increases renal blood flow at doses < 6 µg/kg/min
		High	+ + +	+ +	Moderate arrhythmogenesis
Dobutamine (Dobutrex)	2–10 µg/kg/min (5–10 min)	Low	+	+ +	Predominately stimulates inotropic beta receptors
		High	+ +	+ +	
Ephedrine	5–50 mg IV (5–10 min)		+ +	+ +	Moderate arrhythmogenesis

| Amrinone (Inocor) | 0.75 mg/kg IV loading, then 5–10 µg/kg/min (2.5–12 hr) | Nonsympathomimetic | No arrhythmogenesis; minimal vascular effects |

*Refer to Drug Appendix for drug preparation information.

are stimulated by epinephrine, with beta effects predominant at low doses. This results in profound bronchodilatation, increased cardiac output, and tachycardia at low dosages, without an increase in SVR. As dosages are increased, alpha effects become predominant, eventually eclipsing the peripheral beta effects, resulting in vasoconstriction, hypertension, and tachycardia. As with norepinephrine, epinephrine is useful in settings of myocardial depression and hypotension, but where preservation of cardiac output and peripheral perfusion is of greater concern. As with other mixed agonists, arterial monitoring is mandatory.

c. **Dopamine.** A norepinephrine precursor, dopamine manifests a dose-related combination of alpha, beta, and dopamine receptor effects, as well as indirect sympathomimetic effects. At 1–4 μg/kg/min, renal and splanchnic vessel dopamine receptors are activated, resulting in increased renal cortical blood flow and diuresis. At 5–10 μg/kg/min, beta effects predominate, and cardiac output and heart rate increase. At high dosages (> 10 μg/kg/min), alpha-1 effects are predominant, which increase arterial and venous pressures and may decrease renal blood flow. The tachyarrhythmias, increased $M\dot{V}O_2$, and vasoconstriction seen with high dosages limit the usefulness of dopamine. However, it remains a very useful drug for providing inotropic and vascular support while preserving or augmenting renal blood flow.

d. **Dobutamine.** Initially classified as a selective beta-1 agonist, dobutamine has positive inotropic action with some vasodilatation but less arrhythmogenicity than the mixed agonists already discussed. A racemic mixture, dobutamine's L-isomer has potent alpha-1 and weak beta properties, while its D-isomer produces potent beta-1/beta-2 and minimal alpha-1 activity, resulting overall in a preservation of vascular tone and little chronotropy at low doses. This makes it a useful agent for treating cardiogenic shock, where the goal is to support the failing heart without causing severe tachycardia or vasodilatation. At dosages above 10–15 μg/kg/min, chronotropic and vasodilating effects become evident.

e. **Ephedrine** is an indirect alpha- and beta-sympathomimetic, capable of producing tolerance when given in repeated doses or used as an infusion. Because of tachyphylaxis and its long duration of action, it is used mainly in a bolus fashion. It is often used as a temporizing agent while the underlying cause of hypotension is corrected. It is also the drug of choice for parturients during regional anesthesia, since its beta effect raises MAP without producing uterine vasoconstriction.

C. **Phosphodiesterase inhibitors.** These recently introduced synthetic agents are nonglycoside, nonsympathomimetic positive inotropic agents that work by inhibiting cardiac-specific phosphodiesterase. They are not affected by beta-, alpha-, or histamine-receptor blockade, are independent of baseline sympathetic tone, and are used mainly in patients with end-stage heart failure.

   1. **Amrinone** produces a concentration-dependent positive inotropy and arterial and venous dilatation. A long-acting IV agent, amrinone's elimination half-life varies from 2.5 hours in healthy subjects to 12 hours in patients with impaired cardiac function. Side effects include a dose-dependent reversible thrombocytopenia, liver function test abnormalities, fever, and gastrointestinal distress, which are seen infrequently with the IV preparation.

   2. **Milrinone.** A bipyridine derivative of amrinone, this agent has the same hemodynamic and pharmacologic activities, but is 15 times more potent than its parent compound. Although presently unavailable for use in the United States, no fever or thrombocytopenia has been associated with milrinone use in clinical studies.

III. **Vasodilators** (Table 16-2) are used in anesthesia to induce hypotension electively, treat hypertensive emergencies, and improve organ perfusion. Vasodilating drugs have been shown to improve cardiac performance in patients with heart failure. Properly administered, vasodilators can prevent the potentially deleterious effects of vasoconstriction and reduce $M\dot{V}O_2$ by reducing both preload and afterload. In patients with elevated left ventricular filling pressures, vasodilating drugs can potentially increase stroke volume and cardiac output, decrease SVR, yet not change MAP. In normal persons, decreased SVR produces a marked reduction in venous return, decreasing preload, stroke volume, and MAP, precipitating the need for volume replacement.

A. **Sodium nitroprusside** (SNP). SNP's nitroso moiety acts directly on vascular smooth muscle, producing arterial, arteriolar, and venous dilatation. SNP has no direct effect on myocardial contractility, and its activity is independent of sympathetic innervation. The principal action on ventricular performance is mediated by mechanical unloading of the heart. It is extremely potent, with an instantaneous onset of action and an ultrashort duration after discontinuation of infusions. Induced hypotension with SNP is associated with a compensatory tachycardia and increased plasma renin activity. SNP dilates cerebral blood vessels, increasing intracranial blood volume. Thus, in patients with low intracranial compliance, it should be avoided prior to opening the dura.

Table 16-2. Vasodilator drugs*

Drug (trade name)	Dosage	Mechanism of action	Comments
Sodium nitroprusside (Nipride)	0.1 µg/kg/min, then titrate accordingly	Direct relaxing effect on vascular smooth muscle	May produce reflex tachycardia
Nitroglycerin	0.2 µg/kg/min, then titrate accordingly	Direct relaxing effect on vascular smooth muscle	Can cause methemoglobinemia in very high doses
Hydralazine (Apresoline)	2.5–5.0 mg IV in incremental doses q15min	Direct relaxing effect on arteriolar smooth muscle	Gradual onset (15 min); reflex tachycardia occurs
Phentolamine (Regitine)	1.5–2.0 µg/kg/min, then titrate accordingly	Alpha-receptor blockade and direct effect on vasculature	Tachycardia and hypoglycemia may occur
Trimethaphan (Arfonad)	1–4 mg/min for 5 min, then titrate accordingly	Ganglionic blockade and histamine release	Cycloplegia, mydriasis, and tachycardia may occur
Labetalol (Normodyne or Trandate)	2.5–5.0 mg IV in incremental doses q5min	Alpha- and beta-receptor blockade	

*Refer to Drug Appendix for drug preparation information.

Aqueous SNP solutions are unstable upon standing and with exposure to light. In blood, SNP reacts nonenzymatically with hemoglobin, rapidly liberating five cyanide radicals per molecule. Most of the cyanide is converted enzymatically in the presence of thiosulfate to thiocyanate by tissue and liver rhodanese; the conversion rate is dependent on thiosulfate availability. Therefore, SNP should be used with caution in patients with hepatic insufficiency. **Toxic cyanide levels** ($>$ 100 µg/dl) occur when more than 1 mg/kg is administered within 2.5 hours. The first sign of toxicity may be **tachyphylaxis**: a requirement to increase infusion rates to maintain hypotension. In awake patients, early symptoms of toxicity include fatigue, nausea, muscle spasm, angina, and psychotic behavior. Tachyphylaxis in the absence of toxicity is characterized by the absence of metabolic acidosis. Other adverse effects of SNP infusion include intracranial hypertension; rebound, systemic, and pulmonary hypertension; and increased pulmonary shunting. Metabolic acidosis and death may result from SNP overdosage.

B. Nitroglycerin (NTG) is a potent venodilator that also relaxes ureteral, uterine, gastrointestinal, and bronchial smooth muscle. NTG has a greater effect on venous capacitance than on arteriolar tone; NTG's major mechanism of decreasing MAP is reduction of venous return. It is useful for treating congestive heart failure and the ischemic myocardium by increasing coronary flow and improving left ventricular performance through preloading reduction. It can be used for induced hypotension but may require high doses, especially in young, healthy patients, unless supplemented by other agents such as halothane. NTG is short-acting, is metabolized in the liver, and has no known toxicity in the clinical range. In extremely high doses, it may cause methemoglobinemia in susceptible individuals. As with SNP, low intracranial compliance contraindicates its use. Adverse effects include tachycardia.

C. Hydralazine. A longer acting, direct arterial dilator, hydralazine is administered in bolus fashion to treat hypertensive crises or to augment hypotensive agents. It is frequently used with propranolol, as reflex tachycardia may precipitate myocardial ischemia in susceptible patients. After incremental doses, careful monitoring of the blood pressure is required, as the effects develop gradually over 15 minutes. The elimination half-life of hydralazine is 3 hours, while its duration of action may be shorter.

D. Phentolamine. A very short-acting, competitive alpha antagonist, phentolamine causes vasodilatation both through alpha blockade and direct vascular smooth muscle relaxation. It may precipitate transient endogenous catecholamine release, increasing cardiac output. Both arterial and venous dilatation are seen, resulting in hypotension and tachycardia. Increased intracranial pressure during phentolamine-induced hypotension has not been reported. It is used mainly as an adjuvant drug in induced hypotension and during resection of pheochromocytomas.

E. **Trimethaphan.** The only ganglionic blocker available in the United States, trimethaphan appears to have direct vasodilator and histamine-releasing properties, in addition to its ganglion-blocking properties. Onset of action is rapid and duration is short, due to renal excretion. As with SNP and NTG, infusions should be judiciously titrated against clinical response; dosage requirements may vary widely. There is a high incidence of tachyphylaxis, which develops during continued use, and tachycardia may limit the usefulness of this agent. Desired reductions in vascular tone are accompanied by other manifestations of ganglionic blockade, including mydriasis, and cycloplegia as well as tachycardia. Mydriasis may be extreme, so trimethaphan is contraindicated in patients with known narrow-angle glaucoma and relatively contraindicated where pupil size serves as an indicator of the patient's neurologic condition.

F. **Labetalol.** A mixed adrenergic antagonist, labetalol is a potent hypotensive agent with a beta-alpha blockade ratio greater than 2:1 in humans. It decreases blood pressure by reducing SVR without increasing heart rate. In patients with depressed left ventricular function, labetalol's negative inotropic effect is balanced by decreased afterload, so that ventricular function is not reduced. Metabolized primarily by the liver, its elimination half-life is 2–4 hours, and it is administered in bolus fashion. Although the desired reduction in MAP may be difficult to achieve with labetalol alone, it may be useful in management of pheochromocytomas and clonidine withdrawal. Elevation in intracranial pressure has not been seen after labetalol use in patients with intracranial hypertension.

G. **Nifedipine.** A calcium channel blocker, nifedipine reduces blood pressure by altering extracellular calcium flux, resulting in cardiac depression and vasodilatation. Increases in intracranial pressure have occurred in animals when hypotension is induced by calcium channel blockers, although these agents may have a protective effect during cerebral ischemia. Unavailable in IV form, nifedipine is not useful for induced hypotension.

H. **Adenosine** has been used in clinical trials to induce hypotension in humans. Administered as ATP, adenosine dilates cerebral blood vessels, impairs autoregulation, and is metabolized to uric acid. With its prompt onset and short duration of action, it may be useful for induced hypotension.

I. **Prostaglandin E$_1$** (PGE$_1$) has potent relaxing effects on both systemic and pulmonary arterial smooth muscle; in large doses, it causes severe systemic hypotension. It has been used to treat refractory pulmonary hypertension after mitral valve replacement, but only in conjunction with left atrial norepinephrine infusion. Other clinical uses as a vasodilating agent are under investigation.

J. **Atrial natriuretic peptides** have recently been isolated from cardiac atria and shown to have potent vasodilating, natriuretic, and diuretic effects in normal man. With its ability to increase renal blood flow and GFR, it is also likely to find multiple uses in the future.

IV. Induced hypotension

A. Induced hypotension may benefit patients in the following circumstances:

1. When control of bleeding improves operative conditions and facilitates surgical technique. For example, in middle-ear microsurgery, a single drop of blood can obscure the field.

2. When control of bleeding reduces the need for multiple transfusions and thus lowers the risk of transfusion complications.

3. When reduction in MAP lessens the risk of vessel rupture, as in the treatment of aortic dissection and in the resection or ligation of intracranial aneurysm or arteriovenous malformation.

4. In certain plastic operations, to decrease oozing beneath skin flaps with improved cosmetic results.

B. Induced hypotension is **contraindicated** in the following circumstances:

1. Cardiovascular instability, unless induced hypotension is used to reduce afterload.

2. Severe cerebral or peripheral vascular disease.

3. Uncontrolled hypertension: While autoregulation is altered in hypertensive states, recent data suggest that antihypertensive therapy will partially restore autoregulation. The decision whether to use induced hypotension or allow arterial pressure to decrease significantly for a particular procedure should be based on the adequacy of antihypertensive therapy prior to surgery. If preoperative hypertension is present, it is recommended to postpone elective surgery until antihypertensive therapy can be instituted.

4. Severe renal or hepatic disease.

5. Gross anemia, or hypovolemia, or both.

6. Narrow-angle glaucoma (ganglionic blockers contraindicated).

7. Inexperience of the anesthesiologist with these techniques.

C. **General considerations.** The suitability of induced hypotension for a given patient will depend on the overall metabolic requirements and the length of the planned procedure.

1. Hypotension is not synonymous with inadequate local tissue perfusion. If SVR falls in parallel with MAP, local blood flow may not be adversely affected. Considering the limits of autoregulation, it is reasonable to aim for a MAP of 50–60 mm Hg in

young, healthy individuals and MAPs of 60–70 mm Hg in suitable older patients.

2. All hypotensive techniques abolish normal compensatory mechanisms, so scrupulous volume replacement is critical. Failure of normotension to return when dilators are discontinued is considered to be due to **hypovolemia** until proved otherwise. Similarly, failure of prompt return of urine flow should be treated with generous volume infusion.

3. If ECG evidence of myocardial ischemia appears, induced hypotension should be abandoned.

4. Regardless of the agent used, bleeding may be reduced by positioning the operative site uppermost, preferably above right atrial level, to lower venous and capillary pressures.

5. While controlled ventilation is always indicated during induced hypotension (see sec. **I.E**), positive airway pressure also diminishes venous return and potentiates induced hypotension. However, hyperventilation should be avoided, since cerebral vasoconstriction in the setting of hypotension may lead to cerebral ischemia. This consideration remains valid even though cerebrovascular sensitivity to carbon dioxide is reduced by vasodilators and inhalational anesthetics.

D. Preparation

1. Generous premedication will prevent an excess of circulating catecholamines and may facilitate the hypotensive effects of vasodilators.

2. Aside from routine monitoring (see Chap. 9), a Foley catheter and arterial and central venous pressure catheters should be placed.

3. Vasodilators in appropriate dilutions, as well as resuscitation drugs such as calcium chloride, a catecholamine inotrope, and a vasoconstrictor should be readily available. A separate IV route for hypotensive agent administration should be established so that flow may be reliably regulated without interruption or inadvertant bolus drug administration. Use of an infusion pump or a 60 drop/ml administration set is recommended. A hypotensive drug should not be considered discontinued until the infusion is off and the line cleared.

E. Method. The ideal hypotensive technique should be easy to control, be nontoxic, have a short plasma and biologic half-life, and should not significantly alter vital organ perfusion.

Although general anesthetics alter sympathetic tone and potentiate the effects of vasoactive agents, MAP may be controlled more sensitively by altering the resistance vessels, either with direct-acting vasodilator drugs or indirectly through pharmacologic sympathectomy. Sympathectomy may be induced at a preganglionic level by epidural or subarachnoid block, or at a ganglionic level with trimethaphan.

1. **Sodium nitroprusside** should be used only for the interval when reductions in blood pressure are needed. Administration should start at a very slow rate (10 μg/min) and the dose carefully titrated to the desired response. Should the infusion rate become too rapid, blood pressure may decline precipitously. The total dose should not exceed 1.5 mg/kg, as cyanide toxicity may ensue. Frequent ABG determinations must be made with dosages greater than 6 μg/kg/min; if metabolic acidosis develops, SNP should be discontinued and the patient monitored for cyanide toxicity (see III.A).

2. **Nitroglycerin** is also used at a starting dose of 10 μg/min followed by careful titration.

3. **Trimethaphan** use may be accompanied by tachycardia, which may be overcome by IV propranolol or through the vagotonic effects of fentanyl. The total dose of trimethaphan should not exceed 1000 mg; higher doses are usually not effective. Trimethaphan's effects may take 10–30 minutes to wear off fully.

4. **Trimethaphan and SNP** may be used in **combination** to minimize adverse effects while achieving adequate hypotension. The agents may be mixed in the same bottle (e.g., 250 mg of trimethaphan and 25 mg of SNP in 500 ml of 5% D/W). The infusion should begin at 0.1 ml/min (5 μg/min of SNP and 0.05 mg/min of trimethaphan), then titrated according to blood pressure.

5. Preganglionic sympathectomy is most predictably achieved with **subarachnoid block.** Spinal anesthesia will produce a sympathectomy to a predictable level by means of postural adjustment. At the same time, it provides profound analgesia, excellent skeletal muscle relaxation, and a contracted, flat, vagotonic bowel, ideal for intraabdominal surgery. The use of a **catheter spinal technique** for induced hypotension offers even greater control of both sympathectomy level and analgesia, particularly when the procedure may be prolonged. It may, however, increase the incidence of postoperative spinal headache.

   a. After lumbar puncture with a Tuohy needle, a catheter is advanced 3 cm cephalad beyond the needle tip. The needle is then removed without displacing the catheter, and the catheter taped securely in place. Aspiration of cerebrospinal fluid confirms that the catheter is still in place, and the patient is turned supine. Sterility is scrupulously maintained, since meningitis is a possible complication.

   b. Light general anesthesia is then induced, including 4% lidocaine spray to the trachea, and while spontaneously breathing 70% nitrous oxide via endotracheal tube, the patient is placed in steep (30–40°) Trendelenburg position with the neck flexed. Then an appropriate dose of hyperbaric 0.4% tetracaine (40 mg of 1% tetracaine diluted with 10% D/W to a total of 10 ml), scaled from a typical dose of 16 mg for a patient 6-feet (183 cm) tall, may be injected into the subarachnoid space. The dose and position are intended to obtain a total thoracic sympathetic block, so that all the cardiac accelerator fibers and sympathetic ganglia will be blocked. (It should be very difficult to produce apnea in this dosage range because of the anterior convexity of the cervical curvature and drug dilution at the level of the cervical roots.) Patients should be allowed to continue to breathe spontaneously, so that the degree of motor blockade may be assessed. As the thoracic motor block becomes apparent (the intercostal spaces lose their normal widening and begin to sink on inspiration), the table may be leveled. Hereafter, ventilation should be controlled.

c. Hypotension may now be induced by judicious head-up tilt, allowing venous pooling peripherally. Once the appropriate MAP is established, surgery may begin.

d. After the initial dose of tetracaine provides the desired sympathetic block, top-off doses are about one-half of the starting dose and are given when the heart rate begins to rise. Once MAP has begun to rise, renewal of hypotension may be difficult. Before readministrations, the catheter should be aspirated to confirm patency and the patient repositioned. Infrequently, the effect cannot be reproduced, possibly because the patient cannot be placed in a steep enough tilt for reinjection. The effect may sometimes be recovered by injecting a large volume of 0.5% procaine, achieving spread of anesthesia by volume displacement rather than by gravity.

e. The light general anesthetic is maintained with nitrous oxide, thiopental, and small increments of narcotics.

f. At the conclusion of the requirement for hypotension, blood pressure may be restored by head-down tilt. In long procedures, there may be a loss of inherent vessel tone due to sustained block; in this case, infusion of fluids or use of a peripherally acting pressor, such as phenylephrine, may help.

g. When the procedure is completed, the patient may be extubated and the catheter carefully removed. As with any dural puncture, patients should remain flat in bed for several hours and be kept well hydrated.

6. Potentiation of induced hypotension

   a. **Propranolol** is a nonselective beta-adrenergic blocking drug with negative inotropic and chronotropic effects. It also blocks the renin-angiotensin axis, making it a useful adjuvant with SNP, trimethaphan, and hydralazine. It should be titrated in small IV increments (0.25 mg/dose) against both heart rate and blood pressure.

   b. Deep levels of potent **inhalational agents,** especially halothane, have been used to potentiate vasodilators or ganglionic blockers, especially in younger patients.

   c. **Captopril,** a specific inhibitor of angiotensin I converting enzyme, has been used to potentiate induced hypotension. A fivefold increase in plasma renin activity has been demonstrated in patients undergoing induced hypotension, and the renin-angiotensin axis has been implicated in tachyphylaxis to SNP. By pretreating patients with a single oral dose of captopril (6.25–12.5 mg one hour before surgery), a dramatic reduction in the dose of SNP needed to achieve hypotension can be accomplished.

F. **Reversal of hypotension.** Blood pressure should be allowed to normalize prior to closure in order to facilitate hemostasis.

   1. Provided intravascular volume is sufficient, blood pressure will return spontaneously after these drugs are discontinued:
      a. Trimethaphan, in 10–30 minutes.
      b. SNP, in 1–10 minutes.
      c. NTG, in 1–10 minutes.
      d. Propranolol, in 60–180 minutes.
      e. Hydralazine, in 60–180 minutes.
      f. Tetracaine spinal, in 75–150 minutes.

   2. If hypotension persists, and immediate reversal is necessary in spite of adequate volume repletion, the following can be used:
      a. Ephedrine, 5–10 mg IV.
      b. Phenylephrine titrated to the desired blood pressure; an infusion may be required until the longer acting vasodilators are eliminated.
      c. Calcium chloride in increments of 250 mg IV, to a total of 1 gm.

G. **Complications.** Although induced hypotension has been shown to be a safe procedure, provided patients are properly selected, the following complications may occur in rare instances:

   1. Altered mentation from cerebral ischemia, thrombosis, or edema.
   2. Acute renal failure.
   3. Myocardial infarction, congestive heart failure, and cardiac arrest.
   4. Reactive hemorrhage with hematoma formation.

Suggested Reading

Braunwald, E. Regulation of the circulation. *N. Engl. J. Med.* 290:1124, 1974.

Chernow, B., and Roth, B. L. Pharmacologic manipulation of the peripheral vasculature in shock: Clinical and experimental approaches. *Circ. Shock* 18:141, 1986.

Colucci, W. S., Wright, R. F., and Braunwald, E. New positive inotropic agents in the treatment of congestive heart failure. *N. Eng. J. Med.* 314:290, 1986.

Fahmy, N. R. Nitroglycerin as a hypotensive drug during general anesthesia. *Anesthesiology* 49:17, 1978.

Tinker, J. H., and Michenfelder, J. D. Sodium nitroprusside: Pharmacology, toxicology and therapeutics. *Anesthesiology* 45:340, 1976.

17

Anesthesia for Abdominal Surgery

Charles E. Cook

I. Preoperative considerations

A. Fluid management

1. **Causes of fluid losses**

   a. **Bleeding** from abdominal trauma, peptic ulcers, esophageal varices, Meckel's diverticulum, or angiodysplasia of the colon.

   b. **Vomiting or nasogastric suctioning.**

   c. **Fluid sequestration** in the intestinal lumen or peritoneal cavity, secondary to ileus or peritonitis.

   d. **Diarrhea** from intestinal disease or bowel preparation with cathartics, resulting in depletion of 1–2 liters of extracellular fluid.

2. **Assessment of fluid status**

   a. **History of losses** can sometimes be obtained from the patient or nursing records.

   b. **Physical examination** centers on the vital signs. Although blood pressure and heart rate may appear normal, mild hypovolemia may be unmasked when the patient is placed in a sitting position or inclined head-up 30 degrees on a tilt table. Severe hypovolemia will cause tachycardia and hypotension, even with the patient supine. Dryness of mucous membranes and decreased skin turgor may also indicate the presence of dehydration.

   c. **The mainstays of monitoring fluid status** are urethral (Foley) catheters and central venous pressure (CVP) lines. In the absence of primary renal disease, oliguria (especially with a high urine specific gravity and low urine sodium concentration) indicates renal hypoperfusion, possibly from hypovolemia. CVP measurement quantifies the degree of intravascular volume depletion and guides fluid replacement. Pulmonary artery pressure measurement is even more specific but is not indicated in all patients (see Chap. 2).

3. **Fluid replacement** with colloids (e.g., blood products, albumin, and starch expanders) and crystalloids (e.g., Ringer's lactate and normal saline solutions) is discussed in Chaps. 4 and 27.

B. A full stomach

is often encountered in patients for abdominal procedures and puts them at risk for pulmonary aspiration during induction. Because pulmonary aspiration is life-threatening, full-stomach considerations often dictate the timing of surgery and the anesthetic technique.

1. **Causes of a full stomach** include intake of solid or liquid food within 8 hours prior to surgery or abdominal trauma, obstruction or ileus of the bowel, upper gastrointestinal or pharyngeal bleeding, abdominal masses, pregnancy, and obesity. Patients with incompetence of the lower esophageal sphincter and symptomatic acid reflux (with or without a hiatal hernia) are also considered to be at risk for aspiration and are treated as if they had a full stomach.

2. **The risks from aspiration** are increased if the gastric volume is greater than 0.4 ml/kg, the pH is below 2.5, or the contents include particulate matter.

3. **Management options**

   a. **Delaying surgery** will allow the stomach to empty, provided the bowel is functioning. Delay may involve some surgical risk, which must be weighed against the risks of aspiration.

   b. **Regional or local anesthesia** avoids the period during induction when the airway is unprotected. However, general anesthesia may suddenly be required by a complication or failure of the regional technique.

   c. **Reducing gastric volume and acidity** can be achieved by administering oral, nonparticulate antacids (citric acid solution, 30 ml PO), histamine$_2$-antagonists (cimetidine, 300 mg PO or IV; ranitidine, 150 mg PO or 50 mg IV), and peristalsis stimulators (metoclopramide, 5–10 mg PO or IV). Antiemetics (droperidol, 0.625–1.25 mg IV) may decrease vomiting triggered by narcotics, anesthetics, or airway manipulation but will not prevent passive regurgitation in the presence of an ileus. Practically, particulate food can be removed only with a large-bore nasogastric tube.

   d. **Awake intubation** is mandatory in patients with full stomachs who also have abnormal airway anatomy or a history of difficult intubation. Otherwise, **rapid sequence induction and endotracheal intubation** are appropriate (see Chap. 10).

C. **Metabolic derangements** are frequently found in patients for emergency abdominal surgery. Hypokalemia and metabolic alkalosis can be caused by prolonged vomiting or nasogastric suctioning. Metabolic acidosis may be found with sepsis or diarrhea-induced dehydration.

II. **Regional versus general anesthesia**

   A. **Factors related to performing the procedure**

   1. **Most lower abdominal procedures** can be performed under regional anesthesia; spinal or epidural anesthesia to a T4–T6 level produces excellent operative conditions below the umbilicus. Cau-

dal epidural blocks work well for perirectal and perineal procedures (see Chap. 13).

2. **Upper abdominal procedures** require a T2–T4 level. High thoracic levels may result in vasodilatation, hypotension, and reflex tachycardia. Sympathetic blockade above T2 will block this cardiac accelerator reflex and worsen the hypotension. Free peritoneal air or high abdominal exploration will produce a dull pain referred to a C5 distribution (usually over the shoulders). Furthermore, cough will be limited by motor block of the abdominal musculature, and deep breathing will be reduced by paralysis of the accessory muscles of inspiration. (However, even at this high level, the diaphragm will not be paralyzed.) Thus, regional anesthesia alone is generally unsuitable for procedures high in the abdomen. A technique that is growing in popularity is to place a catheter for continuous epidural anesthesia prior to induction of general anesthesia, which can then be used postoperatively to administer epidural narcotics.

3. **Superficial procedures** (e.g., gastrostomy, herniorrhaphy) can be done with infiltration of local anesthetic.

4. **Procedures of unknown extent and duration** (e.g., exploratory laparotomy) are difficult to approach with a "single-shot" regional technique. Continuous spinal or epidural anesthesia can be adjusted to meet the surgical needs. General anesthesia must always be available to treat complications or failure of regional anesthesia.

5. **Surgeons** often prefer general anesthesia because there are fewer restrictions on duration, extent of exploration, and conversations related to teaching and other matters.

B. **Factors related to the patient**
1. **Informed consent** for regional anesthesia may be withheld by the patient. The patient must be lucid, willing, and physically able to cooperate during induction and the subsequent period (of several hours).

2. **The site of the proposed regional block** must be unobstructed by previous surgery (e.g., spinal fusion). Systemic infection or infection near the block site are contraindications to a regional block, which could spread the infection.

3. **Clotting and bleeding times** should be normal at the time of the block. Anticoagulation after an atraumatic block has been shown to be safe. Anticoagulation after a bloody epidural or subarachnoid puncture carries a theoretical risk of hemorrhage.

4. **Hypovolemia** must be corrected prior to spinal or epidural anesthesia.

C. **Other limitations** to regional anesthesia include the experience of the anesthesiologist with the particular block, the urgency in starting, and the duration of the procedure.

D. **Advantages of regional anesthesia**
   1. Maintenance of **the patient's ability to communicate** problems (e.g., angina or dyspnea).
   2. Avoidance of the **myocardial and cerebral depression** associated with general anesthetics.
   3. **Protection from aspiration.**
   4. Profound **muscle relaxation and contracted bowel** will provide optimal surgical exposure.
   5. **Continuous techniques** are useful into the postoperative period to provide analgesia (see Chap. 33).

E. **Disadvantages of regional anesthesia**
   1. The **discomfort** involved in placing the block.
   2. **Nerve stretch injury and other complications** of regional anesthesia (see Chap. 13).
   3. **Toxicity** of local anesthetics (see Chap. 12).
   4. **Loss of the ability to cough** effectively secondary to motor block of the abdominal muscles, possibly causing atelectasis and retention of secretions.
   5. Blockade of the accessory respiratory muscles, which may lead to **hypercarbia** in patients with severe chronic obstructive pulmonary disease.
   6. **Hypotension,** from decreased systemic vascular resistance due to sympathetic block, which may be profound in hypovolemic patients or those who cannot increase their cardiac output (e.g., mitral stenosis, subaortic stenosis, restrictive pericarditis).
   7. **Hypoxemia** in patients with bidirectional or right-to-left intracardiac shunts (e.g., tetralogy of Fallot, ventricular septal defect), from decreased systemic vascular resistance and worsening of the right-to-left shunt.
   8. **Excessive sedation** may be required by some patients.

III. **Intraoperative management under general anesthesia**
   A. **Additional fluid losses**
      1. **Surgical bleeding** can be measured in the suction traps and by weighing the surgical sponges; the loss on the drapes can only be estimated. Hidden blood losses have been found underneath the drapes, in retroperitoneal hematomas, and within the bowel. Patients with abdominal trauma should also be evaluated for bleeding into the pelvis, thorax, and long bone fractures.
      2. **Tissue edema** may result from direct trauma disrupting the capillary endothelial integrity. The mesentery, omentum, and bowels can sequester liters of fluid as they are manipulated. Edema fluid may also accumulate in areas with low turgor, such as found in the conjunctiva, lips, and dorsum of the hands. Such observations might influence the selection of colloid versus crystalloid to treat hypotension. Although swelling in these areas is not troublesome per se, it does suggest that swelling might

be occurring in other, more sensitive tissues (e.g., the aryepiglottic folds of the larynx).

3. **Evaporation** from the exposed surface of the parietal and visceral peritoneum results in profound losses of both water (10 ml/kg/hr) and heat.

4. **Nasogastric and other enteric drainage** should also be quantified and replaced but usually represents only a small proportion of the fluid lost.

B. **Temperature control**

1. **Causes of heat loss**

a. **Conduction** is the direct transfer of heat from a warm object to a cooler one. The amount of heat lost is proportional to the area of the warm object exposed, the difference in temperature between the two objects, and the thermal conductivity of the medium between the objects. Still gases such as air have low thermal conductivity and are very good insulators. Fluids (e.g., wet drapes) and dense solids (steel operating room [OR] tables) are very poor insulators and can conduct large amounts of heat.

b. **Convection** is the loss of heat by conduction to a moving gas. Despite its low thermal conductivity, the high turnover of air in the OR leads to significant convective heat loss.

c. Heat may also be lost by infrared **radiation.** Radiant heat loss cannot be prevented by insulation, although objects around the source, such as a reflective space blanket, can reflect the radiation back and maintain body temperature.

d. **Evaporative** heat loss is the energy removed from a body when a liquid is vaporized from its surface. There are evaporative losses during sweating and drying of the mucosal membranes and serosal surfaces; these are directly dependent on the relative humidity of the gas and the surface area exposed. Skin can also be cooled rapidly by the evaporation of surgical prep solutions.

2. **The effects of anesthesia** on the generation and conservation of heat are profound. Surgical planes of anesthesia, with or without muscle relaxation, will suppress shivering in skeletal muscle, which is the major mechanism of excess heat production. Vasodilatation warms the skin despite hypothermia, causing even more heat losses by conduction, convection, and radiation.

3. **Temperature measurement** in the OR is usually done electronically with a **thermistor** (a resistor whose resistance changes with temperature). Placing the probe in the axilla or groin will measure skin temperature. Because of the loss of thermoregulation and significant temperature gradients around the OR, skin temperature is the least reliable reflection of core body temperature. Probes measuring the temperature at the pharynx, esoph-

agus, rectum, or tip of a pulmonary artery catheter are much more reliable indicators of core body temperature.

Liquid crystal temperature strips or dots applied to the skin of the forehead are useful to detect hypo- or hyperthermia but are no substitute for accurate core temperature measurements.

4. **Preventing and treating hypothermia**

   a. **Covering exposed surfaces** is the single most important step in conserving heat. A dry blanket completely covering a part of the body will produce a layer of warm, still air around the skin, which will minimize conductive and convective heat loss. As the temperature of the inside surface of the blanket is raised to body temperature, radiation losses will also be minimized. Reflective ("space") blankets reflect infrared radiation and will minimize radiation losses without necessarily being warmed to body temperature; these are used mostly in the recovery room and the intensive care unit.

   b. **A warming blanket** placed under patients can actually raise body temperature because of the high heat capacitance and conductivity of the water pumped through the blanket. Care must be taken not to raise the blanket temperature above 40°C to avoid skin burns. The best warming blankets have feedback loops consisting of temperature probes in both the blanket and patient. Dislodging the patient probe risks overheating the blanket.

   c. **Heated humidifiers** can be added to the anesthetic circuit to warm and humidify inspired gases. Warming assures that the relative humidity is near 100% at physiologic temperature and minimizes evaporative heat loss from the lungs. Since the heat capacities of gases are low, this method **cannot** be used to raise the body temperature by conduction. Furthermore, when inspired temperature exceeds body temperature, "rain" and scald burns of the airway can occur. Other problems associated with heated humidifiers include obstruction or leaks in the breathing circuit and transmission of infectious diseases.

   d. **A closed or low-flow semiclosed circuit** can also be used to decrease evaporative losses. Gases are warmed and humidified by previous transit through the lungs and by the exothermic, water-producing chemical reactions in the carbon dioxide absorber.

   e. **Fluid warmers** are especially useful in cases requiring large fluid replacement. A liter of crystalloid at a room temperature of 20°C will lower a 70-kg patient's body temperature by 0.25°C; a unit of blood (250 ml) at 4°C will lower it by 0.125°C. Warming fluids to 37°C prevents these losses.

   f. Raising room temperature and humidity will aid in warming patients but is limited by the reasonable comfort of the OR staff.

   g. Radiant warmers are especially useful in infants because of the infants' large surface-volume ratios. Servocontrolled temperature regulators are usually used to prevent hyperthermia.

  5. Treating hyperthermia. It is rare for an adult patient to become hyperthermic as a result of maneuvers to conserve body heat in the OR. Hyperthermia usually results from either **systemic sepsis** or **malignant hyperthermia.** Sepsis is often accompanied by high $P\bar{v}O_2$ with normal $P\bar{v}CO_2$ because of arterio-venous shunting, whereas malignant hyperthermia produces a hypermetabolic state with low $P\bar{v}O_2$, high $P\bar{v}CO_2$, and clinical rigidity. Sepsis should be treated with broad-spectrum antibiotics and drainage; the therapy for malignant hyperthermia is discussed in Chap. 28.

In mild cases, hyperthermia can be treated by reversing the principles of treatment used to prevent hypothermia. Extreme hyperthermia can be treated with more extreme measures such as exposing body surfaces (skin, gastric, or bladder mucosa, peritoneum) to cold saline, ice, or a cooling blanket and dousing the skin with volatile liquids (e.g., alcohol or Freon). Conductive heat loss can be accentuated with vasodilators (e.g., acetaminophen or sodium nitroprusside). Phenothiazines (e.g., chlorpromazine, 25–50 mg IV slowly over 30–60 min) will help suppress shivering.

C. Optimizing surgical conditions

  1. Retraction of abdominal contents with soft packs, rigid retractors, or Trendelenburg positioning is often done to improve exposure. These maneuvers may elevate the diaphragm, resulting in atelectasis, diminished functional residual capacity, and possibly hypoxia. Addition of 5–10 cm H_2O of positive end-expiratory pressure (PEEP) and periodic hyperexpansion of the lungs ("sighs") will counter these effects.

  2. Distention of the bowels may be due to edema, fluid sequestration, or gaseous distention from nitrous oxide (N_2O). Nitrous oxide should not be used in cases of total obstruction (e.g., volvulus, incarcerated hernia, toxic megacolon) or in cases where anastomoses may have to be created in unprepared bowels (e.g., penetrating or blunt abdominal trauma, emergency colectomy for bleeding or abscess, partial bowel obstruction). In the latter cases, the expansion of air spaces within the bowels can propel stool into the surgical field.

  3. Biliary tract spasm can be caused by narcotics,

especially morphine, codeine, and their synthetic derivatives. In susceptible patients, morphine premedication may produce painful biliary spasm, which can be reversed with naloxone. Intraoperative spasm of the common biliary duct or sphincter of Oddi can complicate the surgical repair or the interpretation of intraoperative cholangiograms. Traditionally, meperidine or fentanyl has been used in this setting. However, narcotic agonist/antagonists (e.g., butorphanol or nalbuphine) may be the best choice.

4. **Muscle relaxation** is required for all but the most superficial of intraperitoneal operations (e.g., gastrostomy). The clinical use of relaxants is discussed in Chap. 11. Abdominal closure is a particularly difficult phase of each procedure because the peritoneal cavity may be overcrowded from edema, hematoma, intestines inflated by nitrous oxide, or transplanted organs. The need to provide adequate relaxation at this juncture conflicts with the goal of having an "extubatable" patient shortly after the closure is completed. Strategies for resolving these conflicting goals include

   a. **Titrating relaxants** against the train-of-four twitch response (aiming for a single twitch) and avoiding clinical signs of neuromuscular recovery such as swallowing or attempting to breathe. Intermediate-acting agents such as atracurium and vecuronium may be useful in this setting.

   b. **Increasing the depth of anesthesia** with the potent inhalation agents or thiopental. The potent agents block myoneural conduction and are synergistic with relaxants. Thiopental will be most useful in awakening patients who are becoming intolerant of intubation.

   c. **Decreasing the volume of the stomach** with nasogastric suctioning and discontinuing N_2O well in advance of closing.

   d. **Flexing the operating table** to decrease tension on transverse abdominal or subcostal incisions.

   e. **Discontinuing PEEP and decreasing the tidal volume** temporarily to allow the diaphragm to rise in the thorax. It may be necessary to increase the respiratory rate and FIO_2 to compensate.

5. **Hiccoughs** are episodic spasms of the diaphragm that may occur spontaneously or in response to stimulation of the diaphragm or abdominal viscera. Potentially useful therapies include

   a. **Increasing the depth of anesthesia,** especially if the hiccoughs are a sign of intolerance of the endotracheal tube or reflect direct diaphragmatic or other visceral stimulation.

b. **Removing the source of diaphragmatic irritation,** such as gastric distention, retractors, packs, and suprahepatic hematomas or abscesses.

c. **Increasing the respiratory rate,** which might "overdrive" the diaphragm and decrease the frequency of hiccoughs.

d. **Increasing the degree of neuromuscular blockade,** which may decrease the strength of spasms. Complete diaphragmatic paralysis is difficult to achieve, and may be possible only with doses in excess of those required for relaxation of the abdominal muscles.

e. **Chlorpromazine** IV in 5-mg increments, given slowly.

IV. **Emergence from general anesthesia and extubation**

A. **Termination of anesthesia**

1. **Reversal of neuromuscular blockade** with an acetylcholinesterase inhibitor and a vagolytic (see Chap. 11) can begin after the last fascial layer has been closed and all of the surgical sponges have been located.

2. **Termination of volatile anesthetics** is usually started 10–30 minutes prior to the end of the operation to facilitate a timely emergence. Several factors will affect the rate of emergence:

a. **The depot of anesthetic agents** will be increased by a higher tissue/blood partition coefficient, administered concentration, length of the procedure, and mass of fat stores.

b. **The cardiac output** limits the amount of anesthetic that is returned to the lungs for excretion. Patients in low-output states will emerge slowly.

c. **The blood/gas partition coefficient** will determine the equilibration of the agent between the blood and gas in the lungs. Agents with lower coefficients (e.g., isoflurane as compared to halothane) will partition more into gas and can be excreted faster.

d. **Alveolar ventilation** will remove the agent from the lungs. Low ventilation will raise the alveolar concentration and delay emergence.

e. **Fresh gas flow** from the anesthesia machine will clear the agent from the breathing circuit. Low flow rates will allow rebreathing of the agent, raise the alveolar concentration, and delay emergence.

3. **Narcotics** must be titrated to treat pain from the procedure while preserving the ventilatory drive (unless the decision has been made not to extubate the patient). Too little narcotic may result in discomfort, splinting, and decreased ventilation. Excessive narcotic will decrease the respiratory response to hypercarbia. Hypoventilation will delay

emergence from inhalational anesthetics, and respiratory acidosis can interfere with the reversal of relaxants. Ideally, after receiving narcotics, the patient will not spontaneously complain of pain, the respiratory rate will be greater than 12/min, $PaCO_2$ will be less than 50, and the patient will respond to questions appropriately.

Overnarcotization can be treated with **naloxone** (0.05–0.10 mg IV) as long as the hemodynamic consequences of catecholamine release are considered. Since the half-life of naloxone is less than that of most narcotics, patients must be observed for renarcotization and be treated appropriately. Postoperative analgesia is considered in Chap. 33.

B. Extubation after emergence ("awake" extubation)

1. **The main advantage** of awake extubation is that patients have recovered protective airway reflexes. Laryngospasm and aspiration are much less likely, but this maneuver is frequently accompanied by coughing, straining, and hypertension.

2. **Criteria for awake extubation**

    a. **Adequate spontaneous ventilation** must be established prior to extubation and may be defined as demonstrating a respiratory rate greater than 8/min, tidal volume greater than 5 ml/kg, and inspiratory force of greater negative magnitude than -15 cm H_2O. Inadequate ventilation can be caused by

      (1) **Breath holding.**

      (2) **Depression of the respiratory drive** by narcotics, barbiturates, benzodiazepines, general anesthetics, or hypocarbia (from previously controlled ventilation).

      (3) **Inadequate reversal of neuromuscular blockade** due to hypothermia, respiratory acidosis, inadequate dosage of reversal agents, or potentiation of partial blockade by other drugs (e.g., antibiotics).

      (4) **Inadequate pulmonary function** either from preexisting pulmonary disease or from splinting, atelectasis, aspiration, or pneumothorax.

      (5) **Obstruction of the airway** from bronchospasm, secretions, or occlusion of the endotracheal tube or breathing circuit.

    b. **Adequate oxygenation**

    c. **Adequate recovery of protective airway reflexes** will depend on the degree of residual anesthesia and neuromuscular blockade. Spasms of coughing on the endotracheal tube are not evidence of adequate recovery. Recovery of consciousness and purposeful movements are associated with the recovery of protective reflexes.

    d. **Stability** in overall hemodynamics.

C. **Extubation while still anesthetized ("deep" extubation)**
1. **Advantages** of extubating deep are related to the patient's emerging without the stimulation of an endotracheal tube. Prevention of coughing and straining is particularly desirable after herniorrhaphy. Deep extubation will also decrease the likelihood of bronchospasm on emergence in asthmatics and will prevent the tachycardia and hypertension associated with extubating awake.
2. **The risks of laryngospasm and aspiration** are increased by deep extubation. Patients who require awake intubation or rapid sequence induction are not candidates for deep extubation. Similarly, intraoperative events that increase the risk of aspiration (e.g., bowels distended by blood or N_2O, placement of a nasogastric tube) would also preclude deep extubation.

V. **Anesthetic considerations for specific abdominal procedures**

A. **Splenectomy** is often an emergency following blunt or penetrating abdominal trauma or may be performed electively for treatment of idiopathic thrombocytopenic purpura or for staging Hodgkin's lymphoma. In either case, it is not unusual to encounter major blood losses requiring transfusion. General endotracheal anesthesia and muscle relaxation are always required. Occasionally, a transthoracic approach to gain control of the hilar vessels of a very large spleen may be necessary.

B. **Cholecystectomy** is a common operation in the upper abdomen. General endotracheal anesthesia with muscle relaxation is required, although supplementation with right intercostal nerve blocks will improve postoperative pain management. Narcotics must be selected judiciously for premedication and maintenance to minimize spasm in the biliary tract and sphincter of Oddi. Retraction in the right upper quadrant can cause atelectasis at the base of the right lung; postoperative pain and splinting may exacerbate atelectasis and impair ventilation.

C. **Partial hepatectomy** is used to treat hepatoma, solitary metastasis of a gastrointestinal carcinoma, arteriovenous malformation, or echinococcal cyst. Major hemorrhage should be anticipated, as well as postoperative intensive care. The liver has considerable parenchymal reserve, and extensive resection is needed before drug metabolism is clinically impaired. The effects of liver disease on anesthetic management is discussed in Chap. 5.

D. **Orthotopic liver transplantation** is done for large hepatomas without metastases, biliary duct obstruction from biliary atresia or sclerosing cholangitis, genetic diseases such as Wilson's disease, alpha$_1$-antitrypsin deficiency, or hereditary tyrosinemia, and for hepatocellular failure from primary biliary cirrhosis, systemic lupus erythematosus, and chronic active or acute fulminant hepatitis.

1. **The surgical procedure** involves total hepatectomy including the gallbladder, hepatic veins, and a section of the inferior vena cava (IVC). Then transplantation of the donor liver is performed with reanastomoses to the supra- and infrahepatic IVC, portal vein, hepatic artery, and biliary duct (except in cases of biliary duct obstruction, where a Roux-en-Y choledochojejunostomy is done). In adults and larger children, an interim venous shunt connecting the portal and femoral veins to the axillary vein is used while the IVC and portal vein are interrupted. A donor cholecystectomy is then performed, and a common-duct T tube placed.

2. **The major complications** are
   a. **Hemorrhage** (up to 10 blood volumes) due to portal hypertension, peritoneal inflammation, multiple vascular anastomoses, dilutional and consumptive clotting factor deficiencies, and thrombocytopenia.
   b. **Marked hypothermia** usually results because of the prolonged exposure of the bowel, extensive blood transfusions, transplantation of a 3- to 4-kg liver stored in iced saline, and unheated extracorporeal circulation. Every strategy for heat conservation should be applied (see sec. **III.B**).
   c. **Metabolic derangements** may suddenly develop; thus monitoring must be frequent and specific.
      (1) **Metabolic acidosis** occurs from accumulation of lactate and citrate, which are normally metabolized by the liver. Consequently, normal saline is a better choice for fluid replacement than lactated Ringer's solution. Sodium bicarbonate (NaHCO$_3$) may be needed acutely, but postoperative metabolic alkalosis may ensue once the lactate and citrate load is metabolized.
      (2) **Low ionized calcium (Ca^{2+}) levels** are caused by citrate intoxication from anticoagulated blood products and are treated with calcium chloride (CaCl$_2$) IV.
      (3) **Hyperkalemia** accompanies rapid blood transfusion and results from release of cold, acidotic, hyperkalemic saline by the ischemic transplanted liver. Perfusing the graft can cause cardiac arrest, which is treated with CaCl$_2$, NaHCO$_3$, and CPR to move the potassium (K$^+$) bolus out of, and the drugs into, the heart. Insulin and glucose are less useful in lowering plasma K$^+$ because skeletal muscle is cold and rela-

tively poorly perfused and the liver is ischemic. After the transplanted liver is warmed and perfused, its transmembrane K^+ gradients are restored, which may cause hypokalemia. Lactate and citrate metabolism at this point will raise the pH and ionized Ca^{2+}.

(4) **Hyperglycemia** is seen in most cases but usually is not severe enough to require treatment.

d. **Hypoxia** can occur from intrapulmonary arteriovenous shunting, atelectasis (from upper abdominal retraction), or acute respiratory disease, and is best treated with PEEP and a high FiO_2.

e. **Immunosuppression** with steroids and cyclosporine may lead to life-threatening infections. All invasive monitoring catheters should be placed under sterile conditions and maintained with this risk in mind.

f. **Severe hypertension** can develop postoperatively for reasons that remain unclear.

3. **Anesthetic management.** By definition, donor livers are unpredictably available and cannot be supported extracorporeally. Thus, most recipients have full stomachs and will require **rapid sequence inductions.** Maintenance is usually with oxygen, relaxants, narcotics, and low concentrations of isoflurane or enflurane if tolerated. (If not, then scopolamine or a benzodiazepine will be needed to provide amnesia.) Halothane is avoided because it can cause hepatic artery vasospasm. Nitrous oxide can be used in the beginning of cases but may have to be discontinued if right pneumothorax (from diaphragmatic perforation during dissection over the dome of the liver) or air emboli (following resection of the IVC or during venous bypass) are detected. The donor liver is often larger than the recipient's shrunken, cirrhotic one. Thus, closure of the abdomen may be difficult, and a bowel distended with N_2O only compounds the problem.

E. **Heterotopic pancreatic transplantation** is usually done in conjunction with heterotopic renal transplantation in the groin for treatment of diabetes mellitus. Although recipients may undergo a nephrectomy, their native pancreas is left intact. **Anesthetic considerations** are primarily related to renal transplantation and are discussed in Chap. 26. Blood glucose should be determined frequently, since it often falls toward normal within minutes of perfusing the new pancreas. The exocrine pancreatic secretions are diverted through the common bile duct and a small button of duodenum, into the recipient's bladder. Since there is no pepsin present, trypsinogen and chymotrypsinogen are not activated and the bladder and urethra are not damaged by digestive enzyme action. However, a gram-negative urinary tract infection (especially with *Proteus*) can activate these enzymes, leading to bladder damage, and emergency removal of the transplanted pancreas may be necessary. The pancreas will also secrete bicarbonate (HCO_3^-), which will be lost with urine; if the kidney should fail but the pancreas continue to work, severe metabolic acidosis can result.

F. **Pancreatectomy** for hemorrhagic pancreatitis or pseudocyst is a difficult surgical dissection resulting in significant bleeding and third-space fluid loss. The inflammatory nature of these diseases also results in severe peritonitis, ileus, and edema. Release of pancreatic lipases can result in soponification of omental fat, releasing fatty acids that sequester Ca^{2+}, producing hypocalcemia.

G. **Whipple procedure (pancreaticojejunostomy with gastrojejunostomy and choledochojejunostomy)** is done for resection of an adenocarcinoma at the head of the pancreas. These are long and surgically difficult procedures with extensive evaporative fluid and heat losses.

H. **Intraoperative radiation therapy** (RT) for pancreatic or colonic adenocarcinoma usually involves exploratory laparotomy and possibly a primary resection or debulking procedure. Then before wound closure, the anesthetized patient is moved from the OR to the (sometimes distant) RT suite. The route of transportation and the RT suite must be prepared in advance, along with supplies of resuscitation drugs, volume replacement, and intubating equipment to accompany the patient. Anesthesia can be maintained with IV agents until the anesthesia machine in the RT suite is reached.

In the RT suite, the safety of both patient and anesthesiologist must be assured. Patients are positioned so that ventilation can be visualized on remote television monitors. When the sterile cone of the cyclotron is lowered into the abdominal wound, patients are checked for signs of aortic or IVC compression. Ventilation should be done with 100% oxygen to maximize the sensitivity of the tumor to RT. Treatments usually last 5–20 minutes but may be interrupted if ventilatory or cardiovascular instability develops. Wound closure may be performed in the RT suite or after transport back to the OR.

I. **Gastrectomy or hemigastrectomy** with gastroduodenostomy (Billroth I) or gastrojejunostomy (Billroth II) are usually done for gastric adenocarcinoma or for bleeding gastric or duodenal peptic ulcers. Either the presence of blood in the stomach or gastric outlet obstruction from scarring or tumor would indicate that a rapid sequence induction or awake intubation is needed.

J. **Gastrostomy** can be done through a small upper abdominal incision under local anesthesia, particularly in debilitated elderly patients.

K. **Small-bowel resection** may be done for penetrating trauma, Crohn's disease, obstructing adhesions, Meckel's diverticulum, or infarction (from volvulus, intussusception, or thromboembolus). Patients can be hypovolemic from vomiting, diarrhea, ileus, third spacing, or bleeding, and most are to be considered to have "full stomachs." Usually muscle relaxants are required.

L. **Appendectomy** is usually a brief procedure done through a small lower abdominal incision. However, patients with appendicitis may be dehydrated from fever, poor oral intake, or vomiting. Generous IV hydration is usually indicated prior to initiation of anesthesia. In cases where systemic sepsis is absent, hydration adequate, the patient cooperative and calm, and high abdominal exploration is unlikely, then a spinal or epidural anesthetic can be used. Otherwise general anesthesia with a rapid sequence induction or awake intubation is necessary; muscle relaxants are usually required.

M. **Colectomy or hemicolectomy** is used to treat adenocarcinomas, diverticulosis, angiodysplasia, ulcerative colitis, penetrating trauma, and infarctions. Emergency colectomy on an unprepared bowel runs a high risk of fecal spillage with peritonitis. Thus, many colonic emergencies are treated by a diverting colostomy followed by bowel preparation and elective colectomy.

Patients for colectomy must be evaluated for hypovolemia from bleeding, vomiting, overzealous bowel preps, as well as anemia and sepsis. All emergency colectomies or colostomies, and some elective colectomies, should be treated as having "full stomachs."

N. **Perirectal abscess drainage, hemorrhoidectomy, and pilonidal cystectomy** are relatively noninvasive, brief procedures. Pilonidal cysts are usually approached in prone position, the others in prone or lithotomy positions. General anesthesia by mask is possible when in lithotomy; however, intubation is necessary for prone cases. If general anesthesia is selected, deep planes of anesthesia or muscle relaxants may be required to relax the anal sphincter. Hyperbaric spinals can be used for procedures in lithotomy, while hypobaric spinals work well in the flexed prone or knee-chest position, and thus minimal repositioning is needed after induction. After anal surgery, bearing down to void will be painful; thus fluids should be kept to a minimum.

O. **Inguinal, femoral, or ventral herniorrhaphies** can be done under local, spinal, epidural, or general anesthesia. Closure of large fascial defects is facilitated by muscle relaxation, which regional anesthesia provides the best. If general anesthesia is selected, then either a mask technique or deep extubation should be considered to decrease coughing on emergence, which can strain the hernia repair.

Suggested Reading

Borland, L. M., and Cook, D. R. Anesthesia for organ transplantation. *Adv. Anesth.* 3:1, 1986.

Ryan, J. F., and Vacanti, F. X. Temperature Regulation. In J. F. Ryan et al. (eds.), *A Practice of Anesthesia for Infants and Children.* Orlando, Fla.: Grune & Stratton, 1986.

18

Anesthesia for Vascular Surgery

James L. Konigsberg

Patients with significant systemic arterial disease requiring surgery are a challenge, in terms of both risk assessment and intramanagement. As a rule, these patients have coexisting medical problems including atherosclerosis of other systemic arteries supplying the heart, brain, and kidneys; hypertension; metabolic defects including diabetes and hypercholesterolemia; pulmonary disease; and advanced age.

I. **Preoperative assessment** should be aimed at identifying coexistent disease, optimizing specific therapies, and anticipating intra- and postoperative problems.

   A. **Cardiovascular system.** Coronary artery disease (CAD) is present in 40–80% of vascular surgery patients and is their major source of morbidity and mortality. Myocardial infarction (MI) accounts for about one-half of deaths early after operation. Several retrospective studies have sought to identify cardiac risk factors, but when applied prospectively to patients undergoing vascular surgery, these risks are underestimated. Risk factors are listed in Chap. 2.

   1. **Implications of the history and physical examination**

      a. **Hypertension** per se does not predispose to cardiovascular complications after anesthesia. However, uncontrolled hypertension is associated with greater lability on induction and emergence and, when combined with other diseases, may increase anesthetic risks. In general, hypertensive patients have a higher incidence of CAD, stroke, renal failure, and congestive heart failure (CHF). Both treated and untreated patients are more likely to have abnormalities in electrolytes, intravascular volume, and renal function.

         (1) The severity of hypertension and the therapy necessary for control should be ascertained. Hypertension may be asymptomatic unless quite severe; in this case, intervention may be needed prior to surgery. Potential side effects of antihypertensive therapy should be sought through the history, physical examination, and laboratory tests (e.g., orthostatic signs and symptoms, hypokalemia with diuretics, bradyarrhythmias with beta blockers, prerenal azotemia with diuretics and afterload-reducing agents, proteinuria with angiotensin-converting enzyme inhibitors).

         (2) With end-stage hypertensive heart disease, the left ventricle (LV) may be hy-

pertrophied and dilated, with a reduced ejection fraction. Sometimes, hypertrophic cardiomyopathy is characterized by poor LV compliance and poor relaxation during diastole, but a normal or supranormal ejection fraction and exquisite sensitivity to changes in preload and after-load (such pathophysiology resembles idiopathic subaortic stenosis). In general, these patients respond poorly to inotropes or excess afterload reduction.

(3) Secondary causes of hypertension may be masked by treatment but are suggested by severe hypokalemia (hyperaldosteronism), orthostatic hypotension and palpitaions (pheochromocytoma), or, especially in vascular surgery patients, a periumbilical bruit (renovascular hypertension).

b. **CAD and previous MI** are common in patients with systemic vascular disease. History of MI, typical or atypical symptoms of myocardial ischemia, and the stability of symptoms should be ascertained. It may be useful to know whether anginal symptoms occur in tandem with some objective sign (i.e., ECG changes, hypotension, changes in heart rate or rhythm, premature ventricular contractions, or elevations in the pulmonary capillary wedge pressure [PCWP]).

Patients with a history of MI, especially within 6 months of a planned vascular procedure, are at significantly higher risk of reinfarction and death. One type of MI is not necessarily more ominous than another (e.g., a subendocardial MI may be a prelude to further infarction, while transmural MI may indicate that little myocardium is still at risk). Exercise testing, dipyridamole/thallium scanning, and coronary angiography are methods available to define this risk. In those whose workups indicate a high risk of MI, coronary artery bypass surgery should be considered prior to peripheral vascular surgery. This course may result in a much better chance for perioperative, and long-term, survival.

c. **Congestive heart failure.** Patients with reduced cardiac output are more susceptible to the depressant effects of anesthetics. Decompensation may be precipitated by volume overload or increased systemic vascular resistance, and if combined with ischemia, hypotension may be severe. Classic signs and symptoms of CHF seem to be among the most ominous factors predisposing to postoperative cardiovascular complications.

         d. Other cardiac disease. Anesthetic considerations in the presence of valvular heart disease are found in Chap. 20.

    2. Laboratory considerations

         a. Electrocardiogram. Preoperative ECGs are most useful as baselines, because normal ECGs do not necessarily rule out CAD. In some cases, ECG abnormalities may mask ischemia (e.g., left bundle branch block or left ventricular hypertrophy with strain).

         b. Exercise stress testing, gated blood pool scans, thallium scans, and cardiac catheterization are discussed in Chap. 2.

B. Respiratory system. Smoking greatly increases the risk of chronic obstructive pulmonary disease, as well as vascular disease. History of morning cough, sputum production, wheezing, marked dyspnea on exertion, the use of oxygen at home, or a physical examination revealing cyanosis, a barrel-shaped chest, digital clubbing, wheezing, lack of breath sounds, or consolidation suggests a likelihood of perioperative respiratory complications. A chest x-ray should be obtained from all smokers, while pulmonary function tests (PFTs) are indicated in those with abnormal histories or physical examinations. Patients with FEV_1 less than 1.5 liters or less than 20% of predicted, FEV_1 less than 35% of VC, or $PaCO_2$ greater than 45 are more likely to need postoperative ventilation (see Chap. 3). Ventilatory support will almost certainly be required if patients with the above signs or symptoms undergo upper abdominal or thoracic operations. Smoking should be stopped at least 2 weeks before surgery; this has been shown to return PFTs toward normal. If wheezing is noted, or if PFTs are improved by bronchodilators, aminophylline IV and/or a beta-2 agonist by inhaler should be considered.

C. Renal system. Renal insufficiency is often found in patients with atherosclerotic disease of major systemic arteries. When severe, there is a substantially increased risk of death during the postoperative course. Causes of renal failure include atherosclerosis of the renal arteries, hypertensive nephrosclerosis, diabetic nephropathy, inadequate perfusion secondary to low cardiac output, overzealous diuresis, or angiographic dye-related acute tubular necrosis. Blood urea nitrogen (BUN), creatinine, electrolytes, and urinalysis should be routinely obtained before any vascular surgical procedure. With any abnormality, strict attention to volume status and electrolyte balance is mandatory to prevent oliguria and azotemia.

D. Central nervous system

    1. A history of transient ischemic attacks or stroke is highly suggestive of cerebrovascular disease. The neck should be examined for bruits. The presence of asymptomatic carotid bruits prior to a peripheral vascular procedure generally does not indicate further therapy, since it will not prevent stroke. But patients with symptomatic carotid bruits should receive evaluation for possible endarterectomy (see Chap. 22); definitive diagnosis requires carotid arteriography. Unfortunately, angiography itself is associated with a 1% incidence of neurologic deficit and thus should only be done when symptoms are clear-cut. Less invasive procedures such as digital subtraction angiography, Doppler flow studies, and ocular plethysmography offer possible alternatives. Patients with a history of stroke have a higher risk of perioperative cardiac complications.

2. Historical and physical evidence for lower extremity neurologic dysfunction, or low back pain syndromes or operations, may be relative or even absolute contraindications to the use of regional anesthesia.

E. Endocrine system. Diabetes mellitus is a major cause of vascular disease. Diabetics may manifest accelerated large-vessel atherosclerosis, as well as distal small-vessel disease. Long-standing diabetics may have autonomic neuropathy (giving rise to postural symptoms or silent MIs), diabetic nephropathy, and reduced resistance to infection. Preoperative insulin orders and related management recommendations are discussed in Chap. 6.

F. Gastrointestinal system. Vascular surgery on the abdominal aorta may be complicated by postoperative pancreatitis or intestinal infarction.

G. Hematologic system. Vascular surgery patients are often on anticoagulants (heparin, warfarin, dipyridamole, or aspirin). A history of easy bruisability, petechiae, or ecchymosis should be evaluated with a prothrombin time (PT), partial thromboplastin time (PTT), platelet count, and bleeding time. In emergencies, fresh-frozen plasma, whole fresh blood, or platelets may be needed. Facilities for autotransfusion should be arranged if massive blood losses are anticipated.

H. Infection. Patients with any evidence of infection should receive appropriate antibiotics preoperatively and consideration given to postponing cases where heterologous graft materials will be used. The risk of graft infection is 1–2%, even in the absence of any evidence of systemic infection and despite administration of prophylactic antibiotics.

II. Medication prior to surgery

A. Antihypertensives are usually held 24–48 hours prior to surgery. Clonidine withdrawal has been associated with exaggerated rebound hypertension. Chronic reserpine use may induce a "denervation hypersensitivity," leading to exaggerated responses to sympathomimetics. Beta blockers should be continued preoperatively if in use for their antianginal properties.

B. Antianginals. Nitrates, calcium (Ca^{2+}) channel antagonists, and beta blockers should all be continued until the time of surgery.

    C. Digoxin. Unless needed for ventricular rate control, digoxin should be held 24–48 hours prior to surgery. Hypokalemia following intraoperative diuresis will increase the likelihood of digoxin toxicity.

    D. Antiarrhythmics should generally be continued. However, these agents are also myocardial depressants and may act synergistically with inhalational anesthetics.

    E. Anticoagulants. Heparin should be substituted for warfarin preoperatively, allowing the PT to normalize. Generally, heparin is withheld for 4 hours prior to surgery, unless otherwise ordered by surgical staff.

    F. Bronchodilators should be continued when there has been proven benefit.

    G. Premedication. The goals and regimens for sedating premedicants are generally the same as for other patients undergoing major procedures; the presence of CAD may modify these and are discussed in Chap. 2

III. Monitoring requirements are a function of the general health of the patient and the nature, duration, and extent of the planned surgical procedure.

    A. Electrocardiogram. A seven-lead ECG (the limb leads and V5) with a rhythm strip should be obtained prior to starting anesthesia. It should be available for comparison to pre- and intraoperative tracings. The V5 lead monitors the bulk of the LV muscle mass.

    B. Blood pressure. Patients with vascular disease of any major organ (coronary, cerebral, or renal) are intolerant of major blood pressure fluctuations; in procedures where this might occur, intraarterial cannulation is indicated. Blood pressure must be checked in both arms to rule out asymmetry from subclavian or aortic arch atheromas.

    C. Intravascular volume

        1. If ventricular function is normal, a catheter placed in the central venous circulation will reliably reflect cardiac preload and provide central venous access for medication. If however, there is right or left ventricular dysfunction, the central venous pressure (CVP) is not necessarily related to the left ventricular end-diastolic pressure (LVEDP).

        2. Pulmonary artery (PA) catheters allow measurement of both left-sided (PCWP) and right-sided (CVP) filling pressures. Cardiac output may be monitored by thermodilution, allowing calculation of stroke volume and both pulmonary and systemic vascular resistance. Changes in the PCWP often precede ECG evidence of ischemia. The indications for PA catheter placement are reviewed in Chap. 2. The pertinent anatomy, techniques, and complications appear in Chap. 8. Because of the high coincidence of carotid atherosclerosis in vascular surgery patients, it is worth reiterating that the result of carotid compression from hematoma formation near an already narrowed artery could be devastating.

    D. Urine output. A Foley catheter should be placed prior to any major vascular procedure to monitor global renal function.

E. Temperature. Heat loss during prolonged vascular procedures may exacerbate myocardial dysfunction and coagulopathy and should be prevented. Strategies for heat conservation include gas humidification, warming of infusions, adjustment in room temperature, and use of warm irrigation and plastic bowel bags (see Chap. 17).

IV. Procedures in peripheral vascular surgery include bypass procedures such as iliofemoral, femoral-popliteal, femoral-femoral, femoral-tibial, axillofemoral, as well as aneurysmectomies and embolectomies. Although these procedures are generally confined to the more distal branches of the aorta, perioperative cardiac complications may still occur, and appropriate monitoring should be undertaken.

A. Anesthetic considerations. Choice of anesthesia is dictated by the type of surgery planned, the physical and psychological limitations of individual patients, and the skills and preference of the anesthesiologist and surgeon. There is little conclusive evidence that regional anesthesia is safer than general anesthesia.

1. **General anesthesia.** Either balanced or inhalational anesthesia is appropriate, since massive volume shifts are uncommon and hemodynamic stability is the rule.

2. **Regional anesthesia.** Epidural or spinal anesthesia may be tolerated well, provided patients are selected with discrimination. A **continuous lumbar epidural** will provide excellent anesthesia and has the added advantage of providing a route to administer postoperative analgesia (dosage regimens for epidural narcotics are discussed in Chap. 33). However, the suggestion that lumbar sympathetic blockade improves graft patency remains unproved. In some respects, monitoring during regional anesthesia is facilitated (e.g., conscious patients with angina are able to complain of acute chest pain).

   a. Attention to patient comfort is particularly important when using regional techniques during long procedures. Appropriate back and shoulder padding, as well as freedom of the neck and arms, should be provided. Sedation is aimed at reducing patient anxiety without producing respiratory depression or unresponsiveness. A phenylephrine drip should be available during inductions to treat hypotension associated with sympathetic blockade; nausea or light-headedness may be the earliest manifestations.

   b. Large studies support that **heparin** may be safely given after epidural catheters have been placed. Clearly, lower extremity weakness following such maneuvers mandates immediate neurosurgical consultation, but fortunately, such emergencies are exceedingly rare.

3. Regional and general anesthesia may be used in **combination** and has the advantages of overall reduction in anesthetic requirements, relatively rapid emergence, and a route for the administration of analgesics postoperatively.

B. Peripheral embolectomy or aneurysmectomy can usually be performed under **local anesthesia** administered by the surgeon. During such procedures, substantial blood loss may occur, and occasionally, local anesthetics are administered in toxic doses.

V. **Abdominal aortic surgery** may be required for atherosclerotic occlusive disease or aneurysmal dilatation. These processes can involve the aorta and any of its major branches, leading to ischemia or rupture and exsanguination. Three-fourths of all abdominal aortic aneurysms occur below the renal arteries.

A. **Infrarenal abdominal aortic operations.** The overriding physiologic considerations stem from aortic cross-clamping. Even infrarenal cross-clamping diminishes perfusion of the renal cortex, reducing glomerular filtration rate, thus creating the potential for renal failure.

1. **Anesthetic administration.** Either **regional or general anesthesia** may be appropriate. Many of the same considerations mentioned for peripheral vascular surgery apply here as well.

a. **Monitoring.** At minimum, an ECG with V5 lead and arterial and CVP catheters are required to monitor cardiac and hemodynamic function, as well as to provide central circulatory access if vasoactive infusions are required.

b. **Induction of general anesthesia.** In patients with adequate ventricular function, $M\dot{V}O_2$ should be limited by preventing hypertension and tachycardia. Potent inhalational anesthetics are a sensible choice for this group. With poor ventricular function, the goal is to prevent decompensation from myocardial depression and sympathetic blockade (see Chap. 20 for relevant discussion of inducing general anesthesia in patients with poor ventricular function).

c. **Bowel manipulation** is usually necessary to gain access to the aorta and may be accompanied by hypotension, fall in systemic vascular resistance, and skin flushing. Treatment consists in reducing anesthetic depth and, if necessary, infusing additional volume and phenylephrine.

d. **Aortic cross-clamping**
   (1) **Cardiovascular function**
      (a) Increased afterload following aortic cross-clamping is well tolerated by patients with normal hearts but poorly tolerated in those with compromised left ventricles. A rise in

PCWP with a falling cardiac output indicates LV failure, and ischemic changes on the ECG may follow. Deepening anesthesia (to reduce myocardial work and systemic vascular resistance) or afterload reduction with nitroglycerin or sodium nitroprusside often improves the myocardial oxygen supply-demand balance.

    (b) Prolonged aortic occlusion produces peripheral ischemia and accumulation of anaerobic metabolites, with subsequent, profound distal vasodilatation. Consequently, intravascular volume must be maintained in the normal-to-high range, anticipating a fall in systemic vascular resistance following release of the aortic cross-clamp.

  (2) Renal function. Renal cortical blood flow and urine output fall with infrarenal aortic cross-clamping. The mechanism is unknown, although possibilities include microcirculatory derangement, effects on the renin/angiotensin axis, and microembolization. Adequate hydration and maintenance of urine flow seem to reduce the incidence of acute renal failure (ARF). Mannitol (0.25–0.5 g/kg IV) and possibly furosemide should be given prior to aortic occlusion. If the diuresis is inadequate during the cross-clamp period, additional mannitol and furosemide or low-dose dopamine (1–5 μg/kg/min) should be given. Patients with chronically elevated creatinine levels (> 2 mg/dl have substantially higher morbidity and mortality after vascular surgery. Even with normal renal function, there is a 5–10% chance of ARF postoperatively. Patients with ruptured abdominal aortic aneurysms face a 15–25% chance of ARF. In those who do develop ARF, it unfortunately is usually irreversible, and there is a 65–95% death rate.

 e. Aortic unclamping. Cross-clamp release leads to both venous and arterial dilatation, and the negative inotropic effects of anaerobic metabolites can reduce cardiac output. Hypotension should be anticipated and can be prevented by volume loading, "lightening" anesthesia, discontinuing vasodilators, or if need be, infusing a vasopressor. Reperfusion of the lower extremities results in hyperemia with washout of anaerobic products and possibly systemic acidosis. Sodium bicarbonate administration is rarely necessary, although it is indicated if the pH is less than 7.25. Occasionally, cardiac output may rise following cross-clamp release secondary to the reduced afterload.

f. **Blood and fluid replacement.** Intravascular volume is depleted by hemorrhage, third spacing into the bowel and peritoneal cavity, and insensible losses associated with large abdominal incisions. Crystalloid may be used for volume replacement, provided electrolytes, glucose, and osmolarity are monitored. Hematocrit should be maintained in the 30% range for oxygen-carrying capacity, particularly in patients with critical coronary stenoses. With greater blood losses (> 5–10 units), coagulation profiles and appropriate replacement of platelets, clotting factors, and Ca^{2+} become mandatory (see Chap. 27 for diagnosis and management of posttransfusion bleeding diatheses).

Autotransfusion devices should be employed whenever possible. These devices suction blood from the operative field; add heparin; pool, filter, and wash the blood; and then pack it for reinfusion. This blood is low in K^+, free hemoglobin, fibrinogen, fibrin split products, platelets, total protein, and white blood cells. The pH is roughly normal, and the hematocrit may be as high as 40–50%.

g. **Hypothermia.** Massive transfusion, large incisions, and prolonged operating times all conspire to produce hypothermia. Strategies for temperature conservation were mentioned in sec. **III.E.** Hypothermia may be associated with arrhythmias, myocardial depression, coagulopathies, vasoconstriction, and potentiation of anesthetics.

h. **Emergence.** Hypertension and hypothermia are the major problems late in the procedure. Uncomplicated patients under anesthesia for a relatively short time may be extubated in the operating room (OR). Higher-risk patients often remain intubated and are transported directly to an intensive care setting. Prior to departure from the OR, hypertension, pain, shivering, and tachycardia should be prevented or treated. Blood pressure and ECG should be monitored during transport, paralysis maintained to prevent shivering (which sharply elevates oxygen consumption), and ventilation continued.

B. **Ruptured abdominal aortic aneurysms.** Initial management of the patient with a ruptured abdominal aortic aneurysm is dominated by resuscitative measures. Mortality can be limited by restoration of intravascular volume, judicious use of vasoconstrictors and rapid surgical control. Under the best of situations there is a 40–50% mortality, usually resulting from the physiologic consequences of hypotension and massive blood transfusion. The incidence of MI, ARF, respiratory failure, and coagulopathy is high. Survival depends on coordination between the emergency room, OR, surgical, anesthesia, and intensive care unit staffs.

1. **Preoperative considerations**
    a. **Initial volume management.** MAST (Military Anti-Shock Trousers) or "G" suits are often applied in the emergency room, where several large-bore (#14) IV catheters are placed. Blood samples should be sent immediately for crossmatching and any other particularly pertinent studies. Blood components should be ordered immediately, but universal donor-type blood (type O-negative) should be obtained if type-specific blood is unavailable. Crystalloid and pressors should be used to maintain the systolic blood pressure in the 80–100 mm Hg range.
    b. **Before induction.** The G suit should be kept inflated to 20 cm H_2O to compress the abdomen, which may temporarily tamponade a leaking aneurysm. Once the surgeon is scrubbed, the abdomen is prepared and draped and induction begun Foley catheter or nasogastric tube insertion should be delayed until after induction to avoid Valsalva maneuvers that may aggravate bleeding or cause frank rupture.
    c. **Monitoring.** Although time is of the essence in a dire emergency, the minimum monitoring standards (see Chap. 9) should still be applied. Arterial and PA catheters may have to await volume resuscitation.
2. **Anesthetic administration**
    a. **Induction.** In the shocky or moribund patient, intubation may be safest while awake. Oxygen with scopolamine and/or a benzodiazepine for amnesia and a relaxant, may be all that is tolerated. In most other patients, a rapid sequence induction to prevent aspiration is indicated (see Chap. 10). Ketamine may be used in the alert but hypotensive patient. If succinylcholine is to be used, pretreatment with a small dose of a nondepolarizing muscle relaxant will prevent an increase in intraabdominal pressure and avoid exacerbating aneurysm leakage. Clearly, hypertension must be scrupulously avoided, and sodium nitroprusside or trimethaphan are the drugs of choice (see Chap. 16). Trimethaphan offers a theoretical advantage because it is a ganglionic blocker and decreases autonomic tone, thus preventing the dP/dt increases seen with sodium nitroprusside. Sodium nitroprusside may be used, provided the reflex enhance-

ment of contractility is prevented by concurrent beta blockade. Mannitol should be given as early as possible since cross-clamping the aorta above the level of the renal arteries usually follows within minutes of the induction.

b. **Hemodynamics.** Aortic cross-clamping may transiently increase blood pressure. Nevertheless, treatment of hypovolemia should continue unabated. If hypertension is severe, a short-acting vasodilator may be indicated.

c. **Laboratory studies.** Acid-base status, electrolytes, and hematocrit may drastically change and should be monitored closely. Acidosis is often accompanied by hyperkalemia and should be corrected with sodium bicarbonate.

d. **Renal failure.** Urine output should be preserved with transfusion, mannitol, furosemide, and low-dose dopamine to avoid renal failure.

e. **Paraplegia.** When the aorta is cross-clamped above the T10 level, paraplegia may result. This is most likely due to spinal cord ischemia from hypoperfusion or embolization and may possibly be prevented by distal shunt insertion. Cross-clamp periods longer than 30 minutes more than triple the chance of this complication. Somatosensory evoked potential (SEP) monitors (see sec. **VI.C.3** and Chap. 22) are usually unavailable in emergencies.

3. **Postoperative considerations.** Intensive care is required during recovery. Emergence should be gradual, with particular attention to urine output, cardiac output, distal extremity perfusion, respiratory adequacy, hematocrit, and hemostasis. Abrupt withdrawal of anesthesia and muscle paralysis should be avoided. The most frequent complications include acute respiratory distress syndrome, MI, renal failure, bowel infarction, pancreatitis, sepsis, disseminated intravascular coagulation, and peripheral embolization.

VI. **Thoracic aortic surgery.** Disease of the thoracic aorta may result from atherosclerosis, degenerative disorders of connective tissue (Marfan's and Ehlers-Danlos syndromes, cystic medial necrosis), infection (syphilis), congenital defects (coarctation or congenital aneurysms of the sinus of Valsalva), trauma (penetrating and deceleration injuries), and inflammatory processes (Takayasu's aortitis).

The most common problem affecting the thoracic aorta is atherosclerotic aneurysm of the descending portion, accounting for some 20% of all aortic aneurysms. When these dissect proximally, they may involve the aortic valve or the coronary ostia. Distal dissection may involve the abdominal aorta or the renal or mesenteric branches. Next most frequent are traumatic disruptions of the thoracic aorta. Adventitial false aneurysms may form distal to the left subclavian artery at the insertion of the ligamentum arteriosum, as a result of penetrating or decelerating injuries. These false aneurysms may dissect anterograde, involving the arch and its major branches.

A. Preoperative considerations

1. **Ascending aortic aneurysms** are approached by median sternotomy and require cardiopulmonary bypass (CPB) with arterial cannulation through the femoral artery, the distal ascending aorta, or the aortic arch.

2. **Transverse aortic arch repair** requires median sternotomy, CPB, and hypothermic total circulatory arrest to assure CNS protection.

3. **Descending aortic aneurysms** are often approached by left lateral thoracotomy with cross-clamp placement distal to the left subclavian artery.

4. **Thoracic aortic aneurysms may produce**

    a. **Airway deviation or compression,** particularly of the left main stem bronchus, leading to atelectasis.

    b. **Tracheal displacement or disruption,** leading to difficulties with intubation and ventilation. Long-standing aneurysms may damage the recurrent laryngeal nerves, resulting in vocal cord paralysis and hoarseness.

    c. **Hemoptysis** secondary to erosion of the aneurysm into an adjacent bronchus.

    d. **Esophageal compression** with dysphagia and an increased risk of aspiration.

    e. **Distortion and compression of central venous and arterial anatomy,** leading to markedly asymmetric pulses and difficult internal jugular cannulation. A right radial artery catheter is often best because cross-clamping in the arch may occlude flow through the left subclavian artery. However, the arterial pressure monitoring site must be tailored to each anatomic situation.

    f. **Hemothorax and mediastinal shift** from rupture and/or leakage with resultant respiratory and circulatory embarrassment.

    g. **Reduced distal perfusion** secondary to aortic branch vessel occlusion, leading to coronary, cerebral, renal, mesenteric, spinal cord, or extremity ischemia.

    h. **Aortic regurgitation** from retrograde dissection and involvement of the aortic valve.

    i. **Tamponade** from bloody pericardial effusion.

B. Monitoring

1. **Distal perfusion** may be assessed by a second arterial line placed in the dorsalis pedis artery, by pedal Doppler, or by pulse oximeter.

2. **Adverse effects of increased afterload on cardiac function** may necessitate PA catheter placement. Extreme care should be taken during PA catheter insertion because of the potentially disas-

trous results of great artery (e.g., carotid, subclavian) puncture in the presence of preexisting intimal dissection.

3. **Arterial oxygen saturation** should be monitored during one-lung anesthesia using pulse oximetry.

4. **Spinal cord ischemia** may be detected using SEP monitoring (see sec. **C.3**).

C. **Anesthetic management.** The goals are maintenance of adequate oxygen-carrying capacity, cardiac output, and distal perfusion; prevention of myocardial decompensation from increased afterload; protection of vital organs from hypoperfusion; and maintenance of adequate hemostasis and metabolic balance.

1. **Induction.** A double-lumen endotracheal tube will facilitate surgical access and protect the left lung from trauma during left thoracotomy. The method for its placement is described in Chap. 19.

2. **Management of reduced distal perfusion.** During repair of descending thoracic aortic aneurysms in which a proximal and distal aortic clamp isolate the affected aortic segment, distal perfusion may be maintained by one of three methods: (a) perfusion pressure may be allowed to increase (to 160 mm Hg systolic if the LV can tolerate it) to feed collaterals, (b) a shunt may be placed to provide flow across the aneurysm, or (c) partial bypass may be established. Gott shunts are heparin-bonded and therefore obviate the need for systemic heparinization. Pump-assisted partial bypass may be established with inflow from either the left atrium, axillary vein, femoral vein, or pulmonary artery; outflow is then to the femoral artery. However, even with these precautions, tissues that lie between cross-clamps may still suffer ischemic injury.

   a. For short procedures on relatively small segments of the aorta, the method of choice would be cross-clamping without shunt or bypass. Next, Gott shunt placement within the chest (i.e., both proximal and distal insertion is into the thoracic aorta) is best, followed by Gott shunt placement from the proximal aorta (or LV apex) to the femoral artery. Finally, pump-assisted partial bypass is indicated, although clear-cut evidence favoring the use of shunts or bypass in descending thoracic aortic surgery is yet to be presented.

   b. Operations on the ascending aorta usually necessitate full CPB. Aortic arch procedures may require CPB with hypothermia and total circulatory arrest (see sec. **C.5**).

3. **Spinal cord protection and evoked potential monitoring.** The anterior spinal artery branches from the vertebral arteries at the base of the skull and anastomoses with aortic radicular arteries. The latter arise segmentally (a few in the lumbar and lower thoracic regions, but none or one in the

upper thoracic region). The dominant radical is the artery of Adamkiewicz (usually found between T9 and T12); cross-clamping may compromise flow, depriving the anterior spinal artery of flow and producing spinal cord ischemia. Manifestations of the **anterior spinal artery syndrome** are paraplegia, rectal and urinary incontinence, and loss of pain and temperature sensation, but sparing of vibratory and proprioceptive sensation. The incidence of paraplegia resulting from the anterior spinal artery syndrome is 5–15% in patients operated on for descending thoracic aortic disease. Risk factors include the duration of the procedure, the location of proximal and distal cross-clamps, increased body temperature, the length of the involved segment, the degree of collateralization of spinal cord circulation, the underlying severity of atherosclerosis of the collateral vessel, and the success of perfusion of collaterals as well as reperfusion on cross-clamp removal.

   a. Steroids, hypothermia, barbiturates, and assorted free-radical scavengers have all been reported to protect against experimental spinal cord ischemia. However, whether these measures have value during aortic surgery in humans is unproven. It does seem reasonable to avoid hyperthermia and, perhaps, to actively produce mild hypothermia by means of a cooling blanket. It may also be prudent to avoid infusing glucose-containing solutions since experimental evidence indicates that hyperglycemia is detrimental during incomplete ischemia and may worsen neurologic outcome.

   b. It may be possible to detect spinal cord ischemia by monitoring SEPs. Ischemia increases the latency and decreases the amplitude of the potentials (see Chap. 22). Intraoperative loss of the SEP is certainly a worrisome development, but is not always associated with an acquired neurologic deficit. Moreover, since SEPs reflect conduction primarily in the *dorsal* (sensory) spinal cord, motor dysfunction can theoretically occur without an SEP change. The technique is promising, but additional human studies are needed to establish the utility of SEP monitoring during aortic surgery.

4. Aortic unclamping. Management of volume and afterload is complicated when bypass or shunt procedures are employed. When shunts or bypass systems without a reservoir are used, they must be clamped when the aorta is unclamped to prevent a "steal" of flow. Volume may be given from the reservoir when partial bypass is used. Low-dose epinephrine (1–4 µg/min), sodium bicarbonate, and calcium chloride should be available when cross-clamps are released in case of hypotension.

5. **Hypothermic circulatory arrest.** Aneurysms involving the arch may compromise cranial blood flow. Thus, the relevant vessels must either be grafted or reimplanted into the aortic arch. Cerebral protection, avoidance of emboli, control of hemorrhage, and a reasonably bloodless surgical field may be achieved by hypothermic circulatory arrest. Hypothermia is produced by surface cooling, then core cooling on CPB. Patients are placed on cooling blankets, and the head and neck packed in ice. Cerebral protection may possibly be provided by thiopental, dexamethasone, and mannitol administration several minutes prior to total circulatory arrest. (Myocardial preservation is provided by cold cardioplegia.) Cooling is continued until the core temperature is 18–20°C, then flow is arrested and venous lines drained to the pump reservoir. Arrest time should not exceed 60 minutes to avoid neurologic injury. After arch replacement, CPB is reinstituted, warming proceeds, and the patient is weaned from CPB.

6. **Emergence.** If a double-lumen endotracheal tube is used, it should be replaced by a single-lumen model prior to transfer to the intensive care unit.

Suggested Reading

Boucher, C. A., et al. Determination of cardiac risk by dipyridamole-thallium imaging before peripheral vascular surgery. *N. Engl. J. Med.* 312:389, 1985.

Davison, J. K. Anesthesia for major vascular procedures in the elderly. *Clin. Anesth.* 4:931, 1986.

DeBakey, M. E., and Lawrie, G. M. Combined coronary artery and peripheral vascular disease: Recognition and treatment. *J. Vasc. Surg.* 1:605, 1984.

Diehl, J. T., et al. Complications of abdominal aortic reconstruction: An analysis of perioperative risk factors in 557 patients. *Ann. Surg.* 197:49, 1983.

Goldman, L. Cardiac risks and complications of noncardiac surgery. *Ann. Intern. Med.* 98:504, 1981.

Hertzer, N. R., et al. Coronary artery disease in peripheral vascular patients: A classification of 1000 coronary angiograms and results of surgical management. *Ann. Surg.* 199:223, 1984.

Jeffrey, C. C., et al. A prospective evaluation of cardiac risk index. *Anesthesiology* 58:462, 1983.

Laschinger, J. C., et al. Definition of the safe lower limits of aortic resection during surgical procedures on the thoracoabdominal aorta: Use of somatosensory evoked potentials. *J. Am. Coll. Cardiol.* 2:959, 1983.

Rao, T. L. K., and El-Etr, A. A. Anticoagulation following placement of epidural and subarachnoid catheters: An evaluation of neurologic sequelae. *Anesthesiology* 55:618, 1981.

Rao, T. L. K., Jacobs, K. H., and El-Etr, A. A. Reinfarction following anesthesia in patients with myocardial infarction. *Anesthesiology* 59:499, 1983.

Ropper, A. H., Wechsler, L. R., and Wilson, L. S. Carotid bruit and the risk of stroke in elective surgery. *N. Engl. J. Med.* 307:1388, 1982.

Topolo, E. J., Traill, T. A., and Fortuin, N. J. Hypertensive hypertrophic cardiomyopathy of the elderly. *N. Engl. J. Med.* 312:277, 1985.

Vitez, T. S., et al. Chronic hypokalemia and intraoperative dysrhythmias. *Anesthesiology* 63:130, 1985.

19

Anesthesia for Thoracic Surgery

William E. Hurford

I. **Bronchoscopy.** Flexible or rigid bronchoscopy usually is performed to obtain tissue for pathologic diagnosis and to determine the resectability of intrathoracic lesions.

A. **Flexible bronchoscopy under topical anesthesia**

1. **Flexible bronchoscopy** is performed most commonly in the awake, fasting patient under topical anesthesia.

2. **Cough reflexes** must be abolished to permit an adequate examination but must return rapidly at the end of the procedure so that the patient can clear secretions and blood from the airway. Topical anesthesia plus transtracheal lidocaine and superior laryngeal nerve blocks are used with intravenous sedation.

3. The airway is anesthetized by spraying the palate, pharynx, larynx, vocal cords, and trachea with 4% lidocaine using a nebulizer or bronchoscope. If this is done thoroughly, transtracheal or superior laryngeal nerve blocks are not necessary.

4. **Transtracheal injection** of lidocaine is performed by injecting 2 ml of 2% plain lidocaine through the cricothyroid membrane using a 22-gauge needle attached to a small syringe. Proper position of the needle is confirmed by aspiration of air prior to injection of the anesthetic. The needle is quickly withdrawn after the injection, since the patient will begin to cough. Coughing spreads the anesthetic over the surface of the trachea and the inferior surface of the vocal cords.

5. **Superior laryngeal nerve block** is performed by inserting a 25-gauge needle immediately anterior to the superior cornu of the thyroid cartilage until resistance is encountered. The needle is then withdrawn slightly, and after a negative aspiration, 2 ml of 2% lidocaine is injected. The block is then repeated on the opposite side.

6. **Intravenous lidocaine** (0.5–1.5 mg/kg) decreases airway reflexes and is a helpful adjunct to topical anesthesia for bronchoscopy. Small doses of diazepam, midazolam, or fentanyl may be used to provide additional sedation.

B. **Flexible bronchoscopy under general anesthesia**

1. Flexible bronchoscopy is easily performed after induction of general anesthesia and endotracheal intubation. As long as airway reflexes are suppressed, almost any anesthetic technique is acceptable.

2. The endotracheal tube must be large enough to permit the endoscope to pass easily and without unduly limiting the lumen for ventilation. Most bron-

choscopes require an 8-mm or larger endotracheal tube.

C. **Rigid bronchoscopy** permits superior visualization and control of the airway compared to fiberoptic bronchoscopy. Adequate operating conditions require general anesthesia.

   1. **General considerations**

      a. **Hypercarbia** secondary to inadequate ventilation is the most common complication during bronchoscopy and frequently results in ventricular arrhythmias.

      b. The high incidence of **ventricular arrhythmias** mandates that the ECG be continuously monitored and lidocaine be available for immediate use. Most arrhythmias, however, are best treated by increasing ventilation.

      c. **Hypoxemia** secondary to intermittent and uneven ventilation may be minimized by using controlled ventilation with 100% oxygen. Oxygenation should be continuously monitored with a pulse oximeter.

      d. **Anesthesia machines** capable of delivering high flow rates of oxygen (up to 20 L/min) are necessary to compensate for air leaks occurring around the bronchoscope or during suctioning.

      e. **Air leaks** around the bronchoscope may be minimized by having an assistant compress the hypopharynx externally.

   2. **A rigid bronchoscope with a side-arm** permitting positive-pressure ventilation is most commonly used.

      a. This type of bronchoscope permits controlled positive-pressure ventilation and the use of inhalation anesthetics.

      b. Manual ventilation is necessary, since ventilation must be interrupted whenever the surgeon removes the eyepiece of the bronchoscope to suction or perform a biopsy. In addition, manual ventilation can instantly compensate for changes in effective compliance that may occur when the bronchoscope enters a bronchus.

      c. If difficulty in oxygenating or ventilating the patient occurs during bronchoscopy, the surgeon should be instructed to withdraw the bronchoscope back into the trachea. Once adequate conditions are reestablished, endoscopy may continue.

   3. **Sanders bronchoscopes** use a manually or machine-triggered jet of oxygen within the bronchoscope to entrain air through the proximal end of the tube by the Venturi effect.

      a. Several disadvantages limit the use of this bronchoscope. First, balanced anesthesia must be used, since the high fresh gas flow rates may result in unpredictable anesthetic concentrations. Also, the inspired oxygen concentration is uncertain, since the amount of room air entrained cannot be controlled. <u>Muscle relaxation is required for the jet to inflate the lungs adequately.</u>

  b. The advantage of this bronchoscope is that ventilation is not interrupted by suctioning or surgical manipulations, since the proximal end of the bronchoscope is always open. This makes the Sanders bronchoscope suitable for use during laser surgery of the airway.

4. **Anesthetic technique**

  a. **Inhalational anesthetics** are used predominantly during rigid bronchoscopy. For brief procedures, a balanced anesthetic using a short-acting muscle relaxant is acceptable as long as the patient can be ventilated easily by mask.

  b. After preoxygenation, anesthesia is induced with thiopental. A volatile anesthetic is then added progressively until adequate anesthesia is achieved. <u>Ventilation is assisted or controlled as necessary.</u> Muscle relaxants may be used to reduce the requirement for inhalational anesthetics if the airway is easily maintained. While \ <u>we usually use a succinylcholine infusion,</u> atracurium or vecuronium also could be used.

  c. The patient's eyes and teeth should be protected. The airway is then intubated with the rigid bronchoscope. Once the bronchoscope is in place, ventilation may be controlled.

  d. If thoracotomy is to follow the bronchoscopy, the patient is intubated with a double-lumen endotracheal tube immediately after the bronchoscope is withdrawn.

5. **Complications of bronchoscopy** include dental and laryngeal damage from intubation, airway rupture, pneumothorax, and hemorrhage. Airway obstruction may occur as a result of excessive bleeding or by obstruction from a foreign body or dislodged mass. Inadequate ventilation may lead to hypoxemia, hypercarbia, and ventricular arrhythmias.

II. Pulmonary resection

  A. **Endobronchial tubes.** These specialized tubes were initially developed for differential bronchospirometry and the control of unilateral pulmonary hemorrhage and secretions. In current use, they permit selective ventilation of each lung, providing a quiet, collapsed lung upon which to operate while isolating the nonoperative lung from blood and secretions. Most importantly, endobronchial tubes maintain an intact airway during unilateral bronchial resections.

  1. <u>Robertshaw tube</u>

    a. Robertshaw tubes are made of red rubber and are available in left- or right-sided versions. The right-sided version has a slotted bronchial cuff to accommodate the orifice of the right upper lobe bronchus. They have large-diameter, low-resistance lumens and no tracheal hook. Small, medium, and large sizes are available, corresponding to 8-, 9.5-, and 11-mm endotracheal tubes.

b. Disposable, polyvinyl versions of the Robertshaw tube are available in 35, 37, 39, and 41 Fr sizes. The greater variety of sizes may permit a better fit; however, the tubes are expensive and not reusable.

c. Insertion

   (1) Prior to intubation, the cuffs of the tube are checked for leaks, the tube lubricated, and a stylet placed in the bronchial lumen.

   (2) The nonoperative or dependent lung is chosen as the lung to be selectively intubated if at all possible. If this is done, the endobronchial tube will not interfere with resection of the mainstem bronchus should this be necessary. If the nondependent lung is intubated, mediastinal compression or surgical manipulation may displace the bronchial limb and interrupt isolation of the operative lung. Mediastinal compression may also push the tracheal lumen against the tracheal wall, creating a ball-valve obstruction to ventilation.

   (3) For laryngoscopy, a Macintosh blade is preferred over a Miller blade, as it provides more room for manipulating the tube within the pharynx. Double-lumen tubes have a compound curve: the upper shaft of the tube curves anteriorly, while the distal tip curves laterally. Intubation must therefore follow a systematic procedure. First, the tube is placed in the oropharynx with the concavity of the distal tip facing anteriorly. Once the tip of the tube has passed through the cords, the tube is rotated so that the concavity of the shaft faces anteriorly. The tube then is slid off the stylet until it seats with its tip in the bronchus and its bite block at the incisors.

d. Confirming position of the tube. The position of the tube must be checked carefully after insertion and again after positioning the patient to ensure that the correct lung can be isolated.

   (1) Chest movements should be observed and breath sounds auscultated bilaterally prior to the cuffs being inflated. A moderate leak around the tube should be detectable.

(2) The tracheal limb of the Cobb connector is then clamped, the cap of the tracheal limb removed, and the bronchial cuff inflated to produce an airtight seal. The patient then is ventilated only through the bronchial side of the Robertshaw tube. The chest should move and breath sounds should be heard only on that side. No air should leak from the open tracheal port.

(3) Next, the patient is ventilated through both lumens and the tracheal cuff inflated. The bronchial cuff should be left inflated from the time of insertion until differential ventilation is no longer needed. Keeping this cuff inflated minimizes changes in the tube's position.

2. **Carlens and White double-lumen tubes**

   a. The Carlens tube is designed for left-sided endobronchial intubation; the White tube is a right-sided version.

   b. Carlens and White tubes are constructed of red rubber and available in 35, 37, 39, and 41 Fr sizes. They have lumens of smaller internal diameter than the Robertshaw tubes and a carinal hook. The hook, while increasing the stability of the tube, makes the tube difficult to insert. Also because of the hook, the tube must be withdrawn back into the trachea before carinal surgery can be performed.

   c. **Insertion of the Carlens or White tube**

      (1) After laryngoscopy, the tube is placed in the oropharynx so that the concavity of the distal tip is anterior. Once the tip passes through the cords, the tube is rotated so that the carinal hook is anterior and can pass through the cords. Once the hook is beyond the cords, the tube is rotated back 90 degrees so that the concavity of the shaft is anterior. The tube is then slid off the stylet and advanced until the hook engages the carina.

      (2) The position of the tube is checked using the procedure outlined for the Robertshaw tube.

3. **Bronchial blockers.** When endobronchial intubation is impossible, as in a pediatric or laryngectomized patient, a Fogarty catheter, placed with the aid of a fiberoptic bronchoscope and then inflated, may be used to selectively occlude a bronchus. A standard endotracheal tube is then placed, and the position of the Fogarty catheter is confirmed by fiberoptic bronchoscopy if necessary. Once one-lung ventilation is no longer necessary, the Fogarty catheter may be deflated without disturbing the endotracheal tube.

4. Complications of endobronchial intubation

   a. Poor positioning of the endobronchial tube with failure to isolate the operative lung is the most common problem. Usually the tube has not been passed far enough into the bronchus.

   (1) Failure to advance the tube far enough into the bronchus occurs when an inappropriately small tube is selected or when bronchial or tracheal narrowing prevents passage of an appropriate size tube. The inflated bronchial cuff then rests at or above the level of the carina, producing partial or complete obstruction of the non-intubated bronchus. Gas trapping with inability to deflate the operative lung may occur.

   (2) The tube also may be passed too far down the bronchial tree, resulting in obstruction of an upper lobe bronchus.

   (3) When the position of the tube is in doubt, it should be withdrawn and replaced. In questionable cases, the position of the endobronchial tube may be confirmed visually by passing a pediatric fiberoptic bronchoscope through the lumen of the endobronchial tube.

   b. Laryngeal trauma and tracheal and endobronchial rupture may occur secondary to the large size of the endobronchial tube or overinflation of the cuffs.

B. Positioning. Most thoracic procedures are performed with the patient in the full lateral or anterolateral position and the table flexed. These positions can produce nerve injuries, compromise venous return, and impair ventilation.

   1. Peripheral nerve injuries. Stretch or compression injuries, most commonly to the brachial plexus, radial, ulnar, or peroneal nerves, may result from poor positioning. Potential pressure points should be carefully padded. Axillary rolls, however, are not used, as they may increase stretch on the brachial plexus. Pressure points about the face, ears, neck, and arms should be examined periodically during the operation and padded as necessary. Protection of the "down" eye is especially critical, as direct pressure may produce retinal artery occlusion and blindness.

   2. Circulatory effects

   a. With the patient in the lateral position, pooling of blood in the dependent parts of the body may reduce venous return and cardiac output. This effect is exacerbated by hypovolemia and by flexion of the operating table.

   b. Positional changes should be made slowly and as tolerated by the patient. Blood pressure should be checked frequently. Lightening the level of anesthesia during positional changes may reduce the degree of hypotension. Muscle relaxants are used to prevent bucking and movement if necessary.

3. Ventilatory effects

a. Impairment of ventilation is proportional to the degree of impairment to motion of the diaphragm and chest wall. Careful positioning may reduce the deleterious effects of the lateral position on ventilation.

b. Controlled high-volume, positive-pressure ventilation tends to produce a more even distribution of ventilation and is mandatory when the chest is open.

C. One-lung ventilation. General anesthesia, the lateral position, an open chest, surgical manipulations, and one-lung ventilation all contribute to alter ventilation and perfusion relationships.

1. Oxygenation

a. The amount of pulmonary blood flow passing through the unventilated lung (pulmonary shunt) probably is the most important factor determining arterial oxygenation during one-lung ventilation.

b. Diseased lungs often have reduced perfusion secondary to vascular occlusion or vasoconstriction. This may limit shunting of blood through the nonventilated operative lung during one-lung ventilation.

c. Perfusion of the unventilated lung also is reduced by collapse of the lung and hypoxic pulmonary vasoconstriction.

d. The lateral position tends to reduce pulmonary shunting, since gravity will decrease blood flowing to the nondependent lung.

e. Since arterial oxygenation may change rapidly, multiple blood gas analyses and a pulse oximeter are used to monitor the adequacy of oxygenation during one-lung ventilation.

2. Ventilation

a. Carbon dioxide tension should be maintained on one-lung ventilation at the same level as on two lungs as long as minute ventilation remains constant.

b. Controlled ventilation is mandatory during open-chest operations, since spontaneous ventilation is hindered by several factors:

(1) Loss of negative intrathoracic pressure results in collapse of the operative lung from unopposed elastic recoil.

(2) Since the operative lung is exposed to zero rather than negative pleural pressure, a spontaneous inspiratory effort will tend to empty the lung. With a single-lumen tube, expiration will cause the operative lung to be filled from the nonoperative lung, resulting in paradoxical respiration.

(3) The efficiency of the intact hemithorax will also be reduced. Contraction of the diaphragm during spontaneous inspiration will decrease pleural pressure in the intact hemithorax and displace the mediastinum into the dependent lung. During expiration, pleural pressure in the intact hemithorax will increase, causing outward displacement of the mediastinum. A rocking mediastinum and decreased tidal volume result.

c. **Minute ventilation** is maintained while on one-lung ventilation by maintaining tidal volume at 10–15 ml/kg and increasing respiratory rate as necessary.

d. **Peak airway pressure** may increase during one-lung ventilation, since airway resistance is increased by the narrow lumen of the endobronchial tube.

e. **Manual ventilation** is preferable to the use of a ventilator during one-lung ventilation, since manual ventilation can compensate instantly for the rapid changes in lung compliance that may result from surgical manipulations. It is also easier to minimize or momentarily interrupt ventilatory movements during critical surgical manipulations.

3. Management of one-lung ventilation

a. During one-lung ventilation, **100% oxygen** is used, since the PaO_2 may change rapidly and unpredictably during surgery.

b. As one-lung ventilation is begun, the patient is manually ventilated and collapse of the unventilated lung confirmed visually. Large changes in effective lung compliance, oxygen saturation, air trapping, or failure of the operative lung to collapse mandates return to two-lung ventilation until the problem is solved. Usually, the problem is one of tube position. Advancing or withdrawing the endobronchial tube slightly, under bronchoscopic guidance if necessary, often corrects the problem.

c. If the tube is in good position but hypoxemia persists, the nonventilated lung may be briefly inflated with 100% oxygen and the exhalation port to the operative lung capped. In this way, a motionless, partially collapsed lung is maintained. Reinflation of the lung with oxygen will be necessary every 10–20 minutes.

d. If the dependent lung is significantly atelectatic or diseased, oxygenation may improve if positive end-expiratory pressure (PEEP) is provided.

(1) PEEP should increase the functional re-

sidual capacity (FRC) of the dependent
lung and reduce ventilation/perfusion mismatching.

(2) Pulmonary vascular resistance in the dependent lung, however, may increase with PEEP. This would increase shunting of blood through the collapsed lung and worsen oxygenation.

(3) Since the effects of PEEP on FRC and shunt fraction are impossible to predict in these cases, the efficacy of PEEP should be assessed through arterial blood gas measurements.

e. **Continuous positive airway pressure** (CPAP) can also be applied to the operative lung in an effort to improve oxygenation. PEEP may be simultaneously applied to the dependent lung. Systems for delivering one-lung CPAP, however, are cumbersome and not readily available.

f. **High-frequency or jet ventilation** may also be applied to the operative lung. These techniques, however, remain largely experimental.

g. If hypoxemia remains a problem, clamping the pulmonary artery of the collapsed lung will reduce the shunt fraction. PaO_2 may rise dramatically.

h. If these maneuvers are unsuccessful or are not feasible, a return to two-lung ventilation may be the only solution. Proceeding with careful manual ventilation, avoiding excessive lung movement during surgical manipulations, may be an acceptable compromise for many procedures that do not require absolute lung isolation.

D. Anesthetic technique

1. **Preoperative preparation**

a. A detailed preoperative evaluation should be performed with special emphasis on the patient's pulmonary and cardiac function. Preoperative pulmonary function tests and room air arterial blood gas values are helpful in predicting the likelihood of perioperative complications and the probability of postoperative ventilation.

b. Peripheral intravenous and radial artery catheters are routinely used. In a healthy patient undergoing a limited procedure such as a wedge resection or routine lobectomy, a pulse oximeter may be used in place of the arterial cannula. In any event, pulse oximetry appears to be a useful adjunct to routine monitoring and is recommended for all patients undergoing thoracic procedures.

c. If the operation is to be performed in the lateral or anterolateral position, the arterial cannula should be placed in the lower arm so that axillary artery compression can be monitored as well.

d. Central venous catheters are rarely necessary. In a pneumonectomy patient with significant cardiac disease, however, a pulmonary artery catheter is useful, since pulmonary artery pressure may rise significantly as the pulmonary artery is clamped. The pulmonary artery catheter should be placed under fluoroscopic guidance to ensure that it terminates in the non-operative lung and does not interfere with the surgical resection.

2. Anesthetic techniques. The technique chosen must permit the use of high inspired oxygen concentrations to minimize hypoxemia.

a. Potent inhalational anesthetics are recommended, since they permit the use of 100% oxygen and provide for a smooth induction, rapid emergence, and depression of airway reflexes.

b. Muscle relaxants usually are used as adjuncts to inhalational anesthesia.

   (1) Relaxants decrease the incidence and severity of bucking and permit reduced concentrations of inhalational anesthetic to be used.

   (2) Generally, if bronchoscopy is to precede the operation, a succinylcholine infusion is used. This permits a rapid return of muscle strength if the procedure is terminated because of the results of bronchoscopy. If thoracotomy follows, an intermediate- or long-acting muscle relaxant is given to facilitate intubation, positioning, and chest wall incision. Profound muscle relaxation is not required for the procedure. Restriction of muscle relaxants to the early phases of the operation permits a more complete reversal of neuromuscular blockade at the end of the procedure.

c. The use of **balanced anesthesia** during pulmonary resections is limited since

   (1) The requirement for high inspired oxygen concentrations limits the use of nitrous oxide. Complete loss of consciousness and amnesia cannot be assumed.

   (2) If nitrous oxide is used, the margin of safety for avoiding hypoxemia is reduced.

   (3) The use of moderate or high doses of narcotics will reduce ventilatory drive at the end of the procedure and may necessitate postoperative ventilation.

E. Emergence/extubation. The goal of the anesthetic technique selected is to have an awake, comfortable, and extubated patient at the end of the procedure.

1. Prior to closing the chest, the lungs are inflated to

30 cm H_2O pressure to reinflate atelectatic areas and check for significant air leaks.

2. **Chest tubes** are inserted to drain the pleural cavity and promote lung expansion. Chest tubes usually are placed under water seal and 20 cm H_2O suction, except after a pneumonectomy. Following pneumonectomy, a chest tube, if used, should be placed under water seal only. Applying suction could shift the mediastinum to the draining side and reduce venous return.

3. **Prompt extubation** avoids the potential disruptive effects of endotracheal intubation and positive-pressure ventilation on fresh suture lines. If postoperative ventilation is required, the double-lumen tube should be exchanged for a conventional endotracheal tube with a high-volume, low-pressure cuff. Peak inspiratory pressures should be kept as low as possible.

F. **Postoperative analgesia**
   1. **Parenteral narcotics.** To limit respiratory depression in the immediate postoperative period, intravenous narcotics are used sparingly, if at all, during the operation. After the patient is extubated and breathing adequately, small doses of morphine may be administered as necessary.
   2. **Intercostal nerve blocks**
      a. Intercostal nerve blocks are the mainstay of analgesic therapy for post-thoracotomy patients.
      b. Five interspaces are usually blocked: two above, two below, and one at the site of the incision.
      c. **Performing the block.** Under sterile conditions, a 23-gauge needle is inserted perpendicularly to the skin over the lower edge of the rib and along the posterior axillary line. The needle then is "walked" off the rib inferiorly until it just slips off the rib. After a negative aspiration for blood, 4–5 ml of 0.5% bupivacaine with or without 1 : 200,000 epinephrine is injected. The procedure is repeated at each interspace to be blocked. In addition, subcutaneous infiltration with bupivacaine is performed in a V-shaped pattern around each chest tube site to reduce the discomfort of chest tube movement.
      d. Analgesia lasts from 6–12 hours and may be prolonged by the addition of epinephrine to the anesthetic solution. Epinephrine is usually avoided, however, in patients with coronary artery disease.
      e. Since the area blocked is highly vascular, vascular uptake of anesthetic is extensive and the risk of intravascular injection high. Hence, the patient must be monitored closely for toxic reactions to the anesthetic. Also, if a chest tube is not in place, the risk of pneumothorax from the block needs to be considered.
      f. Intercostal blocks are not recommended for

postpneumonectomy patients, since the needle insertions theoretically may introduce infections into the empty hemithorax.

3. Epidural narcotics

   a. When intercostal blocks are contraindicated or inadequate, epidural morphine may provide additional analgesia. Usually, 2–5 mg of preservative-free morphine is injected every 12 hours by a lumbar epidural catheter.

   b. Complications of epidural morphine include urinary retention, which may be treated by catheterization of the bladder; pruritus, which may be treated with small doses of intravenous naloxone; and respiratory depression, which may occur up to 24 hours following epidural narcotics. Patients who are normally hypercarbic as a result of intrinsic lung disease are especially prone to narcotic-induced respiratory depression.

   c. To minimize respiratory depression following epidural morphine, the concomitant use of parenteral narcotics is restricted.

III. Tracheal resection and reconstruction

   A. General considerations

   1. Tracheal resection and reconstruction is potentially one of the most dangerous thoracic operations because of the risk of completely obstructing an already compromised airway and the necessity of intermittently disrupting airway continuity.

   2. The goal of the anesthetic is to be able to extubate the patient at the end of the procedure, since the presence of an endotracheal tube and positive-pressure ventilation may disrupt the suture line.

   3. The surgical approach depends on the location and extent of the lesion. Lesions of the cervical trachea are approached through a transverse neck incision. Lower lesions necessitate a manubrial split. Lesions of the distal trachea and carina may require a median sternotomy and/or single or bilateral thoracotomies.

   B. Preoperative preparation

   1. Patients with stridor at rest or critical airway lesions should not receive preoperative sedation. Healthy patients without compromised airways may tolerate small doses of diazepam preoperatively.

   2. A peripheral intravenous line and a radial artery line should be placed preoperatively, preferably in the left arm. The right arm should be left free of lines, since the right subclavian artery may be occluded by retraction during the procedure. Also, the right arm may be prepped and draped into the surgical field to provide adequate lateral exposure during carinal resections.

   3. Pulse oximetry is helpful in constantly monitoring arterial oxygen saturation during the procedure, especially when continuity of the airway is temporarily interrupted.

C. **Induction** should be attempted only in the presence of the surgeon and adequate staff.

1. Additional equipment required for induction are Macintosh and Miller laryngoscope blades, an assortment of uncut orotracheal tubes (20–34 Fr) with stylets, several sizes of rigid bronchoscopes, and a tracheostomy set.

2. Spontaneous respiration should be maintained throughout induction. An intravenous induction is contraindicated in a patient with a critical airway stenosis, since it may depress respiration unpredictably, resulting in an apneic patient who cannot be ventilated.

3. Halothane and oxygen by mask is the preferred technique for induction. Halothane produces a smooth induction and depresses airway reflexes. In addition, high inspired concentrations of halothane are well tolerated and may be required when a critical stenosis limits the rate of rise of alveolar concentrations of anesthetic.

4. Enflurane and isoflurane are not tolerated as well as halothane in the high concentrations required to induce these patients.

5. Muscle relaxants are contraindicated during induction and maintenance of anesthesia, since ventilation often depends on the patient's spontaneous efforts alone.

6. If a tracheostomy is present below the level of the lesion, respiration can be assisted as necessary.

D. **Anesthetic technique**

1. **Bronchoscopy** is usually performed prior to the operative procedure.

   a. After a mask induction with spontaneous ventilation, the oropharynx, vocal cords, and trachea are carefully sprayed with lidocaine.

   b. Next, rigid bronchoscopy is performed to determine the exact location and size of the lesion. These factors determine whether an attempt should be made to pass an endotracheal tube through the site of the lesion.

   c. Spontaneous ventilation under halothane and oxygen is continued. Assisted ventilation may be used if care is taken not to overcome the patient's respiratory drive.

2. The patient is intubated under halothane anesthesia without the use of muscle relaxants.

   a. If the endotracheal tube can be passed through the lesion, a continuous, patent airway can be maintained until the trachea is divided. Respiration then can be assisted and nitrous oxide used to decrease the concentration of halothane required.

   b. If the tube cannot be passed through the lesion, intermittent airway obstruction may occur at any time during the tracheal dissection. Spontaneous ventilation should be preserved and 100% oxygen used at all times.

   c. <u>For carinal resections, the patient is intubated with an extra-long armored endotracheal tube, which can be directly placed in either mainstem bronchus by the surgeon as he dissects the carina</u>.

   d. Nitrous oxide, if used, should be discontinued prior to the trachea's being divided.

   e. Intravenous lidocaine, 0.5–1.0 mg/kg, may be used to diminish laryngeal and tracheal irritability during the procedure.

3. When the trachea is divided, the surgeon maintains the airway by placing a sterile, armored Tovell tube in the distal trachea while the anesthetist withdraws the original endotracheal tube to a position proximal to the lesion. Sterile breathing hoses are attached to the armored tube by the surgeon, and the free ends are passed under the drapes and connected to the anesthesia machine.

   a. A suture may be placed through the distal end of the endotracheal tube so that it may be easily retrieved and guided back through the anastomosis. If no suture is placed and the endotracheal tube is removed accidentally, a red rubber catheter can be passed retrograde through the cords and into the pharynx. Next, the anesthetist retrieves the proximal end of the catheter and sutures the distal end of the endotracheal tube to it. The surgeon then can reintubate the patient by using the catheter to guide the endotracheal tube through the cords and larynx.

   b. Close attention must be paid to the armored endotracheal tube, as it must be removed frequently as the posterior sutures are placed. It also may be accidentally removed, kinked, or passed into a bronchus.

   c. Prior to reanastomosis of the trachea, the distal trachea should be suctioned to remove blood and secretions that will have accumulated.

   d. After the posterior suture line is completed, the original endotracheal tube is readvanced and substituted for the armored tube. The original breathing hoses are reconnected.

4. <u>To reduce tension on the suture line, the neck is flexed as the tracheal sutures are tied</u>. Two folded blankets placed under the occiput usually produce an adequate amount of flexion. Flexion is maintained for the remainder of the operation and well into the postoperative period.

5. Occasionally during carinal resections, the distal bronchus is too small to permit passage of an endotracheal tube or the tube overcrowds the operative field. In these cases, high-frequency jet venti-

lation using a ventilating catheter held in the distal
bronchus by a surgical assistant may be useful.

   a. If jet ventilation is used, inhalational anesthetics cannot be given reliably. During this
part of the procedure, anesthesia may be maintained using a neuroleptic technique or short-
acting barbiturates.

   b. Muscle paralysis, generally using a succinylcholine infusion, may be necessary if patient
movement becomes troublesome. Muscle relaxants should not be used in these cases without
careful consideration of the potential risks involved. Relaxants are discontinued and the
patient returned to spontaneous ventilation under inhalational anesthesia as soon as technically possible.

E. Emergence/extubation. After the tracheal anastomosis is completed, anesthesia is lightened with the
aim being to extubate the patient immediately upon
conclusion of the surgery.

   1. After skin closure, a heavy suture is placed from
the chin to the chest to help maintain neck flexion.
As the patient awakens, care must be taken to
maintain neck flexion, since pain will cause the patient to extend his neck.

   2. The timing of extubation is important. The endotracheal tube should be left in place until the patient is awake enough to protect his airway but
should be removed before severe bucking or coughing occurs.

   3. Narcotics are not given until the patient is wide
awake and responsive. Usually only small amounts
of morphine are required, since postoperative pain
is not severe.

IV. Intrapulmonary hemorrhage

A. Massive intrapulmonary hemorrhage is usually
due to thoracic trauma or erosion of a major vessel by
an abscess or tumor.

**B. Hemoptysis, hypovolemic shock, and severe hy-
poxemia** are presenting signs. Emergent management
is required.

   1. The patient must be intubated immediately, the
airway suctioned clear, and positive-pressure ventilation with 100% oxygen begun.

   2. If bleeding is coming from only one lung, the opposite lung may be intubated with a double-lumen
tube.

   3. As a temporary measure, the mainstem bronchus of
the bleeding lung may be occluded by passing an
endotracheal tube down the mainstem bronchus of
the uninvolved lung.

C. Obstruction of the endotracheal tube by clot is an
everpresent danger. Frequent suctioning may be necessary to keep the endotracheal tube free of blood. If an
obstruction cannot be cleared quickly, the endotracheal
tube must be changed immediately.

    D. Definitive treatment of intrapulmonary hemorrhage requires a thoracotomy and surgical repair.

V. Esophageal surgery

  A. General considerations

    1. Preoperative evaluation is similar to that for pulmonary surgery, but with the addition of several factors:

      a. Patients with esophageal cancer often have dysphagia and anorexia and may be significantly malnourished and hypovolemic. Anesthesia and surgery may not be well tolerated.

      b. Patients may have had preoperative chemotherapy, which may increase their operative risk. Exposure to doxorubicin (Adriamycin), for example, may produce severe cardiomyopathies. Bleomycin may produce pulmonary toxicity, which may be worsened by exposure to high inspired concentrations of oxygen.

      c. Pulmonary function may be decreased, as many patients with esophageal cancer also have a significant smoking history. Patients with reflux may have decreased pulmonary function secondary to recurrent aspiration pneumonias.

      d. Liver function may be decreased as a result of alcoholic liver disease.

      e. Operative time may be prolonged and blood loss significant. Routine monitoring may need to be more extensive. Foley catheterization is routine. Central venous catheterization is advisable if the anticipated volume requirements are great; pulmonary artery catheterization is indicated in those patients with significant cardiac disease.

    2. Patients with esophageal diverticulum, esophageal cancer, or gastroesophageal reflux are at risk for regurgitation and aspiration during induction.

      a. Preoperative treatment with H_2-antagonists reduces the volume and acidity of gastric contents. Metoclopramide also reduces the volume of gastric contents. Alternatively, a nonparticulate antacid such as sodium citrate may be effective.

      b. These patients should be induced using a rapid sequence technique. If a difficult airway is anticipated, awake intubation should be performed prior to induction.

  B. Operative approach and anesthesia

    1. Upper esophageal lesions are approached through a cervical incision. Lesions of the lower third of the esophagus and gastroesophageal junction may be approached through a laparotomy and diaphragmatic split.

    2. A left or right thoracotomy is used to expose midesophageal lesions. Additionally, a laparotomy may be required for adequate mobilization of the stomach or colon.

3. One-lung anesthesia provides excellent surgical exposure when a thoracic or thoracoabdominal approach is used.
   a. The guidelines for one-lung anesthesia for esophageal surgery are identical to those used during pulmonary resection.
   b. Since the nonventilated lung usually is not diseased, significant pulmonary shunting through the lung may persist after the lung is collapsed. The hypoxemia experienced during one-lung anesthesia for esophageal surgery may therefore be of greater magnitude than that experienced during pulmonary surgery.
4. Extubation at the end of surgery depends on the patient's underlying cardiopulmonary status and the nature of the surgical procedure.
   a. Patients who have relatively limited procedures such as excision of a diverticulum or antireflux procedures may be extubated once they are wide awake and able to protect their airways.
   b. Patients who have undergone thoracoabdominal incisions or esophagogastrectomy require postoperative intubation and ventilation until they are fully awake, comfortable, and able to protect their airways and have adequate return of pulmonary function.

VI. Mediastinal operations
A. **Mediastinoscopy** is indicated to determine extrapulmonary spread of pulmonary tumors and for diagnosis of mediastinal masses.
   1. After endotracheal intubation, either an inhalational or balanced anesthetic may be used. While the procedure is not very stimulating, the patient must remain motionless and airway reflexes blunted at all times. An inhalational anesthetic combined with the use of a short- or intermediate-acting muscle relaxant achieves both these goals.
   2. Complications of mediastinoscopy include airway rupture, perforation of great vessels with possible exsanguinating hemorrhage, airway obstruction from compression by mediastinal masses, and pneumothorax.
B. **Mediastinal tumors** are a common indication for mediastinal surgery.
   1. In descending order of occurrence, the most commonly found tumors are neurogenic tumors, cysts, teratodermoids, lymphomas, thymomas, parathyroid tumors, and retrosternal thyroids.
   2. **Thymoma.** Myasthenia gravis occurs in 10–50% of patients with thymomas, and more than 85% of patients with myasthenia gravis have thymic abnormalities. Thymectomy may be beneficial in these patients.
      a. Oral anticholinesterase agents and steroids should be continued preoperatively. In patients

receiving steroids, full glucocorticoid coverage (the equivalent of 100 mg of hydrocortisone every 8 hours) should be administered on the day of surgery and then quickly tapered postoperatively.

b. Premedication with oral diazepam decreases patient anxiety without excessively reducing airway reflexes. Preoperative narcotics are not recommended.

c. Muscle relaxation is not required for thymectomy, and as these patients may be extremely sensitive to nondepolarizing agents and have a variable response to succinylcholine, the use of muscle relaxants is avoided. Anesthesia is induced with a barbiturate and then deepened with an inhalational agent. Intubation and surgery are performed under inhalational anesthesia alone.

d. Should muscle relaxants be required, very small doses of nondepolarizing agents are given. The response to muscle relaxants should be followed carefully with a twitch monitor. Residual neuromuscular blockade can be reversed with neostigmine.

e. Postoperatively, patients are observed in an intensive care unit. Most can be extubated once fully awake.

f. Anesthesia and surgery often decrease the need for anticholinesterase drugs in the postoperative period. Anticholinesterase agents are begun at half the patient's usual dose for the first several days after surgery, after which the dosage is adjusted. Respiratory weakness is best treated with intubation and mechanical ventilation rather than excessive doses of anticholinesterase agents, which may precipitate a cholinergic crisis.

Suggested Reading

Drachman, D. B. Myasthenia gravis. *N. Engl. J. Med.* 298:136, 1978.

Geffin, B., Bland, J., and Grillo, H. Anesthetic management of tracheal resection and reconstruction. *Anesth. Analg.* (Cleve.) 48:884, 1969.

Kaplan, J. A. *Thoracic Anesthesia.* New York: Churchill Livingstone, 1983.

Kerr, J. H., et al. Observations during endobronchial anaesthesia. *Br. J. Anaesth.* 45:159, 1973.

Rehder, K., Sessler, A. D., and Marsh, H. M. General anesthesia and the lung. *Am. Rev. Respir. Dis.* 112:541, 1975.

Robertshaw, F. L. Low resistance double lumen endobronchial tubes. *Br. J. Anaesth.* 34:576, 1962.

20

Anesthesia for Cardiac Surgery

Fred A. Rotenberg and Leonard L. Firestone

I. General preanesthetic assessment
A. History
1. **Symptoms** of coronary artery disease (CAD), congestive heart failure (CHF), or arrhythmias should be sought. Specifically, has the patient ever experienced
   a. Angina, dyspnea, or palpitations at rest or with exertion?
   b. Limitations to activity? (If so, what is the limiting symptom?)
   c. Syncope, dizziness, or focal neurologic symptoms?
   d. Orthopnea, paroxysmal nocturnal dyspnea, or ankle edema?
2. **Relevant hospitalizations,** diagnostic studies, and treatments should be documented, including dates if known.
   a. Previous myocardial infarctions (MI) (which may reduce ejection fraction, predispose to arrhythmias, or result in ventricular aneurysm or papillary muscle dysfunction producing mitral regurgitation).
   b. Pacemaker implantations, including the indication(s).
   c. Episodes of CHF and successful treatment regimens.
   d. Prior surgery on the thorax, great vessels, or lungs, which may technically complicate cardiac surgery.
   e. Episodes of transient ischemic attacks or stroke; noninvasive and invasive studies of carotid arterial or aortic arch anatomy and flow.
3. **Medications** used to control angina or CHF, including dates when drugs were started or discontinued, must be ascertained.
   a. Adequate **beta blockade** implies that the heart rate is 60–70, with minimal elevation during stress.
   b. **Calcium (Ca^{2+}) channel blockers** are vasodilators and myocardial depressants whose effects may be potentiated by anesthetic agents.
   c. **Digitalis** toxicity is common, especially when medical regimens include potassium (K^+)-wasting diuretics (e.g., furosemide or thiazides). Because of its slow elimination, digitalis is usually held for 24 hours preoperatively unless needed to control a rapid ventricular response to atrial fibrillation.
   d. **Aspirin** and **dipyridamole** (Persantine) inhibit platelet cohesion and are, in general, dis-

continued for 10 days preoperatively. When bleeding times are prolonged (> 10 minutes) and hemostasis is impaired, it may be necessary to transfuse platelets. One or two doses of dipyridamole may be given on the day before surgery, since long-term graft patency rates may be improved by antiplatelet drug therapy.

- **e.** Type I **antiarrhythmics** (quinidine, procainamide, disopyramide, oral lidocaine derivatives) may suppress automaticity and conduction, especially when patients are hyperkalemic; disopyramide has significant negative inotropic effects.
- **f.** High-dose (IV) **nitroglycerin** may cause methemoglobinemia.

4. Permanent pacemakers must be identified with respect to their sensing and pacing modes (see Chap. 2). The ECG will reveal either underlying or paced rates and rhythms.

5. Other systemic diseases may have an impact on the management of patients for cardiac surgery. Symptomatic or documented carotid arterial disease may warrant endarterectomy prior to, or simultaneous with, cardiac operations requiring cardiopulmonary bypass (CPB). Pulmonary symptoms may benefit from therapeutic interventions such as corticosteroids and IV bronchodilators to prevent bronchospasm or chest physiotherapy to prevent pneumonia. Pulsatile perfusion during CPB (see sec. II.G.3.c) may be indicated with chronic renal failure. Because of lengthy mask ventilation during inductions, the possibility of pulmonary aspiration must be considered in patients with symptomatic esophageal reflux or marked obesity.

6. An indication should be made on the record if blood has been donated by the patient (autologous) or family members ("designated donor"), to alert other operating room (OR) personnel involved in the patient's care.

B. Physical examination. Of particular concern is the symmetry of blood pressure measurements in both arms, the collateral blood supply to the hands, and the presence of bruits over the carotid arteries. Note cutdown scars from prior cardiac catheterizations on the arms, as measuring blood pressures distally may give falsely lowered values.

C. Laboratory studies. At minimum, routine studies for patients undergoing CPB include hematocrit, prothrombin time, partial thromboplastin time, platelet count, electrolytes, BUN, creatinine, glucose, AST, LDH, CPK, urinalysis, chest x-ray, and a 12-lead ECG with a rhythm strip.

1. Noninvasive cardiac studies suggest the extent and location of CAD, pump or valvular dysfunction. Exercise tolerance tests can reveal the specific

Table 20-2. Ventricular function indices

Formula	Units	Normal value
$SV = \dfrac{CO}{HR} \times 1000$	ml/beat	60–90
$SI = \dfrac{SV}{BSA}$	ml/beat/m²	40–60
$LVSWI = \dfrac{1.36(MAP - CVP)}{100} \times SI$	gram-meters/m²	45–60
$RVSWI = \dfrac{1.36(PAP - PCWP)}{100} \times SI$	gram-meters/m²	5–10
$SVR = \dfrac{MAP - CVP}{CO} \times 80$	dynes-sec/cm⁵	900–1500
$PVR = \dfrac{PAP - PCWP}{CO} \times 80$	dynes-sec/cm⁵	50–150

Key: BSA = body surface area; CO = cardiac output; CVP = central venous pressure; HR = heart rate; LVSWI = left ventricular stroke work index; MAP = mean systemic arterial pressure; PAP = pulmonary artery pressure; PCWP = pulmonary capillary wedge pressure; PVR = pulmonary vascular resistance; RVSWI = right ventricular work index; SI = stroke index; SV = stroke volume; SVR = systemic vascular resistance.

distention.

    e. Pacing PA and Paceport catheters may be lifesaving during sudden bradyarrhythmias (particularly in patients with aortic regurgitation), during rapid atrial rhythms (which may be suppressed by overdriving), in patients dependent on an atrial "kick" (mitral stenosis), and as a trigger for intraaortic balloon pumps (IABPs). They are often used in patients undergoing "redo" cardiac surgery and where temporary pacemaker insertion may be indicated (Mobitz type 2 and 3 heart block, sick sinus syndrome).

E. Induction

    1. Despite the abundance of sophisticated monitoring devices in the cardiac OR, the **standard anesthesia machine checkout procedure** is still fundamental (see Chap. 8).

    2. Aside from the drugs needed for any safe administration of general anesthesia, lidocaine, calcium chloride, heparin, and positive inotropes and vasoconstrictors should be readily at hand.

    3. A functioning, synchronizable **defibrillator** must be charged and within easy reach, as should an **external pacemaker generator**.

4. **Typed and cross-matched blood** for each patient must be present and checked.
5. Baseline hemodynamics including cardiac output and a 7-lead ECG are recorded immediately prior to induction.
6. The CPB pump should be primed and the surgeon, perfusionist, and circulating nurse in attendance.
7. In general, the **choice of induction and maintenance agents** is based on the underlying disease process (coronary versus valvular disease), the degree of decompensation (good versus poor LV function), and the surgical plan. A systematic, gradual induction with frequent assessments of the degree of cardiovascular depression and depth of anesthesia will minimize hemodynamic instability.
    a. **Coronary artery disease**
        (1) In patients with CAD, the **overriding goal is to minimize O_2 consumption while maximizing O_2 delivery.** Maintaining the diastolic blood pressure and preventing the heart rate from exceeding resting values are the keys to achieving the goal. The cardiovascular responses to intubation and incision should be blocked by an adequate level of anesthesia, supplemented by short-acting beta blockers and vasodilators when necessary.
        (2) **Intravenous narcotics,** particularly fentanyl, produce vasodilatation and bradycardia without significant myocardial depression.
        (3) **Potent inhalation anesthetics** are myocardial depressants but reduce MVO_2 while depressing contractility. **Halothane** is well-known for sensitizing the heart to catecholamine-induced arrhythmias. **Isoflurane** increases heart rate in non-beta-blocked patients and is a potent vasodilator. Current evidence indicates that isoflurane produces "coronary steal" by dilating the coronary bed regardless of local metabolic demands. **Enflurane** is often chosen because it stabilizes myocardium against catecholamine-induced arrhythmias.
        (4) Typically, **fentanyl** (50–100 μg/kg IV) or **sufentanil** (7–20 μg/kg IV) is used with O_2 for induction. Muscle relaxants are administered early to counteract rigidity and facilitate assisted and then controlled ventilation and intubation. Hypercarbia must be avoided to minimize sympathetic stimulation and acidosis; however, hypocarbia may predispose to arrhythmias and coronary vasoconstriction and should also be avoided.

(5) **Nitrous oxide** (N_2O) may produce ventricular wall motion abnormalities, myocardial depression, and increased pulmonary vascular resistance (PVR). Thus it seems prudent to avoid it in patients with ischemic cardiomyopathy and most valvular lesions.

(6) The choice of **muscle relaxant** must be made in light of their hemodynamic side effects (see Chap. 11). **Vecuronium** does little to alter hemodynamics, while **curare** and **metocurine** are vasodilators. **Gallamine** is used to provide graded increases in heart rate without predisposing to nodal rhythms, as may occur with the use of **pancuronium.** **Succinylcholine** often causes bradycardia, particularly when administered after fentanyl or sufentanil.

(7) In debilitated patients with poor ventricular function (ejection fraction < 30%), hemodynamic stability often depends on maximal endogenous sympathetic tone. Therefore, induction may cause profound hypotension, which initiates a vicious downward spiral in vital signs. In these cases, judicious titration with morphine (5 mg/min, up to 1.5 mg/kg) or fentanyl in the presence of 100% O_2 is tolerated best, although support with a catecholamine is frequently necessary (dopamine or dobutamine is preferred if PA pressures are elevated).

b. Valvular heart disease

(1) **Aortic stenosis** patients tolerate systemic vasodilatation and extremes in heart rate poorly. A fentanyl-O_2-vecuronium induction is often used. Volume infusion or a vasoconstrictor may be needed to counterbalance vasodilatation and maintain aortic diastolic (hence, coronary perfusion) pressure, while judicious use of gallamine or pancuronium will prevent bradycardia.

(2) The goals in **aortic and mitral regurgitation** are to avoid bradycardia and high SVR. Induction with IV morphine, supplemented by low concentrations of isoflurane or enflurane or an IV vasodilator, will accomplish these objectives.

(3) With **mitral stenosis,** tachycardia, elevated PVR, hypovolemia, and abrupt loss of sinus rhythm are poorly tolerated. High-dose narcotics (with scrupulous attention to ventilation) have been used with good success. A pacing PA catheter (with an overdriving pacemaker generator) may be lifesaving if paroxysmal atrial tachycardia is accompanied by hypotension. With pulmonary hypertension, dopamine and dobutamine are the positive inotropes of choice.

F. The prebypass period

1. **Supplementation** is sometimes required for major stimuli (incision, sternotomy, sternal spreading, incising the pericardium, and aortic cannulation). Either volatile anesthetics, vasodilators, or beta blockers may be the best choice depending on specific circumstances (e.g., the need for additional anesthesia or muscle relaxation).

2. **Phlebotomy with hemodilution** should be considered before anticoagulation in otherwise healthy patients if the starting hematocrit is greater than 40%. Autologous fresh whole blood will then be available for transfusion following CPB and heparin reversal.

3. **Anticoagulation for cannulation**

   a. Prior to induction of anesthesia, 3 mg/kg of heparin should be drawn up in case emergency initiation of CPB is necessary. Administration is through a **centrally placed catheter only**; blood is aspirated both before and after injection to establish that heparin actually reached the central circulation. Alternatively, in emergencies, the surgeon may inject heparin directly into the right atrium.

   b. Vasodilatation often follows a heparin bolus.

   c. The activated clotting time (ACT), determined about 5 minutes after heparin administration, is used to monitor the degree of anticoagulation. Control values are 80–150 seconds, while "full heparinization" (at ≥ 35°C) implies an ACT of longer than 400 seconds. Patients with unstable angina who are on continuous IV heparin (5–10 mg/hr) preoperatively may be relatively "heparin-resistant" and often require a 4–5 mg/kg bolus to achieve ACTs of more than 400 seconds.

   d. Anticoagulation may be done just prior to incising the left internal mammary artery; cannulation will then follow, as described in the following sections.

4. **Insertion of the aortic cannula** (for CPB) often causes a reflex increase in heart rate and blood pressure. Hypertension must be controlled immediately to avoid inadvertent aortic tearing and dissection during cannulation, or hemorrhage from dislodging side-biting clamps after aortotomy.

5. An improperly placed side-biting clamp or arterial cannula may occlude more than 50% of the aortic lumen and markedly increase afterload, causing myocardial decompensation. The early signs are el-

evation of PA pressures and S–T or T-wave changes on the ECG.

6. The right atrium (or else the superior and inferior venae cavae, individually) is then cannulated. Maintaining the central venous pressure (CVP) will help prevent paroxysmal atrial fibrillation during cannulation.

7. During coronary artery bypass graft procedures, the proximal anastomoses of **saphenous vein grafts** may be sewn onto the ascending aorta prior to initiating CPB. This reduces CPB time (possibly diminishing the risk of post-pump adult respiratory distress syndrome) and facilitates measuring the lengths of vein needed while the heart is still in a normal state of distention. Each application of the aortic side-biting clamp can cause a hypertensive response similar to that encountered during aortic cannulation.

G. Cardiopulmonary bypass

1. A typical **CPB machine** ("pump") consists of an 80-ml stroke volume Silastic double-headed roller pump, a blood oxygenator, and a heat exchanger.

2. **Venous inflow** (from the inferior and superior venae cavae cannulas) into the pump occurs by gravity, which also drives blood through the integrated oxygenator–heat exchanger–reservoir unit.

3. The **large roller-head** pumps arterialize blood from the oxygenator, through a filter to the aortic cannula, providing nonpulsatile flow at a rate directly related to the revolutions per minute.

   a. **Smaller roller pumps** are used to create suction for the LV vent and "pump suction," which returns heparinized blood from the surgical field back into the pump reservoir, and to perfuse cardioplegic solutions.

   b. In **"bubble" oxygenators,** O_2, and sometimes CO_2, is bubbled through the venous blood. **"Membrane" oxygenators** have a gas-permeable membrane that separates blood from the O_2 stream, reducing trauma to the blood cells and eliminating the formation of foam. After long pump runs, patients seem to have less postoperative respiratory complications with membrane oxygenators. However, when CPB lasts less than 2 hours, there appears to be little benefit gained by using the more expensive membrane oxygenator.

   c. **Pulsatile perfusion,** produced by either an intraarterial perfusion line balloon pump or a pulsatile pump-head, may preserve renal function in patients with chronic renal failure.

   d. Two liters of Ringer's lactate ($\pm$ mannitol) is typically used to "prime" the CPB circuit for adults. In full-sized, euvolemic patients, the hematocrit will fall roughly 12 percentage points with hemodilution. If starting hematocrit is low

(< 25), the prime volume may be reduced or blood transfusion prior to, or on, CPB is indicated (otherwise, the hematocrit may be reduced to levels where, even when hypothermic, tissue O_2 delivery is inadequate and metabolic acidosis ensues). For infants and small children, blood is usually required as part of the prime to limit the fall in hematocrit.

4. **Initiation of CPB.** One venous "line" (cannula) is unclamped at a time, and adequate venous drainage is confirmed. Volume permitting (i.e., if venous drainage is adequate), pump speed is progressively increased to a flow of 2.0–2.4 L/min/m² or roughly 50 ml/min/kg for adults (mean arterial pressure [MAP] of 40–140 mm Hg may be achieved by such flows, depending on SVR and intravascular volume).

   a. At this juncture, volatile anesthetics and N_2O from the anesthesia machine, IV fluids, and positive-pressure ventilation are discontinued, while O_2 flows are reduced to 200 cc/min. Muscle relaxants are supplemented to prevent shivering (which increases O_2 consumption and may produce acidosis) during cooling. Anesthesia is maintained by IV agents or by inhalation agents administered through the vaporizer in the O_2 line of the (properly scavenged) CPB machine. It is also advisable to pull the PA catheter back 1–5 cm (in its sterile sheath) to prevent migration of the catheter tip into the wedge position; this in turn may lead to accidental PA rupture during surgical manipulations or inadvertant monitoring of PCWP (rather than mean PA pressure) during bypass.

   b. **Rising superior vena cava pressure** (monitored through the PA catheter introducer sidearm, *not* through the right atrial port, which may be *below* the superior vena cava tourniquet) indicates obstruction of the superior vena cava cannula. Since cerebral perfusion pressure is equal to MAP minus that in the superior vena cava, rising superior vena cava pressure may compromise cerebral perfusion.

   c. **Elevated PA pressures** indicate left heart distention, which may be due to inadequate venting, aortic regurgitation, or inadequate isolation of venous return. Severe distention may result in irreversible myocardial damage.

   d. **Hypotension** during initiation of CPB may be due to inadequate pump flow, vasodilation, acute aortic dissection, or incorrect placement of the aortic cannula (e.g., directing flow toward the innominate artery not supplying the cannulated radial artery). A phenylephrine drip may be required to compensate for a transient vasodilatation. In the presence of carotid stenosis, MAP should be maintained at a higher level than usual (e.g., 80–90 mm Hg), and hypocarbia should be avoided.

e. **Hypertension.** MAP (> 90 mm Hg) may be treated with vasodilators or anesthetics.

f. **A brisk urine flow** should be established during the first 10 minutes of CPB.

   (1) Oliguria (<1 ml/kg/hr) should be dealt with by checking for a kinked or disconnected Foley catheter, a trial of increased perfusion pressure and/or flow, mannitol (0.25–0.5 gm/kg), or dopamine (1–5 µg/kg/min). Patients on chronic furosemide therapy may require their usual dose during CPB to sustain diuresis.

   (2) Hemolysis during CPB is usually due to physical trauma to red blood cells by the "pump suction"; released pigments may cause acute renal failure postoperatively. For hemoglobinuria, diuresis is maintained with mannitol or furosemide, and when severe, the urine is alkalinized by administering 0.5–1.0 mEq/kg sodium bicarbonate.

g. **Hypothermia** is deliberately produced, using the heat exchanger, to minimize O_2 consumption and thereby flow requirements. With cooling, blood viscosity increases, which is why the prime-induced hemodilution is desirable.

h. **Metabolic acidosis or oliguria** suggests inadequate systemic perfusion; additional volume may be needed to maintain adequate flows. Depending on the hematocrit, either blood or crystalloid may be used. (With internal mammary artery dissection, the ipsilateral chest cavity is opened; this pleural space may subsequently become an inadvertent "hiding place" for significant amounts of volume.)

5. **Myocardial protection** during bypass is accomplished by either reducing metabolic demands (hypothermia, cardioplegia) or maintaining coronary flow.

   a. **Cardioplegic solutions** may contain glucose, insulin, K^+, magnesium, nitroglycerin, lidocaine, mannitol, and balanced electrolytes. The low temperatures (4–6°C) and high K^+ concentrations rapidly arrest the electrical and mechanical activities of the heart. However, some anaerobic metabolism continues, and the by-products should be washed away by reinfusion of cardioplegia roughly every 30 minutes, or more often if electrical activity reappears.

   b. **Cold saline irrigation** of the pericardium maintains the heart at less than 25°C after administration of cardioplegia.

   c. **Mean arterial pressure** is maintained between 50 and 90 mm Hg during CPB at 25°C. At 22°C or even lower, adequate flow to vital organs is maintained at MAP of 40–50 mm Hg. At normothermia (i.e., just before terminating CPB), MAP is maintained in the 70–90 mm Hg range, particularly if ischemia or inadequate coronary revascularization is suspected or with hypertrophic ventricles.

6. **Additional heparin** may be needed for prolonged pump runs. Starting 2 hours after the initial dose, a 1 mg/kg reinforcing dose is given hourly or as necessary, as indicated by the ACT.

H. Discontinuing CPB

1. The initial step in weaning from CPB is **rewarming.** The arterial perfusate is warmed to 39°C and the OR table heating blanket connected. A brain temperature of 37°C and a core temperature of at least 35°C should be achieved, and the patient's skin (on an upper arm) should feel warm to the touch.

2. **Volatile anesthetics** are discontinued during rewarming to minimize myocardial depression when CPB is terminated. If MAP rises, sodium nitroprusside may be used for control.

3. **Neuromuscular blockade** is reinforced to prevent both shivering and lurching should electrical cardioversion be necessary.

4. **Blood transfusion** may be required if the hematocrit is below 20.

5. Pressure transducers are recalibrated, and pacemaker generators are rechecked.

6. Inotropes, vasoconstrictors, and vasodilators should be mixed and ready.

7. The ACT is remeasured at 35°C or more to determine whether more heparin will be needed if weaning is prolonged and to estimate the dose of protamine for reversal.

8. Following procedures when the heart has been opened (e.g., valve replacements), "**de-airing maneuvers**" are necessary to prevent air embolism to the cerebral or coronary circulations. Valsalva maneuvers will move air forward from the pulmonary veins. Air in the ventricular trabeculae can be liberated by shifting the OR table from side-to-side and lifting the apex of the heart; it can then be evacuated by needle aspiration of the apex. Deliberately obstructing carotid flow for the first few heartbeats following removal of the aortic cross clamp also may prevent air embolization to the brain. Direct aspiration of air bubbles visible within coronary artery vein grafts will prevent ischemia in the relevant zone of myocardium.

9. **During warming,** the aortic cross clamp is removed, and continuous coronary perfusion is reestablished. A lidocaine bolus (1 mg/kg) is administered while a drip (1 mg/min) is begun.

    a. **Defibrillation** may be spontaneous; ventricular fibrillation is treated with a directly applied 10–30 joule DC countershock. Other treatments for ventricular arrhythmias include epicardial or endocardial (through the PA line) pacing, correcting hypokalemia or ischemia, or additional antiarrhythmics (e.g., procainamide).

    b. With slow rhythms, **atrial pacing** is established through epicardial wires, but if the P–R interval is prolonged or there is complete heart block, ventricular pacing is added. Hypothermia, hypocalcemia, hyperkalemia, and magnesium from cardioplegic solutions may contribute to a high incidence of reversible heart block immediately following CPB.

    c. **Atrial tachyarrhythmias** may be treated with fentanyl, overdrive pacing ("scrambling"), cardioversion, and then, if necessary, antiarrhythmics (propranolol or verapamil if there is no LV dysfunction; otherwise digitalis may be indicated).

10. The ECG should be inspected, particularly for evidence of ischemia, heart block, and pacemaker capture.

11. The **compliance of the lungs** is tested with a few trial breaths (ventilation should be reestablished when LV ejection, even on bypass, occurs). To facilitate expansion of the lungs, the stomach is suctioned, and if previously opened, the pleural cavities are drained. If the lungs are stiff after reinflation, suctioning or bronchodilators may be indicated. Choices in this setting include epinephrine drip (0.5–2 μg/min), metaproterenol (Alupent) or albuterol (Ventolin) by inhaler, aminophylline IV (5 μg/kg/min), or PgE$_1$ (5–30 ng/kg/min).

12. Venous lines are then clamped, the heart fills, and ejection occurs with each ventricular contraction. CPB perfusion is halted, and the heart alone now provides systemic perfusion.

    a. **Transfusion** from the CPB reservoir continues until the left atrial pressure or PCWP is at an "optimal" level. The cardiac output is the best guide to this optimum, and after several such determinations, a Starling-type relationship (cardiac output versus left atrial pressure) is established.

    b. **If cardiac output is low** despite adequate cardiac filling and rhythm, a positive inotrope may be indicated. Myocardial ischemia is commonly the cause of low cardiac output following CPB and may result from inadequate myocardial protection, or air or thromboembolism; coronary dissection; or acute graft occlusion or kinking. Although it is important to identify and treat the cause of myocardial ischemia, it is critical to maintain coronary perfusion pressure to prevent a vicious downward spiral. If inotropes are ineffective, either alone or in combination with vasodilators (see Chap. 16), other options include returning to CPB, or inserting an IABP (see sec. **IV**) or another assist device. If pulmonary hypertension is present, pressors can be administered into the systemic circulation through a left atrial ("med") line.

   c. **If cardiac output is high but blood pressure is low,** a vasoconstrictor is probably needed. Hypotension may also be an artifact of radial artery spasm; the aortic root pressure will establish this diagnosis.

   d. Hypertension with adequate cardiac output should be treated to prevent bleeding at suture lines and cannulation sites. Either vasodilators (e.g., sodium nitroprusside, narcotics) or volatile anesthetics may be appropriate.

I. The postbypass period

1. Once cardiovascular stability has been achieved, **protamine administration** begins. Initially, 25–50 mg is given over 5 minutes in case of an adverse reaction. Varying degrees of systemic vasodilatation and pulmonary hypertension may be seen; some are severe enough to mandate reheparinization and reinitiation of CPB.

   a. Protamine is a mixture of naturally occurring proteins harvested from fish that may trigger **anaphylactoid reactions** after combining with heparin in the circulation.

   b. **Insulin-dependent diabetics** previously treated with protamine-zinc insulin preparations may be particularly prone to developing deleterious hemodynamic responses.

   c. It is advisable to **monitor PA pressure** while administering protamine (even if a left atrial pressure is available).

   d. In general, 1.0–1.5 mg of protamine is administered for each milligram of heparin *remaining in the circulation.* The half-life for heparin at 37°C is 1.5 hours; thus, the heparin remaining is equal to the total dose administered *minus* the amount metabolized. (For simplicity, assume that heparin is not metabolized at 25°C while on CPB.)

   e. After administration, the ACT is repeated and compared to the baseline. Further protamine is administered to return the ACT toward normal.

   f. During transfusion of heparinized "pump blood," additional protamine is administered.

2. **Pulmonary dysfunction** may follow CPB.

   a. **Bronchospasm** may be caused by asthma, allergic reactions, pulmonary edema or hemorrhage, aspiration, or irritation of the carina by the endotracheal tube; pharmacologic treatment was discussed in sec. **II.H.11.** Ventilation is adjusted to deliver large tidal volumes (15 mg/kg) with high peak inspiratory pressures and short inspiratory/expiratory (I/E) ratios.

b. **Adult respiratory distress syndrome** supportive treatment is discussed in Chap. 32.

3. _Pulmonary hypertension_ may be residual from chronic mitral valve disease or appear acutely from drug reaction, hypoxia, or atelectasis. Treatment consists in correcting ventilatory problems, nitroglycerin, sodium nitroprusside beta-adrenergic agonists, or PgE_1 infusions.

4. Strategies for diagnosis and management of **post-CPB (or any intraoperative) bleeding** diathesis, are discussed in Chap. 27.

5. **Sternal closure** is the next major milestone during cardiac cases. The hemodynamics of cardiac tamponade may acutely develop from compression of the heart and great vessels in the mediastinum.

   a. Volatile anesthetics and other negative inotropes are avoided in anticipation of sternal closure. Intravascular volume should be optimized and the stomach reemptied to create more space for lung expansion.

   b. Immediately after sternal closure, the right atrial pressure and cardiac output are compared to preclosure values, and appropriate adjustments in volume or drug infusions are made.

   c. Mediastinal and chest tubes are placed on suction immediately, to prevent tamponade and facilitate assessment of hemostasis.

   d. The left atrium trace and the ability of pacemakers to capture are rechecked, to verify that displacement has not occurred during sternal closure.

J. **Transfer to the ICU**

1. **Before transfer,** it should be verified that the ICU staff is ready to assume care. Monitoring, ventilator, heating blanket, relevant drug infusions, and personnel must be available. Elevators and hallways should be cleared of traffic and equipment. Patients should always be hemodynamically stable prior to transfer; however, essential resuscitation drugs (calcium chloride, lidocaine, and a pressor), O_2 tank, a synchronizable defibrillator, mask and bag, intubation equipment, and some extra crystalloid or colloid should still accompany patients on the journey.

2. **During transfer,** continuous monitoring of at least ECG and arterial blood pressure is maintained. The ECG is carefully checked for loss of pacemaker capture; the arterial waveform may reveal loss of IABP synchrony. Ventilation and vasoactive drug infusions should also be under contin-

uous surveillance; various commercial infusion devices can ensure steady administration rates and avoid the consequences of inadvertent boluses or interruptions.

3. **On arrival in the ICU**
   a. Mediastinal and chest tubes are immediately attached to suction to prevent cardiac tamponade and to monitor bleeding.
   b. The arterial blood pressure is confirmed by cuff, using the occlusion method.
   c. The arterial transducer and ECG are transferred to the ICU monitors. Following this, the PA and left atrial lines are calibrated.
   d. An **anteroposterior chest x-ray** is then obtained, unless already done prior to the transfer process.
   e. Finally, a **thorough report** is provided to the ICU team, including pertinent hemodynamics, drips and dosages, and the problems that are anticipated.

III. Postoperative cardiac surgery care

A. **Cardiac tamponade** is due to accumulation of blood within the mediastinum (the pericardium is rarely closed after cardiac surgery in adults). Inadequate mediastinal chest tube drainage is the most common reason for early postoperative tamponade.
   1. Impaired venous return reduces preload, and cardiac output falls. Equalization of the mean CVP, PA pressure, and PCWP is pathognomonic and is accompanied by compensatory tachycardia, hypotension, and venous congestion.
   2. This diagnosis must be considered first with early postoperative low-output syndrome, particularly in children.
   3. Placing of mediastinal tubes on suction as soon as the sternum is closed and frequent tube "stripping" will prevent the development of tamponade.
   4. Reopening the sternotomy by cutting sternal wires may be lifesaving.

B. **Arrhythmias**
   1. Postoperative cardiac dysrhythmias may be due to trauma to the conduction system during valve replacements or congenital lesion repairs, hypokalemia, myocardial ischemia, hypoxia, hypercarbia, competition with external temporary pacemakers, intermittent loss of pacemaker capture, or sympathetic response to pain.
   2. Alterations in drug regimens (beta blockers, antiarrhythmics, or digitalis) may also produce arrhythmias.
   3. Twelve-lead ECGs and atrial electrograms (from epicardial atrial wires) are often needed to assign the source (atrial versus ventricular) of arrhythmias.
   4. Because of the prevalence of premature ventricular

contractions after cardiac surgery and the consequences of ventricular fibrillation, almost all patients receive lidocaine IV (1–2 mg/min) for prophylaxis.

C. Core temperature returns toward normal in the ICU, and the resulting vasodilatation may produce hypotension. Additional volume or judicious infusion of an alpha-adrenergic agonist may be indicated.

IV. **The intraaortic balloon pump (IABP)**

A. The IABP is indicated in patients with **cardiogenic shock** who are known to have surgically correctable lesions; with **unstable angina** that cannot be stabilized with any medical regimen including high-dose nitroglycerin and heparin; or **following CPB,** where myocardial failure is expected to be relatively transient.

B. **The IABP improves myocardial performance** by augmenting aortic diastolic pressure (a determinant of coronary perfusion pressure; see Chap. 2) and reducing afterload.

1. The IABP is **inserted** through a femoral artery and advanced until the tip is just distal to the left subclavian artery in the descending thoracic aorta. It may occasionally be placed transthoracically if iliofemoral occlusive disease precludes use of a femoral artery.

2. **Inflation** of the IABP is synchronized with either the patient's ECG, a pacemaker potential, or the arterial blood pressure trace. Balloon inflation occurs early in diastole, augmenting aortic pressure by driving blood both proximally (toward the coronary bed) and distally (toward the systemic circulation). Deflation occurs just prior to systole, reducing LV stroke work and hence $M\dot{V}O_2$.

3. **Complications of IABPs** include distal embolization (to kidneys, brain, and the gastrointestinal tract), femoral arterial spasm with lower extremity ischemia, bleeding from heparinization, and consumptive coagulopathies.

V. **Other cardiac procedures**

A. Patients for **"redo" cardiac surgery,** for whatever reason, often manifest the following problems:

1. Multiple previous indwelling catheters may make percutaneous arterial and jugular cannulation difficult.

2. The heart, major vessels, or lungs may be adherent to the underside of the sternum; sternotomy can be complicated by catastrophic lacerations and hemorrhage. Femoral vessels should be isolated prior to sternotomy, since partial bypass may be lifesaving.

3. Diffuse bleeding (from extensive dissection of scar tissue) may occur following CPB, so these patients are more likely to require platelets, whole fresh blood, and/or fresh-frozen plasma.

4. Epicardial pacing may be difficult from scarring on the surface of the heart; Paceport or pacing PA

catheters are frequently useful in this setting.

B. Cardiac tumors (e.g., atrial myxomas) may cause inflow obstruction, valvular dysfunction, arrhythmias, or embolic phenomena. Management depends on the specific anatomy of individual cases.

C. Antiarrhythmia surgery may involve aneurysmectomy (with or without electrophysiologic mapping), cryoablation of accessory bundles responsible for Wolff-Parkinson-White syndrome, endocardial resection, or implantation of an automatic implantable cardiac defibrillator (AICD). Choice of anesthetics and monitoring is guided by the length of the planned procedure and the need for CPB.

1. It is crucial to prevent hyperdynamic responses following aneurysmectomy; stress on the ventricular suture line is life-threatening.

2. Electrically induced ventricular fibrillation is performed to test the function of the AICD; a properly functioning defibrillator (as well as a standby) must be available.

D. Cardiac transplantation

1. **Management of the donor.** The principal goals are to coordinate the activities of the harvesting and implantation teams and to preserve organ function, while maintaining the privacy and respect due to all patients.

   a. Brain death makes anesthesia per se unnecessary, but relaxants and ventilation with 100% O_2 still are administered.

   b. To avoid jeopardizing the donor heart, hemodynamic stability should be maintained, to the extent feasible, with volume administration rather than pressors.

   c. Once the recipient is made ready for anesthesia and surgery, the donor undergoes sternotomy and the heart is examined for size and condition. Dissection of the cavae and the PA proceeds while the abdominal organs are harvested. As the latter are removed, the aorta is cross-clamped, cardioplegia is administered, and the heart is removed.

2. **Anesthetic management of the recipient**

   a. These patients have extremely low ejection fractions, chronically poorly perfused vital organs, and extreme apprehension due to their awareness of mortality.

   b. **Full stomachs** are the rule, since cases are done on an emergency basis. Inductions may be prolonged (to preserve the tenuous hemodynamics), so cricoid pressure is indicated.

   c. All anesthesia machines and monitoring devices, the OR table, defibrillator, and supply carts should be thoroughly cleaned or sterilized prior to coming in contact with patients. **Cyclosporin,** an immunosuppressant, is administered orally or by nasogastric tube prior to in-

arterial lines be placed on the right (see sec. **VII.C.3**).

c. The choice between fentanyl (50–75 µg/kg) and halothane anesthesia hinges on ventricular function and the need for postoperative ventilation. For example, halothane is avoided in patients with poor ventricular function, but it is ideal when early extubation is planned following an atrial septal defect repair.

d. Inhalation inductions will be prolonged when there is diminished pulmonary blood flow.

6. Cardiopulmonary bypass

a. For infants and children, the pump prime consists of colloid and crystalloid solutions, with packed red blood cells added to yield a hematocrit of 25%.

b. The volume of the pump prime depends on the child's weight; the range is between 700 and 1200 ml.

c. Sodium bicarbonate, mannitol, methylprednisolone, and antibiotics may also be added to the prime.

d. Blood *flow* is more important than absolute arterial *pressure* while on CPB. Therefore, flows as high as 150 ml/kg may be used (in infants < 5 kg) while MAP as low as 30 mm Hg is well tolerated (provided a low superior vena cava pressure is maintained).

e. Hypothermic circulatory arrest (to a core and brain temperature of 15–17°C) is tolerated for up to 1 hour by infants weighing less than 10 kg. Vasodilators (e.g., phentolamine 0.1 mg/kg) may be needed prior to arrest, to promote and accelerate uniform cooling.

C. Specific congenital lesions (see also Chap. 2)

1. Atrial septal defects seldom produce severe symptoms. Bidirectional shunting may occur with coughing or Valsalva maneuver; elevated PVR and mitral regurgitation may complicate management.

2. Ventricular septal defects with large left-to-right shunts can cause pulmonary hypertension and respiratory failure from increased pulmonary blood flow and biventricular failure. Airway obstruction, hypoventilation, or anesthesia may reverse the shunt and produce cyanosis. Postoperative complications include conduction block, left or right ventricular outflow obstruction, and residual shunts.

3. Aortic coarctation repair procedures may involve transient occlusions of blood flow to the left arm; arterial lines should therefore be placed on the right. Hypertension in the arteries of the arch may be severe while the trunk (and spinal cord) blood supply is interrupted. Judicious use of vasodilators may be indicated, but lower extremity perfusion must be monitored if spinal cord ischemia is to be prevented. During cross-clamping of the aorta, the MAP should be maintained at 100–120 mm Hg; mild hypothermia (35°C), barbiturates, or dexamethasone may also prevent spinal cord infarction. Surgical access to the aorta is through the left chest, and lung retraction may produce hypoxemia.

4. **Patent ductus arteriosus** may produce a bidirectional shunt but usually presents with symptoms of CHF. Ligation is through a left thoracotomy; lung retraction may adversely affect oxygenation and reverse the shunt.

5. The predominant defect in **tetralogy of Fallot** is pulmonary outflow obstruction. When valvular stenosis is the cause, pharmacologic manipulation has little effect on pulmonary blood flow. Subvalvular (infundibular) obstruction may often be dynamic, and as with idiopathic hypertrophic subaortic stenosis (see Chap. 2), it improves with negative inotropes or sedation. Children with tetralogy of Fallot may have "spells," which are periods of intensified cyanosis due to increased outflow obstruction and associated right-to-left shunting; treatment consists in maneuvers that favor pulmonary rather than systemic flow (e.g., phenylephrine and knee-chest positioning).

D. Anesthesia can be helpful for preoperative **cardiac catheterization** in young children. The goal is to provide sufficient sedation to allow the procedure to be completed without excessive movement, while avoiding sedative-induced hemodynamic perturbations and hypoventilation.

1. An anesthesia machine (fitted with compressed air as well as O_2) and all the minimal monitoring (see Chap. 9), as well as resuscitation drugs and a defibrillator (with appropriately sized paddles) must be available.

2. Premedication is similar to that described for pediatric cardiac surgery (see sec. **VII.B.1**).

3. General endotracheal anesthesia is utilized in children prone to airway obstruction (Down's syndrome, nasopharyngeal defects), in those with severe cyanosis from pulmonary hypertension (which may improve after anesthesia reduces sympathetic tone), or in cases of relative premedication overdose.

Suggested Reading

Atlee, J. L., III. *Perioperative Cardiac Dysrhythmias, Mechanisms, Recognition, Management.* Chicago: Year Book, 1985.

Beynen, F. M., and Tarhan, S. Anesthesia for Surgical Repair of Congenital Heart Defects in Children. In S. Tarhan (ed.),

Cardiovascular Anesthesia and Postoperative Care. Chicago: Year Book, 1982.

Conahan, T. J. *Cardiac Anesthesia.* Menlo Park, Calif.: Addison Wesley, 1982.

Kaplan, J. A. *Cardiac Anesthesia.* (2nd ed.). New York: Grune & Stratton, 1987.

Ream, A. K., and Fogdall, R. P. *Acute Cardiovascular Management, Anesthesia and Intensive Care.* Philadelphia: Lippincott, 1982.

Thomas, S. J. (ed.). *Manual of Cardiac Anesthesia.* New York: Churchill Livingstone, 1984.

21

Anesthesia for Eye, Head, and Neck Surgery

Peter Rosenbaum

I. Anesthesia for eye surgery
A. General considerations
1. The quality of anesthetic management during eye surgery can influence the surgical results. Unexpected patient or eye movements during delicate microscopic intraocular eye surgery can lead to increased intraocular pressure (IOP), choroidal hemorrhage, expulsion of vitreous material, and loss of vision. Therefore, the avoidance of coughing, bucking, or straining is a major priority during anesthesia for ophthalmic procedures.
2. Visually impaired patients will be very apprehensive about surgery and require constant verbal orientation about identities, surroundings, and procedures.
3. Many ophthalmic procedures can be done under local anesthesia following a retrobulbar block. Regardless of anesthesia technique, all ophthalmic patients should have an IV catheter, ECG, and blood pressure and ventilation monitoring.
4. Patients with increased intraocular pressure or penetrating eye injuries are more liable to further damage from sudden changes in IOP.
5. Most ophthalmic medications are highly concentrated solutions that can produce systemic effects when absorbed. **Timolol** and **levobunolol** are beta blockers, and **betaxolol** is a new specific β_1-blocker used to treat glaucoma. Timolol has been reported to cause bradycardia and bronchospasm, but the more specific betaxolol may be less likely to cause bronchospasm in asthmatic patients.

    Glaucoma patients may be using **echothiophate iodide** (Phospholine) eye drops. This long-acting anticholinesterase agent depresses plasma cholinesterase activity for 2–4 weeks. These patients will have a prolonged response to succinylcholine. If succinylcholine must be used, it can be titrated in small incremental doses (0.07 mg/kg IV) while muscle twitch response (train-of-four) is monitored.
6. **Acetazolamide** (Diamox), a carbonic anhydrase inhibitor, is used to control aqueous humor secretions. Patients taking acetazolamide chronically may become hyponatremic or hypokalemic or develop metabolic acidosis.

B. Premedication
1. Ophthalmic patients are often very anxious and are susceptible to changes in IOP and to postoperative nausea and vomiting. Therefore, the ideal premedication for these patients should control anxiety

and postoperative nausea without altering IOP or cooperation.

2. Ophthalmic procedures under local anesthesia require that the patient be sedated and calm yet awake and cooperative and not obtunded and sleeping from heavy premedication.

3. Premedication regimens will not increase IOP. There is no evidence that IM atropine causes increased IOP, even in glaucoma patients.

4. Benzodiazepines such as midazolam and diazepam are effective anxiolytics with good amnestic properties. In very large doses, they may cause mydriasis, which is to be avoided in patients with acute narrow-angle glaucoma. Midazolam is about 2.5 times more potent than diazepam and much shorter acting. Midazolam, 2–4 mg IM 30 minutes preoperatively or 1–2 mg IV immediately before a retrobulbar block, is very effective. Alternatively, diazepam 5–10 mg PO 1 hour preoperatively, is used.

5. Narcotics, if used, should be given in combination with some antiemetic such as promethazine (Phenergan), hydroxyzine (Vistaril), or droperidol.

6. Barbiturates produce a lingering sleepiness of variable reliability and not any analgesia, amnesia, or anxiety control.

C. **Choice of anesthetic technique.** Many ophthalmic procedures can be performed under either local or general anesthesia. The choice of technique reflects a balanced judgment of patient safety, cooperation, and surgical difficulty. While current studies are inconclusive, it seems that a well-conducted regional anesthetic for ophthalmic procedures probably has the least morbidity.

1. **Regional block**

   a. Ophthalmic procedures such as cataract extraction, corneal transplant, and anterior chamber irrigation among others can be done following a retrobulbar block and light intravenous sedation.

   b. The retrobulbar block is achieved in a fully monitored patient by injecting 5–7 ml of a 50 : 50 mixture of 2% lidocaine and 0.75% bupivacaine (both with 1 : 200,000 epinephrine) into the muscle conus behind the globe near the ciliary nerve and ganglion. The facial nerve motor branch to the orbicularis oculi muscle is blocked separately to prevent active squeezing.

   c. Patient cooperation and lack of head motion are important for the success of this technique. Therefore, patients who are unable to understand due to deafness, senility, psychosis, or language barrier or are unable to hold still due to a chronic cough, involuntary tremor, or arthritis may not be good candidates for delicate eye procedures under local anesthesia.

d. During the procedure, fresh air at 10–15 L/min flow is provided for the patient under the drapes using a large face mask. This helps remove exhaled carbon dioxide (CO_2). Oxygen (O_2) may be used for patients with a history of coronary artery disease, but the surgeon should be notified not to use cautery while the O_2 is flowing.

e. Intravenous sedation is needed, if at all, usually just prior to the retrobulbar block injection. Small doses of either midazolam (0.015 mg/kg) or diazepam (0.03 mg/kg) are carefully titrated while the effects are monitored closely. During supplementation, the patient should not become unresponsive. Monitoring includes ECG, blood pressure, precordial stethoscope, either a hand in view for color observation or a pulse oximeter, and observation of ventilations. Undue restlessness may be a sign of hypoxia or oversedation in the elderly.

f. The advantages of a retrobulbar block include a lower incidence of coughing, straining, and emesis at emergence. This technique is useful for ambulatory patients, providing a pleasant immediate postoperative experience and increased safety.

g. The **risks** of retrobulbar block are infrequent but include direct optic nerve trauma, retrobulbar hemorrhage, and transient globe compression with increased IOP. The oculocardiac reflex may be stimulated during injection or by eye compression (see sec. **D.2**). Rarely, intravascular injection may cause seizures or myocardial depression. Also rarely, the local anesthetic may dissect along the neural sheath affecting the central nervous system and cause temporary (15 minutes) loss of consciousness without seizures. The patient may become apneic briefly but usually maintains a strong pulse and blood pressure.

2. General anesthesia

a. The eye is a very sensitive, highly innervated organ. Eye surgery requires the full proper depth of general anesthesia to prevent eye motion, coughing, bucking, or hypertension. General endotracheal anesthesia using a potent inhalational agent is usually satisfactory. This may be supplemented by a short-acting nondepolarizing muscle relaxant during any intraocular aspects of the procedure.

b. The lack of access to the airway during the procedure requires endotracheal intubation. Intravenous lidocaine (1.0–1.5 mg/kg) or 4% lidocaine spray to the larynx and trachea may help prevent bucking. The endotracheal tube should be firmly supported and taped in place to prevent disconnection and stimulation of a cough reflex by motion.

c. Ketamine causes blepharospasm, nystagmus, increased arterial pressure, and vomiting and may increase IOP. For these reasons, it is usually a poor choice for most ophthalmic surgery.

d. Smooth emergence and extubation are especially helpful following ophthalmic surgery. This may be facilitated by thorough posterior pharyngeal suctioning while the patient is deeply asleep, minimal endotracheal tube movement, IV lidocaine (1.0–1.5 mg/kg) 5 minutes before planned extubation, and some IV narcotic to reduce the cough reflex. Extubation under anesthesia is possible but may not guarantee a smooth awakening in the recovery room. Our preference is to follow the above regimen and extubate our patients carefully, awake with protective airway reflexes.

D. Specific problems

1. **Control of intraocular pressure.** Patient movement, coughing, straining, vomiting, venous congestion, hypercarbia, increased muscle tone, hypertension, and endotracheal intubation may cause increased IOP. Attention to the following details may help control IOP during anesthesia:

   a. Proper sedation and antiemetic medication.

   b. Smooth induction, intubation, and emergence; maintaining an adequate depth of anesthesia and good ventilation mechanics.

   c. Patients with increased IOP preoperatively (e.g., glaucoma) may need mannitol, 25–50 gm IV, or acetazolamide, 500 mg IV, preinduction.

   d. Succinylcholine produces a transient rise in IOP. The etiology of this response is unclear, and the reliability of methods for controlling the response is controversial. Pretreatment with a small amount of nondepolarizing muscle relaxants has been shown by some, but not all, investigators to attenuate the rise in IOP following succinylcholine.

   e. Young children with glaucoma need IOP measured from time to time to determine the effectiveness of therapy. These measurements are made under general anesthesia. The same anesthetic technique should be used each time to allow a basis for comparison.

2. **The oculocardiac reflex** (OCR) may be initiated by pain, direct eye pressure, or traction on the extrinsic eye muscles. The afferent pathway involves the ciliary branch of the ophthalmic division of the trigeminal nerve; the efferent impulse arises in the brainstem and is carried by the vagus nerve. The OCR may cause many different arrhythmias, especially bradycardia and even asystole. When it occurs, the OCR should be promptly treated by ces-

sation of the stimulus. Occasionally atropine (0.007 mg/kg IV) and even local infiltration of lidocaine near the extrinsic eye muscles may be necessary. The adequacy of the depth of anesthesia and ventilatory mechanics should be checked. Fortunately, the OCR fatigues quickly with repeated stimulation. All patients having ophthalmic surgery should have continuous ECG monitoring.

3. Patients with a **detached retina** are often anxious about the sudden loss of vision. Many are diabetics with the full range of associated medical problems. Unexpected patient movement during the delicate (sometimes intraocular) retinal repair may result in loss of vision. Therefore, deep inhalational anesthesia, supplemented with an intermediate-acting muscle relaxant during the intraocular part of the procedure, is recommended. Postoperatively, excessive coughing, straining, or vomiting should be prevented.

4. **Malignant hyperthermia** may be more likely in eye patients with strabismus or ptosis. Body temperature, heart rate, and end-tidal CO_2 should be monitored. If there is any question, blood gas analysis should be done. If succinylcholine is used, observe for abnormal reactions as described in Chap. 28.

5. **Ophthalmic eye solutions** are used in the perioperative period to produce vasoconstriction and pupillary dilatation or constriction. These concentrated solutions are absorbed from the lacrimal duct and may cause systemic effects such as hypertension, tachycardia, bradycardia, arrhythmias, angina, bronchoconstriction, hallucinations, or headaches. Patients most at risk for complications are infants, the elderly, and patients with ischemic heart disease.

6. The patient with an **open eye injury** requires a carefully conducted anesthetic to prevent further eye damage. A sudden increase in IOP can cause loss of vitreous or global contents and permanent loss of vision. Both succinylcholine and endotracheal intubation will increase IOP, but the mechanisms involved are not clear. The efficacy of pretreating with a nondepolarizing muscle relaxant to control increases in IOP from succinylcholine fasciculations is controversial (see sec. **D.1**). However, this rapid sequence induction method using pretreatment and succinylcholine has been used in many open eye/full stomach situations without evidence of causing further eye damage. Alternatively, an intermediate-duration nondepolarizing muscle relaxant such as atracurium or vecuronium may be used, allowing at least 90 seconds for satisfactory muscle relaxation conditions to develop to permit a smooth, easy intubation. Atracurium and vecuronium are neither marketed nor approved by the

FDA for rapid sequence inductions. Endotracheal intubation itself raises IOP, but this response may be attenuated by injecting lidocaine (1.0–1.5 mg/kg IV) 2–4 minutes before laryngoscopy.

7. During retina surgery, the surgeon may inject an intravitreal gas bubble containing an inert, high molecular weight, low diffusivity gas such as SF_6 or C_3F_8. Continuation of nitrous oxide (N_2O) at this time will result in rapid expansion of this bubble and possibly increase IOP. Subsequent cessation of N_2O at the end of the case will result in rapid shrinkage of this bubble and loss of its mechanical advantage. Thus, if the surgeon intends to use an intravitreal bubble, the anesthesiologist should be aware and discontinue N_2O prior to bubble injection. This intravitreal gas bubble will remain for about 5 days, and N_2O should be avoided in these patients during this time.

II. Anesthesia for ear, nose, and throat surgery
A. General considerations

1. During ear, nose, and throat (ENT) surgery, the anesthesiologist must frequently share the patient's airway with the surgeon. This airway may be limited due to bleeding, pathology, or surgical manipulation, and it may not always be accessible. Thoughtful, preoperative evaluation, intraoperative planning, and surgical cooperation are essential to avert management problems.

2. Besides standard monitoring, oxygenation and ventilation status should be under continuous surveillance by pulse oximeter and capnograph. Major head and neck procedures also mandate monitoring urinary output, response to relaxants, and intraarterial blood pressures.

3. Extubation following any upper airway surgery must be carefully planned. Posterior pharyngeal packs are removed, the pharynx is suctioned and inspected for blood, the patient is fully oxygenated, and only then, the patient may be extubated when full protective laryngeal reflexes return. Immediately following extubation, the patient's face is turned to the side (maintaining 100% O_2 by mask) and closely observed to confirm adequacy of the ventilation and the absence of laryngospasm.
Excessive upper airway bleeding, edema, or pathology may preclude a safe extubation attempt.

B. Specific procedures
1. Ear surgery

a. Inhalation anesthesia is the best technique for ear surgery. There is no need for muscle relaxation, N_2O may be safely discontinued if necessary, and hypertension is not likely.

b. Ear surgery often involves dissecting and preserving the facial nerve. The surgeon depends on muscle response to direct nerve stimulation to locate the facial nerve. If a muscle relaxant must be used, close monitoring of partial paralysis is essential. The facial nerve response to direct stimulation should not be hindered while at least one of the train-of-four twitches is visible.

c. Delicate microsurgery of the ear requires diminished bleeding for accurate surgery. Agents administered with controlled ventilation work well to lower blood pressure. In addition, a 15-degree head-up tilt to decrease venous congestion and topical epinephrine in small amounts will provide satisfactory operating conditions. A formal controlled hypotension technique is not without risk and is usually not necessary during routine ear surgery.

d. The use of N_2O causes increased middle-ear pressure, especially in the presence of a malfunctioning eustachian tube. Rarely, hemotympanum, tympanic rupture, and disarticulation of artificial stapes have been attributed to the effects of N_2O on the middle ear. The negative middle-ear pressures developed subsequent to the cessation of N_2O can lead to serous otitis media. During tympanoplasty surgery, the graft may be displaced by the N_2O pressure in the middle ear. Nitrous oxide concentration should be limited to 50% for ear surgery and may even need to be discontinued for surgical convenience.

2. **Nasal surgery**

a. Nasal surgery may be performed under either local anesthesia or general anesthesia. Even during general anesthesia, ENT surgeons will inject 2% lidocaine with epinephrine and place 4% cocaine nasal packs for vasoconstrictive effect. The painful stimuli of surgery are attenuated by these measures; hence, general anesthesia is needed mainly for amnesia, patient cooperation, and the toleration of the endotracheal tube.

b. **Cocaine** has sympathomimetic effects by blocking the synaptic reuptake of norepinephrine. The synergistic effect of cocaine and epinephrine may cause tachycardia, hypertension, or tremulousness in an otherwise comfortable patient. If necessary, these reactions can be attenuated with increments of propranolol (0.008 mg/kg IV).

c. Following nasal cosmetic surgery, the nose is unstable and face mask application is not desirable. A smooth, painless rapid awakening and extubation are important to decrease postoperative bleeding and avoid laryngospasm and use of the face mask. Neuroleptanesthesia or a N_2O-narcotic method with awake extubation are thus the techniques of choice.

d. Blood loss during nasal surgery may be substantial and difficult to estimate because blood drains posteriorly into the pharynx or esophagus. A posterior pharyngeal pack helps prevent gastric aspiration of blood and decreases postoperative vomiting.

e. Patients with **chronic epistaxis** presenting for internal maxillary artery ligation are often anxious, tired, uncomfortable, and hypertensive and may be hypovolemic and anemic. A posterior nasal pack may cause edema and hypoventilation. These patients need reassurance, rehydration, and careful sedation. They are assumed to have a full stomach (blood) and should be induced and intubated accordingly. The extent of the preoperative blood loss is deceptive; therefore a large-caliber (16 gauge) IV, several units of blood, and good suction are important. If a posterior nasal pack is in place, its removal during surgery can be followed by substantial bleeding.

3. Upper airway surgery

    a. Tonsillectomy and adenoidectomy

        (1) Anesthetic management for this brief operation, even in healthy patients, is not in any sense minor. Major problems of airway bleeding, obstruction, and cardiac arrhythmias can occur. Preoperative evaluation should seek a history of bleeding disorders and loose teeth and confirm that coagulation studies are normal.

        (2) **Light premedication** using a narcotic and antiemetic will provide postoperative comfort in a wakeful patient. Heavy premedication, especially with barbiturates, will result in slow awakening and contribute to postoperative airway problems.

        (3) A successful anesthetic technique for tonsillectomy in adults and older children is N_2O-fentanyl with either succinylcholine drip or an intermediate-acting nondepolarizing muscle relaxant. The tonsillar area is sprayed with 4% lidocaine, and a volatile agent is used only in small amounts, if necessary, to prevent hypertension. The advantage of this method is rapid, comfortable awakening with protective airway reflexes and good airway maintenance.

        (4) Intraoperative arrhythmias are not uncommon (due to light anesthesia or hypoventilation), and inadvertent endotracheal tube displacement can occur during head and mouth gag manipulations.

Therefore, continuous ECG, pulse oximetry, and precordial stethoscope are essential monitors. A well-functioning IV line is important in case there is sudden bradycardia or excessive bleeding.

(5) At the end of the operation, the posterior pharynx should be carefully suctioned and inspected for active bleeding. After breathing 100% O_2 for at least 3 minutes, the patient should be extubated awake when protective airway reflexes have returned. Mild bucking is acceptable, but may be reduced with IV lidocaine (1.0–1.5 mg/kg). Deep extubation after upper airway surgery may "look good" in the operating room, but patients may have more airway problems in the recovery room upon emergence with an irritated airway. After extubation, patients are placed on their side, head lower than hips, while breathing 100% O_2, and are observed for unobstructed breathing. Occasionally (especially in children anesthetized with volatile agents), there is a brief breath-holding episode upon extubation.

(6) Transport to the recovery room is in the "tonsillar" position (head down, turned to side). Once in the recovery room, patients are given humidified O_2 by mask, observed for at least 90 minutes, and checked for a dry pharynx before discharge. Restlessness may be due to pain or hypoxia and should be evaluated before being treated. If necessary, analgesics such as meperidine (0.5 mg/kg IV) may be titrated carefully.

b. **Rebleeding** following a pediatric tonsillectomy usually occurs within 2 hours after surgery. Expectoration of bright red blood, persistent swallowing, and tachycardia all suggest an ongoing blood loss. The extent of blood loss is often underestimated until the patient vomits a large amount of swallowed blood.

A large IV cannula must be inserted if not already present, and patients should be hydrated before reoperation. Coagulation parameters should be rechecked, and transfusion may be necessary. The rush to induce general anesthesia in a bleeding, hypovolemic child can result in severe hypotension and even cardiac arrest. An assistant and good suction are essential to ensure a view for intubation. These patients are considered to have full stomachs (blood), so rapid sequence inductions are indicated. The stomach can be then aspirated before extubation.

c. **Tonsillar abscess** may present with painful trismus, dysphagia, and a distorted, compromised airway. Before induction, the surgeon may be able to reduce the abscess size by needle aspiration. This will decrease the risk of rupture and aspiration during intubation. Careful instrumentation is required, since an abscess may be friable and partially block an upper airway. Anesthetic management and extubation procedures are similar to those discussed for adult tonsillectomies.

d. **Direct laryngoscopy** procedures for therapeutic (vocal cord polyp removal) or diagnostic (tumor biopsy) purposes may involve potentially compromised airways. The anesthesiologist should be as fully informed as possible about what pathology to expect in these patients. A good history and physical examination concentrating on the airway and head and neck area, information from the surgeon (indirect laryngoscopy), the old chart, and x-ray studies should ellucidate the nature, size, and location of the airway pathology. An informed anesthesiologist can then decide the safest approach (e.g., awake examination, intubation, mask induction, conventional induction, fiberoptic laryngoscopy, tracheostomy under local).

Problems may include a large vocal cord polyp causing a ball-valve obstruction during induction, a large supraglottic soft-tissue tumor obstructing any view of the vocal cords, a tumor displacing or distorting the trachea, and limited mandibular mobility due to fibrotic tumor or trismus. A patient with **inspiratory stridor** at rest has a severely limited airway (4 mm). If possible, these patients should have an awake direct laryngoscopy examination and either be intubated awake or undergo a tracheostomy under local anesthesia before receiving general anesthesia.

(1) **Intubation** preparation requires that several endotracheal tube and laryngoscope sizes be available. Stylets should be used cautiously, especially when advanced blindly into unknown pathology. Preoxygenate prior to all instrumentation. Monitor O_2 saturations by pulse oximeter, and evaluate the airway at each step of induction. A small (5.0–5.5 mm ID) microlaryngoscopy endotracheal tube is used for direct laryngoscopy procedures. It allows the surgeon a good view of the larynx in 95% of cases. Patients should be ventilated actively to overcome the increased endotracheal tube resistance. The anesthetic technique for direct laryngoscopy

under general anesthesia is similar to that used for adult tonsillectomies to ensure an awake extubation with good airway reflexes.

   (2) In the recovery room, the patient is observed for at least 90 minutes, placed head-up 45 degrees, and given humidified O_2 by mask. If airway edema is anticipated, **dexamethasone** (Decadron), 8 mg IV, may be given prior to extubation. **Racemic epinephrine** (0.5 ml in 1.5 ml saline) may be given by nebulizer every 2–4 hours if stridor develops to reduce laryngeal swelling.

e. Laser is light amplification by stimulated emission of radiation. A laser produces a high-energy density beam of coherent light that generates a focused thermal effect on contact with tissue. The emission media used to produce the monochromatic coherent light determines the wavelength.

   (1) Short wavelength (1 μm) lasers (Argon gas, ruby, yttrium aluminum garnet) in the red-green visible part of the electromagnetic spectrum are poorly absorbed by water but well absorbed by pigmented tissues such as retina and blood vessels.

   (2) The infrared (10 μm) CO_2 laser is well absorbed by water and superficial surface cells. The CO_2 laser is commonly used for laryngeal lesions. It cannot be transmitted through fiberoptics.

   (3) Eyes must be protected from the laser beam. Operating room personnel must wear appropriate safety goggles, and the patient's eyes should be taped closed and covered with wet gauze.

   (4) The most serious complication of laser surgery of the upper airway is airway fire. The likelihood of fire depends on the gas environment in the airway, the laser energy level, the manner in which the laser is used, the presence of moisture, and the type of endotracheal tube. Nitrous oxide supports combustion as well as O_2. A safe gas mixture during laser upper airway surgery is 25–30% O_2 in N_2. Helium (60–70%) is a fire quencher but is only protective at laser energy less than 12.5 watts.

   (5) Lasers should be used intermittently, in the noncontinuous mode, at moderate wattages (10–15 watts). Surgeons should not use the laser as a cautery and should share responsibility for fire prevention by limiting the energy input, allowing time for heat dispersal, packing aside nontarget tissue and endotracheal tube cuffs with moist gauze, and maintaining moisture (as a heat sink) in the field.

(6) Endotracheal tube options during laser surgery of the airway include wrapped, metal, impregnated, and none. Red rubber tubes are more flame resistant than PVC tubes and, when properly wrapped with metallic tape, are safe in a 25% O_2-N_2 environment at moderate beam energy levels. Metal endotracheal tubes are available but can be cumbersome. A special impregnated, disposable, fire-resistant endotracheal tube is available but is expensive. The use of a jet-Venturi technique eliminates the need for an endotracheal tube, but dry tissue can still spark and enflame, causing a blowtorch effect with the jet O_2. Endotracheal tube cuffs can be filled with saline as a precaution against an inadvertent hit by the laser beam.

(7) If an airway fire occurs, pour saline into the pharynx to absorb the heat, temporarily discontinue the O_2 source, then extubate, and reintubate with a new endotracheal tube. Follow up with chest x-ray, bronchoscopy, steroids, and arterial blood gases. Tracheal and/or laryngeal granulation tissue formation or stenosis may be a late complication.

(8) The anesthetic technique for laser surgery of the upper airway is similar to that described for direct laryngoscopy under general anesthesia. Goals include adequate surgical view, decreased laryngeal reflexes, absence of vocal cord motion, and rapid return of airway reflexes for awake extubation. Most often, a small (5.0–5.5 mm ID), wrapped red-rubber endotracheal tube is used in an environment of 30% O_2-N_2. Since airway edema may occur, the patient is given humidified O_2 and observed closely in the recovery room. Steroids or racemic epinephrine may also be necessary.

f. Many patients with carcinoma of the larynx scheduled for **laryngectomy** are heavy smokers with chronic bronchitis and frequently are alcohol abusers as well. Inhalation anesthesia is preferable, allowing high FIO_2 if necessary and spontaneous breathing during tracheal transection and insertion of a Tovell tube from the operative field. At equipotent dose levels, enflurane seems to obtund tracheal reflexes less well than other volatile agents, so topical tracheal lidocaine or deeper anesthesia may be required to obliterate cough reflexes.

4. **Difficult intubations**

   a. ENT surgical patients are often the most difficult of patients to intubate. Causes of difficulty include facial or tracheal deformities (congenital or trauma), trismus (tumor, irradiation, inflammation), foreign body in the airway, cleft palate, supraglottic tumors, and infection.

   b. Informed management decisions will avert acute airway emergencies. The anesthesiologist should gather information from previous intubation notes, indirect laryngoscopy diagrams, and upper airway x-rays. Patient examination includes neck flexibility, patency of nasal passages, mandible size and mobility, tracheal location and mobility, dental conditions, voice quality, presence of stridor, and respiratory pattern. The extent and location of lesions should be ascertained to the extent possible before deciding on anesthetic management. Often, a direct laryngoscopy examination under light IV sedation (e.g., 2 ml of Innovar) with topical laryngeal block is very informative. Lack of visibility of pharyngeal or glottic structures (uvula, faucial pillars, arytenoids) may portend a very difficult airway management situation and indicate awake intubation or even preoperative tracheostomy.

   c. A carefully performed awake oral or nasal intubation in a spontaneously breathing, cooperative patient is usually safe. Light sedation (fentanyl, 1–3 µg/kg, plus droperidol, 0.05–0.10 mg/kg IV) may be needed for patient cooperation. Copious nasal bleeding can be prevented by applying a topical nasal vasoconstrictor (cocaine 4%, or oxymetazoline), then using a small, well-lubricated nasal endotracheal tube inserted slowly, parallel to the turbinates.

   d. Experienced personnel may opt to use a fiberoptic laryngoscope or bronchoscope when limited airway access due to trismus or cervical spine injury is present (see Chap. 10).

   e. Intubation in the presence of upper airway tumor or polyps should proceed carefully with a well-lubricated, small endotracheal tube passed gently under direct vision. Blind instrumentation or intubation attempts will quickly cause tumor bleeding or displacement of tissue or polyps into the trachea.

   f. In especially difficult situations, if there is any doubt about the ability to maintain an adequate airway, an experienced surgeon and tracheostomy set should be ready before proceeding.

g. A difficult intubation will most likely also be a difficult extubation that requires careful consideration of consequences. Such patients are best extubated fully awake.

5. **Emergency tracheostomies**

a. When upper airway manipulations cannot clear the airway and intubation seems impossible, a tracheostomy or cricothyroidotomy is required. These patients are in acute respiratory distress, stridorous, anxious, tachypneic, and tachycardic and may be hypoxic, acidotic, hypercarbic, and hypertensive as well. Do not try to calm these patients with sedatives. Giving 100% O_2 by mask with gentle assisted respirations can calm and reassure many patients.

As a last resort, a percutaneous cricothyroid puncture can be performed using a 12- or 14-gauge IV needle. The hub can then be connected to the anesthesia machine by a 3-mm pediatric endotracheal tube adapter or a 3-ml syringe barrel connected to a universal 15-mm endotracheal tube adapter.

b. Once the airway is reestablished, there may be a sudden return to normocarbia with decreased endogenous catecholamine levels and lessened anxiety. These tired patients may then become sleepy and hypotensive.

c. In the recovery room, an obturator is kept at the bedside and the tracheostomy site checked for bleeding. A chest x-ray should be obtained to confirm proper positioning of the tracheostomy tube and absence of pneumothorax.

III. Anesthesia for maxillofacial trauma

A. In the **acute situation,** there may be extraoral, intraoral, and nasal bleeding with facial swelling. The patient is assumed to have a full stomach of swallowed blood and may even have aspirated blood or gastric contents when unconscious. Head trauma and cervical spine fracture are often associated with facial trauma, and therefore, skull and cervical spine x-ray and neurologic evaluations should be done before administering general anesthesia. Suction with a tonsil tip should be available during induction.

1. A rapid induction and oral intubation with cricoid pressure may be considered if there is no intraoral bleeding and airway anatomy is undamaged. If any doubt exists, an awake oral intubation will be safest. Nasal intubation in patients with severe midface trauma requires careful assessment and is often contraindicated. However, if the nasal passages are intact and trauma is limited to the mandible, an awake nasal intubation may not only be safest but also the best tolerated.

2. An isolated mandibular fracture should not worsen with jaw manipulation during laryngoscopy, but the anesthesiologist should be aware of the possibility of avulsion and aspiration of loose teeth at this time.

3. If the mandible has limited motion, it is important to know whether the cause is pain, swelling, or mechanical (e.g., a depressed zygoma impinging on the mandibular coronoid process). A mechanically obstructed mandible may make it difficult to view the glottic opening during a rapid sequence induction. In severe midface trauma with intraoral bleeding and jaw motion limitation, an elective tracheostomy under local anesthesia is absolutely the safest way to secure the airway.

4. Awake oral intubation is a useful, safe technique that can be simplified by considering the following details:

   a. Patient cooperation can be recruited by explanations, rapport, and judicious IV sedation with narcotics. Instrumentation should always proceed slowly and gently.

   b. Topical laryngeal nerve block, including superior laryngeal nerve block and possibly transtracheal lidocaine injection, is often useful in this setting.

   c. Topical laryngeal anesthesia is a double-edged sword and depresses protective airway reflexes, which increases the risk of aspiration.

   d. Mandibular nerve block (intraoral or external approach) can be used to relax the mandible in especially uncooperative patients.

   e. Using a small (7 mm) oral endotracheal tube with stylet is helpful.

5. The choice of anesthetic technique will depend on individual patient needs. Significant muscle relaxation is not required, and assisted ventilation may often be desirable.

6. Occasionally it may be necessary to perform an oral intubation and then change to a nasal endotracheal tube during the procedure to facilitate surgical access and postoperative care. During the exchange, the patient still has a full stomach and is subject to risk of aspiration. Therefore, exchange should still be done quickly under direct vision with cricoid pressure.

7. In patients with midface fractures, the nasal passages must be assessed carefully and the mucosa treated with vasoconstrictors before attempting nasal intubation. Two cotton-tipped applicators soaked in 4% cocaine are passed gently, as a unit, down each nasal passage into the nasopharynx. During slow withdrawal, the applicators should be rotated slowly to contact the mucous membrane. Obstructions and deviated septa should be appreciated at this time. Initially, a small (5 mm) endo-

tracheal tube may be passed into the nasopharynx to dilate the nasal passage gently. Then a properly sized endotracheal tube may be inserted, with the aid of direct oral vision or intranasal fiberoptics if necessary.

8. Patients with **interdental fixation** of maxillary fractures should be extubated when wide awake, given an antiemetic (e.g., droperidol, 0.02 mg/kg IV), humidified O_2 by mask, and observed closely for 24 hours for signs of upper airway problems. A clamp and scissors should be taped to the bedside to cut the interdental attachments in case of an airway emergency.

B. **Elective surgery** on a patient with facial trauma resembles the acute situation with two exceptions: there is no full stomach, and most facial swelling and nasal bleeding have subsided. However, painful trismus may still be present.

1. Patients with isolated mandibular fractures may be a challenge only when there is a mechanical obstruction to mandible mobility, decreasing the view of the larynx. These patients may be nasally intubated (awake or asleep), blindly while breathing spontaneously, or with the aid of a nasal fiberoptic view.

2. Patients with **midface trauma** should first be intubated orally to allow thorough evaluation of the nasal passages under general anesthesia. Midface trauma is classified by LeFort types. LeFort I (isolated maxillary fracture) may be safely nasally intubated if necessary. The LeFort II (pyramidal fracture around the nose) and LeFort III (craniofacial disarticulation fracture including the orbits) are of greater concern because of possible ethmoid cribriform plate disruption (rare), cerebrospinal fluid leak, nasal mucosal tear, and intracranial placement of the nasal endotracheal tube. If present, palate disruption may obstruct the view and make laryngoscopy more difficult. Occasionally, tracheostomy may be indicated for optimal care of severe midface trauma patients.

C. Patients with **zygomatic fractures** (elective or emergent) not associated with maxillary or mandibular fractures may be intubated orally with the tube on the side contralateral to the fracture. Nasal intubation includes the risk that Kirschner fixation wire (passed through the attached zygoma and nasal passages into the unstable zygoma) may pass through the nasal endotracheal tube and make extubation impossible.

IV. **Anesthesia for head and neck procedures**

A. A primary anesthetic concern during this surgery is establishing and maintaining a **secure airway** while sharing the airway with surgeons.

1. An armored (Tovell) endotracheal tube may be necessary to prevent kinking.

2. Following thyroid or parathyroid surgery, operative

site bleeding may compress the trachea, causing difficult breathing. A sterile hemostat placed through the incision opens the wound to allow egress of trapped blood. Emergency endotracheal intubations may be difficult due to tracheal displacement.

3. Injury to one recurrent laryngeal nerve causes unilateral vocal cord paralysis, a benign condition limited to hoarseness and a weak voice. Bilateral vocal cord paralysis, however, is more serious and causes signs of increasing upper airway obstruction and stridor. Obstruction may be relieved by positive-pressure face mask ventilation but requires immediate reintubation.

   Partial obstruction caused by vocal cord edema may be treated by humidified O_2, nebulized racemic epinephrine (0.5 ml in 1.5 ml saline), and head-up position.

4. **Teflon injection** of the vocal cords must be done during awake laryngoscopy so that the patient can cooperate and phonate while the quality of the voice is assessed. Therefore, these procedures should be done with a good topical laryngeal block and light sedation.

B. Radical neck dissection

1. Radical neck dissections, especially in previously radiation-treated patients, may elicit unappreciated large blood loss. Controlled hypotensive anesthesia (see Chap. 16) may be considered but is not usually needed if a 15-degree head-up tilt and positive-pressure ventilation with a potent volatile agent are used to keep systolic blood pressures at 90–100 mm Hg.

2. During dissection, traction or pressure on the carotid sinus may cause arrhythmias such as bradycardia or cardiac arrest. Treatment includes immediate cessation of surgical stimulus. If necessary, the surgeon may use lidocaine to block the carotid sinus reflex, or atropine (0.07 mg/kg IV) may be used as a vagolytic.

3. **Air embolism** through large open veins during neck surgery is possible but infrequent.

4. An elective tracheostomy may be performed at the end of the procedure if soft-tissue edema or neck bleeding is expected to cause airway compromise during the first 48–72 hours postoperatively. Alternatively, a nasotracheal tube may be left in place during this period.

Suggested Reading

Donlon, J. V. Anesthetic management of patients with compromised airways. *Anesth. Rev.* 7:22, 1980.

Donlon, J. V. Anesthesia for Eye, Ear, Nose, and Throat. In

R. D. Miller (ed.), *Anesthesia*. New York: Churchill Livingstone, 1985. Pp. 1837–1894.

Hermens, J. M., Bennett, M. J., and Hirshman, C. A. Anesthesia for laser surgery. *Anesth. Analg.* 62:218, 1983.

Latto, I. P., and Rosen, M. *Difficulties in Tracheal Intubation.* Philadelphia: Saunders, 1985.

Lopez, N. R. Mechanical problems of the airway. *Clin. Anesth.* 3:8, 1978.

McGoldrick, K., Bruce, R. A., and Oppenheimer, P. *Anesthesia for Ophthalmology*. Birmingham, Ala.: Aesculapius, 1982.

Morrison, J. D., Mirakhur, R. K., and Craig, H. J. *Anaesthesia for Eye, Ear, Nose and Throat Surgery* (2nd ed.). New York: Churchill Livingstone, 1985.

Murphy, D. T. Anesthesia and intraocular pressure. *Anesth. Analg.* 64:520, 1985.

Murphy, T. Somatic Blockade for Head and Neck. In M. J. Cousins and P. O. Bridenbaugh (eds.), *Neural Blockade*. Philadelphia: Lippincott, 1980. Pp. 420–432.

Patil, V., Stehling, L., and Zauder, H. (eds.). *Fiberoptic Endoscopy in Anesthesia*. Chicago: Year Book, 1983.

Symposium on anesthesia for eye surgery. *Br. J. Anaesth.* 52, July 1980.

22

Anesthesia for Neurosurgery

Richard A. Miller

Anesthesia for intracranial surgery depends on understanding the physiology and pharmacology of cerebral blood flow (CBF) and intracranial pressure (ICP).

I. Physiology

A. Cerebral blood flow

is equal to cerebral perfusion pressure (defined as the difference between mean arterial pressure [MAP] and ICP or central venous pressure [CVP], whichever is higher) divided by cerebral vascular resistance. Cerebral blood flow varies regionally in response to changes in cellular metabolic activity; it averages about 50 ml/100 gm of brain/minute in humans. When CBF is inadequate to support aerobic metabolism, ischemia develops and infarction may ensue.

1. Control of CBF (Fig. 22-1)

a. Autoregulation.

Cerebral blood flow remains essentially constant between 50 and 150 mm Hg MAP in the normal person. This phenomenon, termed *autoregulation,* is a consequence of changes in vascular smooth muscle tone in response to changes in transmural pressures. Many conditions alter the limits of autoregulation. Chronic hypertension shifts the autoregulatory curve to the right, rendering patients susceptible to cerebral ischemia at blood pressures considered normal in healthy individuals. Cerebral ischemia, head trauma, hypoxia, severe hypercarbia, edema surrounding brain tumors, and volatile anesthetics also impair autoregulation. When the limits of cerebral autoregulation are exceeded, or when there is no autoregulation, CBF varies directly with MAP.

b. $PaCO_2$.

Cerebral blood flow is altered by about 4% for every 1 mm Hg change in $PaCO_2$ between 25 and 100 mm Hg. Since there is little additional decrease in CBF below 25 mm Hg $PaCO_2$ and biochemical evidence of cerebral ischemia may develop, excessive hyperventilation should be avoided. The effect of $PaCO_2$ on CBF diminishes with time due to adaptive changes in cerebrospinal fluid (CSF) bicarbonate (HCO_3^-) concentration; this process takes 12–24 hours to develop. Within regions of fixed vascular resistance, $PaCO_2$ may produce paradoxical CBF effects. For example, hypercarbia will dilate normal vessels and consequently "steal" blood flow from areas supplied by stenotic vessels. Conversely, by constricting normal vessels, hypocarbia can divert blood toward regions with fixed vessel diameters.

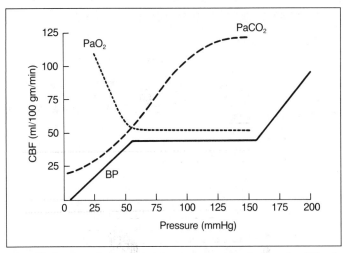

Fig. 22-1. Autoregulation maintains a constant level of cerebral blood flow (CBF) over a wide range of carotid artery mean blood pressure (BP). Independent of this effect, CBF is elevated by hypercarbia ($PaCO_2$) and hypoxemia (PaO_2); hypocarbia diminishes CBF.

    c. PaO_2 has little effect on CBF under normal circumstances. However, if PaO_2 falls below 50 mm Hg, CBF increases markedly.

  2. Effects of anesthetics on CBF

    a. Inhalation agents in common use (halothane, enflurane, isoflurane) produce cerebral vasodilatation and increase CBF, but at equianesthetic doses, halothane increases CBF the most. Hyperventilation blunts this effect to some extent with all these agents but predisposes to seizure activity with enflurane. Isoflurane decreases cerebral metabolism to a greater extent than do halothane or enflurane. Consequently, isoflurane is often selected when an inhalation anesthetic is needed during intracranial surgery. Nitrous oxide (N_2O), either alone or when combined with inhalation agents, increases CBF, but this effect is eliminated by prior administration of thiopental.

    b. Intravenous anesthetics (barbiturates, narcotics, benzodiazepines, butyrophenones, etomidate, lidocaine) decrease CBF. Ketamine is the exception; it markedly increases CBF and should not be used in patients with space-occupying intracranial lesions. Thiopental is a potent cerebrovasoconstrictor and will reduce CBF by as much as 50% when doses that produce an isoelectric EEG are given.

c. **Muscle relaxants** may indirectly alter CBF. Rapid administration of curare causes histamine release, which decreases cerebral perfusion pressure and produces cerebral vasodilatation. Laudanosine, a metabolite of atracurium, is a central nervous system (CNS) stimulant but does not increase CBF significantly at concentrations resulting from clinical doses of atracurium. Succinylcholine increases CBF, possibly by increasing cerebral metabolic rate ($CMRO_2$).

3. **Effects of vasoactive agents on CBF**

a. **Vasopressors.** Phenylephrine, epinephrine, and norepinephrine do not cross the blood-brain barrier and have little direct effect on cerebral vasculature. However, they may increase CBF indirectly by increasing arterial perfusion pressure. When the blood-brain barrier is disrupted, epinephrine stimulates cerebral metabolism and increases CBF.

b. **Vasodilators.** The ganglionic blocker trimethaphan (1–4 mg/min titrated to blood pressure) is often used to control blood pressure in the neurosurgical patient because it does not increase CBF or ICP as much as direct vasodilators. It does, however, cause cycloplegia and mydriasis, which may confuse the postoperative neurologic assessment. Sodium nitroprusside, nitroglycerin, and hydralazine are direct cerebral vasodilators that increase CBF if arterial perfusion pressure is maintained.

B. **Intracranial pressure** is normally 5–15 mm Hg and reflects the volume of brain, CSF, and blood within the cranial vault. Increased ICP reduces cerebral perfusion pressure and may produce cerebral ischemia and ultimately brain herniation.

1. **Pressure-volume dynamics.** The cranium is rigid, and its capacity to accommodate volume increases is limited. A developing intracranial mass (e.g., tumor, hematoma, edema, or hydrocephalus) initially displaces CSF and blood from the cranial vault, the net volume is constant, and ICP remains normal (Fig. 22-2A). As the mass enlarges, intracranial compliance decreases, and small increases in intracranial volume result in large increases in ICP (Fig. 22-2B). Patients with decreased compliance may develop marked increases in ICP when cerebrovasodilatation, which increases cerebral blood volume, occurs. The symptoms and signs of increased ICP include headache, nausea, vomiting, papilledema, coma, and finally, hypertension, bradycardia, and irregular respirations.

2. Two methods are commonly used to **measure ICP.**

a. **The subarachnoid bolt** is a hollow screw placed through a burr hole and connected to a pressure transducer through saline-filled tub-

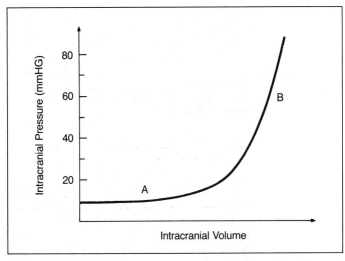

Fig. 22-2. The intracranial compliance curve. See text for details.

ing. The device is technically easy to place but is prone to clogging and infection, and, because CSF cannot be withdrawn through a subdural bolt, it cannot be used to treat intracranial hypertension.

b. Alternatively, ICP can be measured by a catheter inserted through a burr hole into a lateral ventricle. Although more accurate than a subdural bolt and useful for draining CSF, placement of a catheter is difficult in a patient with compressed ventricles. Complications include infection and hemorrhage.

3. **Treatment.** The goal is to improve intracranial compliance or reduce ICP.

a. **Hyperventilation** causes cerebral vasoconstriction and rapidly decreases CBF and cerebral blood volume. The maximal effect occurs at a $PaCO_2$ of about 25 mm Hg; after about 12–24 hours of hyperventilation, CBF returns to normal levels. With sustained hyperventilation, CSF HCO_3^- production decreases, allowing CSF pH gradually to decrease as well.

b. **Diuretics.** Osmotic diuretics (e.g., **mannitol, 0.5–1.5 gm/kg IV**) increase plasma osmolality and draw water from the intracellular and interstitial spaces into the vasculature. This decreases intracranial volume, lowers ICP, and improves intracranial compliance. The osmotic diuretics are only effective in regions where the blood-brain barrier is intact, and they act more slowly than hyperventilation to reduce ICP. Serum osmolality should be followed and maintained at less than 320 mOsm/L to prevent neurologic and renal complications. Mannitol initially increases intravascular volume and may precipitate congestive heart failure in susceptible patients; it may also cause hypokalemia from renal excretion of potassium. Loop diuretics (furosemide, ethacrynic acid) lower ICP by their dehydrating effects and by decreasing CSF production. They do not increase intravascular volume and are thus safer in patients with cardiac dysfunction.

c. Steroids reduce edema associated with tumors (vasogenic edema) but appear to be ineffective in treating edema secondary to trauma or hypoxia (cytotoxic edema). Because their effects occur slowly (over about 12 hours), steroids are not useful for treating acute elevations in ICP.

d. Barbiturates are potent cerebral vasoconstrictors and may be used to decrease ICP in patients resistant to other modes of therapy.

e. To improve **cerebral venous drainage,** patients with increased ICP should be kept in a 30-degree head-up position, and factors that impair venous drainage (e.g., coughing, straining, and elevated airway pressures) should be avoided.

C. Cerebral metabolism. The brain requires a constant supply of substrate to meet its relatively high metabolic demands. Glucose is the usual fuel for nerve tissue, although ketone bodies can also serve as energy-producing substrates during periods of fasting and ketoacidosis.

1. Cerebral blood flow and cerebral metabolic rate are coupled: regional increases in $CMRO_2$ elicit a corresponding increase in CBF, possibly mediated by metabolic by-products.

2. Anesthetic effects

a. Potent inhalation anesthetics produce dose-dependent increases in CBF and decreases in $CMRO_2$ (e.g., uncoupled CBF and $CMRO_2$). Of the volatile anesthetics, isoflurane is the most potent cerebral metabolic depressant, reducing $CMRO_2$ by 50% at an end-tidal concentration of about 2.5%. High doses of enflurane may induce seizures and consequently stimulate brain metabolism.

b. With the exception of ketamine, **IV anesthetics** decrease $CMRO_2$. Barbiturates depress $CMRO_2$ (and CBF) the most; at the point of EEG isoelectricity, $CMRO_2$ is approximately 50% of normal.

3. Temperature effects. Hypothermia decreases $CMRO_2$ 7%/1°C, and hyperthermia increases it. Temperatures above 42°C may cause neuronal cell death.

4. Seizures increase $CMRO_2$ and CBF.

II. Electrophysiologic monitoring
A. Electroencephalography. Brain electrical activity correlates with CBF, and therefore, the EEG is a useful monitor during procedures that jeopardize cerebral perfusion such as carotid endarterectomy and cardiopulmonary bypass (CPB). Electroencephalographic monitoring can also serve as a guide to drug therapy for cerebral protection (where an isoelectric EEG is sought).

1. **The electrical activity measured by EEG** is generated largely by neurons of the cerebral cortex but is also strongly influenced by subcortical pacemakers such as the thalamus and reticular activating formation. The EEG is a plot of voltage versus time and is described by wave frequencies, amplitudes, and patterns.

   a. Alpha activity (8–13 Hz) predominates in awake patients with closed eyes and is most evident over the occipital region. Beta activity (13–30 Hz) is predominant anteriorly and is seen in awake patients during mental tasks. Slower frequencies (delta: 1–3 Hz; theta: 4–8 Hz) appear during slow-wave sleep and in pathologic states such as metabolic encephalopathies.

   b. Electroencephalogram changes that may reflect inadequate CBF during surgery include loss of fast activity, loss of amplitude, and increased slow-wave activity. These classic patterns are not always observed during cerebral ischemia, however, and may be produced by other conditions (e.g., hypothermia, drugs) as well.

   c. When CBF decreases below roughly 20–25 ml/100 gm/min, slowing occurs; in the vicinity of 15 ml/100 gm/min, the EEG becomes isoelectric ("flat"). Tissue infarction occurs when flow is less than 8–10 ml/100 gm/min. Thus, EEG changes can warn of ischemia before CBF becomes insufficient to maintain tissue viability.

2. **Anesthesia-related effects on the EEG**

   a. As a general rule, **"light" anesthesia** increases beta activity, whereas slower frequencies (theta, delta) are seen during "deeper" anesthesia. Anesthetic effects are generally global, which helps distinguish them from the often focal changes of ischemia.

   b. By causing EEG slowing, **deep inhalation anesthesia** may make detection of superimposed ischemic changes difficult. Thus, "balanced" (N_2O-narcotic-relaxant) or light inhalational anesthesia is often selected for carotid endarterectomies (see sec. **IV.C**). In addition, it is helpful to maintain a *constant* level of anesthesia during crucial periods of surgery (e.g., during carotid cross-clamping) to minimize EEG interpretation problems.

  c. Hypoxia produces EEG slowing. Hypocarbia, on the other hand, has little effect on the EEG.

  d. Hypothermia depresses EEG activity and may limit the usefulness of EEG monitoring during CPB.

 3. Intraoperative 16-lead EEG monitoring is difficult for nonexperts to interpret. Consequently, commercial devices have been developed that process raw EEG data and display it in a simplified format. In general, these devices process the amplitude and frequency data from the raw EEG to facilitate detection of trends toward lower frequencies; however, the raw data still must be examined to ensure that processing of artifacts (e.g., from muscle) does not obscure interpretation. These devices also use fewer channels and therefore sample fewer discrete areas of the brain, making it less likely that small areas of ischemia will be detected.

B. Evoked potential monitoring

 1. Sensory evoked potentials (EPs) are obtained by stimulating a peripheral nerve and recording the resulting electrical signal as it travels toward the brain. A normal response implies that the conduction pathway being monitored is intact, but an abnormal response does not necessarily mean that the pathway is threatened. The aim of EP monitoring is to detect significant changes early enough to institute corrective measures before irreversible neural damage occurs. Evoked potentials may be classified according to the sensory system being evaluated:

  a. Somatosensory evoked potentials are obtained by electrically stimulating a mixed-function peripheral nerve (e.g., median or posterior tibial) and recording electrical signals over the brachial or lumbar plexus, spinal cord, and cerebral cortex. Somatosensory EPs are used to monitor spinal cord function during spinal column (e.g., Harrington rodding) or spinal cord surgery and may also be used during peripheral nerve, brachial plexus, or thoracic aortic surgery (when spinal cord blood supply is in jeopardy).

  b. Auditory EPs have been used during posterior fossa surgery in attempts to avoid brainstem or eighth (acoustic) cranial nerve damage. The stimulus is a click produced by a small speaker inserted into the external auditory canal. Preoperatively, an audiogram is necessary to verify that acoustic nerve function is intact.

  c. Visual EPs, generated by light flashes to the eyes, have been used during surgery around the optic nerve and tracts (e.g., pituitary surgery). Technical problems (i.e., inability to deliver patterned stimuli) currently limit their utility during surgery.

2. **Principles.** Evoked potentials result from incompletely characterized generators located along the neural pathway and are of lower voltage than the background EEG. To detect them, numerous elicited responses are summed, then averaged and amplified as a waveform that has both positive and negative peaks. (Background EEG activity is randomly positive or negative and will average to zero.) Damage to a neural pathway is manifest, in general, as a decrease in amplitude and an increase in latency (i.e., time from stimulus to response) of the peaks.

3. **Problems associated with EP monitoring**
   a. Factors other than nerve damage can change EP responses. These include
      (1) **Anesthetics and other centrally acting drugs.** Cortical potentials are more sensitive to anesthetic effects than signals arising from subcortical structures or the spinal cord. Consequently, when recording cortical potentials, use of inhalation anesthetics should be minimized. In addition, identification of EP changes specific to surgical manipulation is clearer when a constant level of anesthesia is maintained at crucial points in an operation.
      (2) Changes in **blood pressure, temperature, hematocrit,** and **arterial blood gases.**
   b. Data acquisition and interpretation are complicated and expensive and require the involvement of specially trained personnel.
   c. **False negatives.** Because somatosensory EPs are conducted primarily by the posterior columns (sensory), they may not detect changes in anterior (motor) spinal function. Although cases have been reported where intraoperative somatosensory EPs were normal in patients who nevertheless developed a motor deficit, the true incidence of such false negatives is not known. Proponents of somatosensory EP monitoring argue that the test is useful because most intraoperative insults are not selective and will cause dysfunction of all spinal pathways.
   d. **False positives.** Changes in somatosensory EP occur more frequently than the rate of postoperative complications would predict. These changes may represent functionally insignificant phenomena, which nevertheless, cause anxiety in the staff, unnecessarily narrow the surgical options, or otherwise alter the conduct of surgery or anesthesia. More work is necessary to establish the nature, magnitude, and duration of EP changes associated with irreversible damage.

III. **Anesthetic management of elective intracranial surgery**

  A. **Preoperative considerations**

    1. Intracranial compliance is likely to be decreased from intracranial mass lesions. Signs and symptoms that suggest elevated ICP were discussed in sec. **I.B.1.** A midline shift and compressed ventricles on CT scan also indicate poor intracranial compliance.

    2. Fluid and electrolyte imbalances and glucose intolerance are common, due to fluid restriction, diuretics, poor oral intake, steroids, and occasionally centrally mediated endocrine abnormalities. Severe hypovolemia, hypokalemia, hyponatremia, and hyperglycemia should be corrected preoperatively.

    3. Patients may depend on anticonvulsants for seizure control and steroids for treatment of edema. These drugs should be continued into the morning of surgery.

  B. **Sedating premedication** should be prescribed cautiously, since patients with intracranial disease may be extremely sensitive to the effects of CNS depressants. **Narcotics,** which may cause carbon dioxide retention or vomiting and thereby increase ICP; **scopolamine,** which may cause delirium; and **long-acting sedatives** should all be avoided. If premedication is needed, diazepam (0.15 mg/kg PO) or an even shorter-acting benzodiazepine such as midazolam (0.025–0.05 mg/kg IM) may be the best choice. Additional sedation can be given IV once the patient arrives in the OR.

  C. Besides routine **monitoring** (see Chap. 8), intraarterial catheters are used in all patients undergoing craniotomy. Capnography is particularly useful when controlling ICP by hyperventilation. For cases in the sitting position, a precordial Doppler and right atrial catheter are used to diagnose and treat venous air embolism. Pulmonary artery catheters are often indicated for patients with severe cardiac or pulmonary disease, since marked volume shifts may result from mannitol and furosemide administration. A second IV catheter for drug infusions may be necessary.

  D. **Intraoperative management.** The goals of anesthesia for neurosurgical procedures include immobility and unconsciousness, adequate CPP, a "slack" brain (i.e., optimal surgical conditions), avoidance of high ICP, and an awake, extubated patient who can be evaluated neurologically at the conclusion of the case. Anesthetic techniques that facilitate these goals follow.

    1. **Induction of anesthesia** must be accomplished without increasing ICP or compromising CBF. Hypertension, hypoxia, hypercarbia, and coughing must be avoided.

      a. Thiopental (3–7 mg/kg) produces unconsciousness rapidly and decreases $CMRO_2$, CBF, and ICP. Etomidate (0.3–0.4 mg/kg) and midazolam

(0.2–0.4 mg/kg) have similar effects and may cause less cardiovascular depression.

b. A patent airway is essential to allow hyperventilation by mask immediately after induction of anesthesia.

c. A **muscle relaxant** is given in an intubating dose. Succinylcholine use presents two problems: it may elevate ICP, and it may cause hyperkalemia in patients with upper motor nerve lesions. *D*-tubocurarine releases histamine, which can decrease MAP and increase ICP (hence decreasing CPP).

d. **Narcotics** are administered to minimize the cardiovascular responses to intubation. The advantages of fentanyl (5–10 μg/kg IV) and sufentanil (0.5–1.0 μg/kg IV) are rapid onset (1 minute), brief duration of action, and minimal cardiovascular effects. In contrast, morphine reaches its peak effect in 10–20 minutes, making it a less suitable choice for blocking the hemodynamic response to laryngoscopy and intubation. **Lidocaine** (1.5 mg/kg) will also attenuate the cardiovascular responses to intubation.

e. Low concentrations of a potent **inhalational anesthetic** are frequently necessary to prevent hypertension during the initial surgical stimulation. Trimethaphan (1–4 mg/min) may also be used to treat hypertension during this phase of the procedure.

f. **After intubation,** the position of the endotracheal tube is checked, and it is taped securely, since access to the head will be limited. Eyes are protected with watertight patches to prevent "prep" solutions from causing irritation, and an oral airway, esophageal stethoscope, and temperature probe are placed.

2. Maintenance

a. After craniotomy and opening of the dura, anesthetic requirement is lower, since brain parenchyma is devoid of sensation. To prevent movement (which could have disastrous results), muscle relaxants are frequently administered. If supplemental narcotics are needed, morphine (0.1–0.2 mg/kg IV) or fentanyl is a suitable choice; however, narcotics or long-acting sedatives are usually avoided during the last 1–2 hours of the case, to facilitate neurologic examination in the recovery room and prevent prolonged obtundation postoperatively. Low doses (< 0.5 MAC) of an inhalational anesthetic (generally isoflurane) help to control hypertension and prevent awareness; a vasodilator (sodium nitroprusside, trimethaphan) is an acceptable treatment alternative if amnesia and analgesia have already been provided.

   b. Hyperventilation is continued to minimize cerebral blood volume; $PaCO_2$ should be maintained in the 25–30 mm Hg range.

   c. Mannitol (0.5–1.5 gm/kg in a 20% solution) is administered IV over 30 minutes before the craniotomy is completed. Mannitol initially increases intravascular volume, so in patients prone to congestive heart failure, furosemide (10–20 mg IV) may be substituted.

3. Emergence should occur promptly and without coughing or straining. Lidocaine (1.5 mg/kg IV) suppresses cough reflex and may be helpful prior to extubation. Hypertension must also be controlled to minimize bleeding; rapidly-acting IV agents such as sodium nitroprusside or hydralazine are good choices.

E. Perioperative fluid management. The overall objectives are to decrease brain water content, optimize surgical conditions, and reduce ICP, while maintaining cardiovascular stability and CPP.

   1. The **blood-brain barrier** is selectively permeable, so gradients will develop for various substances between blood and brain. Such gradients for osmotically active substances ultimately determine the distribution of fluids between the brain extracellular and intravascular spaces.

   a. Water freely passes through the blood-brain barrier and moves from areas of low to areas of high osmotic pressure. Intravascular infusion of free water will thus increase brain water content and may elevate ICP. Isoosmotic glucose solutions (e.g., 5% D/W) have the same effect, since the glucose is metabolized and free water remains.

   b. Large, polar substances cross the blood-brain barrier poorly. Albumin has little effect on brain extracellular fluid (ECF) content but may increase ICP if given rapidly (perhaps by increasing intravascular volume or CBF). The efficacy of mannitol depends on an intact blood-brain barrier limiting its access to the brain. Thus, mannitol increases intravascular osmolality relative to that of brain ECF and decreases cerebral water content.

   c. If the blood-brain barrier is disrupted (e.g., by hypoxia, head trauma, or tumor), permeability to mannitol, albumin, and saline increases such that these molecules have equal access to brain ECF. From the point of view of minimizing development of cerebral edema, therefore, there seems to be no advantage of albumin over saline therapy in such patients.

   2. Marked hypovolemia can lead to hypotension, a fall in CBF, and cerebral ischemia; hypervolemia may cause hypertension and cerebral edema.

3. **Specific treatment recommendations**
   a. **The fluid deficit** incurred by an overnight fast is usually not replaced, and a significant fluid deficit is tolerated until the dura is "slack" and brain relaxation is adequate. Thereafter, intra-operative urine output is replaced with 2 ml of isotonic crystalloid (preferably 0.9% saline solution) per 3 ml of urine. If signs of hypovolemia develop, additional fluid is administered.
      (1) Patients with infiltrating malignant tumors are particularly prone to postoperative brain swelling and usually receive even less fluid.
      (2) After a cerebral aneurysm is clipped, patients should receive enough fluid (saline, albumin, or blood) to achieve a mildly positive fluid balance, in order to reduce the likelihood of postoperative vasospasm.
   b. **Blood replacement** is guided by hematocrit; the criteria for transfusion are generally similar to those for other types of surgery.
   c. Serum sodium, potassium, glucose, and osmolality are measured about every 2 hours.
      (1) **Hypokalemia** may develop from the use of potassium-wasting diuretics and is exacerbated by hyperventilation.
      (2) **Hyperglycemia** has been shown in animals to exaggerate neurologic deficits after incomplete cerebral ischemia. However, it has not been established that hyperglycemia is detrimental in humans nor has some critical level of plasma glucose been determined. Thus hyperglycemia should not be treated aggressively intraoperatively solely to reduce neurologic risk. Nevertheless, it seems prudent to avoid using dextrose-containing IV solutions in patients at risk for CNS ischemia.
      (3) Marked **hyperosmolality** (> 325 mOsm/L) may produce obtundation or even seizures postoperatively and should be treated with judicious infusion of a hypotonic solution (e.g., 0.25% saline or 5% D/W).

F. **Immediate postoperative care.** Following craniotomy, close patient observation in an intensive care setting is required to detect and treat complications promptly. The general routine to be followed upon arrival in the **recovery room** is described in Chap. 29; the specific features of recovery room care following craniotomy include
   1. Informing the recovery room staff of the patient's preoperative neurologic condition, extent and site of surgery, intraoperative problems, and anticipated postoperative neurologic deficits.

2. **Elevating the head** to 30 degrees to promote venous drainage.

3. Frequent assessment of the level of consciousness, orientation, pupillary size, and motor strength. Deterioration in level of consciousness or focal neurologic signs may indicate development of brain swelling or hematoma; oculomotor (third cranial) nerve dysfunction (evidenced by a unilaterally dilated pupil) heralds transtentorial herniation. In contrast, respiratory arrest is often the first sign of a hematoma in the posterior fossa.

4. **Hypotension** impairs cerebral perfusion pressure and should be treated by leg elevation, fluid administration, or vasoconstrictors. **Hypertension** may increase intracranial bleeding or aggravate edema and should be controlled.

5. Adequate ventilation, oxygenation, and respiratory toilet are particularly important in patients with reduced level of consciousness. Coughing and deep breathing are encouraged; in somnolent patients, aggressive chest physical therapy helps prevent pulmonary complications.

6. **Intracranial pressure** should be monitored if the dura is tight at the time of closure or if signs of intracranial hypertension develop. Either a subarachnoid bolt or an intraventricular catheter may be installed by the neurosurgeon.

7. **Serum electrolytes** should be measured frequently, since hyponatremia, hypokalemia, and marked shifts in serum osmolality may be encountered in the postoperative period from syndromes such as inappropriate antidiuretic hormone secretion or diabetes insipidus.

8. **Seizures** may occur but are best prevented by prophylactic treatment with phenytoin. If a seizure occurs, adequate oxygenation and ventilation must be assured. Diazepam (5–20 mg IV, for adults) is usually effective acutely, and phenytoin (1.5 mg/kg IV over 20 minutes followed by 300–500 mg/day, PO or IV for adults) prevents recurrence.

9. **Diabetes insipidus** may occur after any intracranial procedure but is most common after pituitary surgery. Polyuria is associated with hypernatremia, serum hyperosmolality, and urine hypoosmolality. Treatment is not essential in conscious patients who can compensate by increasing their fluid intake; otherwise strict IV replacement is mandatory. Vasopressin (5–10 USP U SQ) will decrease urine output and maintain serum osmolality; doses are repeated as needed, based on relevant laboratory measurements.

10. **Tension pneumocephalus** may occur after intracranial operations and should be suspected after failure to awaken from anesthesia. Skull x-rays confirm the diagnosis; treatment consists in opening the dura to release the air.

IV. Specific procedures

A. Patients with an **intracranial aneurysm** or **arterio-venous (AV) malformation** may present for surgery either electively (some time after an initial bleed) or acutely following a subarachnoid hemorrhage. Patients requiring immediate surgery (e.g., to evacuate a hematoma) may have markedly elevated ICP; the management principles were discussed in sec. **III.** In particular, blood pressure must be meticulously controlled because hypertension can precipitate bleeding or rebleeding, and hypotension can cause infarction in patients with vasospasm.

   1. The optimal timing of surgery after subarachnoid hemorrhage is controversial. Early surgery (< 48 hours after hemorrhage) can be associated with suboptimal surgical conditions but may reduce the incidence of major complications such as rebleeding and vasospasm, which are most common 1–4 and 5–9 days after hemorrhage, respectively. Delaying surgery provides time for swelling to subside and the aneurysm to "firm" but involves the risks of prolonged bed rest (pulmonary embolism, pneumonia) and increases the chances of rebleeding or vasospasm. At the Massachusetts General Hospital, the neurosurgeons prefer to operate early if the patient is neurologically intact and stable after the initial episode of hemorrhage.

   2. The presurgical treatment of aneurysm patients is designed to reduce the risk of (re)bleeding and prevent vasospasm. The regimen includes sedatives, bed rest, antifibrinolytics and volume expansion, as well as pressors to produce moderate hypertension (or vasodilators to treat severe hypertension). The ramifications of such measures include occult atelectasis or pneumonia, incipient congestive heart failure, thrombophlebitis, and electrolyte abnormalities.

   3. Premedication should not obscure signs of coincidental neurologic deterioration. However, some sedation is advisable to prevent anxiety and hypertension.

   4. The specific anesthetic goals are

      a. To avoid hypertension, which can precipitate rebleeding, using narcotics, hypotensive agents (e.g., sodium nitroprusside, nitroglycerin) or deeper anesthesia with a volatile anesthetic.

      b. To provide a "slack" brain, thereby optimizing surgical conditions. However, since interventions that lower ICP (e.g., hyperventilation, diuresis) might also reduce the tamponade effect of the hematoma and precipitate hemorrhage, these agents should not be started until about 30–45 minutes prior to opening the dura.

      c. To prevent increases in ICP.

      d. To avoid hypotension if vasospasm is present.

   5. Controlled hypotension may be indicated to decrease transmural pressure across the aneurysm and reduce the risk of rupture. A MAP of 50–60 mm Hg is acceptable in healthy patients but may not be tolerated by patients with cerebral or cardiovascular disease (see Chap. 16).

    6. Intraoperative aneurysm rupture or AV malformation hemorrhage can produce rapid and massive blood loss. To facilitate definitive treatment (surgical control), hypotension or, occasionally, manual pressure on the ipsilateral carotid artery in the neck may be helpful. These patients are already volume depleted and may be extremely sensitive to hypotensive agents.

B. Posterior fossa surgery may be complicated by problems related to patient positioning or the proximity of surgery to cranial nerves and brainstem structures regulating respiratory and cardiovascular function.

    1. Tumors of the posterior fossa may cause cranial nerve abnormalities, cerebellar dysfunction, and hydrocephalus due to obstruction of the fourth ventricle. For example, tumors or surgery around the glossopharyngeal and vagus nerves (ninth and tenth cranial nerves) may cause dysphagia, which increases the risk of aspiration; resection of tumors in the floor of the fourth ventricle may damage respiratory centers and necessitate mechanical ventilation postoperatively.

    2. Cardiovascular instability resulting from surgical manipulation is common. Sudden severe bradycardia and hypertension occur if the trigeminal (fifth cranial) nerve is stimulated, while bradycardia and hypotension may follow stimulation of the ninth or tenth cranial nerve. The surgeon should be notified immediately so that permanent damage is avoided. Treatment, other than cessation of the stimulus, is usually unnecessary.

    3. In some cases, partial lateral or prone position may be substituted for the sitting position; air embolism and hypotension in these positions occur less frequently than with the latter.

        a. The mechanism of venous air embolism in the sitting position involves the development of subatmospheric pressure in dural venous sinuses at the surgical site when tethered open by supporting tissues because the dural venous sinuses are well above the level of the heart. Entrained air follows the pressure gradient and embolizes to the right atrium and pulmonary vasculature. Arterial embolization may occur through a patent foramen ovale.

        b. Monitoring for venous air embolism includes precordial Doppler ultrasound, capnography (preferably with trend recording), pulmonary artery pressure, mass spectroscopy, and cardiac echo, although the latter two modalities are not generally available. A "mill-wheel" murmur heard with an esophageal stethoscope is a classic but late sign of massive air embolism.

(1) The Doppler probe is placed at the right sternal border in the third to sixth intercostal spaces. Proper positioning is confirmed when injection of 10 ml of saline through the CVP catheter produces a "roaring" sound. The Doppler is very sensitive and can detect even clinically insignificant amounts of air.

(2) Air embolism is evident on capnography as a decrease in end-tidal carbon dioxide due to increased dead-space ventilation. Trend monitoring is useful to detect the often insidious, continuous entrainment of small volumes of air.

(3) The optimal position for the tip of the right atrial catheter is probably the mid–right atrium, but a multiorificed catheter will cover a larger area and may be preferable. Proper positioning is confirmed by chest x-ray, pressure tracings (i.e., advancing into the right ventricle and then withdrawing slightly to a right atrium trace), or by a "catheter ECG" (the saline-filled catheter functions as lead II; a biphasic intraatrial P wave is sought).

c. Successful **treatment of venous air embolism** depends on early recognition. Bubbles as small as 0.5 ml may be detected by Doppler and warn of the potential for larger, hemodynamically significant emboli. Other characteristic changes (in order of decreasing sensitivity) include a decrease in end-tidal carbon dioxide, an increase in pulmonary artery pressures, a millwheel murmur heard through the esophageal stethoscope, and finally, cardiovascular collapse. When air embolism is suspected, the surgeon must be notified immediately; the operative field is flooded with saline, and potential sites of air entrainment are sought. Because of its ability to enlarge air bubbles, N_2O must be discontinued immediately (N_2O may be avoided in sitting-position cases by maintaining anesthesia with a volatile anesthetic). The right atrial line is aspirated continuously; elevation of intrathoracic pressure (in an effort to decrease air entrainment) is avoided as it decreases venous return and cardiac output. If cardiovascular instability is severe, the operative site is lowered to the level of the heart, and pressors and closed-chest cardiopulmonary resuscitation are used as needed.

C. **Carotid endarterectomy** is performed to prevent stroke in patients with stenotic or ulcerative lesions of the extracranial portions of the carotid arteries. As with other vascular surgical patients (see Chap. 18), atherosclerotic disease in the vasculature to other vital organs (including the heart) is often present. In general, the goals of anesthesia are to maintain a favorable myocardial oxygen supply/demand balance (since the risk of myocardial infarction during carotid endarterectomy is substantial), assure an adequate CPP, and have a conscious patient who can cooperate for a neurologic examination postoperatively.

1. **Preoperative assessment** should focus on the organs affected most by atherosclerosis: the brain, heart, and kidneys.

   a. Preexisting neurologic deficits should be documented so as to distinguish new deficits.

   b. The normal ranges of blood pressure and heart rate for each individual should be defined and asymmetries in blood pressure between arms should be identified.

   c. Diabetes mellitus, hypertension, chronic obstructive pulmonary disease, and chronic renal failure must be optimally controlled prior to elective surgery.

2. **Premedication**

   a. Heavy sedation may prolong emergence from anesthesia; diazepam (0.15 mg/kg PO) is usually adequate.

   b. Antianginal and other related medications may be continued until the time of surgery (see Chap. 2).

3. **Specific monitoring**

   a. The EEG (see sec. **II.A**) is used to assess the effects of altered CPP during carotid clamping. If the EEG suggests that distal perfusion is inadequate and MAP is normal or high, the surgeon may install a shunt to divert blood to the distal carotid. Shunting, however, can dislodge emboli and consequently is not used in every case.

   b. "Stump" pressure (e.g., the internal carotid artery pressure measured distal to the clamp) depends on collateral flow through the circle of Willis but does not reliably predict the adequacy of cerebral perfusion.

   c. Regional CBF can be measured by Xenon 133 clearance after carotid arterial injection, but this technique is available at few institutions.

4. **Anesthetic management**

   a. **Regional anesthesia** (cervical plexus block) allows for continuous neurologic assessment during carotid artery clamping. Development of deficits may be detected without delay and are almost always reversed by unclamping the carotid artery or by placing a shunt.

   b. However, **general anesthesia** is preferred by many surgeons and offers the advantages of patient comfort, control of ventilation and oxygenation, and reduced cerebral metabolic demand.

  (1) Balanced anesthesia (N_2O-narcotic-relaxant) produces a "light" EEG, predominantly fast activity, which makes ischemia-induced EEG slowing easier to detect. However, blood pressure lability often requires treatment with a vasodilator or volatile anesthetic.

  (2) High concentrations of potent inhalation agents slow the EEG and may confound the effects of ischemia. In addition, emergence may be prolonged, delaying postoperative neurologic assessment.

D. Transsphenoidal resections of the pituitary gland, through either nasal or labial incisions, obviate the need for frontal craniotomy. However, this approach is reserved for small tumors that have little or no suprasellar extension and do not influence intracranial pressure dynamics.

  1. Although nonfunctioning pituitary adenomas are the most common tumor type, some patients have endocrine deficiencies due to hypothalamopituitary compression. Various hyperpituitarism syndromes may accompany a functioning adenoma (see Chap. 6).

  2. Access to the patient's head is obstructed by the operating microscope, so the endotracheal tube must be firmly secured. Continuous monitoring of ventilation (e.g., esophageal stethoscope, end-tidal carbon dioxide) is essential.

  3. Insertion of a throat pack will prevent blood from accumulating in the stomach and may reduce postoperative vomiting; it must be remembered to remove the pack prior to extubation.

  4. Cocaine 4%, or a dilute epinephrine-containing local anesthetic solution, is applied to the nasal mucosa to decrease bleeding during dissection near the nasal septum. In this setting, halothane may predispose to ventricular ectopy.

  5. At the conclusion of surgery, nasal breathing will be obstructed by packs and drip pads. Therefore, the patient must be conscious and the pharynx suctioned well before the endotracheal tube is removed.

  6. **Diabetes insipidus** may occur after transsphenoidal hypophysectomy. Diabetes insipidus may develop intraoperatively but more often begins 24–48 hours after surgery when patients are able to self-regulate fluid intake. Treatment with IV fluids or vasopressin may be necessary (see sec. **III.F.i** and Chap. 6).

E. Surgery on the spinal column is undertaken for a variety of conditions, including intervertebral disk disease, spondylosis, traumatic injury, scoliosis, and tumors. The major issues include patient positioning and the specific location and duration of pathology.

1. **The prone position** is frequently used. Most patients can be anesthetized on a stretcher and "log-rolled" onto the operating room table after endotracheal intubation. Awake intubations should be considered for patients with tenuous neurologic conditions that could be worsened by the transfer (e.g., patients with unstable cervical or thoracic spine injuries). Awake intubation may be prudent in patients with symptomatic cervical spine disease, a "tight" cervical spinal canal, or morbid obesity. An abbreviated neurologic examination of deep tendon and withdrawal reflexes and motor function should be performed after intubation and transfer to ensure that injury has not occurred.

2. Surgery is occasionally performed after **acute spinal cord injury** for decompression and stabilization of the spinal cord. Hypotension and cardiovascular instability occur during the period of "spinal shock" and may aggravate the neurologic injury; pressors and/or fluids are used to maintain reasonable spinal cord perfusion.

3. Problems associated with chronic spinal cord injuries are discussed in Chap. 26.

4. Evoked potentials may be monitored intraoperatively in an effort to detect surgical damage to the spinal cord (see sec. **II.B**).

F. **Stereotactic surgery** is performed through a burr hole, using a three-dimensional reference grid attached to the head with pins placed in the outer table of the skull. This approach allows localization of a discrete area of brain for biopsy or ablation (by cryoprobe, proton beam, or radiofrequency). In most cases, the procedure can be performed under local anesthesia with IV sedation. Since the stereotactic apparatus precludes full access to the airway, sedation must be given with extreme caution. Should general anesthesia become necessary, awake oral, nasal, or fiberoptic intubation (see Chap. 10) may be indicated if the stereotactic frame interferes with the mask airway.

G. Anesthesiologists may be asked to consult on patients with head trauma, stroke, or tumor who need **endotracheal intubation,** hyperventilation, and other treatments aimed at decreasing ICP. With head trauma, it is important to ascertain the mechanism and extent of injury. Cervical spinal cord injury must be suspected and the neck stabilized until cervical vertebral fracture is ruled out by lateral neck x-rays (which must include C7–T1).

1. Patients who are responsive and ventilating adequately should receive **supplemental oxygen** and be observed closely for evidence of neurologic deterioration.

2. Comatose patients require immediate endotracheal intubation for **airway protection.** In addition, hy-

percarbia and hypoxia must be corrected, since these can exacerbate increases in ICP and contribute to secondary brain injury.

3. If **endotracheal intubation** is necessary, it should be accomplished rapidly (assuming a full stomach), with minimal blood pressure lability, and without coughing or straining. If a cervical spine fracture has not been ruled out, it is safest to assume instability and have an assistant (preferably the neurosurgeon) maintain axial traction on the neck. If intubation following smooth induction of general anesthesia and neuromuscular blockade is chosen, flexion or extension of the neck is scrupulously avoided. The remainder of the "rapid sequence" intubation routine is described in Chap. 10.

   a. **Facial fractures** limit the ability to open the mouth, and severe facial swelling may make intubation impossible. In these situations, emergency tracheostomy may be indicated.

   b. **Blind nasal intubation** may produce coughing, straining, and hypertension (which increases ICP) in uncooperative or combative patients. In addition, nasal intubation is contraindicated in patients with clinical or radiographic evidence of a basilar skull fracture (e.g., CSF rhinorrhea), since the endotracheal tube could further traumatize the cranial vault.

   c. A **short-acting induction agent** such as methohexital (1–3 mg/kg IV), thiopental (2–4 mg/kg), or etomidate (0.3–0.4 mg/kg) is used to induce anesthesia; lidocaine (1.5 mg/kg IV) may also be helpful. A **muscle relaxant** with rapid onset and short duration is preferable; vecuronium (0.15 mg/kg) satisfies both of these conditions, while pancuronium (0.1–0.2 mg/kg) will produce much longer neuromuscular blockade. Since succinylcholine may elevate ICP in some patients, its use in this setting is controversial.

4. After induction, **hyperventilation** should proceed while an assistant maintains cricoid pressure until intubation is accomplished.

5. Additional **narcotics or sedatives** should be limited so as to promote postoperative neurological evaluation, and muscle relaxants should be monitored.

H. Anesthesia for **electroconvulsive therapy** (ECT) must be brief, produce amnesia, minimize undesirable effects of convulsions (e.g., intense muscle contractions and autonomic stimulation), and not inhibit the cerebral seizure activity thought to be essential for ECT's efficacy.

   1. **Preoperative evaluation.** Since ECT involves general anesthesia, medical problems such as recent myocardial infarction, cerebral aneurysm, or intracranial mass lesion are contraindications to its

use. Also, the presence of long-bone or vertebral fractures, or possible severe osteoporosis, is a relative contraindication, since convulsions may exacerbate skeletal trauma. Although antipsychotic agents may compound the sedating properties of anesthetics, they are frequently necessary and are usually not discontinued prior to ECT. Monoamine oxidase inhibitors, however, predispose to hemodynamic instability—hypertensive crisis as well as occasional hypotensions. In addition lithium may prolong the action of succinylcholine.

2. **Premedication** is unnecessary, but an anticholinergic drug may be used to decrease airway secretions.

3. **Anesthetic management**
   a. The minimum monitoring standards (see Chap. 8) apply to anesthesia for ECT. Typically, a small IV is inserted on the morning of ECT, but it is removed soon after recovery.
   b. Methohexital (0.75–1.0 mg/kg IV) is the usual induction agent, since its redistribution is more rapid than that of thiopental, thus decreasing recovery time (see Chap. 10); etomidate (0.3–0.4 mg/kg IV) may be a suitable alternative.
   c. If ventilation by mask is adequate, succinylcholine (1 mg/kg IV) is then administered. A tourniquet previously applied to one arm and inflated to occlude arterial flow prevents succinylcholine from reaching that arm and allows the ECT-induced seizure activity to be visualized.
   d. While an electrical charge is then applied to the head, contact with the patient and stretcher is avoided. Ventilation continues by mask with 100% oxygen; an oral airway is inserted to prevent tongue and tooth damage.
   e. Severe hypertension occasionally ensues; appropriate treatment with short-acting IV agents is indicated for patients intolerant of cardiovascular stresses.
   f. Following ECT, mask ventilation is resumed until spontaneous recovery occurs. Patients are then placed in the lateral position and recovered in the manner appropriate after general anesthesia.

Suggested Reading

Donegan, J. H. Anesthesia for Carotid Surgery. In R. D. Miller (ed.), *Anesthesia*. New York: Churchill Livingstone, 1986.

Grundy, B. L. Intraoperative monitoring of sensory-evoked potentials. *Anesthesiology* 58:72, 1983.

Messick, J. M., et al. Principles of neuroanesthesia for the non-neurosurgical patient with CNS pathophysiology. *Anesth. Analg.* 64:143, 1985.

Newfield, P., and Cottrell, J. E. (eds.). *Handbook of Neuroanesthesia: Clinical and Physiologic Essentials*. Boston: Mosby, 1983.

Shapiro, H. M. Anesthesia Effects on Cerebral Blood Flow, Cerebral Metabolism, Electroencephalogram, and Evoked Potentials. In R. D. Miller (ed.), *Anesthesia*. New York: Churchill Livingstone, 1986.

Shapiro, H. M. Neurosurgical Anesthesia and Intracranial Hypertension. In R. D. Miller (ed.), *Anesthesia*. New York: Churchill Livingstone, 1986.

Smith, D. S. Fluid management of the neurosurgical patient. In *ASA Refresher Course Lectures*. Park Ridge, Ill.: American Society of Anesthesiologists, 1986. P. 122.

23

Anesthesia for Pediatric Surgery

Susan L. Streitz

I. **Anatomy and physiology.** Understanding the physiologic and anatomic differences between adults and children is the key to safe administration of anesthesia to the pediatric age group.

A. **Upper airway**

1. Infants are **obligate nasal breathers** until age 3–5 months. Twenty-five percent of the work of breathing is needed to overcome the resistance of the nasal passages. Occlusion of the nares by secretions, bilateral choanal atresia, or lymphoid tissue can cause complete airway obstruction. In such cases, simply placing an oral airway will establish airway patency.

2. The relatively large size of the **tongue** can easily obstruct the airway and makes laryngoscopy more difficult.

3. Deciduous **teeth** start to erupt at about 6 months of age and begin shedding from ages 6–8 years. Loose teeth should be noted, since they can become dislodged and aspirated during airway manipulations.

4. The **epiglottis** of a child is narrower, longer, and angled away from the axis of the trachea, making it more difficult to lift during intubation.

5. In children, the **larynx** is located more cephalad and anterior (C3–C4) than it is in adults (C4–C5).

6. The narrowest portion of a child's trachea is subglottic (at the level of cricoid cartilage), not at the glottis as in adults. Therefore, an oversized endotracheal tube can pass through the vocal cords only to meet obstruction distally.

7. The length of the **trachea** (vocal cords to carina) in neonates and children up to 1 year of age is 5–9 cm.

8. Resistance to airflow varies inversely with the radius to the fourth power (Poiseuille's law), so that small decreases in airway size (i.e., edema from inflammation or trauma) will result in a *large* increase in resistance.

B. **Respiratory system**

1. Absolute values for the **tidal volume** (V_T) and **dead space** (V_D) in infants are very small, approximately 15 ml and 5 ml, respectively. Therefore, the increase in V_D from masks and circuit tubing is significant. Newborns under anesthesia must always be managed with controlled ventilation.

2. The small **functional residual capacity** (FRC) in neonates results in more rapid inductions with inhaled anesthetics. The presence of **anatomic shunts** (e.g., patent ductus arteriosus) leads to $\dot{V}A/\dot{Q}$ abnormalities. Both contribute to the rapid onset of hypoxia during periods of apnea.

3. The neonate's <u>increased **closing volume**</u> and decreased FRC make them particularly prone to atelectasis and hypoxia during anesthesia.

4. Newborns have <u>fewer type I muscle fibers in the **diaphragm,**</u> which support prolonged repetitive efforts; therefore, fatigue begins earlier after the work of breathing is increased.

5. Infants who are premature, asphyxiated, stressed by cold or sepsis, or have central nervous system (CNS) damage can manifest immature **respiratory control,** leading to an increased incidence of postanesthetic apnea.

6. Neonates have high metabolic rates, which elevate oxygen (O_2) consumption and carbon dioxide (CO_2) production. <u>Resting oxygen consumption in healthy infants is 7 ml/kg/min, which is twice that of an adult.</u> A newborn's metabolic rate may increase several fold from cardiorespiratory disease, fever, exposure to cold, and light anesthesia; the greater metabolic needs must then be met by an increase in minute ventilation ($\dot{V}E$) per kilogram.

7. The age-dependence of typical respiratory parameters in neonates, infants, and children is presented in Table 23-1.

C. **Cardiovascular system**

1. <u>**Cardiac output** is 180–240 ml/kg/min in newborns, which is two to three times that in adults.</u> The relatively high cardiac output is necessary to meet the high metabolic demands.

2. The **cardiac ventricles** are noncompliant and have a relatively smaller muscle mass in newborns and infants; therefore, there is minimal compensatory reserve. <u>Increases in cardiac output are accomplished largely by increasing heart rate.</u> Bradycardia is the most deleterious arrhythmia in infants, resulting in direct, proportional decreases in cardiac output.

3. **Heart rate** and **blood pressure** vary with age (Table 23-2).

D. **Fluid and electrolyte balance**

1. The **glomerular filtration rate** (GFR) at birth is <u>15–30% of normal adult values.</u> Adult values are reached by age 1 year.

2. Newborns tolerate water or salt loads poorly because of low GFR and decreased **concentrating ability.**

3. The **total body water** (TBW) in the preterm infant is 90% of body weight. In term infants, it is 80%; at 6–12 months, it is 60%. This increased percentage of TBW affects drug volumes of distribution and therefore the dosages of some drugs (e.g., thiopental, pancuronium) are 20–30% greater than the equally effective dose for adults.

4. **Hypocalcemia** is common in infants who are <u>preterm,</u> small for gestational age, asphyxiated, offspring of diabetic mothers or who have received

Table 23-1. Age-dependence of typical respiratory parameters

Variable	Newborn	1 Year	3 Years	5 Years	Adult
Respiratory rate (breaths/min)	40–60	20–30	Gradual decrease to	18–25	12–20
Tidal volume (ml)	15	80	110	250	500
Minute ventilation (L/min)	1	1.8	2.5	5.5	6.5
V_D/V_T	0.3	Gradual decrease to →			
Functional residual capacity (ml)	80	Gradual increase to →			3000
Closing volume as a % of vital capacity	55			20	4
Hematocrit (%)	47–60	33–42			40–50
Arterial pH	7.30–7.40	7.35–7.45			→
$PaCO_2$ (mm Hg)	30–35	30–40			→
PaO_2 (mm Hg)	60–90	80–100			→

Table 23-2. Cardiovascular variables

Age	Heart rate (beats/min)	Blood pressure (mm Hg)	
		Systolic	Diastolic
Preterm neonate	120–180	45–60	30
Term neonate	100–180	55–70	40
1 year	100–140	70–100	60
3 years	85–115	75–110	70
5 years	80–100	80–120	70

transfusions with citrated blood or fresh-frozen plasma. Serum calcium (Ca^{2+}) concentration should be monitored and $CaCl_2$ administered if the ionized Ca^{2+} is less than 1.0 mmol/L (see Chap. 30).

E. **Hematologic system**
  1. The **blood volume** in preterm infants is 90–100 ml/kg; it is 80 ml/kg at term.
  2. Normal values for **hematocrit** are listed in Table 23-1. The nadir of physiologic anemia is at 3 months of age and may reach as low as 28% in an otherwise healthy infant.
  3. At birth, **fetal hemoglobin** (HbF) is predominant but is largely replaced with the adult type by 3–4 months. Fetal hemoglobin has a higher affinity for O_2 (left shift of O_2/Hb dissociation curve), but this does not produce any clinically significant problems under normal circumstances.
F. **Liver**
  1. Newborns have fewer selective hepatic mechanisms with which to metabolize drugs.
  2. Jaundice, which is common in neonates, can be physiologic or have pathologic causes. Hyperbilirubinemia and displacement of bilirubin from albumin by drugs can result in **kernicterus.** Premature infants develop kernicterus at lower levels of bilirubin than do those at term.
G. **Endocrine system**
  1. Newborns, particularly prematures, have decreased glycogen stores and thus are more susceptible to hypoglycemia.
  2. Infants of diabetic mothers are also prone to **hypoglycemia.**
H. **Gastrointestinal system.** Infants often have incompetent lower esophageal sphincters, leading to gastroesophageal reflux and pulmonary aspiration. Such episodes can present as apnea and bradycardia during feedings.
I. **Temperature regulation**
  1. Compared to adults, infants and children have a **greater surface area to body weight ratio.** This results in greater losses of body heat by radiation, evaporation, convection, and conduction.

2. Infants less than 3 months old **cannot compensate** for cold by shivering.
3. Infants respond to **cold stress** by increasing norepinephrine production, which enhances metabolism of brown fat. While increasing body heat production, norepinephrine also produces pulmonary and peripheral vasoconstriction. If profound, right-to-left shunting, hypoxia, and metabolic acidosis can result. Sick and preterm infants have limited stores of brown fat and therefore are more susceptible to cold. Strategies to prevent cold stress include warming the operating room (OR), keeping infants covered with a blanket *and* hat, and using both heating blankets and overhead radiant heaters.

II. **The preanesthetic visit.** General principles of the preanesthetic visit are discussed in Chap. 1. Specific concerns include the following:

A. **History**
 1. Gestational age and weight.
 2. Events during labor and delivery including APGAR scores.
 3. Neonatal hospitalizations.
 4. Congenital anatomic or metabolic anomalies or syndromes.
 5. Recent upper respiratory infections, croup, or asthmatic episodes.

B. **Physical examination**
 1. **General appearance.** Toxic or critically ill children may appear "floppy" preoperatively.
 2. Baseline **vital signs.**
 3. **Weight** must be known to calculate appropriate drug dosages and fluid requirements. Note whether the measurement is in pounds or kilograms.
 4. Examine the **upper airway** for signs of a respiratory infection. Acute rhinitis may predispose the child to a stormy induction and bronchospasm as well as postoperative respiratory complications. When elective surgery is planned, it may be prudent to postpone the procedure for 3–4 weeks. Airway irritability persists for 4–6 weeks after an upper respiratory infection.
 5. Potentially **loose teeth** should be identified, as well as congenital anomalies of the mouth or face that might complicate mask ventilation or intubation.

C. **Laboratory data** that are appropriate for the child's illness and proposed surgery should be obtained. However, a hematocrit and urine analysis are routine.

D. **Communicating with the child and parents**
 1. Infants less than 6 months old generally tolerate short periods of separation from parents well and require no premedication.
 2. Children 6 months–5 years cling to their parents and, when feasible, should be sedated prior to the induction of anesthesia (see sec. **III.B**).

Table 23-3. Preoperative orders for oral intake

Age	Hours NPO prior to anesthesia
Prematures and newborns	2
1–6 months	4
6–36 months	6
> 36 months	8

    3. Children older than 6 years are more independent and may be allowed to express their preferences regarding the type (IV versus mask) of induction.
    4. Reassuring the parents is often the best way to relieve a child's anxiety.
    5. It is important to be honest about procedures, including those that will be painful. Any contradiction in what a child is told, and what is actually done, may lead to a breakdown of trust.

III. Preanesthetic orders

A. Oral intake

    1. No milk, formula, or solid foods should be given after midnight.
    2. The last feeding should consist of clear liquids or sugar-water. The child should be awakened and clear liquids offered at a specified time depending on the **required fasting period** (Table 23-3).
    3. If there are scheduling delays, additional clear liquids may be ordered or hydration maintained with IV fluids.

B. Premedication

    1. For children less than 18 months old, premedication is not necessary and, if used, may lead to respiratory depression.
    2. Older children usually only need reassurance. However, for a particularly frightened child, sedation may simplify induction and relieve anxiety. Oral premedication is preferable, since it avoids the trauma of an injection.
        a. Diazepam (0.2–0.3 mg/kg PO) may be given 2 hours prior to surgery.
        b. Barbiturates, such as secobarbital or pentobarbital (2–4 mg/kg IM), may be given 1 hour preoperatively.
        c. Narcotics are seldom indicated in young children because of their respiratory depressant effects. However, in children with congenital heart disease, they are useful to minimize O_2 consumption and cardiovascular stress during induction (see Chap. 20).
    3. Mentally handicapped or hypokinetic children require little or no sedation, while the reciprocal is true in some hyperkinetic children.
    4. Anticholinergics are used to block the vagotonic ef-

fects of succinylcholine and intubation, but are best given IV at the time of induction.

5. In the presence of a hiatal hernia or gastroesophageal reflux, cimetidine, 7.5 mg/kg PO 1.5–2.0 hours prior to surgery, can be used to raise gastric pH and reduce gastric volume.

6. Children on medication for control of chronic systemic illnesses such as asthma, seizures, or hypertension should continue to take these medications preoperatively.

IV. Preparation of the operating room
A. Anesthetic circuit

1. The **semi-closed circuit** normally used in adults cannot be used in infants because
   a. The mask, metal connectors, and large-bore tubing significantly increase V_D.
   b. The inspiratory and expiratory valves increase the work of breathing.
   c. The large volume of the absorber system acts as a reservoir for anesthetic agents.

2. In children 10 kg or less, the nonrebreathing, open circuit solves these problems.
   a. **The Mapleson D circuit,** which we use most often, consists of a corrugated tube with a reservoir bag at one end. Fresh gas enters at the patient's end of the tubing, and the expiratory valve is located near the reservoir bag. The expiratory valve is kept open during spontaneous respiration and partially closed during assisted or controlled ventilation. The **Bain circuit** is a subtype of the Mapleson D. One source for a full discussion and comparison of the Mapleson-type systems is given in Suggested Reading.
   b. Rebreathing is prevented by using fresh gas flows 2.0–2.5 times the V_E to wash out CO_2. (These flows are only guidelines because individual responses vary widely.) **Capnography** is helpful in recognizing rebreathing ($FiCO_2 > 0$) and avoiding excessive hyperventilation.
   c. The fresh gas flow comes directly from either central supply or tanks; both sources supply *cold* and *dry* gases. It is therefore essential to use a **heated humidifier** in the circuit to prevent drying the airway, which causes inspissation of secretions and excessive heat and water losses.
   d. **Reservoir bag volume** should be at least as large as the child's vital capacity, but small enough so that a comfortable squeeze does not overinflate the chest. General guidelines are newborns, 500-ml bag; 1–3 years, 1000-ml bag; and over 3 years, 2000-ml bag.

3. In children 10–12 kg or more, the semi-closed circle–absorber system can be utilized with a smaller reservoir bag and a circuit with small-caliber wire-reinforced tubing.

B. Airway equipment

1. Choose a **mask** with minimum dead space. A clear plastic type is preferred, since it allows observation of the lips (for color) and mouth (for secretions or vomitus).

2. An appropriate size of **oral airway** can be estimated by holding the airway in position next to the child's face. The tip of the oral airway should reach to the angle of the mandible.

3. Laryngoscope

a. A narrow handle is preferred for comfort and dexterity.

b. A straight blade (Miller or Wis-Hipple) is recommended for children less than 2 years old. The smaller flange and long tapered tip of the straight blade provide better visualization of the larynx and manipulation of the epiglottis in the confined spaces of a small oral cavity.

c. Curved blades are generally used for patients over 5 years.

d. **Guidelines for laryngoscope blade sizes:**

Miller 0	neonate and premature
Miller 1	up to 6–8 months
Wis-Hipple 1.5	9 months–2 years
Miller 2	2.5–5.0 years
Macintosh 2	Child over 5 years old

4. Endotracheal tubes

a. Disposable clear-plastic endotracheal tubes are used routinely. Tubes with premolded curves are also available for nasal or oral use when surgery involves the mouth or pharynx.

b. Uncuffed tubes are used for children under ages 6 or 7 years (5.5-mm endotracheal tube). The ideal size will have a leak at 15–20 cm H_2O airway pressure. If the leak is present at less than 10 cm, the endotracheal tube should be changed to the next larger size. At the time of intubation, endotracheal tubes that are one size larger and smaller than the guesstimated size should be available. Special techniques of endotracheal intubation are discussed in sec. **VI.**

c. **Guidelines for endotracheal tube sizes:**

Age	Size (mm internal diameter)
Premature–newborn	2.5–3.0
Full-term newborn–9 months	3.5
12–20 months	4.0
2 years	4.5
Over 2 years	$4.5 + \dfrac{age\ (years)}{4}$
French size	Age (years) + 18
Tube length at mouth (cm)	$10 + \dfrac{age\ (years)}{2}$

C. Temperature control

1. The OR should be warmed to 80–90°F prior to the child's arrival, and a heating blanket placed on the OR table.

2. A servocontrolled radiant warmer will keep infants warm while monitoring is being applied. However, skin temperature should not be allowed to exceed 39°C as measured by a skin thermistor. The servocontrol from a core thermistor should never be used.

3. Gases should be heated and humidified; humidifiers can *actively* warm a child weighing ≤ 10 kg (0.5 m²) and prevents *passive* losses in larger children.

4. Fluids and blood should also be warmed.

D. Monitoring

1. A **precordial or esophageal stethoscope** (12 Fr) should be used at all times.

2. **Electrocardiogram.**

3. **Blood pressure.**

   a. A blood pressure cuff should cover at least two-thirds of the upper arm but not encroach on the axilla or antecubital space. For children less than 2 years old, a Doppler flow probe will provide more reliable blood pressure readings.

   b. Blood pressure can also be obtained by using a pediatric model automated blood pressure device.

4. **Pulse oximeters** are particularly useful because infants and small children desaturate rapidly; they also aid in avoiding hyperoxic complications in prematures.

5. **Capnographs** are helpful when using a nonrebreathing circuit to assure the adequacy of ventilation.

6. **Temperature** should always be monitored because so many factors conspire to produce hypothermia during anesthesia. Axillary temperatures are generally 1°C lower than oral and rectal temperatures.

7. **Urine output** is an excellent reflection of volume status in children. In newborns, 0.5 ml/kg/hr is adequate; for infants over 1 month of age, 1.0 ml/kg/hr usually indicates that renal perfusion is not impaired.

E. Intravenous catheters

1. For children under 40 kg, a control chamber (buret) should be used to prevent inadvertent overhydration.

2. For older children, a pediatric infusion set is used where 60 drops equal 1 ml.

3. The "standard" solution for the healthy child is 5% dextrose in lactated Ringer's solution. Prematures, septic neonates, infants of diabetic mothers, and those on total parenteral nutrition will require additional glucose. Ten percent dextrose solutions can be used in these cases.

4. Extension tubing is used so that injection ports are

not draped out of reach, but drugs should be administered as close to the IV insertion site as possible to avoid the use of excess fluid volumes.

5. Extra care should be taken to purge IV tubing of air, since, in principle, it is possible for infants to shunt right-to-left through a patent foramen ovale. Neonates and children known to have intracardiac shunts should always have air filters in the IV tubing.

V. Induction techniques

A. Infants less than 6–8 months old can be transported to the OR without sedation; anesthesia can then be induced by an inhalation technique (see sec. **V.C**). The vessel-rich parenchymous organs are proportionately larger and the muscle and fat groups smaller in neonates than in adults. This will affect uptake and distribution of inhalational agents (see Chap. 10).

B. **Rectal methohexital** (Brevital) can be used for children 8 months–5 years; older children may be offered the choice between rectal methohexital and an inhalation induction. To administer rectally:

1. Mix a 10% solution (500 mg dissolved in 5 ml of sterile water).

2. Fill a 5-ml syringe, and attach 3–5 cm of a soft plastic tubing (14 Fr tubing fits on the end of a syringe, e.g., the tip of an O_2 catheter).

3. The syringe should be concealed in a towel, reassuring the child that no injection will be given. Older children can be told that it will feel like "taking a temperature."

4. The tubing should be inserted through the external sphincter and advanced approximately 1 inch; the solution is instilled into the lower two-thirds of the rectum so that the methohexital is absorbed into the *systemic* circulation (not the *portal* circulation, which perfuses the upper one-third of the rectum). Administer 25–30 mg/kg followed by 2–3 cc of air to ensure delivery of the full dose. If the child expels the solution, the procedure is repeated from the beginning with the *full* dose.

5. Peak effect usually occurs after 10–15 minutes. If there are no results after 20 minutes, a second full dose is given.

6. An anesthesiologist should remain in attendance after the drug has been administered. Once the child is asleep, inhalation anesthesia may be added.

C. **Inhalation induction**

1. This is the method of choice for most pediatric patients, except when rapid sequence induction is required. In older children, placement of an IV catheter makes IV induction an option.

2. An "excitement stage" of anesthesia is often encountered during inhalation induction. For this reason, stimulation (from noise and activity in the OR) should be minimized during this period.

3. Methods

a. Children 9 months–5 years may be induced after profound sedation with rectal methohexital (called a "steal" induction). Specifically, the face mask is held near, but not touching, the child's face, and low flows (1–3 L) of O_2 and nitrous oxide (N_2O) are begun. Then, the volatile agent (halothane is the least irritating to the airways and is best tolerated) is gradually increased from 0.5–4.0% in 0.5% increments. When the lid reflex disappears, the mask can be applied to the child's face and the jaw gently lifted.

b. Children 6 years–teens (with/without oral sedating premedication) may be induced from the awake state with a "single breath" induction.

   (1) The minimum alveolar concentration of halothane necessary to cause loss of consciousness can be achieved with a single vital capacity breath of 4% halothane in 70% N_2O:O_2.

   (2) The circuit should be prefilled with N_2O-O_2 (3 : 1) and 4–5% halothane. The end of the circuit should be occluded with a plug or another reservoir bag and the pop-off valve left open to minimize nonscavenged anesthetic spillage.

   (3) Painting the mask with flavor extracts will increase acceptance by the children.

   (4) The child is instructed to take a deep breath (vital capacity) of room air, blow it all out (forced expiration), and then hold his/her breath. At this point, the anesthesiologist gently places the mask on the patient's face. Then the child takes a deep inspiration (vital capacity) and again *holds his/her breath*.

   (5) Most children will be asleep in 30–60 seconds; a few children will need more than one breath.

D. Intramuscular induction

1. For the uncooperative or retarded child who is not otherwise controllable, anesthesia may be induced with ketamine (4–10 mg/kg IM), which takes effect in 3–5 minutes. Atropine (0.02 mg/kg IM) should be administered at the same time.

2. Alternatively, methohexital (10 mg/kg IM) may be used.

E. Intravenous induction.
For children over 10 years old, the option of having an IV placed should be offered and anesthesia induced as it is in adults; children may require up to 6 mg/kg of thiopental.

F. Induction of children with full stomachs

1. **Rapid sequence induction.** In general, the same principles apply to infants and children as were dis-

cussed for adults in Chap. 10. In addition:

- **a.** Atropine (0.02 mg/kg, minimum dose 0.1 mg) must be given IV prior to administration of succinylcholine to prevent bradycardia.
- **b.** Children require larger doses of thiopental (4–6 mg/kg) and succinylcholine (2 mg/kg).
- **c.** Infants with gastric distention should have their stomachs decompressed by orogastric tubes placed prior to induction, to minimize the chance of aspiration.
- **d.** Cimetidine (7.5 mg/kg PO or IV) can be used to decrease gastric volume and raise gastric pH.
- **e.** Rapid sequence inductions are usually preferable for vigorous infants, to avoid the risks of traumatizing the airway and gastric distention from air swallowing.

2. **Awake intubations** are often preferable for very sick infants. Those with anatomically abnormal airways also should be intubated awake.

VI. Endotracheal intubation
A. Oral approach

1. Older children are placed in the "sniffing" position using a blanket. Infants and small children have large occiputs, and blankets are often not necessary.
2. The larynx is located during laryngoscopy as in adults, but the tip of the blade is used to elevate the epiglottis.
3. The distance from the glottis to the carina is about 4 cm in a term neonate. Pediatric endotracheal tubes have a single black marking located 2 cm from the tip and a double mark at 3 cm; these markings should be observed as the tube is passed beyond the glottis.
4. The narrowest portion of the trachea is at the cricoid cartilage; therefore, if resistance is met during intubation, the next smaller (by one-half size) tube should be tried.
5. Following intubation, the chest should be examined for bilaterally equal expansion and the lungs auscultated for equal breath sounds. There should be a leak around the uncuffed tube when 15–20 cm H_2O positive-pressure is applied.
6. Flexion of the head can result in extubation, while extension can cause advancement of endotracheal tubes into the right mainstem bronchus. Therefore, the chest should be auscultated to assure the presence of equal breath sounds *every* time an intubated child is repositioned.
7. Endotracheal tubes should be securely taped using benzoin or else by circumferential taping around the head. Once correctly positioned, the numerical marking on the tube closest to the gingiva should be noted; migration of the endotracheal tube will be apparent from any change in this relation.

B. Nasal approach

1. The method for nasotracheal intubation is generally similar to that for adults (see Chap. 10).

2. The anterior position of the infant larynx makes an unaided pass difficult; Magill forceps are almost always needed to guide the tip of the tube through the vocal cords.

3. Nasal intubation should be performed only when specifically indicated (e.g., oral surgery), due to the risk of epistaxis from swollen adenoids and tonsils.

4. Apneic infants will become hypoxic within 30–45 seconds, even after preoxygenation. If bradycardia, cyanosis, or desaturation occurs, intubation attempts should cease immediately and 100% O_2 administered until recovery is complete.

VII. Fluid management. The calculations that follow can be used to estimate fluid requirements for infants and children. Other reflections of volume status, including blood pressure, heart rate, urine output, central venous pressure, and pulmonary artery pressure may suggest that adjustments are needed in individual patients.

A. Maintenance fluid requirements

1. Administer 4 ml/kg/hr for the first 10 kg of body weight (100 ml/kg/day); 2 ml/kg/hr for the second 10 kg (50 ml/kg/day), then add 1 ml/kg/hr for more than 20 kg (25 ml/kg/day) (e.g., maintenance fluids for a 25-kg child: $[4 \times 10 \text{ kg}] + [2 \times 10 \text{ kg}] + [1 \times 5 \text{ kg}] = 65$ ml/hr.)

2. Children may require supplemental glucose to avoid hypoglycemia after hours of fasting. Therefore, initial fluid replacement should be with 5% D/LR. Sick neonates and premature infants may require the use of 10% dextrose solutions; blood sugar levels should be periodically checked with Dextrostix.

B. Estimated blood volume (EBV) and blood losses

1. EBV = 90 ml/kg in neonates
   = 80 ml/kg in infants up to 1 year
   = 70 ml/kg thereafter

2. Estimated red cell mass (ERCM) = EBV × Hct/100

3. Acceptable red cell loss (ARCL) = ERCM − $ERCM_{30}$, which is the ERCM at a hematocrit of 30%.

4. Acceptable blood loss (ABL) = ARCL × 3

   a. If the amount of the blood loss is less than one-third of the ABL, it can be replaced with Ringer's lactate.

   b. If the amount of blood loss is greater than one-third of the total ABL, it should be replaced with colloid, preferably 5% albumin.

   c. If the amount of blood loss is greater than ABL, replace with frozen packed cells and an equal amount of colloid.

C. Estimated fluid deficit (EFD)

EFD = (maintenance fluid/hr)

× (hours since the last oral intake)

The entire EFD is replaced during all major cases; the first half is given during the first hour, and the remaining deficit is divided over the next 1–2 hours.

D. Third-space losses may require up to an additional 10 ml/kg/hr of Ringer's lactate or normal saline if there is extensive exposure of the intestine or a significant ileus.

VIII. Specific pediatric anesthesia problems

A. The compromised airway

1. Airway obstruction may be secondary to
   a. Congenital abnormalities (e.g., choanal atresia, Pierre Robin syndrome, tracheal stenosis, laryngeal web).
   b. Inflammation (e.g., croup, epiglottitis, cervical abscess).
   c. Foreign bodies in the trachea or esophagus.
   d. Neoplasms (e.g., congenital hemangioma, cystic hygroma, thoracic lymphadenopathy).
   e. Trauma.

2. Presenting symptoms include stridor, wheezing, retractions, and tachypnea.

3. **Management principles**
   a. Administer 100% O_2 by mask.
   b. Keep the child as calm as possible. Evaluation should be kept to a minimum, since it may increase agitation and cause further airway compromise. Parents are invaluable in their ability to pacify their children and should remain with them as long as feasible.
   c. An anesthesiologist must be present during transport to the OR. Oxygen, a Hope-type resuscitation bag and mask, laryngoscope, atropine, succinylcholine, and an appropriate sizes of endotracheal tubes must also be available.
   d. **Induction of anesthesia**
      (1) Minimize manipulation of the patient. A precordial stethoscope and pulse oximeter are all the monitoring that is necessary during the initial phase of induction.
      (2) A gradual inhalation induction in a sitting position with the parents present is begun using 100% O_2 and halothane. Airway obstruction with poor air exchange will prolong induction.
      (3) Parents are then asked to leave when the child becomes unconscious, and an IV is started and atropine administered.
      (4) Patients with croup may benefit from gentle application of continuous positive airway pressure (CPAP), but positive-pressure can cause acute airway obstruction in patients with epiglottitis or a large foreign body.
      (5) The oral endotracheal tube chosen should be smaller than the one predicted from the child's age and size.

(6) At this point, patients are usually hypercarbic (end-tidal CO_2 50–60 mm Hg), but it is generally well tolerated provided they are not also hypoxic. <u>Bradycardia is an indication of hypoxia</u> and requires immediate establishment of a patent airway.

(7) Perform laryngoscopy only when the patient is deeply anesthetized. <u>Muscle relaxants are contraindicated, except as a true last resort.</u> Orotracheal intubation should be accomplished before any further airway procedures are attempted, except in cases of large upper airway foreign bodies or friable subglottic tumors (e.g., hemangiomas), when bronchoscopy is indicated prior to intubation.

(8) <u>For illnesses that require several days of intubation (e.g., epiglottitis), a nasal tube may be more comfortable.</u> Orotracheal tubes are changed to nasotracheal tubes at the end of the procedure, provided the oral intubation was easily accomplished.

(9) After airway emergencies, the endotracheal tube should be taped absolutely securely. Children should be sedated for the transport to an intensive care unit (ICU); a combination of morphine and a benzodiazepine is particularly effective. Breathing may be spontaneous or assisted during transportation and in the ICU.

B. Intraabdominal malformations

1. These include <u>pyloric stenosis, gastroschisis, omphalocele,</u> atresia of the small intestine, and volvulus.

2. Whatever the cause, these patients have similar physiologic disturbances, which include hypovolemia, electrolyte abnormalities, sepsis, and often respiratory compromise due to abdominal distension.

3. Management

a. Gastrointestinal emergencies frequently lead to marked <u>dehydration</u> and <u>electrolyte abnormalities</u>. It is always possible to delay pyloric stenosis repair as long as necessary to replenish intravascular volume and correct hypochloremic alkalosis. However, the situation is more urgent with the other lesions, and rehydration may need to be accomplished intraoperatively.

b. Abdominal distention in infants and young children rapidly causes respiratory compromise, so <u>nasogastric drainage is mandatory</u>. Even so, many patients require intubation prior to the induction of anesthesia; awake intubation is often all that is tolerated.

c. Children with less severe physiologic disturbances and only mild or moderate distention can be managed with rapid sequence inductions.

d. In very toxic children, arterial and CVP catheters and a Foley catheter may be necessary to monitor volume status and organ perfusion. Two peripheral IV catheters may be needed for infusion of volume.

e. Anesthetics with minimal cardiac depression and vasodilatation are the safest agents for such cases; oxygen/air mixtures, narcotics, and relaxants are usually better tolerated than the potent inhalation agents. Nitrous oxide should be avoided, since it will add to the abdominal distention.

f. When the bowel is exposed and manipulated, third-space losses may be excessive, and remarkable fluid volumes may be needed to maintain blood pressure. Even when employing all the possible warming strategies, heat loss is usually unavoidable.

g. Postoperative ventilatory support is often indicated until abdominal distention is diminished, body temperature normalizes, and fluid shifting ceases.

C. Thoracic emergencies

1. Tracheoesophageal fistula

a. Tracheoesophageal fistula and esophageal atresia can present in several combinations.

(1) Esophageal atresia with a fistula between the trachea and the distal segment of the esophagus is the most common of these lesions (87–90%). Neonates with this anomaly choke and become cyanotic during their first feeding. The diagnosis is confirmed by the inability to pass a feeding tube into the stomach, and chest x-ray demonstrates the feeding tube curled in the proximal esophageal ("blind") pouch. Air in the stomach and bowel confirms the presence of a fistula.

(2) The H-type fistula without esophageal atresia is the next most common of these lesions. Children usually present somewhat later in life with a history of frequent pulmonary infections.

b. The most common **complication** in all forms of tracheoesophageal fistula is pneumonitis secondary to pulmonary aspiration.

c. Preoperative management

(1) Neonates should be kept NPO when this diagnosis is suspected.

(2) Maintaining the upright position minimizes the chance of gastric reflux and pulmonary aspiration of gastric fluid.

(3) Saliva in the proximal pouch is frequently aspirated. Thus, a nasogastric tube should be placed in the pouch and continuously suctioned.

 (4) Pulmonary complications are present in nearly all patients and should be treated before surgery is scheduled. Surgical intervention is urgent, but not emergent.

 d. Intraoperative management

  (1) Prior to tracheoesophageal fistula repair, a gastrostomy tube may be placed to decompress the stomach, preventing aspiration of gastric fluid and perforation. Frequently this can be accomplished under local anesthesia.

  (2) After gastrostomy, either an awake or rapid sequence intubation is done. Narcotics or inhalation agents may be used as tolerated; muscle relaxants are usually necessary to facilitate access to the abdomen or chest.

  (3) The endotracheal tube should be positioned below the fistula, which usually enters 1–2 cm above the carina. One technique for placement is deliberately to intubate endobronchially, then withdraw until bilateral breath sounds are first heard. In this position, the endotracheal tube will almost always be below the fistula.

  (4) After the fistula is ligated, the esophagus is primarily repaired. However, the gastrostomy is left in situ, since esophageal motility is usually abnormal. Gastroesophageal reflux is commonly encountered postoperatively, ultimately requiring fundoplication in about half these patients.

 e. The postoperative course is usually dominated by the presence of pulmonary complications or associated anomalies.

2. Congenital lobar emphysema

 a. Congenital lobar emphysema is overdistention of a lobe of the lung from obstruction of the bronchus supplying the lobe. The most common location is the left upper lobe.

 b. Obstruction of a bronchus can be extrinsic (e.g., blood vessels), intraluminal (e.g., intrinsic web), or secondary to malformation of the bronchus.

 c. Overdistention of the affected lobe from a "ball-valve effect" results in compression of normal lung tissue and displacement of the mediastinum, producing effects like a tension pneumothorax.

 d. Severe cases present in the neonatal period

with respiratory distress and cyanosis. The mediastinal shift can produce kinking of the great vessels with cardiovascular embarrassment and arrest.

    e. Chest x-ray will demonstrate a hyperlucent area with mediastinal shift.

    f. Anesthetic considerations

        (1) Oxygen (100%) should be administered, but infants should be allowed to _breathe spontaneously_ until the thorax is open. Positive-pressure ventilation may cause further distention of the emphysematous lobe(s).

        (2) _Nitrous oxide is contraindicated,_ since it will cause further overinflation of the affected lobe, magnify mediastinal shift, and lead to cardiovascular collapse.

        (3) A nasogastric tube should be placed and connected to continuous suction to avoid distention of the stomach, which may further compromise ventilation.

        (4) Even with these precautions, some infants will require emergency intubation and decompression of the emphysematous lobe (with a chest tube). This procedure is dangerous and should be reserved for those in whom conservative support measures have failed.

        (5) Anesthesia should consist in 100% O_2, muscle relaxants, narcotics, and inhalation agents if tolerated. If arterial blood gases are satisfactory after the emphysematous lobe is decompressed, air should be mixed with O_2 to prevent "absorption atelectasis."

        (6) Postoperatively, many infants will need ventilatory support, but weaning and extubation are usually accomplished in the first 48–72 hours.

3. _Congenital diaphragmatic hernia_

    a. Pathogenesis. In congenital diaphragmatic hernia, incomplete development of the diaphragm results in herniation of the abdominal contents into the chest. It occurs most commonly on the _left_, through the _foramen of Bochdalek._ Traumatic rupture during delivery is a rare cause.

    b. _The lung tissue on the ipsilateral side will be atelectatic or, if herniation occurred early during fetal development, hypoplastic._ Lung development on the contralateral side may be similarly affected.

    c. Neonates usually present shortly after birth with respiratory distress, cyanosis, a scaphoid abdomen, and a shift in heart sounds toward the contralateral side. Arterial blood gases demonstrate marked hypoxia, hypercarbia, and acidosis (e.g., PaO_2 25–50, $PaCO_2 > 100$, pH 6.8).

d. Chest x-ray reveals bowel gas shadows in the chest, but the clinical picture may be indistinguishable from congenital lobar emphysema.

e. **Pathophysiology**

(1) Mechanical compression of lung tissue.

(2) Abnormal pulmonary parenchymal development with diminished numbers of diffusing surfaces (alveoli).

(3) Right-to-left shunting: In neonates, hypoxemia and acidosis inhibit normal closure of the ductus arteriosus and at the same time cause pulmonary vasoconstriction (pulmonary hypertension). The net result is a return to fetal circulation in which most of the cardiac output bypasses the lungs; this is the cause of the intractable hypoxia associated with congenital diaphragmatic hernia. Severe right-to-left shunting may intermittently appear during surgery and is also the most frequent cause of death in the postoperative period.

f. **Anesthetic considerations**

(1) Congenital diaphragmatic hernia is a true surgical emergency, so little or no preparation or placement of monitoring catheters may be possible. Consequently, pulse oximetry and capnography are invaluable in these cases.

(2) A nasogastric tube should be placed to relieve distention and minimize respiratory compromise.

(3) Positive-pressure ventilation by mask should not be applied, since it can cause inflation of the bowel and precipitate decompensation.

(4) Most of these patients require emergency intubation prior to arrival in the OR. After intubation, ventilation should be controlled using minimal positive pressure to prevent overinflation of the contralateral lung. If there is a sudden deterioration, a pneumothorax of the contralateral side should be suspected.

(5) Nitrous oxide is contraindicated, since it will cause bowel distention.

(6) Initially, 100% O_2 and muscle relaxation may be all that are tolerated until the thorax is decompressed. Afterward, judicious doses of narcotics are desirable, since anesthesia seems to prevent episodic right-to-left shunting. In fact, postoperative management calls for main-

tenance of anesthesia with (high-dose) infusions of narcotics.

(7) Acidosis and hypercarbia must be corrected with hyperventilation and sodium bicarbonate to avoid elevations in pulmonary vascular resistance.

(8) Hypothermia and light anesthesia should be vigorously treated, since they too can precipitate a return to fetal circulation.

g. Postoperative care

(1) These infants have atelectatic and/or hypoplastic lungs and continue to require ventilation postoperatively. When possible, high airway pressures should be avoided.

(2) Due to the frequency of pneumothorax, bilateral chest tubes are frequently placed prophylactically.

(3) Pulmonary artery hypertension persists in 40% of cases. A "preductal" arterial (see Chap. 20) catheter and often a pulmonary arterial catheter are needed for optimal postoperative management.

(4) Prognosis is poor in patients with severely hypoplastic lungs. Despite aggressive therapy, most patients die of intractable hypoxia and acidosis.

D. Congenital heart disease. For relevant physiologic and anesthetic considerations, see Chap. 20 and references cited therein.

Suggested Reading

Dorsch, J., and Dorsch, S. The Breathing System II: The Mapleson Systems. In *Understanding Anesthesia Equipment* (2nd ed.). Baltimore: Williams & Wilkins, 1984. Pp. 182–196.

Gregory, G. (ed.). *Pediatric Anesthesia.* New York: Churchill Livingstone, 1983.

Klaus, M., Fanaroff, A., and Martin, R. The Physical Environment. In M. Klaus and A. Fanaroff (eds.), *Care of the High-Risk Neonate.* Philadelphia: Saunders, 1979. Pp. 94–112.

Klaus, M., Fanaroff, A., and Martin, R. Respiratory Problems. In M. Klaus and A. Fanaroff (eds.), *Care of the High-Risk Neonate.* Philadelphia: Saunders, 1979. Pp. 173–204.

Ryan, J., et al. (eds.). *A Practice of Pediatric Anesthesia.* Orlando, Fla.: Grune & Stratton, 1986.

Wald, M. Problems in Metabolic Adaptation: Glucose, Calcium and Magnesium. In M. Klaus and A. Fanaroff (eds.), *Care of the High-Risk Neonate.* Philadelphia: Saunders, 1979. Pp. 224–242.

24

Anesthesia for Ambulatory Procedures

Paul Alfille

A variety of surgical and diagnostic procedures that require anesthesia can be done without subsequent hospitalization. Advantages include lower costs, reduction in nosocomial infection, less disruption of patients' routines, and in children, less separation anxiety. These benefits may be safely realized as long as the special needs of ambulatory patients are considered.

I. **Milieu.** Whether ambulatory procedures requiring anesthesia are performed in freestanding units or hospital-based facilities, equipment for resuscitation should be readily available. In addition, a mechanism must exist for admitting patients to the hospital should the need for postoperative care arise.

II. **Patient selection**
   A. **The guiding principle** is that patients are expected to return to their preanesthetic level of function soon after the procedure. In addition, pain must be controllable by nonparenteral medications.
   B. Patients requiring **postoperative monitoring,** such as adults with cardiac arrhythmias or premature infants with a history of apneic spells, are more appropriately admitted to the hospital.
   C. Patients with **logistical problems,** such as living alone or far from an emergency medical center, may also need hospitalization.
   D. Besides healthy patients, those with **stable or well-compensated systemic diseases** are often appropriate candidates for ambulatory procedures.
   E. Elective procedures in **pregnant women** are avoided because there is a theoretical risk of teratogenicity with anesthetic agents, as well as an increased incidence of spontaneous abortion associated with, although not necessarily due to, anesthesia.
   F. In a given facility, **criteria for appropriate patient selection and preparation** must be mutually developed by surgeons and anesthesiologists. In certain cases, even physically or mentally handicapped patients need not be excluded from the outpatient operating room as long as there is advanced planning and coordination by both surgeon and anesthesiologist to minimize disruption of the facility.

III. **Procedures**
   A. The **range of procedures** successfully performed on an outpatient basis continues to expand. The following lists some of the more common outpatient procedures; it is not meant to be exhaustive and will vary among institutions.

1. **General surgery.** Breast surgery; hemorrhoidectomy; uncomplicated inguinal, femoral, or umbilical herniorrhaphy; endoscopy of esophagus, stomach, and colon; excision of pilonidal sinus; lipoma excision; esophageal dilatation.
2. **Gynecology.** Dilation and curettage; cone biopsy; examination under anesthesia; laparoscopy for tubal ligation, endometriosis, or infertility.
3. **Ophthalmology.** Cataract extraction, examination under anesthesia, laser treatments.
4. **Oral surgery.** Odontectomy, extractions, reduction and fixation of uncomplicated fractures of the mandible and zygoma.
5. **Orthopedic surgery.** Removal of wires and hardware; release of tendons and nerves; arthroscopy of knee, shoulder, elbow, wrist, and ankle.
6. **Otorhinolaryngology.** Pharyngoscopy, laryngoscopy, turbinectomy, submucuous resection, myringotomy tubes, Caldwell-Luc procedure.
7. **Plastic surgery.** Augmentation mammoplasty, suction lipectomy, carpal tunnel release, excision and biopsy of cutaneous lesions, revision of scars.
8. **Urology.** Cystoscopy, retrograde pyelography, circumcision, vasectomy, hydrocelectomy, varicocelectomy, transurethral bladder biopsy, extracorporeal shock-wave lithotripsy (ESWL).
9. **Radiology.** Painful procedures such as angiography, procedures for young children who are unable to cooperate.

B. The procedures performed should be limited by the **availability of facilities** to handle possible complications.

IV. **Patient preparation**

A. **Prior to the day of surgery,** a history and physical examination must be performed by a physician.

B. An elaborate "routine" laboratory evaluation has not been found to be cost-effective; however, hematocrits are obtained from all patients, as are ECGs from those over 40 years old. Pregnancy tests are not obtained from women of child-bearing age unless the history reveals that pregnancy is likely.

C. For adult patients, specific instructions to remain NPO after midnight are delivered both verbally and in writing, as are instructions regarding chronic medications and the need for a responsible escort postoperatively.

D. If the preoperative history or physical examination suggests a medical problem, the planned procedure is postponed and reevaluated after relevant laboratory studies and consultations are obtained.

E. **Special arrangements** are sometimes required; warfarin (Coumadin) should be discontinued for several days prior to most procedures and a prothrombin time determined on the day of surgery. Diabetics are usually scheduled early in the day and, if they live near the facility, are instructed to take half their usual insulin dose prior to leaving home. They are also instructed to eat if they feel symptoms of hypoglycemia (but in this case, the procedure will be postponed). Diabetics living at a distance are given half their usual insulin dose subcutaneously upon arrival at the ambulatory care center, after a glucose-containing infusion is begun.

V. **The day of surgery.** On arrival, patients undergo

   A. **Reinterview** by an anesthesiologist to investigate any interim changes since their preoperative evaluation (e.g., acute upper respiratory infections [URI], to verify that the patient has followed NPO instructions and arranged for a responsible adult companion to escort them home, to explain the anesthetic procedure, and to obtain informed consent.

      1. A developing URI with cough and fever is cause for postponement of the surgical procedure. Once the URI is in the resolving stage, a patient with otherwise normal respiratory status is felt to be able to tolerate general anesthesia without incurring risks of pulmonary complications.

      2. **Last-minute cancellation** of outpatient surgery is most commonly caused by patients not complying with NPO requirements. It is prudent to ask about oral intake several times during the admitting procedure to be certain that an outpatient has not had any food or other oral intake.

   B. **A physical examination,** including the airway, main organ systems, and the site of a regional technique, if planned.

   C. **IV placement** in patients scheduled for general, regional, or monitored anesthesia care. The IV is useful for repletion of an overnight fluid deficit and administration of drugs if necessary. In small children, the IV may be placed after an induction with rectal methohexital or mask inhalation anesthesia; however, in extremely brief cases (e.g., insertion of myringotomy tubes), an IV may be unnecessary.

   D. **Premedication.** Small doses of short-acting sedating premedicants are useful and have not been found to prolong postanesthetic recovery. Typically, benzodiazepines and narcotics are chosen; relevant doses and guidelines for clinical use are found in Chap. 10.

VI. **Anesthetic management**

   A. **Local anesthesia** by infiltration is often used for relatively superficial procedures such as excision of cutaneous lesions or carpal tunnel releases. In these cases, an IV, sedation, NPO status, recovery period, escort home, and even involvement of an anesthesiologist are usually superfluous. Occasionally, the anesthesiologist will be called to help manage the complications of local anesthetic toxicity or oversedation. More extensive procedures under local anesthesia (e.g., inguinal herniorrhaphy) usually require "monitored anesthesia care," which means that an anesthesiologist is in attendance should IV sedation, general anesthesia, or resuscitation become necessary. These patients require the same workup and considerations as patients receiving regional and general anesthesia.

B. Regional anesthesia usually has the advantage of less postoperative drowsiness and nausea than that seen with general anesthesia but often requires a longer induction period. Commonly, regional techniques are supplemented with IV sedation.

1. **Upper extremity procedures** can be done under IV regional (Bier block), brachial plexus, or peripheral nerve blocks. Intravenous regional blocks are quick in onset and recovery, but their duration is limited by the time the tourniquet can be tolerated. Since the supraclavicular approach to the brachial plexus runs the risks of phrenic nerve block and pneumothorax, the axillary approach is favored. After receiving an axillary, wrist, or elbow block, the patient's arm should be placed in a sling and the patient warned about the risk of inadvertent injury while the limb is still insensate.

2. **Lower extremity procedures** can be performed with specific peripheral nerve blocks. Intravenous regional blocks of the leg are more difficult because of the large volume of local anesthetic required and thus the higher risk of systemic toxicity. Further, discharging a patient who may have residual leg weakness is more of a problem. Spinal and epidural anesthesia can be used as long as there are contingency plans for dealing with complications, including spinal headaches.

3. **Other regional techniques** include intraoral, retrobulbar, and paracervical blocks. These blocks are commonly performed by the surgeon, with monitored anesthesia care.

C. General anesthesia is frequently employed for outpatient procedures. Various techniques have been championed, including balanced, inhalational, and continuous IV infusions. Clearly, agents with short duration due to rapid redistribution or elimination are preferred, but the ideal management for outpatients is a matter of some debate. For example, in one study, fentanyl–nitrous oxide (N_2O)–oxygen (O_2) anesthesia was associated with faster awakening and orientation that was isoflurane, but no differences were found in time to oral intake, ambulation, or discharge. Continuous drug infusions have the theoretical advantage of a more steady plasma drug level, leading to less total drug required and faster awakenings. Indeed, such were the findings made in a study comparing bolus injection and continuous infusion of either fentanyl or alfentanil. Further, alfentanil promoted faster awakening and less respiratory depression than did fentanyl.

1. Typically, for adults, a small dose of fentanyl (25–50 µg IV) plus droperidol (1.25 mg IV) is administered just before thiopental induction, and anesthesia is maintained with an inhalation agent. Succinylcholine or a short-acting nondepolarizing

muscle relaxant is used if necessary. The preoperative dose of narcotic reduces the requirement for the inhalation agent and helps to control postoperative pain.

2. Endotracheal intubation is used as necessary; intubation of infants is discussed in sec. **IX.A.2.**

VII. **Complications.** Just as for inpatients, complications from anesthesia range from minor to life-threatening.

A. **Pulmonary aspiration** is the major threat to patient safety in the outpatient setting. Obese patients and those with symptomatic esophageal reflux are more prone to aspiration. Larger volumes of gastric fluid are also found in smokers and often in very anxious patients. Severe anxiety may also lead to low gastric pH, so these patients are most appropriately treated as if they have a full stomach. Specifically, we begin to reassure these patients even before they have changed their clothes and follow this by treating with oral or IV H_2 blockers.

B. **Postoperative vomiting** is experienced by 10–60% of outpatients; the average is about 30%. Predisposing factors are sex (female), age (young), obesity, and previous history of perioperative vomiting. Narcotics, N_2O, and inflation of the gastrointestinal tract by mask ventilation may also play a role, along with postoperative pain. Routine prophylactic use of antiemetic medications is gaining popularity; we often use droperidol (1.25 mg IV) as part of our anesthetic regimen. Orogastric suctioning is sometimes employed. Patients recovering from anesthesia are prone to vertigo, and therefore transfer to the recovery room is done both slowly and gently.

C. **Myalgias** from succinylcholine-induced fasciculations are relatively common and vary widely in severity. Such muscle cramps are usually, but not always, short-lived, which has led some ambulatory units to substitute short-acting nondepolarizing relaxants when brief periods of relaxation are desired. Pretreatment with small doses of nondepolarizing relaxants may lessen the incidence of myalgias, although this has never been conclusively demonstrated.

D. Avoiding **"minor" complications** is particularly important in the ambulatory setting. Nausea, somnolence, sore throat, myalgias, spinal headaches, and phlebitis are often perceived by patients as more inconvenient, even incapacitating, than the procedure itself.

VIII. **Postanesthetic recovery and discharge.** All patients who receive general anesthesia or significant IV sedation require a postoperative recovery period.

A. As alertness increases, patients are gradually elevated to a sitting position and given **PO fluids.**

B. Once PO fluids are tolerated, the IV can be removed and **solid food** (such as dry or jellied toast) offered.

C. In adults, **pain** may be treated with small doses of fentanyl (12.5–25.0 µg IV every 5 minutes until relief begins), topical ice, or even nonsteroidal anti-inflammatory drugs (see Chap. 33).

D. Patients are **discharged** when an anesthesiologist judges them to be sufficiently "alert" and comfortable. It is clear from psychomotor tests such as driving simulators, light-flicker discrimination, and pencil and paper tasks that memory, judgment, and motor skills are impaired after sedation and general anesthesia. Specifically, **diazepam** causes at least 6–10 hours of psychomotor impairment; **halothane** reduces driving simulator performance below control for at least 5 hours. As expected, impairment after combinations of agents is longer than that after the agents singly. Thus, it is made explicitly clear that driving, operating dangerous machinery, and making important decisions are forbidden for the remainder of the day of surgery.

E. It is best to issue both verbal and written **instructions** for potential complications, wound care, and follow-up appointments to both the patient and the patient's escort.

IX. Special considerations for pediatrics. Children benefit from the ambulatory setting, since separation from parents and familiar surroundings is minimized. Additional problems specific to pediatrics include small airway caliber, frequent URIs and otitis, and inability to cooperate.

A. Patient selection

1. Almost all healthy children, even as young as several days old, are suitable candidates for ambulatory procedures. However, healthy children who have a history of apnea and are under 46 weeks of conceptual age may experience postoperative apneic episodes requiring ventilatory support. In one study, 6 of 13 such infants manifested apneic episodes, so it is recommended that such infants be monitored for 24 hours postoperatively in a hospital with suitable facilities.

2. It is safe to intubate young infants without fear of late respiratory compromise; in fact, all but the briefest anesthetics in infants should employ endotracheal intubation. Controlled ventilation is preferred in neonates and very young infants because of their tendency to become atelectatic when breathing spontaneously under anesthesia, due to their highly compliant chest walls and high airway resistance.

3. The most common outpatient procedures for infants and children are congenital, inguinal, femoral, and umbilical herniorrhaphies; eye examinations under anesthesia; cystoscopies; and placement of myringotomy tubes.

B. Preoperative preparation. Children fear unknown surroundings and can sense their parents' uneasiness as well. Consequently, making parents comfortable with the procedures will also reassure the child. Families are oriented with booklets and tours of the facility prior to the day of the procedure.

C. **The day of surgery**
1. Both children and parents are reinterviewed by the anesthesiologist; particular attention is paid to NPO status, since children often innocently feed themselves.
2. Appearance of a new URI, fever, or loose tooth is ruled out. Children with URIs may have a higher incidence of laryngospasm and/or atelectasis. Consequently, anesthesia is postponed until the URI symptoms resolve. However, seasonal allergic rhinitis is *not* a contraindication to proceeding with anesthesia.
3. Postpubescent girls should be asked about the possibility of pregnancy.
D. **Anesthetic management**
1. **Infants under 8 months old** are generally induced by mask and, after IV insertion, are intubated with an uncuffed endotracheal tube. **Children under 5 years old** can be sedated with rectal methohexital (25–30 mg/kg in 10% solution) before separation from parents, followed by inhalation anesthesia. **Children more than 5 years old** are allowed to exercise their preference for either mask or IV induction. Oral premedication in this age group may reduce crying (and secretions) without delaying discharge.
2. If possible, a local block is performed by the surgeon with bupivacaine 0.5% (maximum of 3 mg/kg) prior to the end of surgery to facilitate a smoother emergence and minimize the need for postoperative pain medication.
3. **Computerized tomography scans** are frequently done on an outpatient basis; since these procedures are not painful, sedation with rectal methohexital is usually sufficient to perform the study. Close audiovisual observation is maintained through leaded glass and with microphones, as well as monitoring by pulse oximeter and ECG.
E. **Postanesthetic recovery.** After anesthesia, children are observed for a minimum of 1 hour. When the child becomes alert and is not vomiting, the IV is removed and the family reunited.
1. Any signs of stridor, hoarseness, respiratory distress, or weak crying merit further observation and treatment with humidified cool O_2, nebulized racemic epinephrine, or IV dexamethasone.
2. Young children have difficulty articulating that they are in pain. A stormy emergence, crying, or refusal to take food or fluids may be symptoms of pain. Either an intraoperative field block, IV narcotics, or rectal acetaminophen may be the appropriate therapy, depending on the circumstances. It is also important to realize that parental expectations of the degree of discomfort will condition those of the child.

Suggested Reading

Brzustowicz, R. M., et al. Efficacy of oral premedication for pediatric outpatient surgery. *Anesthesiology* 60:475, 1984.

Korttila, K. Recovery and driving after brief anesthesia. *Anaesthetist* 30:377, 1981.

Liu, L. M. P., et al. Life-threatening apnea in infants recovering from anesthesia. *Anesthesiology* 59:506, 1983.

Palazzo, M. G. A., and Strunin, L. Anesthesia and emesis: Part I. Etiology. *Can. Anaesth. Soc. J.* 31:178, 1984.

Philip, B. K. Supplemental medication for ambulatory procedures under regional anesthesia. *Anesth. Analg.* 64:1117, 1985.

Pollard, J. Clinical evaluation of intravenous vs. inhalational anesthesia in the ambulatory surgical unit: A multicenter study. *Curr. Therap. Res.* 36:617, 1984.

White, P. F., et al. Comparison of alfentanil with fentanyl for outpatient anesthesia. *Anesthesiology* 64:99, 1986.

Wright, D. J., and Pandya, A. Smoking and gastric juice volume in outpatients. *Can. Anaesth. Soc. J.* 26:328, 1979.

25

Anesthesia for Obstetrics and Gynecology

Robert E. Tainsh, Jr.

I. **Maternal physiology**
   A. **Respiratory system.** Anatomic and physiologic changes lead to alterations in pulmonary function, ventilation, and gas exchange.
   1. The functional residual capacity (FRC) is decreased by 15–20%, leading to an increased shunt fraction and less O_2 reserve. In fact, airway closure exists in 30% of women during tidal ventilation. These factors contribute to a rapid decrease in PaO_2 during anesthesia induction, even with denitrogenation.
   2. Minute ventilation increases 50%, accounting for rapid anesthesia induction in this population.
   B. **Cardiovascular system**
   1. At term, increases in stroke volume (30%), heart rate (15%), and cardiac output (40%) are seen.
   2. A 45% increase in plasma volume coupled with a 20% increase in red cell volume produces the "dilutional anemia of pregnancy."
   3. In spite of the significant increase in blood volume, compression of the aorta and inferior vena cava by the gravid uterus can lead to the **supine hypotension syndrome.** Ten percent of pregnant women become hypotensive and diaphoretic when supine; decreased uterine blood flow and fetal asphyxia may result if not corrected.
   4. The average blood loss for a normal vaginal delivery is 400–600 ml and 1000 ml during a cesarean delivery, but transfusion is usually not necessary. **Clotting** factors VII, VIII, X, XII, and fibrinogen increase with pregnancy, leading to a hypercoagulable state.
   C. **Renal system**
   1. Renal blood flow and glomerular filtration rate (GFR) increase up to 150% in the first trimester of pregnancy, but drop to 60% above the nonpregnant state by term. These effects are thought to be caused by progesterone.
   2. Creatinine, BUN, and uric acid levels may also be reduced but are usually normal. Preeclamptic patients may be on the verge of renal failure in spite of "normal" laboratory values.
   D. **Gastrointestinal system**
   1. Anatomic and hormonal changes in pregnancy predispose the parturient to esophageal **regurgitation and pulmonary aspiration.** The gravid uterus causes increased intragastric pressure and alters the normal obliquity of the gastroesophageal junction. In addition, lower esophageal sphincter tone decreases and gastric acid secretion increases.

Progesterone inhibits gastric motility and food absorption, resulting in decreased gastric emptying.

2. Serum levels of the **liver enzymes** alkaline phosphatase, AST, and LDH all rise slightly during pregnancy.

3. Plasma cholinesterase levels decrease as much as 28%, probably due to such factors as decreased synthesis and hemodilution. Although moderate doses of succinylcholine are usually readily metabolized, patients with decreased cholinesterase activity are at risk for slightly prolonged neuromuscular blockade.

E. **Central nervous system**

1. Concentrations of inhalation agents required for anesthesia (measured in MAC units) decrease during pregnancy: halothane by 25%, isoflurane by 40%, and methoxyflurane by 32%. Decreased requirements are likely to be due to increased serum progesterone and endorphins.

2. Intrathecal and epidural local anesthetic requirements are also decreased. Epidural venous engorgement decreases the volume of the subarachnoid and epidural spaces. Other factors include the increased sensitivity of nerve fibers or the enhanced diffusion of local anesthetics to membrane receptor sites.

II. **Evaluation of the obstetric patient**

A. **Stages of labor and pain pathways**

1. **Labor** can be divided into three stages. The **first stage** commences with the onset of regular contractions and ends with full cervical dilatation. The **second stage** extends from full cervical dilatation to the delivery of the infant. The **third stage** begins with delivery of the infant and ends with expulsion of the placenta.

2. **Pain** during the first stage of labor is primarily due to cervical dilatation and uterine contractions. Afferent pain fibers from the cervix and uterus enter the spinal cord through the posterior roots of T10–L1. Second-stage pain is from distention of the vulva and perineum. These areas are innervated by the pudendal nerve through S2–4.

B. **Physiologic changes** of pregnancy are often accentuated during active labor. Oxygen demand increases up to 100%, and cardiac output rises 80% above prelabor values due to placental autotransfusion of 300–500 ml of blood during uterine contractions. Central venous pressure (CVP) is also elevated 4–6 cm H_2O by these transient increases in maternal blood volume.

C. **Fetal monitoring.** Changes in baseline fetal heart rate (FHR) during labor occur in the form of accelerations or decelerations. The normal range of FHR is 110–160 beats/min. Accelerations are a normal response to stimuli and are usually indicative of fetal well-being, whereas decelerations may herald fetal distress.

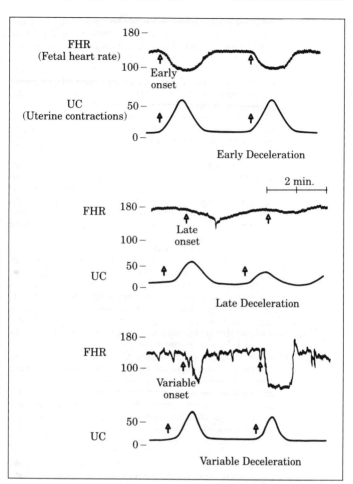

Fig. 25-1. Patterns of periodic fetal heart rate (FHR) decelerations in relation to uterine contractions (UC). See text for details.

1. **Early decelerations (type I)** usually mirror the uniform uterine pressure curve, beginning with onset and ending on completion of a uterine contraction (Fig. 25-1A). This type of FHR slowing is caused by **fetal head compression** leading to a reflex (vagal) bradycardia. Early decelerations are not associated with low Apgar scores and usually do not require intervention.

2. **Late decelerations (type II)** begin after the onset of a contraction and persist after a contraction is completed (Fig. 25-1B). The cause is believed to be due to **uteroplacental insufficiency** with de-

creased intervillous space blood flow. The decrease in maternal-fetal oxygenation results in fetal hypoxia and acidosis. Late decelerations are ominous, particularly when associated with a loss of baseline ("beat-to-beat") variability. Recurrent late decelerations are an indication for **fetal scalp blood sampling** (described in sec. **D**).

3. **Variable decelerations (type III)** lack consistency in configuration or time relationship to contractions (Fig. 25-1C). They are the most common type of deceleration and are usually due to **umbilical cord compression.**

4. **Prolonged decelerations** represent a decline in the fetal heart rate of > 30 beats/min that persist for > 2 minutes. Most instances of prolonged bradycardia will resolve spontaneously, but, in the absence of apparent resolution, preparation for intervention (low outlet forceps or cesarean delivery) should be made.

D. **Fetal scalp blood sampling** is utilized when abnormal fetal heart rate patterns cannot be corrected or the significance of the pattern cannot be determined. The normal range of fetal scalp blood pH is 7.25–7.40. A scalp pH of 7.20–7.24 is "preacidotic," and necessitates close monitoring and repeat sampling every 15–20 minutes until delivery. A fetal scalp blood pH of less than 7.20 is "acidotic," suggestive of significant asphyxia. Immediate delivery is recommended.

III. Regional anesthesia and analgesia

A. Lumbar epidural analgesia is often used for labor and vaginal delivery, whereas either epidural or spinal anesthesia may be used for cesarean delivery. For labor and delivery (in most cases), epidural block should not be administered before active labor is achieved (cervix 3–5 cm dilated with vigorous, regular uterine contractions). The progress of labor may be retarded or arrested from premature administration of local anesthesia, and augmentation of labor by oxytocin may then be necessary. Similarly, spinal anesthesia may prolong the second stage of labor by interfering with the urge to "bear down" and the abdominal strength necessary for expulsion of the infant.

B. **Advantages**

1. Epidural analgesia decreases the need for systemic narcotics and lessens drug-induced neonatal depression.

2. Mother is awake and able to participate in labor/delivery.

3. Risk of pulmonary aspiration is reduced (compared with that of general anesthesia).

4. Regional route of anesthesia has been established for cesarean delivery, if needed.

C. **Disadvantages**

1. Hypotension.

2. Long onset time.

3. Possible postdural puncture headache.

D. Contraindications
  1. Patient refusal.
  2. Uteroplacental insufficiency.
  3. Hypovolemic shock.
  4. Infection at site of injection or septicemia.
  5. Coagulation disorder (see Chap. 13).
  6. Certain neurologic disorders (see Chap. 13).
E. Recommended technique
  1. A large-bore IV (16 gauge) should be placed, and 1.5–2.0 liters of isotonic crystalloid infused prior to beginning cesarean delivery; 0.5–1.0 liters prior to vaginal delivery.
  2. Thirty milliliters of nonparticulate antacid (citric acid solution) should be administered within 15–30 minutes of anesthesia.
  3. Baseline vital signs must be obtained.
  4. **Epidural**
     a. With the patient in a lateral decubitus or sitting position, an interspace between L2 and L5 is entered with a 17-gauge Tuohy-Weiss needle. Using hanging drop and/or loss-of-resistance techniques, the epidural space is identified (see Chap. 13). A catheter inserted through the needle may be threaded either cephalad or caudad.
     b. **Anesthetics**
        (1) For either analgesia (labor and delivery) or anesthesia (cesarean delivery) lidocaine 1–2%, chloroprocaine 2–3%, or bupivacaine 0.25–0.5% is used.
        (2) In any case, a 3-ml test dose of 1.5% lidocaine with epinephrine (1 : 200,000) is given to rule out subarachnoid or intravascular injection.
        (3) Incremental doses of 3–5 ml of the selected local anesthetic are administered every 3–5 minutes, until the desired effect is reached (sensory level of T4–T6 for cesarean delivery, or T10–T12 for labor and delivery).
        (4) Bupivacaine 0.75% is no longer approved for use during obstetrical anesthesia, due to an association with cardiac arrest in these patients.
        (5) "Top-off" epidural doses are one-half to two-thirds of the initial total dose.
  5. **Spinal**
     a. A lumbar puncture is performed in the lateral decubitus or sitting position with a 25- or 26-gauge spinal needle.
     b. **Anesthetics.** Local anesthetic requirements in the obstetric patient are lower (by 30–50%) than those of nonpregnant patients. A dose of 35–50 mg of 5% lidocaine in 7.5% dextrose, 5–7 mg of 1% tetracaine with 10% dextrose, or 3–5 mg of 0.75% bupivacaine in 8.25% dextrose may

be used for vaginal delivery. For cesarean delivery, 50–80 mg of 5% lidocaine in 7.5% dextrose, 7–11 mg of 1% tetracaine with 10% dextrose, or 5–10 mg of 0.75% bupivacaine in 8.25% dextrose is used.

6. Patients should then be positioned with left uterine displacement.

7. Blood pressure and pulse are then recorded every 1 to 2 minutes for 15 minutes.

8. If blood pressure decreases by 30%, or if the systolic drops to less than 100 mm Hg, crystalloid infusion should be initiated. Persistent hypotension is immediately treated with 5–15 mg of ephedrine IV.

F. **Complications**

1. Inadvertent subarachnoid injection of local anesthesia intended for the epidural space may produce **total spinal anesthesia.** Nausea, hypotension, and unconsciousness may be followed by respiratory and cardiac arrest. The patient should be placed supine, with left uterine displacement, ventilated by mask with 100% O_2 using cricoid pressure, and then intubated. Hypotension should be treated with intravenous fluids and ephedrine.

2. **Intravascular injections** are heralded by garrulousness, visual disturbances, tinnitus, and loss of consciousness. The incidence of convulsions from local anesthetics in obstetrics is 0.03–0.5%. Seizures may be terminated by 50–150 mg of thiopental IV; 100% O_2 by mask is used to maintain oxygenation should a seizure occur. It is usually necessary to intubate the patient, using 1.0–1.5 mg/kg of succinylcholine, and hyperventilate to offset metabolic acidosis.

3. **Neurologic complications.** The most common neurologic complication is postdural puncture headache. Initial treatment consists of bed rest, hydration (> 3 L/day), analgesics, and an abdominal binder. If symptoms persist for 24–48 hours, an **epidural blood patch** may be performed by injecting 10 ml of autologous blood into the epidural space at the level where the dura was punctured.

IV. **General anesthesia for cesarean delivery**

A. **Indications**

1. Acute fetal distress.

2. Regional anesthesia contraindicated or refused.

3. Need for uterine relaxation.

B. **Advantages**

1. Rapid induction.

2. Optimal control of airway and ventilation.

3. Less hypotension and cardiovascular instability.

C. **Disadvantages**

1. Increased risk of maternal aspiration.

2. Fetal depression from drugs.

3. Maternal hyperventilation leading to fetal hypoxemia and acidosis.

        4. Inability to intubate remains a major cause of maternal morbidity and mortality.

D. Recommended technique

    1. A large-bore IV (16 gauge) is placed; 30 ml of nonparticulate antacid is administered 15–30 minutes prior to induction. Standard monitoring is applied and the patient positioned with left uterine displacement.

    2. The patient is preoxygenated with 100% O_2 for 3 minutes, or the patient should take at least 5–10 deep breaths.

    3. Once the abdomen has been prepared and draped and the surgeons are ready to begin, induction proceeds with 4 mg/kg IV of thiopental and 1.5 mg/kg IV of succinylcholine.

    4. Cricoid pressure is applied, intubation performed, and the endotracheal tube cuff is inflated before administering positive pressure.

    5. Fifty percent O_2–50% N_2O and a succinylcholine infusion are administered. Add 1.0% enflurane, 0.75% isoflurane, or 0.5% halothane until delivery to prevent maternal recall.

    6. Potent inhalation agents are discontinued once the umbilical cord has been clamped; thereafter maintenance anesthesia may consist in a balanced (N_2O/narcotic/relaxant) technique, or a low concentration of a potent inhalation agent may be continued to control hypertension.

    7. Extubation should be performed when the patient is fully awake.

E. When general anesthesia is required for relaxation of uterine hypertonus, rapid sequence induction and administration of a potent inhalation agent is indicated.

V. Vasopressors

A. The most common complication of regional anesthesia in obstetrics is hypotension, which may occur during general anesthesia as well.

    1. Decreased systemic vascular resistance results from **sympathetic blockade** due to interruption of transmission from preganglionic sympathetic fibers. This inability to constrict peripheral arterioles also causes a decrease in venous return (preload) and a decline in cardiac output.

    2. The **supine hypotension syndrome,** also known as the **aortocaval compression syndrome,** is the result of aortic and inferior vena cava compression by the gravid uterus, thus decreasing venous return, cardiac output, and systemic blood pressure.

B. Prevention

    1. Left uterine displacement during labor.

    2. Insertion of a large-bore IV before regional anesthesia, and infusion of the following:

        a. Vaginal delivery: 1000 ml of crystalloid.

        b. Cesarean delivery: 1500–2000 ml of crystalloid.

C. Treatment

    1. Relieve aortocaval compression.

2. Bolus infusion of crystalloid.

3. Oxygen by face mask.

4. A vasopressor, preferably ephedrine, 5–15 mg IV.

D. Vasopressors act on the sympathetic nervous system through adrenergic receptors. In general, alpha-adrenergic receptors mediate vasoconstriction by smooth muscle contractions. Beta-1 receptors mediate sympathetic stimulation of the heart (rate and contractility), while the beta-2 receptors are responsible for smooth muscle relaxation (bronchial, vascular, and uterine). The **uteroplacental circulation** is regulated by vasoconstrictive alpha-adrenergic receptors which reduce uteroplacental blood flow in spite of an increase in systemic blood pressure. The ideal vasopressor for obstetrics should therefore have predominant beta and limited alpha effects. Such drugs augment cardiac output yet produce only a modest increase in systemic vascular resistance.

1. **Ephedrine** stimulates both alpha and beta receptors but is a beta-predominant agent. It increases blood pressure in part by vasoconstriction, but major actions are from cardiac stimulation with subsequent increased peripheral and uterine blood flow. Ephedrine is the drug of choice for treatment of maternal hypotension.

2. Pure **alpha-adrenergic agents** such as phenylephrine and methoxamine, or predominantly alpha agonists such as epinephrine or norepinephrine, are vasoconstrictors that will increase maternal blood pressure but decrease uteroplacental blood flow.

VI. Oxytocics

A. The primary uses for agents that stimulate uterine contraction are

1. To induce or augment labor.

2. To control postpartum bleeding and uterine atony.

3. To cause uterine contraction after cesarean delivery or other uterine surgery.

4. To induce therapeutic abortion.

B. The most frequently used drugs include the synthetic posterior pituitary hormone oxytocin (Pitocin) and the ergot alkaloids ergonovine (Ergotrate) and methylergonovine (Methergine).

1. **Oxytocin** acts on the uterine smooth muscle to stimulate both the frequency and force of contractions. Its effect on the cardiovascular system include a decrease in systolic and especially diastolic blood pressure as well as tachycardia and arrhythmias. In high doses, an antidiuretic effect can be seen, leading to water intoxication, cerebral edema, and convulsions in the presence of overzealous IV hydration.

2. **Ergot alkaloids** in small doses increase the force and frequency of uterine contractions, followed by normal uterine relaxation. At higher doses, contractions become more intense and prolonged. Rest-

ing tonus is increased, and tetanic contractions occur. For these reasons, the use of ergot alkaloids is restricted for use in the third stage of labor to control postpartum bleeding. Effects on the cardiovascular system include vasoconstriction and hypertension, especially in the presence of vasopressors. Intramuscular or oral administration is recommended, as intravascular injection has been associated with severe hypertension, convulsions, stroke, retinal detachment, and pulmonary edema.

VII. Tocolytics

A. Premature birth accounts for a large percentage of neonatal morbidity and mortality. Up to 85% of early neonatal deaths not due to congenital abnormalities are associated with premature labor. In general, tocolytics are used for fetuses with gestational ages between 20 and 34–36 weeks. Cervical dilatation of less than 4 cm and cervical effacement of less than 80% are associated with a greater likelihood of terminating premature labor.

B. **Indications**
   1. To delay or prevent labor.
   2. To slow or arrest labor to initiate other therapeutic measures (e.g., steroid therapy to mature fetal lungs).

C. **Contraindications**
   1. Chorioamnionitis.
   2. Fetal distress.
   3. Preeclampsia or eclampsia.

D. **Terbutaline, ritodrine, and isosuprine** are "selective" beta-2 agonists used to inhibit preterm labor and produce myometrial inhibition, bronchodilatation, and vasodilatation. Their undesirable beta-adrenergic activities may produce tachycardia, hypotension, and restlessness. Metabolic effects include hyperglycemia, hyperinsulinemia, hypokalemia, and metabolic acidosis. Pulmonary edema occurs in up to 5% of patients using terbutaline or ritodrine, especially when used with steroids. Correction of preexisting anemia, hypokalemia, and hyperglycemia should be considered in these patients, and the drug should be discontinued for a maternal heart rate above 140 beats/min. A baseline ECG is required before treatment.

E. **Magnesium sulfate** is more commonly used in the treatment of preeclampsia but it is also an effective tocolytic agent. The frequency and force of uterine contractions are decreased by uncoupling of the excitation-contraction sequence in the myometrium. Magnesium sulfate also increases the patient's sensitivity to depolarizing and nondepolarizing muscle relaxants by decreasing the amount of acetylcholine released at the neuromuscular junction and lowering the sensitivity of the end plate to it.

F. **Calcium channel blockers** such as nifedipine are being investigated for their promising tocolytic properties.

VIII. Placental transfer of drugs

  A. Placental transport of anesthetics occurs primarily by passive diffusion as described by Fick's law of diffusion. Briefly, drugs with a high diffusion constant more readily cross the placental membranes. Factors that promote rapid diffusion include the following:

    1. Low molecular weight (< 600 daltons).

    2. High lipid solubility.

    3. Low degree of ionization (the more drug in the "free" nonionized form at physiologic pH, the more diffusable).

    4. Low protein binding.

  B. Most of the agents used to produce sedation, analgesia, or anesthesia are of low molecular weight, of high lipid solubility, relatively nonionized, and minimally protein bound, accounting for their easy passage across the placenta.

  C. Muscle relaxants are water soluble and ionized, have high molecular weights, and therefore tend not to cross the placenta.

  D. Damage to the placenta, as seen in hypertension, diabetes, and toxemia, may lead to loss of placental capillary integrity, resulting in nonselective transfer of materials across the placenta.

IX. Obstetrics for high-risk parturients

  A. Preeclampsia and eclampsia

    1. Hypertensive disorders of pregnancy account for 25% of maternal deaths and 15% of perinatal mortality in the United States. Hypertension is defined as a systolic pressure above 140 mm Hg or a diastolic pressure above 90 mm Hg. A rise in baseline systolic (≥ 30 mm Hg) or diastolic (≥ 15 mm Hg) pressure is also considered to be hypertension. Preeclampsia is the syndrome of hypertension, proteinuria, and/or edema. When seizures occur, the condition is known as eclampsia. Predisposing conditions include nulliparity, hydatidiform mole, multiple pregnancy, diabetes, and Rh incompatibility.

    2. Pathophysiology. Symptoms of preeclampsia usually appear after the 20th week of pregnancy and are thought to be related to immunologic rejection of fetal tissues, causing placental vasculitis and ischemia. Decreased placental perfusion results in increased renin, angiotensin, and aldosterone, which cause vasoconstriction and endothelial damage. Increased platelet adherence, coagulopathies, and disseminated intravascular coagulation (DIC) may ensue. Generalized vasoconstriction with a shift of intravascular fluids to extravascular spaces leads to hemoconcentration and hypovolemia. Glomerular filtration rate, renal blood flow, and urinary output are reduced, and hyperreflexia due to hyperexcitability of the central nervous system is not uncommon.

3. **Management.** The best treatment of preeclampsia is prompt delivery of the fetus, and symptoms usually abate within 48 hours of delivery. Management is symptomatic; immediate goals are prevention of convulsions, improvement of organ and uteroplacental perfusion, reduction of blood pressure, and correction of clotting abnormalities. In severe cases, monitoring of arterial, CVP, and pulmonary artery pressures may be necessary.

a. **Hypertension**

(1) **Hydralazine** (Apresoline) increases both uteroplacental and renal blood flows and is the most commonly used vasodilator. Incremental doses of 5–10 mg IV have an effect within 15 minutes and last up to 6 hours. The associated tachycardia may be treated with beta blockers such as propranolol.

(2) **Sodium nitroprusside** (Nipride) is a vasodilator with a rapid onset and short duration; it is ideal for preventing dangerous increases in blood pressure during induction of general anesthesia or treating a hypertensive crisis.

b. **Central nervous system**

(1) **Magnesium sulfate** is a mild central nervous system depressant and vasodilator. By relaxing the myometrium, it also causes an increase in uteroplacental blood flow. After an initial IV loading dose of 4 gm, continuous infusion of 1–2 gm/hr is used to maintain therapeutic blood levels of 6–8 mEq/L. Deep tendon reflexes diminish at 10 mEq/L, and respiratory paralysis and heart block may ensue above 12–15 mEq/L. Because magnesium potentiates both depolarizing and nondepolarizing muscle relaxants, placental transfer of the drug causes neonatal weakness and respiratory depression. Intravenous calcium may be given to offset the neuromuscular blockade of mother or newborn.

(2) Treatment of **seizures** consists in oxygenation, ventilation, and anticonvulsant administration. Although diazepam usually abolishes seizures, it readily crosses the placenta to cause neonatal hypotonia, lethargy, respiratory depression, and hypothermia. Therefore, thiopental (50–150 mg IV) is the preferred anticonvulsant. Succinylcholine will control motor activity if airway maintenance or ventilation is difficult.

(3) **Intravascular depletion** is corrected with fluid therapy. Prehydration increases uri-

nary output and decreases the incidence of hypotension associated with sympathetic blockade in regional anesthetics. Generally, the CVP is a reliable indicator of left heart filling, since there is no significant myocardial depression associated with preeclampsia. The aim is to raise the CVP to 6–8 mm Hg, which improves cardiac index and mean arterial pressure. The use of colloids may be useful in severely toxemic patients, especially when the CVP is less than 0.

c. **Coagulopathies.** Disseminated intravascular coagulation may occur in severe preeclampsia; administration of platelets, fresh-frozen plasma, and red cells often becomes necessary. Regional anesthesia is contraindicated in this setting.

d. **Anesthesia**

   (1) **Epidural anesthesia** is recommended for cesarean delivery in the preeclamptic patient who is volume repleted and has normal clotting. A reduction in endogenous epinephrine and norepinephrine is seen with regional techniques, thus improving uteroplacental blood flow. Decreased pain and anxiety lessen swings in blood pressure and the need for narcotics. **Spinal anesthesia** is associated with sudden severe hypotension from sympathetic blockade, which may lead to diminished uteroplacental perfusion and fetal asphyxia.

   (2) **General anesthesia** may be necessary for emergency cesarean deliveries in the event of fetal distress. Soft-tissue edema can make a rapid sequence induction difficult due to periglottic swelling. Systemic and pulmonary hypertension increase the incidence of stroke and pulmonary edema. The sensitizing effect of magnesium on muscle relaxants mandates the use of a peripheral nerve stimulator. Up to 0.67 MAC of enflurane, halothane, or isoflurane with nitrous oxide is recommended. Ketamine should be avoided.

B. **Obstetrical hemorrhage**

  1. The major cause of maternal mortality is hemorrhage. The most common causes of peripartum bleeding are placenta previa and abruptio placenta.

  2. **Placenta previa** occurs when the placenta is implanted at or very near the cervical os. During cervical dilatation, the placenta prematurely separates from the myometrium, often resulting in massive bleeding. Pelvic examinations can aggra-

vate bleeding, thereby necessitating the use of a **"double setup"** examination in the operating room in the event an emergency cesarean delivery is required. General anesthesia (rapid sequence induction) should be performed in the case of active bleeding. If the patient is hypotensive, ketamine (1 mg/kg) should be used for induction. Blood, plasma expanders, and crystalloids should be infused as needed. If the patient is not actively bleeding and is euvolemic, a subarachnoid or epidural block may be performed.

3. **Abruptio placenta** is the premature separation of the placenta prior to birth and is the most common cause of DIC in pregnancy. Placental abruption occurs in as many as 3% of pregnancies and is associated with a perinatal mortality of as much as 50%. Etiologic factors include trauma, short umbilical cord, sudden decompression of the uterus, and particularly, hypertension. The anesthetic management is the same as that for placenta previa. Regional techniques may be used only in the case of a mild abruption with no fetal distress, uteroplacental insufficiency, hypovolemia, or coagulopathy. Consumption of coagulation factors and activation of the fibrinolytic system occur frequently and should be treated with balanced blood product and crystalloid replacement as needed.

C. **Amniotic fluid embolism**

1. Amniotic fluid embolism occurs in 1/20,000–30,000 deliveries and most cases are fatal. As many as 10% of the maternal deaths from all causes results from amniotic fluid embolism. The pathogenesis of this disorder involves a tear through the amnion or chorion, opening uterine or endocervical veins and pressure sufficient to force the fluid into the venous circulation. The typical signs and symptoms of amniotic fluid embolism include respiratory distress, shock, hemorrhage (from DIC), and coma. Pulmonary edema, cyanosis, altered mental status, and seizures may be presenting symptoms. If the initial insult is survived, coagulopathies and/or renal and respiratory failure may impede recovery.

2. **Predisposing factors** include a tumultuous or oxytocin-stimulated/augmented labor, meconium in the amniotic fluid, intrauterine fetal death, abruptio placenta, advanced maternal age, multiparity, and vaginal manipulation or cesarean section. The diagnosis may be confirmed by the presence of fetal squamous cells, lanugo hair, vernix, or mucin in the buffy coat of heparinized maternal blood sampled from a pulmonary artery catheter. A rising pulmonary capillary wedge pressure is ominous. Further diagnostic work consists of serial arterial blood gases, coagulation studies, chest x-rays, and ECGs.

3. **Treatment** consists in cardiopulmonary resuscitation and immediate delivery of the fetus. Endotra-

cheal intubation and a high FIO_2 using positive end-expiratory pressure, furosemide diuresis, and blood-product transfusions are used to correct pulmonary edema and hematologic derangements.

X. Epidural and intrathecal opiates

A. The use of epidural or spinal narcotics is an effective means of obstetrical analgesia both during labor and following cesarean delivery. Drugs such as fentanyl (see Chap. 33 for the opiates used epidurally with FDA approval) are highly lipid soluble and relatively nonionized (low pK_a). These properties cause a rapid onset, short duration, and rapid clearance from the CSF. In contrast, morphine is polar and less lipid soluble, resulting in slower onset but longer duration of action.

 1. Labor. The use of epidural or spinal narcotics is promising in theory due to lack of hemodynamic effects seen with local anesthetics. **Intrathecal morphine,** 0.5–1.0 mg in 1–5 ml of preservative-free saline, provides excellent analgesia in the first and second stages of labor. However, the slow onset, lack of perineal analgesia, need for special monitoring, and numerous side effects make it less desirable. The greatest use of intrathecal opiates occurs when local anesthetics are contraindicated (e.g., known allergy or patients whose heart cannot tolerate the hemodynamic changes associated with sympathetic blockade). **Epidural** administration offers the advantage of accessibility should multiple doses of **narcotics** or, later, local anesthetics (for cesarean delivery) be needed. Epidural morphine (7.5 mg) or fentanyl (100 µg) results in satisfactory analgesia during labor.

 2. Post-cesarean analgesia. Epidural morphine, 5.0–7.5 mg, provides effective analgesia for 24–36 hours. Epidural fentanyl, 50 µg in 9 ml of saline, provides analgesia for 2–3 hours.

B. Side effects are most commonly seen with intrathecal narcotics, especially morphine, but any of the following may be seen regardless of the technique:

 1. Pruritus.

 2. Nausea/vomiting.

 3. Drowsiness.

 4. Dizziness.

 5. Urinary retention.

 6. Respiratory depression.

Some of these side effects become manifest quite late (> 12 hours) after administration (i.e., when surveillance is low). Almost all side effects can be treated with **naloxone,** 0.04–0.2 mg IV bolus or by infusion.

XI. Nonobstetrical surgery during pregnancy

A. Approximately 1.5% of pregnant women in the United States undergo nonobstetrical surgery each year. Although maternal mortality is not significantly different from that in surgery on nonpregnant women, perinatal mortality ranges 5–35%. The objectives for providing anesthesia for nonobstetrical surgery are

1. Maternal safety.
2. Maintenance of pregnancy.
3. Maintenance of normal uteroplacental physiology.
4. Avoidance of teratogenic substances.

B. Several anesthetic drugs have been shown to have effects on DNA synthesis, and reproduction in animal studies. For example, **N_2O** inactivates vitamin B_{12}, the cofactor for methionine synthetase, which is an enzyme involved in folate metabolism and hence thymidine synthesis. **Halothane** produces anomalies in rat fetuses and also inhibits DNA synthesis in vitro. Yet **no anesthetic drug** (e.g., premedication, IV induction agent, inhalational agent, or local anesthetic) **has been demonstrated to be teratogenic in humans.** Nevertheless, fetal exposure to any drugs should be minimized, particularly during the first trimester.

C. **Recommendations**

1. Elective surgery postponed until 6 weeks postpartum (when the physiologic changes of pregnancy have returned to normal).
2. Semi-urgent surgery postponed to second or third trimester.
3. Regional techniques preferred, especially spinal anesthesia (less fetal exposure to local anesthetic).
4. Minimal premedication: barbiturates preferred to benzodiazepines; narcotics used for pain.
5. Consider pretreating patients who are to receive N_2O with folinic acid.
6. Employ continuous fetal heart rate monitoring after the 16th week of gestation and uterine tocodynamometry to detect preterm labor, especially in the postoperative period.

XII. **Gynecology**

A. **Laparoscopy**

1. Laparoscopy is a diagnostic and therapeutic tool used in gynecology with unique anesthetic ramifications. Laparoscopy differs from other surgical procedures because of the need for pneumoperitoneum, occasional extreme Trendelenburg positioning, and use of electrocoagulation in sterilization procedures. The anesthetic goals for laparoscopy are to offset the rise in $PaCO_2$ associated with carbon dioxide (CO_2) insufflation, minimize the arrhythmic potential of hypercarbia and acidosis, maintain cardiovascular stability in the presence of increased intraabdominal pressure, and provide muscle relaxation for adequate operating conditions.
2. Insufflation of the peritoneal cavity with CO_2 causes an elevation in $PaCO_2$ unless ventilation is controlled. Hypercarbia results from decreased pulmonary compliance, decreased FRC, and absorption of the CO_2 used for pneumoperitoneum. Excess CO_2 may be eliminated with controlled ventilation 1.5 times the basal requirements. Increased intraabdominal pressure secondary to gas insuffla-

tion at pressures of 20–25 cm H_2O produces increases in CVP and cardiac output secondary to central redistribution of blood volume. Pressures greater than 30–40 cm H_2O produce a decrease in CVP and cardiac output by decreasing right heart filling.

3. While virtually all anesthetic techniques have been used for laparoscopy, the preferred method in most instances is a light N_2O (70–75% inspired)–O_2-narcotic muscle-relaxant anesthetic. The additional use of an inhalation agent in low concentrations such as 0.5–1.0% isoflurane or enflurane may also be employed. Local anesthesia consisting of a periumbilical field block with 10–15 ml of 0.5% bupivacaine and light sedation (fentanyl 50 μg IV) may also be used in appropriate patients. Spinal or epidural techniques are generally not tolerated well because of the increased ventilatory load associated with pneumoperitoneum, unless the laparoscopist agrees to insufflate less than 2 liters of CO_2 into the peritoneum.

B. **In vitro fertilization**

1. **In vitro fertilization** and **embryo transfer** have become increasingly popular for the treatment of infertility. The indications for these procedures have been broadened to include infertility due to tubal disease, "male factor" infertility, endometriosis, and idiopathic infertility. While the fertilization rate of oocytes retrieved in vitro averages 70–80%, the current low pregnancy rate of 16–20% emphasizes the need for safe and efficient anesthesia, as most couples need many attempts before a pregnancy is achieved.

2. There are two basic techniques for oocyte retrieval.

    a. **Laparoscopically guided oocyte aspiration** is the most common technique. A total of two or three abdominal trochar or needle punctures are performed for stabilization of the ovaries and aspiration of the follicles. Many infertility patients have pelvic adhesions from previous abdominal surgery or pelvic pathology such as pelvic inflammatory disease or endometriosis. The risk of bowel, bladder, or other organ injury during laparoscopy is increased in these patients. Although general anesthesia is usually utilized, regional techniques may be employed.

    b. **Ultrasonically guided follicle aspiration** is a rapidly growing alternative approach to laparoscopy for oocyte retrieval. The procedure involves percutaneous puncture and aspiration of the follicles under real-time ultrasound through a transabdominal, transvaginal, or transurethral approach. These procedures are often performed under local anesthesia consisting of a suprapubic wheal of 10–15 ml of 0.5% bupivacaine. Benzodiazepines combined with small doses of fentanyl, meperidine, or morphine usually provide satisfactory analgesia and sedation.

Suggested Reading

Cohen, S. E. The anesthetic implications of the physiologic changes of pregnancy. In *1986 ASA Annual Refresher Course Lectures*. Park Ridge, Ill.: American Society of Anesthesiologists, 1985.

DeCherney, A. H., and Levy, G. Oocyte recovery methods in invitro fertilization. *Clin. Obstet. Gynecol.* 29(1):171, 1986.

Drummond, G. B., and Martin, L. V. H. Pressure-volume relationships in the lung during laparoscopy. *Br. J. Anaesth.* 50:261, 1978.

Fishburne, J. I. Anesthesia for laparoscopy: Considerations, complications and techniques. *J. Reprod. Med.* 21(1):37, 1978.

Killam, A. Amniotic fluid embolism. *Clin. Obstet. Gynecol.* 28(1):32, 1985.

Ostheimer, G. W. *Manual of Obstetric Anesthesia.* New York: Churchill Livingstone, 1984.

Ostheimer, G. W. (ed.). Obstetric analgesia and anaesthesia. *Clin. Anaesthesiol.* 4(1), 1986.

Ostheimer, G. W. (ed.). Obstetric analgesia and anaesthesia. *Clin. Anaesthesiol.* 4(2), 1986.

Pritchard, J. A., MacDonald, P. C., and Gant, N. F. *Williams Obstetrics.* Norwalk, Conn.: Appleton-Century-Crofts, 1985.

Shnider, S. M. Epidural and subarachnoid opiates in obstetrics. In *1985 ASA Annual Refresher Course Lectures.* Park Ridge, Ill.: American Society of Anesthesiologists, 1985.

Shnider, S. M., and Levinson, G. *Anesthesia for Obstetrics.* Baltimore: Williams & Wilkins, 1987.

Weinberger, S. E., Weiss, S. T., and Cohen, W. R. Pregnancy and the lung. *Am. Rev. Respir. Dis.* 121:559, 1980.

26

Anesthesia for Urologic Surgery

Thomas L. Higgins

I. **The urologic patient.** Patients undergoing urologic surgery may be young and healthy, but often they present with complicating problems such as extremes of age, atherosclerotic heart disease, hypertension, renal failure, and paraplegia. Specific preanesthetic considerations for such complicated patients have been discussed in earlier chapters.

   A. **Paraplegic and quadriplegic patients**

      1. There is a biphasic response to complete spinal cord transection. **Spinal shock,** total absence of peripheral neural activity, lasts for 1–3 weeks. Characteristics are complete loss of visceral and somatic sensation and absence of sweating below the level of the lesion, a zone of hypesthesia immediately above the level of the lesion, absent deep tendon reflexes with a plantar response to stroking the sole of the foot, paralytic ileus with urinary and fecal retention, and postural hypotension.

      2. **Reflex autonomism** develops following the period of spinal shock. Impulses arising from peripheral nerves in the skin, tendons, muscles, ligaments, joints, and viscera are transmitted to the spinal cord, which is no longer restrained by supraspinal inhibitory influences. The cord now reacts with complex efferent responses, characterized by

         a. Motor hyperreflexia, clinically evident as muscle rigidity and spasticity.

         b. Flexor responses, initiated by pain, bladder distention, and surgical stimulation.

         c. The late return of extensor reflexes.

         d. Autonomic hyperreflexia.

      3. **Autonomic hyperreflexia**

         a. Since transverse lesions of the cord leave the sympathetic outflow functionally disconnected from the brainstem and hypothalamus, sympathetic integration is lost. Uncontrolled sympathetic discharge occurring in response to stimulation such as distention of the bladder or bowel can be life-threatening in the paraplegic undergoing a cystoscopy or other transurethral procedure.

         b. The higher the lesion, the more unmodulated vasculature there is that can constrict uncontrollably and the less remaining innervated vasculature left to compensate. Thus, the syndrome is rarely seen with lesions below T7, but it is common with cervical and high thoracic lesions.

         c. **Manifestations** of autonomic hyperreflexia include

            (1) Hypertension, which, if uncontrolled, may lead to severe headache, loss of conscious-

ness, convulsions, or death from cerebral hemorrhage.

   (2) Bradycardia, ventricular arrhythmias, and cardiac arrest (from intact vagal reflex in the face of hypertension).

   (3) Flushing of the face and neck, congestion of mucous membranes, and sweating and pilomotor erection below the level of the lesion.

   (4) Nausea and apprehension.

   d. The syndrome reaches a peak some time after spinal injury and subsides, but it may recur at any time, even after years of quiescence.

4. Repeated operative intervention may be necessary in paraplegic patients because of urinary retention, infection, or calculi. They may require operations for other complications of the original injury as well as plastic surgery for decubitus ulcers and infection. Their medical status may be complicated by anemia, sepsis, hypoproteinemia, electrolyte imbalance, adrenocortical insufficiency, hypovolemia, emotional instability, and sometimes drug dependency.

   a. Evidence for autonomic lability should be sought preoperatively. Patients may report headache or sweating brought on by bladder catheter obstruction, bladder calculi, or cystitis.

   b. **Spinal and epidural anesthesia** prevents reflex muscle spasm and autonomic hyperreflexia by blocking afferent visceral pathways. **Saddle block** to a T10 level is sufficient to block afferents from the bladder. However, testing the level of the block is difficult. Proper positioning limits spread of the anesthetic, and adequate volume loading will prevent severe hypotension.

   c. **General anesthesia** must be deep enough to prevent mass reactions from taking place.

   (1) Often, a fall in blood pressure occurs during induction, followed by an abrupt rise as instrumentation begins, to such an extent that the operation may have to be halted. Deepening of anesthesia or using ganglionic blocking drugs, vasodilators, or adrenergic-blocking drugs may be needed for blood pressure control.

   (2) Muscle spasms but not contractures may be eliminated by administration of nondepolarizing neuromuscular blockers. Succinylcholine must not be used because of excessive release of potassium from denervated muscle. Ventricular fibrillation following succinylcholine administration has been reported up to 18 months after the original injury.

(3) Intubation, if required, may be accomplished with the patient awake after topical anesthesia, or under a moderately deep level of general anesthesia with a nondepolarizing agent.

d. Paraplegics and quadriplegics may not require anesthesia for surgery performed below the level of the lesion. However, the absence of autonomic hyperreflexia during a previous operation performed without anesthesia does not guarantee that mass reaction will not occur.

e. Careful transfer and positioning are required to avoid hypotension resulting from autonomic insufficiency and to avoid fracturing osteoporotic bones. Decubitus ulcers are common in this population and can develop from 2 hours of continuous pressure on the operating room table. The incidence of pressure sores is twice as high in the quadriplegic as in the paraplegic patient. All pressure points should therefore be carefully padded and constant changing of position performed in the perioperative period.

f. Paraplegic and quadriplegic patients have deficient **body temperature regulation.** Warming the OR as well as IV and irrigation solutions helps prevent hypothermia.

g. Respiratory muscle compromise and kyphoscoliosis, particularly in quadriplegics, result in decreased vital capacity and expiratory reserve volume. Controlled or assisted ventilation maintains oxygenation and helps prevent atelectasis. Chest physiotherapy and postural drainage are useful postoperatively.

B. **Elderly patients**

1. Even minor surgical procedures are more complicated in the elderly population because of the high incidence of congestive heart failure, cardiac ischemia, emphysema, cerebrovascular insufficiency, renal failure, and general debilitation.

2. The preanesthetic assessment should include the patient's baseline mental status as an aid in evaluating postoperative dementia, confusion, or lethargy.

3. The dose of premedication should be adjusted to avoid obtundation, respiratory depression, and hypotension. Anesthetic dosages must also be adjusted, since the elderly have lower anesthetic requirements.

4. Patients in this age group have decreased vascular tone and may be unable to compensate for falling blood pressure. Fluid loading is required before giving vasodilating anesthetics; vasopressors may also be needed. Preparation of a phenylephrine infusion may be advisable before administration of subarachnoid block.

5. Lack of teeth and loss of facial muscle tone make it difficult to achieve a good mask fit but tend to make intubation easier. Gastroesophageal sphincter incompetence or hiatus hernia with esophageal reflux predisposes to pulmonary aspiration.

6. Electrocautery can interfere with the function of demand **pacemakers.** Most, but not all, devices revert to fixed asynchronous pacing in cases of electrosurgical interference (see Chap. 2).

II. Special considerations for urologic procedures
A. Positioning

1. Positioning should be done slowly and in stages with blood pressure monitoring. Volume pushes and vasopressors may be necessary, particularly in patients with cardiovascular compromise.

2. The **lateral decubitus position,** often with the kidney bar raised and the table in flexion, is used for kidney and upper ureteral surgery.

   a. Lateral positioning may produce a $\dot{V}_A/\dot{Q}$ imbalance, with most perfusion going to the dependent lung and preferential ventilation of the upper lung. Larger tidal volumes partially compensate for this mismatch.

   b. The left flank position (right side down) may cause vena caval compression and limitation of venous return from the abdominal viscera and lower extremities. This situation can result in low cardiac output and hypotension.

3. The **lithotomy position,** used for transurethral surgery, and the **extreme lithotomy position,** used for perineal prostatectomy, deserve special consideration.

   a. Ventilation is limited by restriction of the diaphragm. This effect is exaggerated in obese patients and in those with chronic lung disease. The longer the operation and the more extreme the flexion of the legs, the worse the tendency to atelectasis and hypoxia.

   b. Placing the patient in these positions will return considerable volumes of blood (as much as 1500 ml) and interstitial fluid to the heart, which may result in left ventricular failure, though most of the time it tends to help maintain blood pressure. Restoring patients to supine position after completion of the operation should be performed slowly to avoid pooling blood in the lower extremities and thus greatly dropping the blood pressure.

   c. Hypotension is occasionally caused by poor vascular tone secondary to regional or general anesthesia. For this reason, changing the patient's position under anesthesia is hazardous. If necessary, change of position should be done under light anesthesia, with adequate fluid and blood replacement and with vasopressor support as required.

    d. The extreme lithotomy position, which produces a gravitational gradient between the wound and the heart, may rarely lead to air embolism.

    e. The lithotomy position may be precluded by the presence of degenerative joint disease of the hip.

4. Pressure necrosis may be prevented by gentle movement to decrease abrasion, removal of pooled cleaning solution, and even weight distribution. With the patient in the supine position, bony prominences that must be padded include the sacrum, scapulas, elbows, heels, and occiput. In the lithotomy position, the fibular head should always be protected. In the lateral position, the iliac crest, greater trochanter, fibular head, lateral malleolus, deltoid tubercle, lower rib cage, and ear should be cushioned.

5. The **brachial plexus** should not be stretched. Risk is particularly great when the humerus is abducted more than 90 degrees, when the humerus is posteriorly displaced or externally rotated, and when shoulder braces are used in the Trendelenburg position. In the extreme lithotomy position, the required shoulder braces should be placed on the acromion, not the clavicle. The head should never be rotated to the side opposite the abducted arm. If both arms are abducted in the supine position, the head must remain midline. Armboards that lock are preferable, as they are less likely to slip into abduction with the table in Trendelenburg position. Arms can still slip into abduction if not carefully secured to the boards. With the patient lying in decubitus position, the upper arm is best managed in a sling device that prevents extension of the humerus.

B. Diagnostic dyes

    1. Indigo carmine dye 0.8% (5 ml) may be given IV to color the urine so that the ureter can be identified during cystoscopy or open prostatectomy. Indigo carmine has alpha-sympathomimetic effects, causing an increase in systemic vascular resistance and arterial blood pressure. It should be given judiciously to patients with hypertension or cardiac ischemia.

    2. Methylene blue 1% (1 ml) may be used for the same purposes and can cause hypotension.

III. Endoscopic procedures

    A. Cystoscopy

        1. Description. An operating cystoscope may be used in the workup of hematuria, stricture, and tumor; for basket removal of stones; for endoscopic placement of stents; and for follow-up of therapy. Retrograde pyelography and other dye studies may be part of the procedure.

2. Considerations.

   a. Anesthetic requirements are minimal, and simple cystoscopy can be carried out in the sedated, awake patient with topical anesthesia. In anxious patients, general anesthesia may be administered by mask, since patient movement during bladder instrumentation can result in perforation.

   b. Persistent erection is more common in younger males, prevents manipulation of the cystoscope, and almost always responds to deepening the anesthesia with thiopental, ketamine, or an inhalation agent.

   c. Water or irrigation solution may be used to distend the bladder (see sec. **III.B**).

   d. Allergic reactions to radiographic dye are rare, since systemic absorption does not normally occur.

   e. Bacteremia from instrumentation of an infected urinary tract is a possibility, but the complication of septic shock has been essentially eliminated by use of prophylactic antibiotics.

B. Transurethral resection of the prostate

   1. Description. Transurethral resection of the prostate (TURP) is performed by application of a high-frequency current to a wire loop. Obstructive tissue is removed by successive cuts under direct endoscopic vision. Hemostasis is effected by sealing the vessels with the coagulating current.

   2. Considerations. An optically clear, nonconductive, nonhemolytic, nontoxic solution is required to distend the bladder. Glycine 1.5% or Cytal 3.2% (a mixture of mannitol and sorbitol) meets these requirements. Complications of TURP include

   a. Blood loss, which is variable and difficult to quantify. Average loss of about 4 ml/min of resection time or 8.3 ml/gm of tissue resected has been reported, but the amount lost by an individual patient is impossible to predict.

   b. Venous absorption of irrigating fluid may occur during resection of the prostatic bed; open venous sinuses provide direct communication with the circulation. Principal determinants of fluid absorption are height of the irrigation container and exposure duration of open sinuses. Absorption ranges from none to more than 4 liters but is less of a problem with the newer resectoscopes. Increased intravascular volume and dilutional hyponatremia may occur. Early signs include hypertension and tachycardia; central venous pressure (CVP) may rise as cardiac decompensation begins to occur. Awake patients may complain of dyspnea or nausea. Hypoxia and/or hyponatremia may result in apprehension, disorientation, convulsions, and coma.

c. **Perforation with extravasation of irrigation fluid** may occur with deep dissection in the prostatic bed. If perforation into the periprostatic space takes place, the awake patient will experience suprapubic fullness, abdominal spasm, and pain. Hypertension and tachycardia are usually seen early after perforation and may be followed by sudden and severe hypotension.

d. **Bacteremia.** See sec. **III.A.2.c.**

e. **Hypothermia.** Cool irrigation solutions intended to produce local vasoconstriction may produce systemic cooling; solutions warmed to body temperature have a lesser effect. A temperature drop of 1.5°C/hr has been reported as typical.

f. **Coagulopathy.** Severe postoperative hemorrhage following TURP may be due to disseminated intravascular coagulation triggered by release of prostatic thrombogenic substances, particularly with carcinoma of the prostate. Pronounced hematuria may occur due to release of urokinase. Finally, BUN greater than 60 is associated with platelet dysfunction and increased risk of postoperative hemorrhage.

3. **Management.** Close communication with the urologist is essential to estimate blood loss and irrigation fluid absorption. An awake patient will provide the earliest warnings of the problems noted above.

a. **Spinal anesthesia** has the following advantages:

   (1) The bladder is atonic with large capacity; thus infusion pressure can be low, and emptying is less frequent, facilitating resection.

   (2) Postoperative bladder spasm is prevented, allowing for a period of quiescence for clots to contract well. Thus, spinal anesthesia promotes patient comfort and minimizes bleeding.

   (3) An awake patient can provide early warning for complications.

b. A major disadvantage of **general anesthesia** is coughing, which predisposes to bleeding. "Bucking" on the endotracheal tube can be minimized by well-timed extubation and judicious use of narcotics or IV lidocaine.

c. Because of the inevitable gain of salt-free fluid, normal saline or Ringer's lactate (*not* 5% D/W) should be given IV from the outset at no more than 50 ml/hr unless hypovolemia is present. Procedures should be postponed, if possible, when the serum sodium (Na^+) is low ($\leq$ 128 mEq/L). While CVP monitoring may show a marked increase with hypervolemia, positioning and other factors confound interpretation. Pulmonary artery monitoring may have to be used in patients with borderline cardiac function.

  d. When significant **venous absorption** of irrigating fluid is suspected, the surgeon should be asked to control bleeding and quickly terminate the resection. A blood sample should be sent for serum electrolytes; an acute change in serum Na^+ to less than 120 mEq/L is serious when symptoms begin to occur. As the cause is hypervolemia, **hyponatremia** can usually be corrected by fluid restriction and diuretics (furosemide, 10–20 mg IV). If hyponatremia is severe, hypertonic (3%) saline solutions should be given. The correction is calculated as follows:

$$Na^+ \text{ deficit (mEq)}$$
$$= (140 - \text{serum } Na^+) \times 0.6 \times \text{body weight (kg)}$$

  e. The possibility of an open surgical procedure necessitated by bladder perforation or other complications should be anticipated.

  f. If hemolysis occurs, the circulation should be supported, urine output maintained at 1 ml/kg/hr or greater, and blood transfused as needed. Consumption coagulopathy may require IV heparin infusion; consultation with a hematologist is appropriate. The current treatment of TURP-induced fibrinolysis involves administration of aminocaproic acid (Amicar) in a 5-gm initial dose (PO or IV) followed by 1 gm/hr until bleeding is under control. Rapid IV administration may cause hypotension, bradycardia, and arrhythmias. Fortunately, such treatment is rarely necessary.

C. Transurethral resection of the bladder

  1. Description. Endoscopic resection and electrodessication are used in the treatment of superficial bladder tumors.

  2. Considerations. Blood loss, hypothermia, and bacteremia may occur. In contrast to TURP, an atonic bladder is a liability, since a large distended bladder is thin and more easily perforated. Perforation may occur with fulguration of bladder tumors or with patient movement. When the peritoneal cavity is entered, discomfort in the shoulders as well as nausea and vomiting may be noted. Perforation in the presence of high-grade malignancy risks seeding of the peritoneum. In addition, tumors at the anterior dome of the bladder are harder to reach with distention.

  3. Management. The discussions in sec. **III.B.3.c–f** apply here as well. **General anesthesia** is preferable to spinal, with the caveat that coughing or straining increases risk of perforation. Anesthesia should be of satisfactory depth so as to prevent straining.

D. Percutaneous ultrasonic lithotripsy

1. **Description.** The procedure begins with placement of a ureteral catheter by cystoscopy to distend and opacify the renal pelvis. The patient is then placed prone on a C-arm table, and the stone is disrupted by a percutaneous ultrasound probe. Irrigation solution is used to flush away stone fragments and blood. Advantages include reduced blood loss and morbidity compared to conventional surgical techniques.

2. **Considerations.** A Foley catheter is needed to drain the irrigation solution, which passes down the ureter. Reported complications include metabolic acidosis, hypothermia, pneumothorax, urinary obstruction, intravascular coagulation, retroperitoneal bleeding, and accidental rupture of the renal pelvis with extravasation of irrigation fluid into the retroperitoneal space.

3. **Management.** General anesthesia is most commonly employed; however, epidural anesthesia to T8 or above can be used. In patients with high spinal cord lesions, local anesthesia and sedation may suffice, although the possibility of autonomic hyperreflexia exists. Oxygen saturation should be monitored. Instillation and recovery of irrigation fluid should balance; a deficit of more than 2 liters suggests extravasation, which may lead to sepsis and hyponatremia, depending on the nature of the irrigant solution (see sec. **III.B.2**). Retroperitoneal bleeding is suggested by a drop in hematocrit and may call for renal angiography and surgical exploration.

IV. Open procedures

A. Cystectomy and ileal or colonic loop

1. **Description.** Also known as cutaneous ureteroileostomy and ileal or colon conduit, this procedure provides supravesical urinary diversion for treatment of pelvic malignant tumors, neurogenic bladders, and chronic lower urinary tract obstruction or infection with deterioration of renal function.

2. **Considerations.** Patients are often debilitated and usually volume depleted from bowel preparations. Surgery is generally prolonged and extensive, with major blood loss and "third-spacing," yet quantification of urine output is lost throughout most of the procedure. Further complications include bowel distention and difficulty in maintaining normothermia.

3. **Management**

   a. Assume volume depletion (1–3 liters) despite overnight IV infusion. After repletion of fluid deficit, use 7–10 ml/kg/hr as a guide to maintenance during the operation. The presence of urine output into the field is another indicator of adequate volume status. Arterial, central venous, and pulmonary artery pressure monitoring may be used whenever volume status is unclear.

b. Blood loss ranges from 0–15 liters (typically 2–4 units) and occurs early in the procedure. It is often worse in patients who have had radiation therapy.

c. Maintenance of body temperature by the usual strategies avoids vasoconstriction and accompanying low urine output.

d. Establish urine flow early in the procedure, and reestablish that it is adequate at the time of implantation of the ureters. If not, reassess fluid management, and consider use of mannitol or furosemide.

e. A nitrous oxide–free technique results in a small, peristaltic bowel at the conclusion of the procedure and facilitates closure and postoperative ventilation.

f. With very careful management, the intensive care unit may be avoided, except for patients with significant cardiac or respiratory risk.

B. Open renal surgery. The retroperitoneal approach to the kidney through a flank incision is the traditional surgical approach, although the transabdominal route may be chosen when access to the renal vessels is required. A kidney bar is used to place the involved (upper) side on stretch for incision. The upper extremities are at risk for neurovascular injury unless carefully positioned. Staged, gradual positioning will maintain cardiovascular stability and avoid hypotension due to compression of the inferior vena cava.

C. Renal transplantation

  1. Anesthesia for the living donor usually requires general endotracheal anesthesia with particular attention to maintaining adequate renal blood flow. Foley catheters are rarely used in these patients. Urine output should be maintained by administering 100 ml/hr IV of crystalloid overnight preoperatively and 2 or more liters of 0.45% D/W with 12.5 gm of mannitol intraoperatively. Prevention of hypotension during positioning (flexion of the torso and raising the kidney bar) requires close attention to monitoring. Nondepolarizing muscle relaxants may be administered as necessary. The remaining kidney can usually maintain normal renal function despite diminished excretory reserve.

  2. Anesthesia for organ donors who have been declared brain-dead includes positive-pressure ventilation with 100% oxygen, fluid administration, and muscle relaxation to facilitate harvesting. As the cadaver is by definition unresponsive to pain, analgesia is not needed. Homeostasis and blood pressure regulation are maintained until harvesting of the kidney and other organs is accomplished; the anesthesiologist may then leave the room.

3. **The transplant recipient** may be young and in good condition following hemodialysis or chronically ill, anemic, and hypertensive.

   a. **Vascular access** may be limited because of repeated hemodialysis and venipunctures. The extremity with the arteriovenous shunt or fistula is not used for IV access or blood pressure measurement.

   b. Metabolic acidosis, hypertension, heart failure, pericardial effusion, pleural effusion, and pulmonary edema are common in the undialyzed recipient.

   c. **Bilateral nephrectomy** through the abdomen may be performed prior to kidney transplantation for severe hypertension or recurrent infection. Unilateral nephrectomy is sometimes performed to allow end-to-end anastamosis of the ureter.

   d. Packed or frozen washed red cells are generally given during the procedure if the hematocrit is less than 30%; studies suggest that **transfusion** improves survival of the transplanted kidney. However, the risks of hepatitis and other infections remain.

   e. **Hemodialysis** is generally performed prior to transplantation. Normal bleeding time, serum creatinine concentration less than 10 mg/dl, BUN less than 60 mg/dl, and serum potassium between 4.0 and 5.0 mEq/L should be sought. A postdialysis reduction in body weight of 2 kilograms or more, accompanied by an increase in hematocrit, suggests marked fluid shifts and the possibility of hypovolemia. Therefore, volume expansion may be needed in advance of the transplant anastomosis.

   f. There is usually time to prepare the patient, but sudden availability of a cadaver kidney may necessitate a precipitous intervention. Potassium 5.8 mEq/L or greater should be corrected with a glucose-insulin solution or rectally administered cation exchange resin. Sodium bicarbonate is often used to correct metabolic acidosis partially (to a serum HCO_3^- of 20mEq/L). The sodium load from sodium bicarbonate, however, can precipitate or worsen congestive heart failure.

   g. If routine **monitoring** can suffice, central venous catheters should be avoided to diminish the risk of infection.

   h. **General or regional anesthesia** may be used for transplantation. Clotting abnormalities may contraindicate the use of regional anesthesia.

(1) Anesthesia consists of nitrous oxide–narcotic-relaxant technique and use of inhalation agents for blood pressure control. (The theoretical risk of renal damage following enflurane in this situation has led to increased use of isoflurane.) If a pressor is needed, dopamine is a better choice than norepinephrine or phenylephrine.

(2) Succinylcholine raises serum K^+ by 0.5–1.0 mEq/L; in the presence of hyperkalemia, non–renally eliminated nondepolarizing muscle relaxants are better choices.

   i. A marked **diuresis** (500–700 ml) usually follows successful transplantation. If "warm" ischemia time is more than 45 minutes, a variable period of oliguria may occur; aggressive fluid challenge and mannitol or furosemide administration are indicated to promote diuresis.

   j. **Immunosuppressive therapy** with methylprednisolone (Solu-Medrol) is begun at operation. Cyclosporin may or may not be administered IV. When given IV, cyclosporin is a pressor and causes immediate vasoconstriction and hyperkalemia; it must be given slowly (2 mg/kg IV over 1 hour). Long-term toxicities include hepatic necrosis, chronic renal failure, and hyperkalemia.

   k. The **perfusion solution** for a living donor kidney after removal contains Ringer's lactate, mannitol, and heparin. Collins' solution, which is a high-osmolality, high-potassium solution, is used to perfuse a cadaver kidney after harvesting. Subsequently, an alcohol-denatured plasma protein fraction with 200,000 units/L of penicillin G is used as the perfusate for transport in vitro. While penicillin-allergic patients may develop a rash and wheezing at the onset of graft perfusion, anaphylactic reactions are uncommon, possibly because of prior administration of high-dose steroids.

  4. **Pancreatic and renal transplantation** may be combined in diabetics with chronic renal failure. Arterial catheters are useful to facilitate frequent blood glucose determinations. This operation is longer than renal transplantation alone and fluid shifts are generally greater (see Chap. 17).

D. Anesthesia for shunt and fistula placement. Patients may have an arteriovenous fistula created or a synthetic cannula permanently implanted in the forearm or lower leg for hemodialysis access. Such patients are often severely uremic with associated fluid and electrolyte abnormalities (see Chap. 4). These procedures may be done under regional or general anesthesia. Limbs designated for dialysis access should not be used for IV catheters or blood pressure monitoring.

V. Anesthesia for extracorporeal shock wave lithotripsy. Extracorporeal shock wave lithotripsy (ESWL) disintegrates upper urinary tract stones by focusing shock waves that set up vibrations at the tissue-stone interface. The procedure requires immersion of the patient in a large tub of degassed water, which acts as a transmission medium from the electrode to the patient's skin. There are numerous physical difficulties when administering anesthesia to a patient submerged in a tub, strapped to a frame suspended from the ceiling.

At the Massachusetts General Hospital, approximately 80% of patients undergoing ESWL receive epidural anesthesia. General endotracheal anesthesia is recommended for patients with a contraindication to, or who decline, a regional approach; patients who are not able to fully cooperate; and outpatients when there is concern for complications following inadvertent dural puncture. Contraindications to ESWL include body weight greater than 135 kg, height less than 130 cm, coagulopathy, uncontrolled dysrhythmia, severe scoliosis, and pregnancy.

A. Preparation

1. The lithotripsy suite may be located in an area removed from the main ORs, requiring continuous presence of more than one anesthetist in the event of an emergency. Since cystoscopy and stent placement are often carried out prior to ESWL, arrangements for transfer from cystoscopy facilities must be made.

2. Units for ESWL must be as fully equipped for anesthetizing purposes as any OR anesthetizing location (see Chap. 9).

3. IV catheters and monitoring cables are kept together for "tangle-free" transfers. Automated blood pressure monitors are used to obtain blood pressures since the patient's arms are inaccessible and noise makes auscultation difficult.

4. The ESWL machine is triggered by the patient's ECG, to avoid producing extrasystoles when the shock wave occurs during cardiac repolarization. Problems may be encountered when ECG leads become wet and with certain older ECG monitors. Interference is minimized by abrading the skin with the plastic electrode cover and covering the electrodes with a transparent adhesive dressing. Less interference is noted when leads are placed on the trunk, rather than on the shoulders or extremities.

5. The electrically generated shock wave may interfere with certain monitoring units. Newer units with interference suppression circuitry and a square-wave output seem to perform better than older units.

6. Use of an esophageal or precordial stethoscope is impractical due to the noise generated by the shock discharge. Close observation, pulse oximetry, and capnography are advised during general anesthesia.

7. A Foley catheter is placed in most patients following induction.

8. Fluoroscopy exposes the anesthetist to radiation; a lead apron is recommended for proper shielding, and radiation badges are mandatory. X-rays are generated underwater and aimed at the image intensifiers. In the Massachusetts General Hospital unit, at typical fluoroscopy settings of 100 kV and 6 mA, the anesthesiologist is exposed to a maximum of 0.4 mR/hr at 5 feet from the tub, 3.5 mR/hr at the patient's head, and 4.5 mR/hr if standing at the image intensifier.

B. Induction

1. **Epidural anesthesia** is performed as described in Chap. 13.

   a. Lidocaine 1.5% is generally used. We prefer to add 0.1 ml of 1 : 1000 epinephrine to each 20-ml vial of plain lidocaine to produce the desired solution (1 : 200,000) at neutral pH.

   b. If "loss-of-resistance" to air technique is used, air may spread into paravertebral spaces and along the paths of adjacent nerves, creating air-water interfaces. Trauma could theoretically result to the spinal cord and nerves if shock waves focus on such interfaces. Therefore, "hanging drop" or loss-of-resistance to saline is a better method of localizing the epidural space.

   c. Two layers of vapor-permeable transparent dressing (Tegaderm) are applied over the catheter entry site. The catheter may be left in overnight as a route for anesthesia during subsequent stent removal, cystoscopy, or contralateral ESWL. The risk for development of epidural catheter-associated infection is low.

   d. Sensory levels below T4 are insufficient for ESWL, and additional epidural doses of local anesthetic may be needed during the procedure. Patients may require supplemental IV narcotics or diazepam.

   e. Patients are prone to vomiting and bradycardia during the procedure. Atropine, 0.4–1.0 mg IV, is the treatment of choice. Low-dose droperidol may also be helpful.

2. **General endotracheal anesthesia**

   a. Patients are induced on a surface that can be placed in Trendelenburg position. Mask anesthesia is not practical because of the patient's position and limited anesthesia access once the patient is in the tub.

   b. As with other transfers, endotracheal tube placement must be rechecked once the patient is suspended in the frame.

   c. Neuromuscular blockade is not needed, and spontaneous respiration is preferred.

   d. High-frequency ventilation has been successfully employed and may have certain advantages. With decreased respiratory excursion and movement of the stone, the number of shock waves required may be decreased by 15–25%.

C. Positioning
1. Patients must be properly padded while in the suspension frame. Straps prevent buoyancy from floating the patient out of position. Inflatable "water wings" keep the arms out of line of the fluoroscope and partly above water. Brachial plexus injury can result if the arms are secured above the head.
2. Once the patient is lowered into the tub, fluoroscopy arms are rotated into place over the flanks. The suspension frame moves in three axes so that stones can be placed in the second focus of the generating electrode by 2-D fluoroscopy. Care must be taken to secure all lines and prevent disconnections as the frame moves.
3. A stretcher should be nearby, in the event emergency transfer out of the tub is necessary.

D. Special considerations
1. Patients may become hypotensive shortly after transfer to the tub from a fall in systemic vascular resistance produced by the warm water. This response may be attenuated by an increased venous return caused by hydrostatic pressure generated by submersion. In fact, central blood volume may increase by approximately 700 ml, increasing cardiac output. Loss of this "MAST suit" effect when the patient is removed from the water may also lead to hypotension; thus, a phenylephrine infusion should be available.
2. Temperature monitoring of both the patient and the water bath is essential. Hyperthermia (>40° C!!) can result if the inflow water temperature rises and may present as increasing anesthetic requirements because of augmented cardiac output.
3. Shock waves are generated by an underwater spark discharge between two closely placed electrodes. The element must be changed every 700 discharges; during the changeover, hypotension may occur from lack of stimulation.
4. Full treatment requires some 1000–2000 pulses delivered in volleys of 50–100 and may take from 30–90 minutes.
5. Hydration should be sufficient to prevent a significant fall in blood pressure from anesthesia, but overhydration will interfere with dye studies. Then, after the stones are disrupted, a high urine volume is desirable.
6. Furosemide (20 mg IV) is generally administered when hematuria is detected to promote diuresis and expulsion of the stone fragments.
7. Visualization of the stone may require administration of an iodine-containing contrast material (50

ml of Renografin-60 or Conray 60%). Diphenhydramine and epinephrine should be readily available in the event of an allergic reaction.

8. Most patients are given prophylactic **antibiotics** prior to the start of the procedure.

9. General anesthesia should not be terminated until the patient has been transferred from the suspension frame to the stretcher.

10. If transfer to the recovery room involves an elevator ride, the patient should be allowed to regain consciousness before travel and should be accompanied by both the surgeon and the anesthesiologist.

Suggested Reading

Abbott, M. A., Samuel, J. R., and Webb, D. R. Anesthesia for extracorporeal shock wave lithotripsy. *Anaesthesia* 40:1065, 1985.

Arborelius, M., et al. Hemodynamic changes in man during immersion with the head above water. *Aerospace Med.* 43:592, 1972.

Chaussey, C., et al. Extracorporeal shock-wave lithotripsy (ESWL) for treatment of urolithiasis. *Urology* 23:59, 1984.

Colman, R. W., and Robboy, S. J. Postoperative disseminated intravascular coagulation and fibrinolysis. *Urol. Clin. North Am.* 3:379, 1976.

Cooper, G. L., et al. Microbial examination of kidney lithotripter tub water and epidural anesthesia catheters. *Infect. Control* 7:216, 1986.

Desmond, J. Complications of transurethral prostatic surgery. *Can. Anaesth. Soc. J.* 17:25, 1970.

Desmond, J. Paraplegia: Complications confronting the anaesthesiologist. *Can. Anaesth. Soc. J.* 16:435, 1970.

Marsland, A. R., and Bradley, J. P. Anaesthesia for renal transplantation—5 years experience. *Anaesth. Intens. Care* 11:337, 1983.

Miller, J. D., and Katz, R. L. Anesthetic considerations in urologic surgery. *Urol. Clin. North Am.* 2:301, 1976.

Peterson, G. N., Krieger, J. N., and Glauber, D. T. Anesthetic experience with percutaneous lithotripsy. *Anaesthesia* 40:460, 1985.

Rabke, H. B., Jenicek, J. A., and Khouri, E. Hypothermia associated with transurethral resection of the prostate. *J. Urol.* 87:447, 1962.

Riehle, R. A., Fair, W. R., and Vaughan, E. D. Extracorporeal shock-wave lithotripsy for upper urinary tract calculi: One year's experience at a single center. *J.A.M.A.* 255:2043, 1986.

Wickstrom, I. Enflurane anesthesia in living donor renal transplantation. *Acta Anaesth. Scand.* 25:263, 1981.

27

Anesthesia for Trauma and Burns

Alex Mills

Trauma

I. Initial evaluation

   A. ABCs

      1. The airway is secured by intubation, cricothyroidotomy, or tracheostomy. If an endotracheal tube is already in place, its proper position and function should be confirmed by auscultation and inspection. If an esophageal obturator airway (EOA) has been used, the trachea should be intubated prior to EOA removal, as withdrawal is often followed by regurgitation. Relief of airway obstruction takes first priority in any emergency; resuscitation cannot be successful if the airway is occluded.

         a. Obstruction at the level of the hypopharynx should be relieved by an oropharyngeal or nasopharyngeal airway.

         b. Obstruction at the glottic or subglottic level requires endotracheal intubation.

         c. Obstruction of the trachea can be relieved only by passage of a bronchoscope or tracheostomy below the level of the blockage.

      2. Breathing is instituted, if necessary, by positive-pressure ventilation with 100% oxygen (O_2).

      3. Circulation is restored using volume, vasopressors, closed-chest cardiac compression, and/or electrical conversion as necessary.

   B. Define life-threatening injuries. The following should be ruled out as soon as possible:

      1. Cervical spine fracture or subluxation.

      2. Pneumothorax.

      3. Cardiac tamponade.

      4. Aortic or major vascular injury.

      5. Perforated viscus.

      6. Renal injury.

   C. Preexisting medical conditions. Traumatic injury may be due to conditions such as

      1. Hypoglycemia or hyperglycemia in diabetics.

      2. Cardiac arrhythmias with syncope.

      3. Drug overdose, including alcohol.

      4. Stroke.

II. Anesthetic implications of trauma to specific systems

   A. Cranial trauma. About 70% of all serious accidents involve injury to the central nervous system (CNS); the majority of all trauma fatalities result from injury to the brain or spinal cord. The initial neurologic examination establishes a baseline and is useful to compare for early signs of deterioration. The **Glasgow Coma Scale** is simple, brief, and relatively accurate in prognosis; it grades each of three criteria over a range of 1–5 for (1) ability to open the eyes, (2) best verbal response, and (3) best motor response. Scores may range from 3 (deeply comatose) to 15 (fully oriented and responsive).

1. **Airway**
   a. Comatose patients will often obstruct their airway when supine and aspirate if vomiting occurs. The stomach should be emptied by a nasogastric or orogastric tube after the airway has been secured.
   b. Hypoventilation produces hypercarbia, which increases cerebral blood flow and intracranial pressure (ICP). This response is magnified if hypoxia is also present.
2. **Convulsions.** Seizures may accompany direct cerebral injury or signal the expansion of an intracranial hematoma.
   a. To prevent seizures, patients with severe head injury may be treated with phenytoin (15 mg/kg by slow IV infusion; elderly patients require less).
   b. To treat seizures, the drug of choice is diazepam (5–10 mg IV).
   c. Barbiturates can be used if other agents fail.
3. **Diagnostic tests**
   a. Computed tomography (CT) scan has largely replaced other radiologic procedures.
   b. Rule out metabolic and other medical reasons for alteration in neurologic status.
   c. Observe for rhinorrhea or otorrhea, which indicates a communication from the subarachnoid space into the sinuses, nasopharynx, or middle ear.
4. **Acute epidural hematoma** most commonly results from a skull fracture and laceration of a branch of the middle meningeal artery. Classically, head injury results in a brief loss of consciousness, followed by a variable period of recovery, then symptoms of headache, vomiting, and finally, coma. Ligation of the bleeder and early evacuation of the hematoma are essential for a favorable outcome.
5. **Acute subdural hematoma** is usually the result of a vehicular accident, assault, or fall and is 30-fold more common than epidural hematoma. Subdural hematomas are often accompanied by severe impact-produced brain injuries, such as intracranial contusion or hemorrhage. Here too, immediate surgical drainage is mandatory.
6. **Penetrating brain injuries.** Treatment consists in early debridement with removal of bone fragments, hematoma, and devitalized brain tissue.
7. **Anesthetic management** is directed at lowering ICP and treating cerebral edema, as discussed in Chap. 22

B. **Spinal cord injuries** may be either open or closed and may result from physical trauma, vascular compromise, or even electrical shock.

1. **Immobilization** of the spine with immediate attention to the airway is required. Injury to the cervical spine should be presumed in any patient who is unresponsive after a fall, diving injury, or motor vehicle accident. A **soft cervical collar with sandbags** on either side of the head joined by tape across the forehead is an effective way to prevent injurious movement in conscious patients. Once a fracture or subluxation is confirmed, skull tongs or a halo external fixation ring should be applied using local anesthesia.

2. In injuries of the lumbar and thoracic spine, patients should be transported on a firm surface and turned with a "logrolling" technique until placed on a turning (Stryker) frame. Compression fractures, especially at L1–L2, may result from accidents in which the victim lands on his feet after falling from a height.

3. Respiratory insufficiency may be expected with high cervical spine lesions. Assisted ventilation is usually required for a C4, or higher, cord transection.

4. **Spinal shock** indicates complete loss of sensory, motor, and autonomic function below the level of the lesion. Loss of sweating and shivering will produce a tendency toward poikilothermia. Hypotension may be manifested without the other findings of circulatory shock, and although blood pressure may not respond to transfusion, pressors are effective. This state may completely reverse within minutes or days, or there may be a permanent loss of autonomic function (see Chap. 26).

5. The urinary bladder may be paralyzed, even in incomplete cord transections.

6. Paralytic ileus with poor gastric emptying may lead to regurgitation and pulmonary aspiration. Thus, a nasogastric tube should be passed prior to induction.

7. **Anesthetic considerations.** After stabilization, it is important to prevent any further neurologic damage. The utmost care must be exercised when intubating or positioning these patients (see Chap. 22). Patients with spinal cord or major plexus denervation injuries may exhibit acute hyperkalemia in response to succinylcholine. However, this response takes several days to evolve following the injury.

C. **Facial trauma.** Facial injuries sustained during high-velocity impact are associated with other life-threatening injuries, particularly airway obstruction, in more than 30% of cases. Brisk oral or nasal bleeding, broken teeth, or vomitus may occlude the larynx and make intubation difficult or impossible. Emergency cricothyroidotomy or tracheostomy in such cases may be lifesaving.

1. **Maxillary fracture**
   a. Maxillary fractures are usually grouped by the **Lefort classification;** in all of these, a "free-floating" jaw is encountered, and intubation may be extremely difficult.
      (1) **Type I (transverse or horizontal).** The body of the maxilla is separated from the base of the skull above the level of the palate and below the level of the zygomatic process.
      (2) **Type II (pyramidal).** Vertical fractures through the facial aspects of the maxilla extend upward to the nasal and ethmoid bones.
      (3) **Type III (craniofacial dysjunction).** Fractures extend through the frontozygomatic suture lines bilaterally, across the orbits, and through the base of the nose and the ethmoid region.
   b. Lefort and related fractures are often associated with skull fractures and **cerebrospinal fluid rhinorrhea** (by definition, a Lefort III includes a basilar skull fracture).
   c. Nasal intubation or rapid sequence induction is **contraindicated** in almost all cases.

2. **Mandibular fracture**
   a. Malocclusion, limitation of mandibular movements, missing or loose teeth, sublingual hematoma, or swelling at the fracture site will complicate securing the airway.
   b. Posterior displacement of the tongue causing airway obstruction is frequently seen in association with bilateral condylar or parasymphyseal fractures of the mandible. Simple forward traction on the tongue should provide relief.
   c. Awake nasal intubation is recommended if the nose has not been traumatized.

3. **Ocular trauma.** Most injuries require general anesthesia for repair. Special consideration must be given to open eye injuries, as discussed in Chap. 21.

4. **Anesthetic considerations.** Most displaced facial fractures require general anesthesia for repair. Many soft-tissue injuries can be treated using local anesthesia, although children usually require general anesthesia. Airway compromise is the principal concern, and induction may require awake nasal intubation, fiberoptic laryngoscopy, or tracheostomy under local anesthesia, as discussed in Chaps. 10 and 21.

D. **Trauma to the neck and upper airway**
   1. With any head trauma, cervical spine injury should also be suspected.
   2. Airway injuries may be manifested by obstruction, subcutaneous emphysema, hemoptysis, change in

voice, or hypoxemia. In severe laryngotracheal trauma, early tracheostomy is essential. Endotracheal intubation and endoscopy should be avoided to prevent further trauma to the larynx.

3. **"Clothesline" injuries** occur from direct trauma to the laryngotracheal complex caused by striking a barrier and may not be accompanied by an open wound in the neck. Injuries include complete laryngotracheal transection, laryngeal fractures, esophageal tears, thrombotic occlusion of major vessels, contusion or stretching of the brachial plexus, and subluxation of the cervical spine.

   a. With severe neck trauma, paraplegia or quadriplegia with sensory deficits indicates trauma to the spinal cord, whereas hemiplegia, obtundation, or expanding hematoma indicates aortic arch or carotid injury.

   b. Hemorrhage into the **thyroid gland** may lead to respiratory distress.

   c. With **penetrating injury,** patient survival usually depends on control of hemorrhage. Initial treatment is compression of vessels against the cervical spine and securing the airway.

4. Associated **thoracic injuries** such as pneumothorax may occur.

E. **Chest injuries.** Wounds of the base of the neck and of the upper part of the thorax may involve the trachea or larynx, the great vessels, the thoracic duct, esophagus, or lung. Wounds of the midthorax are likely to damage the heart, aorta, or lung. Wounds lower in the chest often involve lung, diaphragm, spleen, liver, stomach, or colon. The lung is the viscus most commonly injured in falls from a height; injury to the lung can lead to adult respiratory distress syndrome (see Chap. 32).

1. When ribs are fractured, **pneumothorax** should be ruled out by chest x-ray. Three or more rib fractures on the same side may produce a **"flail chest"** with respiratory embarrassment, necessitating positive-pressure ventilation.

2. **Subcutaneous emphysema** may indicate the presence of tension pneumothorax; however, laryngeal or tracheal trauma can also cause crepitus.

3. Pneumothorax and hemothorax may lead to both respiratory and cardiovascular collapse. If there is any hemodynamic instability, chest tubes should be placed, under local anesthesia, prior to induction of general anesthesia. Subclavian catheter insertions should be avoided on the side opposite of an injury because of the consequences of bilateral pneumothorax.

4. Rupture of the diaphragm may occur, causing lung collapse, herniation of viscera, and intractable hypoxia.

5. **Anesthetic considerations.** Patients with significant chest injuries almost always require general anesthesia. Intubation may have to be prolonged

into the postoperative period. If there is any suspicion of a pneumothorax, nitrous oxide (N_2O) must be avoided, as it can produce air-space expansion leading to cardiac arrest (see Chap. 10). A hemorrhaging lung must be isolated before blood floods the uninjured side. Double-lumen endotracheal tube placement under these circumstances may be lifesaving; its use is described in Chap. 19.

F. Injuries of the heart and great vessels. Fractured sternum, pericardial tamponade, recurrent hemothorax, changes in ECG, and widened mediastinum all may be signs of cardiac trauma.

   1. Electrocardiograms should be obtained routinely on all trauma victims; arrhythmias are treated as indicated.

   2. A widened mediastinal profile on chest x-ray mandates emergency angiography to rule out **traumatic aortic dissection.**

   3. Myocardial contusion must be considered in patients with multiple injuries and depressed cardiac output.

   4. The **subclavian arteries** are subject to injury with hyperextension of the neck and shoulder.

   5. With major injuries of the heart and great vessels, cannulation of large peripheral veins for transfusion is absolutely essential. However, femoral vessels should be spared if possible, since they may be the access site for emergency angiography or cardiopulmonary bypass. Intravenous catheters should not be placed in the lower extremities if there is suspicion of injury to the inferior vena cava.

   6. Anesthetic considerations. These patients are often desperately hypovolemic and may have compromised cardiac pump function as well. Anesthetic agents that depress the myocardium or cause vasodilatation must be avoided; thus, ketamine, 0.5–1.0 mg/kg IV, is often the best choice for induction.

G. Abdominal trauma

   1. Penetrating abdominal trauma is often followed by surgical exploration. An upright chest x-ray or a left lateral decubitus film should be obtained to check for free air prior to abdominal paracentesis and peritoneal lavage. If significant blood is present, operation is mandated. All gunshot wounds of the abdomen are explored, whether or not penetration is evident, because shock waves may injure intraabdominal structures. With impalement injuries (e.g., stab wounds), the penetrating object, if still present in the wound, will usually be removed in the operating room after anesthesia has been induced and the patient stabilized.

   2. Blunt trauma may produce intraabdominal or retroperitoneal bleeding. Patients may be hypotensive without a demonstrable source of blood loss.

      a. The **spleen** is the abdominal organ most frequently injured by blunt trauma. Symptoms include abdominal or referred shoulder pain; signs include abdominal rigidity, falling hematocrit or hypotension, and a "filling defect" on liver-spleen scan.

b. The **liver** frequently fractures in blunt trauma to the abdomen. Massive blood losses in the perioperative period are not unusual.

3. Fractures of the lower ribs or pelvis are often associated with abdominal injuries.

H. **Injuries of the genitourinary tract.** All traumatized patients undergo urethral catheterization when Foley catheters are placed in their bladders. However, if perineal, pelvic, or lower abdominal injury has occurred, retrograde urethrography should be performed before urethral catheterization. All patients with significant blunt or penetrating injury to the lower chest, flank, or abdomen should undergo radiologic kidney-ureter-bladder (KUB) examination and intravenous pyelography (IVP). Renal scans may be substituted in patients allergic to iodinated contrast media. If these reveal significant injury, or if the patient has an enlarging flank mass or refractory hypotension, renal arteriography is indicated.

1. **Renal.** Eighty-five percent of renal injuries can be managed nonoperatively. However, surgical repair of an injured kidney is indicated when there is

a. Loss of function (confirmed by arteriography).

b. Massive or continued blood loss, or major penetrating injury.

c. Significant extravasation of contrast media.

2. **Ureteral** laceration is usually managed by surgical exploration after locating the lesion by retrograde urography.

3. **Bladder.** Seventy percent of patients with blunt injury of the bladder have an associated pelvic fracture (but only 15% of pelvic fractures have an associated bladder injury). Contusion may be treated nonoperatively, but rupture requires exploration unless the leak is small and the urine uninfected.

4. **Urethra.** Injury is indicated when blood is present at the meatus or in the voided specimen after trauma, or if the patient is unable to void. Diagnosis is by urethrography, and treatment consists in suprapubic cystotomy for urinary diversion and control of hemorrhage. Most disruptions can have delayed repair.

5. **Autonomic dysreflexia.** The pertinent characteristics of this syndrome are discussed in detail in Chap. 26.

I. **Trauma to the peripheral vascular system.** The key to successful management of acute vascular injuries is prompt and accurate diagnosis. Peripheral pulses in all extremities should be checked routinely in all trauma patients. Early arteriography is advisable when any doubt exists. For the anesthesiologist, the most relevant problem with these injuries is hypovolemia secondary to uncontrolled hemorrhage; regional anesthesia may cause acute decompensation and cardiovascular collapse.

J. Orthopedic trauma. Fractures or dislocations that compromise nerve and/or vascular function must be reduced immediately; they constitute bona fide surgical emergencies.

1. **Upper extremity**

   a. Severe depression or hyperadduction of the shoulder girdle can stretch or tear the brachial plexus. Horner's syndrome may be evident if the cervical sympathetic chain is damaged.

   b. When the shoulder is struck hard from the side, the inner end of the clavicle may be dislocated upward or retrosternally; pressure on the trachea in a retrosternal dislocation may cause life-threatening airway compromise.

   c. Dislocation of the glenohumeral joint can cause axillary nerve injury.

   d. Fractures of the humeral shaft, especially the middle or distal part, are frequently associated with radial nerve injury.

   e. Neurovascular compromise of the forearm can occur with fracture or dislocation of the elbow.

   f. Median nerve compression is a possibility with fractures at the wrist.

   g. Fractures about the elbow or direct trauma to the forearm may cause edema of the anterior compartment of the forearm. The anterior compartment is a closed space, and pressure on the blood vessels will result in ischemic necrosis; early fasciotomy is indicated.

2. **Lower extremity**

   a. Fractures of the **tibia** and **fibula** are the most common major skeletal injuries.

      (1) **Fat embolism** can occur with major long-bone fractures. Treatment consists in oxygenation and support of vital signs.

      (2) **Hyperkalemia** and **myoglobinemia** can occur with crush injuries if large amounts of muscle tissue are devitalized. As with burns (see next section), patients may exhibit aberrant responses to muscle relaxants starting several days, and lasting for up to a year, after severe muscle trauma.

      (3) Fracture of the neck of the fibula may damage the peroneal nerve.

   b. Whenever a fracture of the **femur** or **pelvis** is present, blood loss may be much greater than evident from superficial inspection.

   c. **Hip fractures** are common in the elderly. Traction is used initially for pain relief, but most fractures require open reduction and internal fixation to ensure adequate healing and function and to avoid the complications of immobilization. The clinical picture is often dominated by other complicating medical illnesses. Spinal or epidural anesthesia is usually an excellent choice for these patients.

3. **Extremity reimplantation.** In general, these procedures are performed only on the upper extremities and only if patients are otherwise stable. An amputated arm, hand, or digit will not be replanted if it has sustained severe crush injury or been torn from attachments to major nerves and blood vessels. Reimplantations may be extremely lengthy, in some cases (e.g., multiple digit reimplantation) in excess of 24 hours.

   a. **Regional anesthesia** with brachial plexus block is usually chosen, as it avoids the risk of aspiration in patients with a "full stomach," provides optimal operating conditions, and offers postoperative analgesia. Even if general anesthesia becomes necessary for psychological or other reasons, regional blocks will reduce the total dosages of general anesthetics.

      (1) Catheter placements, rather than "single shot" brachial plexus blocks, are preferable due to the potentially lengthy operative times and surgical uncertainties.

      (2) Intravenous sedation will almost certainly be required for such long operations.

   b. If **general anesthesia** is chosen, an inhalation technique is frequently used due to length of procedure. The possibility of bromism from halothane or fluoride intoxication from enflurane is, at least, a theoretical consideration.

      (1) To avoid pressure-induced scalp ulceration and hair loss, the head must be repositioned at frequent (e.g., 1 hour) intervals. Patients should be placed on water blankets to avoid pressure on peripheral nerves (e.g., ulnar, sciatic, sural).

      (2) Inhaled gases should be humidified and all strategies for heat conservation employed (see Chap. 17).

      (3) Controlled ventilation with large tidal volumes will help prevent atelectasis.

Burns

I. **Pathophysiology.** Deep thermal injury destroys skin and thus the body's barrier to the external environment. Skin is the first defense against entry of bacteria and other pathogens and is in large part responsible for thermal regulation as well as fluid and electrolyte homeostasis.

   A. **Thermal loss.** Following major burns, warmth and humidity must be provided to minimize heat loss.

   B. **Fluid loss** is a function of the total body surface area burned and depth of burn. In thermal injury, the total body vascular compartment becomes permeable to both protein and crystalloid. There is also a diffuse alteration in the permeability of cell membranes to sodium, resulting in generalized cellular swelling. Microvascular injury results from local damage by heat and from the release of vasoactive substances from the burned tissue. Therefore, edema occurs not only in burned, but also unburned, tissues.

C. **Caloric supplementation** is needed to balance the massive protein losses and to compensate for catabolism.

D. **Infections** are best prevented, so burned areas are dressed with topical antibacterial agents. Excision of nonviable tissue and substitution by temporary or permanent skin grafts must be attempted as soon as the patient's condition has been stabilized. Multiple anesthetics for excision and grafting are usually required for extensive burns.

II. **Origin of burns**

A. The majority of burns are **thermal injuries,** either from open flame or heat.

B. In **electrical burns,** it is thermal energy that actually destroys tissue, particularly those with high resistances like skin and bone. It is impossible to predict the precise location and extent of tissue damage; periosseous muscle may be destroyed even though the superficial tissues are viable. **Myoglobin release** is a frequent complication of electrical injury. Patients often present with associated injuries such as fractures of the spine (due to arching), long-bone fractures, subdural hematomas, and damaged internal organs. Vital organs that are particularly sensitive to electrical injury include **myocardium,** where damage may present as arrhythmias (including ventricular fibrillation), and the **spinal cord,** which may demyelinate after electrical trauma. As a rule, injured extremities require emergency **fasciotomies** even if the skin appears intact; surgical exploration and debridement are mandatory.

C. In **chemical burns,** the degree of injury depends on the particular chemical, its concentration, duration of contact, and the penetrability and resistance of the tissues involved. For most chemical burns, the immediate treatment is irrigation with water to dilute the causative agent. Some substances that cause chemical burns (e.g., phosphorus) are absorbed systemically, producing symptoms of poisoning.

III. **Clinical picture**

A. **Initial evaluation**

1. After establishing that a patent airway exists and that ventilation and blood pressure are adequate, attention should be directed toward the burn. First, an estimate of the **burn size** is made, expressed as a percent of the total body surface area (%TBSA). The **rule of nines** guides estimations in adults: the head and both of the upper extremities each repre-

sent 9% TBSA; the anterior trunk, posterior trunk, and both of the lower extremities each represent about 18%; and the perineum 1%. Another practical method to estimate %TBSA is that the area of the patient's hand will cover about 1% TBSA. In children, these rules must be modified, since the surface areas of the head and trunk are proportionally larger than the extremities.

2. The **depth of burn** determines the nature of therapy (i.e., excision and grafting versus conservative management). Burn depth is difficult to determine visually; however, in general, the area under a partial-thickness burn should have normal or increased sensitivity to pain and temperature and should blanch with pressure but refill. A full-thickness burn will be anesthetic and will not blanch.

B. **Acute management**
  1. **Cardiovascular system**
      a. Without aggressive fluid repletion, sustained hypotension, hypoperfusion, and shock will develop during the first 24–48 hours because of massive evaporative losses and sequestration of fluid in extracellular spaces.
      b. The composition of lost or sequestered fluid is essentially that of plasma; thus, the protein content of the exudate is usually high.
      c. Fluid resuscitation consists of balanced salt solutions and colloid when indicated. Protocols for fluid replacement factor in body weight (BW) in kilograms and %TBSA burned. Generally, half the calculated amount should be given during the first 8 postburn hours and the remainder over the next 16 hours, in addition to the patient's daily maintenance fluid requirement. Colloid used may be hetastarch, plasma, 5% albumin, or 5% purified protein fraction (PPF). Standard protocols include
          (1) **Parkland** Ringer's lactate, 4 ml × BW × %TBSA (preferred at the Massachusetts General Hospital).
          (2) **Brooke** (0.5 ml colloid + 1.5 ml Ringer's lactate) × BW × %TBSA.
      d. The end point of fluid therapy is maintenance of urine output and hemodynamic stability. In extensive burns, it is imperative that fluid management be followed with appropriate invasive monitoring and laboratory assessments.
      e. A fall in cardiac output and arterial blood pressure may occur in the immediate postburn period despite apparent adequate intravascular volume. The etiology remains uncertain but may be due to circulating factors that depress contractility.
      f. By 36–72 hours after initial injury, capillary integrity begins to return, allowing resorption of

fluid from the interstitial space and decreasing the need for fluids. At this juncture, a "diuretic phase" may begin.

g. Chronic postburn hypertension may be seen in young children (usually boys) who have had extensive injuries. It usually develops within 2 weeks of injury and may result from elevated catecholamines.

h. Circumferential burns of the abdomen may produce increased intraabdominal pressure, which can effect cardiac output by impeding venous return.

2. Respiratory system

a. Circumferential full-thickness burns of the thorax can cause hypoventilation and decrease functional residual capacity, leading to hypoxia. Treatment consists in increasing the FIO_2 and positive-pressure ventilation if necessary. Emergency **escharotomies** are indicated.

b. Thermal injury of the face and upper airway is a common occurrence, but burns in the lower respiratory tract are less frequent. However, during fire in a closed space or when heated noxious vapors are inhaled, **inhalation injury** may occur. This should be suspected in the presence of burns of the head or neck, singed nasal hairs, swelling of the mucosa of the nose, mouth, lips, or throat, a brassy cough, or soot in the sputum. Both upper airway and pulmonary parenchyma may be severely affected, leading to adult respiratory distress syndrome.

c. **Carbon monoxide** (CO) poisoning occurs when CO combines with hemoglobin, displacing O_2 (CO has more than a 200-fold higher affinity for hemoglobin) and shifting the oxyhemoglobin dissociation curve to the left. In essence, toxic effects are due to tissue hypoxia. Carbon monoxide poisoning can be difficult to diagnose because carboxyhemoglobin (COHb) is visually the same as oxyhemoglobin and PaO_2 measurements show normal values. Thus, one must have a high index of suspicion. The half-life of COHb is directly related to inspired O_2 concentration; it is 4 hours when breathing room air, but 30 minutes breathing 100% O_2. Therefore, treatment consists in O_2 therapy and support of the vital signs until the CO is eliminated.

d. The ambient atmosphere during a fire is low in O_2 and high in CO, so all burned patients, especially those burned within a closed space, may have suffered some degree of **hypoxia** with their thermal injury. Ideally, O_2 administration should begin at the scene.

3. Central nervous system. A high incidence of encephalopathy occurs in burned children. The syndrome consists of systemic hypertension, lethargy, disorientation, and CNS irritability and is sometimes accompanied by seizures. Although of uncertain etiology, contributing factors may include electrolyte and metabolic derangements and multiple drug therapy.

4. **Kidneys.** Renal blood flow may be decreased from
   a. **Prerenal factors,** including hypovolemia, myocardial depression, and renal vasoconstriction from stress hormones (e.g., catecholamines, antidiuretic hormone, renin, and angiotensin).
   b. **Intraparenchymal factors,** including toxic damage from myoglobinuria following rhabdomyonecrosis and hemoglobinuria from hemolysis. Renal function can be protected in the presence of these pigments by administration of fresh-frozen plasma, which contains haptoglobin to bind the free hemoglobin; maintenance of urine output with either osmotic or loop diuretics (mannitol or furosemide); or bicarbonate administration to alkalinize the urine.

5. **Gastrointestinal system**
   a. Serum enzyme changes indicative of **liver damage** are sometimes evident in the early postburn period. Paradoxically, metabolic studies suggest enhanced liver activity during the same period; for example, in cytochrome P450-dependent drug metabolism. Thus, depending on the drug and latency since injury, doses of anesthetics and adjuvants may require adjustment.
   b. **Curling's ulcers** (mucosal erosion) will occur at variable times after major burns, leading to life-threatening hemorrhage or perforation. These seem to be more common in children than adults. Therapy consists of antacids and H₂-blocking agents. Metastatic *Pseudomonas aeruginosa* lesions can also lead to ulceration but are usually ameliorated with systemic treatment of the infection.
   c. Other gastrointestinal complications of burns include esophagitis, tracheoesophageal fistula (from prolonged intubation and presence of a nasogastric tube), acalculus cholecystitis, and mesenteric artery thrombosis.

6. **Bacterial infection**
   a. Infection of burned areas delays healing and prevents successful skin grafting. Bacterial invasion of underlying tissues may result in septicemia.
   b. The most common organisms involved are staphylococci, beta-hemolytic streptococci, and the gram-negative rods such as *Pseudomonas* and *Klebsiella*.
   c. Local treatment consists of topical antimicrobials applied to the burned areas:

(1) **Silver nitrate** (0.5%) soaked in several layers of wide-mesh gauze may be wrapped around the wound. Rarely, methemoglobinemia may occur in association with silver nitrate therapy because some organisms (*Aerobacter cloacae*) can convert the nitrate ion to the nitrite, which in turn converts hemoglobin from the ferrous (Fe^{2+}) to the ferric (Fe^{3+}) form, reducing O_2-carrying capacity. Chloride depletion may also result from chloride's reaction with the silver ion. Although silver nitrate decreases evaporative loss, it does not penetrate eschar.

(2) **Mafenide** cream (10%) penetrates tissues readily (including eschar) and is effective against *Pseudomonas* colonization. It can cause metabolic acidosis if absorbed, as it is a carbonic anhydrase inhibitor.

(3) **Silver sulfadiazine** (1%) is more slowly absorbed and longer lasting than either silver nitrate or mafenide and is not associated with electrolyte abnormalities. Leukopenia is the main disadvantage but reverses with discontinuation.

(4) **Povidone-iodine** is easy to apply; however, it elevates serum I^- levels and is contraindicated in any patient with renal dysfunction.

d. Sepsis may also be inhibited by using temporary biologic dressings, which may be allografts (cadaver skin, amnion) or xenografts (porcine). "Artificial skin," which is manufactured from collagen, and cultured epidermis, grown in vitro from a patient's own cells, are being tested at the Massachusetts General Hospital.

e. The use of systemic antibiotics is limited to treatment of documented systemic sepsis (as opposed to colonization) and as prophylaxis prior to surgical procedures.

7. **Endocrine system.** The stress of burn injury causes marked changes in catecholamine, corticosteroid, and glucagon levels. Increases in these catabolic hormones result in loss of muscle and nitrogen breakdown, the severity of which is generally proportional to the extent of the injury. Early hyperalimentation is indicated, but hyperosmolar coma may result from overzealous use.

8. **Musculoskeletal system.** Circumferential burns of the extremities can lead to vascular compromise. Escharotomy is required to prevent ischemic necrosis of distal structures, particularly the digits.

9. **Hematologic system**
   a. Microangiopathic hemolytic anemia can occur.
   b. Sepsis can lead to disseminated intravascular

coagulation (DIC) as well as bone marrow suppression.

   c. The massive blood losses occurring during escharotomy, excision, and grafting are associated with complications discussed under **Transfusion.**

IV. Anesthetic considerations

   A. General considerations. Early excision and grafting of burned areas is now widely accepted. Thus, patients are brought to the operating room in the **acute phase** of injury, when they may still be unstable. Special emphasis should be placed on correcting acid-base and electrolyte disturbances, as well as coagulopathies. Adequate colloid and blood products should be ordered in advance; it is *difficult to overestimate* the volumes that will be needed.

   In the **chronic phase** of burns, when reconstructive procedures are performed, altered pharmacokinetics, drug tolerance, and extremely difficult airways are the main considerations.

   B. Monitoring and IV catheters. Often IV access will still be in situ from the initial resuscitation.

      1. In massive burns, there may be no place to stick **ECG pads.** However, after induction, electrodes can be stitched onto the skin or needle electrodes used.

      2. Arterial catheters are indispensable for continuous blood pressure monitoring and to facilitate frequent sampling. Almost any artery may be used; the site will depend on the availability of unburned areas. If all appropriate sites are burned, the line may have to be placed through the burn wound, after the area has been sterilely prepared.

      3. Central venous pressure (CVP) catheters are useful, both for monitoring central volume and as central access for drug infusions. In massive injuries in elderly patients, a pulmonary artery catheter may be required for optimal management.

      4. Large-bore IVs are mandatory to prevent exsanguination.

   C. Airway. Mask fitting may be poor because of edema in the early phases of burn injury or because of scars and contractures later on. These processes also render *burn patients among the most difficult intubations an anesthesiologist will ever face.*

   D. Muscle relaxants

      1. Succinylcholine and other depolarizing muscle relaxants are absolutely contraindicated any time after major burns, as they can produce profound hyperkalemia and cardiac arrest. If they are given inadvertently, calcium chloride can antagonize the cardiac effects of hyperkalemia (although large amounts may be required); administration of glucose and insulin may also be indicated.

2. **Nondepolarizing relaxants** are used when muscle relaxation is required. Burn patients show a "resistance" to these drugs (diminished response to conventional doses), in some cases requiring three- to five-fold higher doses than are sufficient in non-burned patients. This finding has been made with all nondepolarizing agents studied, but the reason remains uncertain. Possibilities including increased metabolism, alterations in volume of distribution/protein binding, and increased density of muscle membrane acetylcholine receptors near the burn injury have been proposed and are under investigation. Because of the large increase in relaxant requirements, it is advisable to use a blockade monitor whenever administering these agents to patients following major burn injury.

E. **Anesthetics.** There is no single preferred agent, or combination of agents, for use in burn patients. **Ketamine** may have advantages in patients with extensive burns whose volume status is continuously fluctuating. The use of **halothane** in adults has not been associated with a hepatitis-like syndrome, even after multiple uses over short time periods. For dressing changes, N_2O-O_2 can be used as an analgesic, with small amounts of ketamine (0.1 mg/kg IV) for supplementation.

These patients may have greatly increased **narcotic** requirements due to tolerance and increases in apparent volumes of distribution for drugs. It is important to provide adequate analgesia; narcotic dependence is not an issue in the acute setting.

F. **Temperature regulation.** The most comfortable body temperature for a burn patient is about 100°F (38°C), higher than that for normals. Every effort should be made to maintain normothermia during transport and surgery. The operating room, IV fluids, and blood products should be warmed and inspired gases heated and humidified. Place pediatric patients under a radiant heat source and on a warming blanket whenever possible.

G. **Immunosuppression.** The immune system is suppressed for weeks to months after burn injury, and unfortunately, the wound itself serves as an excellent medium for bacterial growth. Thus, every attempt should be made to practice antiseptic technique when handling patients or inserting lines.

H. **Postanesthetic care.** It is important to maintain normothermia while transporting patients back to the intensive care unit, since shivering may contribute to graft loss. Supplemental O_2 should be given until the patient is fully recovered from anesthesia because of high metabolic rate (O_2 consumption) and, often, intrapulmonary shunting.

Transfusion

I. Indications

A. Maintain O$_2$-carrying capacity, since erythrocytes deliver essentially all the O$_2$ to tissues.

    1. Healthy individuals can tolerate a hematocrit (Hct) in the 20–30% range, provided intravascular volume is maintained.

    2. Preoperative anemia may be secondary to decreased production (blood dyscrasia) or increased loss (hemorrhage) or destruction (hemolysis). Ideally, transfusion should be performed 24 hours prior to surgery to allow stabilization of fluid balance, to reverse the "storage defects" of decreased 2, 3-diphosphoglycerate (2,3-DPG) and adenosine triphosphate in the circulation, and to increase O$_2$-carrying capacity of the transfused blood.

    3. One unit of packed red blood cells (RBCs) (Hct about 70%, volume about 250 ml) will usually raise the Hct of a euvolemic adult by 2–3% once equilibration has taken place.

B. Maintain normal coagulation function.

C. Maintain intravascular volume. Blood volume is about 7% of total lean body mass, or 70 ml/kg, in average adults. It is about 80 ml/kg in neonates and can be in excess of 90 ml/kg in premature infants.

    1. Volume to transfuse =

$$\frac{(Hct_{desired} - Hct_{present}) \times (blood\ volume)}{(Hct\ of\ transfused\ blood)}$$

    2. Intraoperative blood losses are estimated by sponge and drape weights and suction volumes. Most healthy individuals can tolerate a gradual loss of at least 20% of total blood volume before vital signs are affected, provided replacement occurs with appropriate volumes of crystalloid.

II. Blood typing and cross-matching

A. Donor and recipient blood is typed in the ABO and Rh systems and screened for antibodies to other RBC antigens. The **cross-match procedure** directly mixes patients' serum with donors' RBCs to establish that hemolysis does not occur from undetected antibodies.

B. Uncross-matched blood transfusion may be lifesaving in very anemic patients when emergency blood replacement outweighs the risk of reactions. Type-specific (ABO and Rh) blood is the most reasonable to use, especially if the recipient has had a negative screen for antibodies.

C. If type-specific uncross-matched blood is unavailable, O negative blood should be used—preferably as packed RBCs rather than as whole blood, since O plasma may contain anti-A or anti-B antibodies, which could cause hemolysis in an A, B, or AB patient. Acutely, O positive blood can be used in males, or females in whom Rh-sensitization will never pose a threat to a fetus (e.g., following menopause or hysterectomy).

   D. If a substantial proportion of the patient's blood volume is replaced with uncross-matched blood (e.g., more than 4 units) without signs of adverse reaction, in the acute situation it is recommended to **continue transfusing the same blood,** rather than switching to properly cross-matched blood when available. This is because the transfused uncross-matched blood could contain antibodies capable of producing an adverse reaction to the newly transfused properly cross-matched blood.

III. Choice of RBC preparation (Table 27-1)

   A. Autologous blood can be stored preoperatively, either during the month prior to surgery, or it can be frozen years in advance. This is especially useful in patients with rare blood types and is the best way to prevent blood-borne viral infection.

   B. In healthy patients, **phlebotomy and hemodilution** can be done at the beginning of surgery when the starting Hct is high. Blood is removed through an arterial line or large-bore IV catheter and anticoagulated with CPD (citrate-phosphate-dextrose), and the volume is replaced with crystalloid. Then, later in the procedure, fresh whole blood is available for retransfusion.

   C. Blood shed into sterile cavities (thorax or abdomen) can be harvested (via "cell-savers") for **autologous transfusion.** This is especially useful in trauma, cardiac, or vascular surgery (see Chap. 18).

   D. It is likely that whole blood will become increasingly hard to obtain. Blood banks require specific blood components for most patients they serve; with few exceptions, transfusions for the surgical patient should also be guided by these principles.

   E. Mandatory antibody testing of donated blood means that most preparations are at least 24 hours old before they can be used.

IV. Technical considerations

   A. To facilitate transfusion, packed RBCs (pRBCs) may be **diluted.** However, only isotonic saline or plasma should be used: calcium (Ca^{2+}) contained in Ringer's lactate will combine with the citrate anticoagulant, leading to clotting; hypotonic solutions will cause lysis; hypertonic solutions will cause dehydration and crenation of RBCs; and dextrose-containing solutions decrease the survival of transfused RBCs. Dilution is usually necessary only during rapid transfusion and when transfusing through small IVs, such as are used in infants.

   B. Filtering of blood for microaggregates is recommended; 80 or 170-µm macrofilters are typically used. Finer filters (20–40 µm) remove smaller aggregates and fibrin strands, but their clinical value remains to be established, even in massive transfusion situations. In fact, increased shear force through fine filters during transfusion may damage RBCs and definitely impedes rapid transfusion.

Table 27-1. Preparations used for blood transfusion

Preparation	Components contained	Advantages/disadvantages
Whole blood	RBCs, WBCs, plasma, platelets	If < 24 hours since donation, contains clotting factors, platelets. If > 24 hours old, clotting factors and platelets are diminished. Limited shelf-life: 48 hours if heparin is used as the anticoagulant (to avoid citrate). Increased volume required to give unit of RBCs.
Packed RBCs	RBCs, WBCs	Less volume per unit than whole blood (Hct 60–80%). Less plasma components that can cause hemolysis. Shelf-life is about 35 days.
Buffy coat–poor RBCs	RBCs, decreased WBCs	Useful in preventing nonhemolytic febrile transfusion reactions.
Frozen deglycerinated RBCs	RBCs	Able to store for years. No WBCs to cause febrile reactions Takes several hours to thaw and deglycerinate, after which must be used within 24 hours.

V. Complications

A. **Volume overload** can be corrected by diuretics, phlebotomy, or surgical losses.

B. **Hemolytic reactions.** Acute intravascular hemolysis is marked by fever, chills, dyspnea, chest pain, hemoglobinemia, and hemoglobinuria. Unfortunately, many of these clinical signs are masked by anesthesia. Intraoperatively, an increase in temperature with a change in vital signs and urine color may be indicative of a reaction. If reaction continues, it may progress to shock and DIC.

   1. **If a reaction is *suspected*:**
      a. Stop transfusion.
      b. Send unused donor blood and a blood sample from the patient back to the blood bank to be recross-matched.
      c. Obtain an anticoagulated blood sample for free hemoglobin, haptoglobin, and direct Coombs test. Inspect the plasma of a spun Hct; it may be pink/red in the presence of free hemoglobin.
      d. Maintain a saline infusion.
   2. **If a reaction is *confirmed*:**
      a. Begin treatments aimed at minimizing the effects of intravascular hemolysis.
         (1) Give fluids to increase intravascular volume and pressors to support hemodynamics if necessary.
         (2) Prevent renal failure from pigment toxicity by forced diuresis with mannitol or furosemide.
         (3) Consider alkalinizing the urine.
      b. Monitor the urine and plasma for free hemoglobin concentration.
      c. Monitor fibrinogen and fibrin split products, prothrombin time (PT), partial thromboplastin time (PTT), and thrombin time for early diagnosis of DIC.

C. **Febrile, nonhemolytic reactions** are caused by antibody to donor white blood cell (WBC) antigens. The incidence can be decreased by using WBC-poor, or frozen, RBCs.

D. **Urticaria.** If there are no other adverse effects, judiciously continue transfusion but treat with antihistamines.

E. The incidence of **anaphylaxis** is about 1 : 800. Treatment is supportive, but future transfusions should only use plasma-free, washed RBCs.

F. **Infection.** Reactions to bacterial toxins are marked by high fever and often shock. Viral infections (including hepatitis B; non-A, non-B hepatitis; human immunodeficiency virus (HIV); cytomegalovirus; Epstein-Barr virus) may have substantial latencies (see Chap. 7).

VI. Massive transfusions (> 1 blood volume)

A. Accurate **monitoring** is vital; blood volume loss should be replaced on the basis of sponge weight, suction bottle volumes, and estimated losses on surgical drapes, and so on.

B. Blood **warming** helps prevent generalized hypothermia. Overwarming must be prevented, since RBCs lyse at greater than 40°C.

C. Coagulopathy may be caused by decreased numbers (dilutional) or poorly functioning platelets, inadequate clotting factors, or DIC.

    1. Platelets

        a. Unless fresh (< 24 hours since donation), RBC products contain essentially no active platelets.

        b. Monitor platelet count and transfuse if less than 50,000/mm³.

    2. Coagulation factors

        a. Banked blood 3 weeks old contains only 10–15% of normal levels of factors V and VIII.

        b. Transfusion of 2 units of **fresh-frozen plasma for every 8–10 units of transfused banked blood** is recommended. This ratio should increase as transfusions continue.

    3. During active **DIC,** the use of heparin to interrupt the consumptive coagulation cycle remains controversial. Treatment of cause (sepsis, low output states, hypoxia, acidosis) is essential if therapy is to be successful. In the operative setting, transfuse with platelets and fresh-frozen plasma to attempt to maintain hemostasis until coagulopathy has resolved. Unfortunately, therapy is often unsuccessful.

D. Citrate is an anticoagulant in banked blood products (fresh-frozen plasma and pRBCs) that can produce ionized hypocalcemia when blood is administered rapidly (≥ 1 unit/5 min in an adult). This can lead to profound hypotension and cardiac arrest. Ionized Ca^{2+} levels and the Q–T interval of the ECG should be monitored; Ca^{2+} should be administered prophylactically during massive transfusion. Calcium chloride, 1 mg/kg IV every 15–20 minutes during periods of rapid transfusion, may prevent hemodynamic compromise.

E. The pH of banked blood falls with storage (by 3 weeks, metabolic acids are increased by 25–30 mEq/L). This is partially compensated by the citrate anticoagulant. There is also excess free potassium in banked blood, which increases with storage time.

F. Red blood cell function is affected by storage; there is a decrease in 2,3-DPG levels, which results in decreased tissue O_2 delivery. After transfusion, RBC 2,3-DPG level returns to normal within 24 hours.

G. DDAVP (desmopressin), a vasopressin analogue, is currently being studied as a possible means of decreasing transfusion requirement in surgery with major blood losses (e.g., cardiac surgery, spinal fusion).

VII. Intraoperative coagulopathy

    A. Differential diagnosis

        1. Decreased platelet number or function.

2. Coagulation factor deficiency (particularly V and VIII.

3. Coagulation factor consumption (DIC) or hemolytic transfusion reaction.

4. Anticoagulation (heparin or coumadin therapy).

5. Chronic disease: liver (decreased coagulation factor production); kidney (platelet dysfunction).

B. **Initial workup.** PT, PTT, fibrinogen, fibrin split products, thrombin time, bleeding time, and platelet count should be obtained. A clot should be observed for size, stability, and lysis, and the plasma observed for evidence of hemolysis.

1. If **thrombocytopenia** is found, the therapy is specific.

   a. Usually 6–10 units of platelets in adults; bring the platelet count to 50,000–100,000.

   b. One unit of platelets should raise the platelet count 5000–10,000 in adults.

   c. Etiologies
      (1) Dilutional.
      (2) Increased destruction (DIC, idiopathic thrombocytopenic purpura).
      (3) Sequestration (hypersplenism).

2. If **PT/PTT** is prolonged, but fibrinogen/split products are normal:

   a. These findings may be due to drug therapy or chronic disease.

   b. Fresh-frozen plasma should be administered while a screen for individual clotting factors is performed; specific factor therapy can then be instituted if a specific diagnosis is made.

   c. Vitamin K deficiency should be considered with liver disease, although acute administration of vitamin K will not be therapeutic immediately (see sec. **D**).

3. If **bleeding time** is prolonged, with platelet count and other clotting parameters normal:

   a. Indicates a functional platelet defect, such as von Willebrand's disease or chronic renal failure.

   b. Treat with platelet transfusions as needed while complete diagnosis is being made.

4. Prolonged **PT/PTT** with elevated **fibrin split products and thrombocytopenia** is compatible with a diagnosis of DIC (see sec. **VI**).

C. If the patient is known to be on **heparin,** hemostasis for surgery can be obtained by reversing heparin with protamine sulfate, generally 1 mg of protamine to reverse 90–100 units (0.9–1.0 mg) of heparin.

D. For emergency surgery on patients receiving **coumadin,** clotting factors may be acutely replaced with fresh-frozen plasma. Vitamin K takes at least several hours to reverse coumadin's effects.

1. Hypercoagulability can occur following reversal of coumadin effects by vitamin K.

   2. Postoperative reanticoagulation must be done with heparin.
   3. Vitamin K administration may prevent reanticoagulation with coumadin for some time.

VIII. Hemophilia
   A. These patients are very difficult to manage; in general, a hematologist should always be consulted preoperatively.
   B. **Factor VIII deficiency** (classical, hemophilia A). One unit of factor VIII/kg of body weight should increase activity by 2%. Heat-treated VIII concentrate and cryoprecipitate are the replacement products most commonly used.
   C. **Factor IX deficiency** (Christmas disease, hemophilia B). One unit of factor IX/kg should increase IX activity by 1%. Overreplacement can lead to thrombosis.
   D. For surgery, one should *attempt* to replace to 100% activity. However, peak levels and factor survival can be much less than calculated by replacement amount, as inhibitor antibodies may be present. Monitoring of levels is necessary, and full and consistent replacement may be difficult to achieve.
   E. DDAVP increases factor VIII levels. In patients with mild hemophilia or some types of von Willebrand's disease, DDAVP may be considered as an alternative to specific factor therapy or cryoprecipitate.

Suggested Reading

American Medical Association. *General Principles of Blood Transfusion.* Chicago: American Medical Association, 1985.

Demling, R. H. Fluid resuscitation after major burns. *J.A.M.A.* 250:1438, 1983.

Demling, R. H. *N. Engl. J. Med.* 313:1389, 1985.

G. R. Schwartz et al. (eds.). *Principles and Practice of Emergency Medicine* (2nd ed.). Philadelphia: Saunders, 1986. Pp. 1297–1421.

Martyn, J. A. J., and Szyfelbein, S. K. Pathophysiology and management of burn trauma in children. *Semin. Anesth.* 2:75, 1984.

Mollison, P. L. *Blood Transfusion in Clinical Medicine.* Oxford, Engl.: Blackwell, 1983.

Moncreif, J. A. Burns. *N. Engl. J. Med.* 288:444, 1973.

Petz, L. D., and Swisher, S. N. (eds.). *Clinical Practice of Blood Transfusion.* New York: Churchill Livingstone, 1981.

Steinbronn, K., and Huestis, D. W. Rationale for Blood Component Therapy. In B. R. Brown (ed.), *Fluid and Blood Therapy in Anesthesia.* Philadelphia: Davis, 1983. Pp. 151–168.

E. W. Wilkins (ed.). *M.G.H. Textbook of Emergency Medicine* (2nd ed.). Baltimore: Williams & Wilkins, 1983. Pp. 463–786.

28

Emergencies Complicating Anesthesia

Philip W. Lebowitz

I. Laryngospasm

A. Laryngospasm is most often brought about by an **irritative stimulus to the airway** during a light plane of anesthesia. Common noxious stimuli that are capable of eliciting this reflex include secretions, vomitus, or blood in the airway; inhalation of irritative anesthetics; oropharyngeal or nasopharyngeal airway placement; laryngoscopy; attempted endotracheal intubation; and positive-pressure ventilation. Movement of the head or neck, painful peripheral stimuli, and peritoneal traction can all cause laryngospasm during light anesthesia.

B. **Reflex closure of the vocal cords,** causing partial or total glottic obstruction, may be manifested in less severe cases by crowing respirations or stridor and, when complete, by "rocking," an obstructed pattern of breathing. In this situation, the abdominal wall rises with contraction of the diaphragm during inspiration, but because air entry is blocked, the chest sinks or fails to expand. During expiration, the abdomen falls as the diaphragm relaxes, and the chest returns to its original position. With complete obstruction, the anesthetist will not be able to ventilate the patient, even with a good mask fit.

C. The hypercarbia, hypoxia, and mixed acidosis that result will reflexively cause hypertension and tachycardia. Hypotension, bradycardia, and ventricular arrhythmias leading to cardiac arrest will ensue from hypoxia unless an open airway is restored within minutes. The greater amount of body oxygen stored, the longer will be the "protected" period until cerebral and myocardial hypoxemia develop. Small children, because of their small functional residual capacity and relatively high cardiac output, are particularly prone to these complications and require intervention within seconds.

D. **Treatment** must be prompt but not panicky. Deepening the anesthesia intravenously and removing the stimulus (e.g., by suction, withdrawal of an artificial airway, stopping peripheral stimulation) while administering 100% oxygen and watching expectantly are often adequate to permit normal breathing to resume. If, however, laryngospasm is not relieved within 1–2 minutes, steady positive pressure on the airway with a good mask fit may "break" the spasm. If this is still insufficient, a small dose of succinylcholine (e.g., 10–20 mg in an adult) will relax the striated muscles of the larynx. The patient should then be ventilated with 100% oxygen and the anesthesia deepened before the noxious stimulation is allowed to be resumed. If muscle relaxants are not available and spasm persists, ventilation through an emergency tracheostomy or a cricothyroid puncture with a large-bore needle must be accomplished as quickly as possible.

E. Care to avoid irritation of the pharynx, larynx, and trachea during light anesthesia will avert these difficulties under most circumstances. Topical application of local anesthetics (e.g., 4% lidocaine spray) prior to instrumentation and anesthetizing the trachea and larynx with 2% lidocaine injected into the trachea through the cricothyroid membrane are prophylactic measures. Extubation should be carried out either while the patient is relatively deeply anesthetized or after he has awakened; extubation during the intervening time increases the risk of laryngospasm.

II. Bronchospasm

A. Reflex bronchiolar constriction may be centrally mediated, as in asthma, or it may be a local response to airway irritation. Anaphylactoid drug and blood transfusion reactions are also characterized by bronchospasm. Cigarette smokers and those with chronic bronchitis have basically irritable airways and react more strenuously to stimulation. Like laryngospasm, bronchospasm may be elicited by noxious stimuli, such as secretions, vomitus, or blood in the pharynx, larynx, or trachea; artificial airways; laryngoscopy; endotracheal or inadvertent endobronchial intubation; positive-pressure ventilation; and surgical stimulation, traction, or head and neck movement during light anesthesia. Unilateral or localized wheezing is pathognomonic of aspiration during anesthesia.

B. Bronchospasm can be detected by characteristic wheezing (usually more pronounced on expiration) and is associated with tachypnea, dyspnea in the patient who is awake, decreased compliance during positive-pressure ventilation, tachycardia, and a lowered PaO_2. The anesthetized patient may, in fact, be unventilatable. The marked increase in airway pressure required for ventilation may, in addition, lead to wide changes in venous return and a lowering of cardiac output.

C. Drugs that predispose to bronchoconstriction through cholinomimetic stimulation include physostigmine, neostigmine, pyridostigmine, edrophonium, and barbiturates. Morphine, *d*-tubocurarine, metocurine, and atracurium may potentially promote bronchospasm through histamine release, but clinical significance is dubious. Propranolol, which blocks bronchodilation, is relatively contraindicated. Atropine tends to bronchodilate.

D. The **prevention** of bronchospasm, through care to achieve sufficiently deep levels of general anesthesia or topical local anesthesia prior to instrumentation, is usually easier than treating this reflex once it occurs. Good preoperative sedation in the susceptible patient is advised. A smooth induction followed by halothane (like diethyl ether, a direct bronchodilator) maintenance anesthesia may be safest; and should bronchospasm develop, deepening the anesthesia provides ready therapy.

E. It may be advisable, however, to use bronchodilators, such as aminophylline (5 mg/kg IV over 20–30 minutes as a loading dose, followed by infusion of 0.9 mg/kg/hr IV), particularly when already infusing and effective; isoproterenol or epinephrine infusions may have to be titrated to effect or hydrocortisone (100 mg IV) added in unrelenting cases. Worth noting, exogenous catecholamines given during halothane anesthesia are likely to cause ventricular irritability. All other factors being equal, extubation should be performed while the patient is deeply anesthetized, to avoid a bronchospastic reaction to the endotracheal tube.

III. Aspiration

A. The passage of vomited or regurgitated gastric contents or other foreign substances into the trachea and down to the smaller air units does not occur in patients with normal protective airway reflexes. In anesthetized or comatose patients and in awake elderly patients or debilitated patients of all ages, however, glottic closure and the cough mechanism do not function properly in response to foreign material in the airway. Aspiration is also more likely to take place during anesthesia in patients with a full stomach and in those with an incompetent lower esophageal sphincter.

B. **Effects** range from undetectable changes to sudden death, depending on the amount aspirated and its acidity (more severe effects with pH < 2.5). Clinical signs of aspiration include tachypnea, wheezing, tachycardia, hypotension, and hypoxia; apnea and bradycardia may also occur. Arterial blood sampling may support the diagnosis by revealing a low PaO_2. The radiologic picture may be one of pulmonary edema, though lobar consolidation (right lower lobe is the most common location) may be the only evidence; in fact, there may be no x-ray change, immediate or otherwise.

C. Prophylaxis and treatment

1. Prevention of aspiration may be approached by performing intubation with the patient awake, using rapid induction or regional anesthesia, or postponing surgery until gastric emptying has occurred, if feasible. Cimetidine or ranitidine (H_2-receptor blockers that inhibit basal gastric secretion, thereby raising the gastric pH to > 5.0) may be given PO or IV preoperatively to prevent acid aspiration. Nonparticulate antacids (e.g., citric acid solutions) are routinely given prophylactically to parturient patients undergoing anesthesia; metoclopramide, which promotes gastric emptying, may be of value in the same regard.

2. If **vomiting or regurgitation** is seen to occur and the airway is not sealed off by an endotracheal tube with an inflated cuff, the patient should immediately be placed head down (Trendelenburg position) with the head turned to one side. If possible, the patient's entire body should be turned on one side. The upper airway should be suctioned clear of foreign material; Magill forceps may help to remove solid particles. At the same time, the patient must be rapidly evaluated for laryngospasm, bronchospasm, and cardiovascular instability.

3. **If aspiration is suspected:**
   a. The patient should be intubated and ventilated with 100% oxygen, and the trachea suctioned clear; the pH of the suctioned material should be tested on litmus paper for prognostic purposes.
   b. Positive-pressure ventilation with positive end-expiratory pressure should be instituted to prevent atelectasis and hypoxia.

4. **In severe cases of aspiration:**
   a. Bronchoscopy may be required to remove particulate foreign material.
   b. Intravenous fluids as well as pressor and/or inotropic drugs should be given as needed to maintain cardiovascular stability.
   c. A chest x-ray and arterial blood sampling should be performed.
   d. Bronchodilators such as aminophylline may be required in the presence of hypoxia or poor pulmonary compliance.

5. Treatment with **steroids** remains controversial but is not recommended except in severe hypoxia and cardiovascular collapse.

6. **Antibiotics** are not used prophylactically. However, if sputum culture indicates the development of a bacterial infection, specific antibiotic therapy should be given.

IV. **Pneumothorax and pleural effusion**
   A. The presence of air, fluid, or both within a pleural space, compressing lung volume and occasionally causing mediastinal shift and rotation, is not a rare occurrence in patients undergoing anesthesia. These conditions may occur in the following situations:
      1. As a result of **chest trauma,** either blunt or penetrating.
      2. From **surgical violation of the visceral pleura** during intrathoracic surgery, surgery on the anterior triangle of the neck, radical mastectomy, tracheostomy, and upper abdominal or retroperitoneal surgery impinging on the diaphragm. A pneumothorax may appear after chest surgery because of a malfunctioning chest tube (e.g., one with a kink, lost connection, or lost water seal) or the development of a bronchopleural fistula.
      3. From **errant pleural puncture** during thoracentesis, pericardiocentesis, supraclavicular and intercostal nerve blocks, and subclavian and internal jugular venous catheterization.
      4. From **spontaneous rupture** of blebs, bullae, and subpleural foci of tuberculosis.

5. From **high inspiratory pressure** during positive-pressure ventilation. Pneumothorax may result from either alveolar rupture and eventual dissection through the visceral pleura or from direct rupture of an emphysematous bleb.

6. **Hemothorax** alone can be found with pleural metastases, pulmonary infarction, aneurysmal rupture, and rarely endometriosis of the pleura. Perforation of a great vein or pulmonary artery during catheterization may also occur.

7. **Pleural effusion** (hydrothorax when no blood is present) may be caused by congestive heart failure, pleural tumor or infection, and intrathoracic, extravascularly administered IV fluids.

B. **Small amounts of air or fluid** in the pleural space may cause no symptoms, although pleuritic chest pain and dyspnea occur commonly. Compression of the heart and great vessels causes hypotension and even cardiovascular collapse secondary to restricted stroke volume; tachycardia will be seen until bradycardia supervenes preterminally. With lung compression comes atelectasis, hypoxia, and cyanosis.

C. Decreased breath sounds, wheezing, and the presence of a sucking chest wound should raise clinical suspicion of **tension pneumothorax.** Increased difficulty in ventilating the patient, due to worsened compliance, should likewise evoke great concern. A chest x-ray, upright if possible, may confirm the diagnosis, although initially a small pneumothorax may not be evident.

D. In the **acute situation,** when cardiovascular collapse is imminent, a large-bore needle (or catheter) should be placed immediately to relieve air buildup; this may be inserted at the midclavicular line in the second or third intercostal space just above the rib (to avoid the neurovascular bundle). A syringe should be placed to cap the needle (or catheter) and prevent air entry. As soon as possible, a chest tube should be inserted and placed on water seal and suction, replacing the original needle (or catheter). For fluid drainage, the chest tube should be placed in the eighth intercostal space at the posterior axillary line.

E. From the standpoint of anesthesia, inspired nitrous oxide will equilibrate between its partial pressure in blood and that in the gas of the pneumothorax. Since nitrous oxide is approximately 31 times more soluble in blood than is nitrogen, movement of nitrous oxide into this closed gas space will not be balanced by movement of nitrogen into the blood. The net result is a marked increase in the volume of the pneumothorax, which worsens pulmonary and mediastinal compression. Consequently, **when pneumothorax is suspected, nitrous oxide should not be used.**

V. **Cardiac tamponade**

A. The presence of fluid (often blood) within the pericardial sac in amounts large enough to prevent cardiac filling and emptying is an unusual event in the anesthetized patient. However, cardiac tamponade

1. May be seen after sharp or blunt trauma to the chest.
2. Must always be considered in the postcardiac surgery patient.
3. Can occur in the presence of pericardial tumor or tuberculosis.
4. May be caused by myocardial perforation by a pulmonary artery or central venous pressure (CVP) catheter.

B. Decreased cardiac output, either sudden or gradual, may often present with tachycardia and hypotension. Pulse pressure decreases, an accentuated pulsus paradoxicus appears, heart sounds become muffled, neck vein distention is seen, and cyanosis may develop. The finding of a high right atrial pressure or high CVP is suggestive of tamponade. Further monitoring reveals near-identical values for mean CVP, mean pulmonary artery pressure, and mean pulmonary capillary wedge pressure. Other diagnostic tools include chest x-rays (showing widening of the mediastinal shadow), ECG, and echocardiography.

C. In the acute situation of a failing circulation and the clinical suspicion of cardiac tamponade, prompt **pericardiocentesis** (inserting a long needle between the xiphoid process and the left costal margin and directing it toward the left clavicle) can be both diagnostic and curative. If nonclotting blood is withdrawn, the patient's cardiovascular function should improve immediately.

If a second pericardiocentesis is needed, thoracotomy should soon follow. If the cardiac tamponade has been produced by pulmonary artery or CVP catheter perforation, treatment initially consists of withdrawing blood through the catheter rather than removing the catheter.

VI. Air embolism

A. Air may be drawn into the venous circulation during surgery involving large veins of the head, neck, thorax, abdomen, or pelvis. It may occur also during large-vein catheterization, during pneumoencephalography, and because of autotransfuser or cardiopulmonary bypass malfunction. It is to be watched for particularly during posterior fossa craniotomy with the patient in the sitting position. The danger of air embolism is more likely when the CVP is low.

B. Air in the venous circulation passes through the right side of the heart to enter the pulmonary circulation, where it blocks the movement of blood at the capillary level. Acute cor pulmonale may develop with hypotension, cardiac arrhythmias, hypoxia, and, when severe, cardiac arrest. A Doppler ultrasound, when the sensor is placed over the right atrium, is the most sensitive detector of air embolism. Other early findings include <u>decreased end-tidal carbon dioxide</u> concentration (or partial pressure) due to increased V_D/V_T and <u>increased pulmonary artery pressure</u>. A <u>millwheel murmur (caused by the turbulent mixing of blood and air)</u> or metallic heart sounds may be heard with an esophageal stethoscope, but these <u>are late results</u>.

C. **As soon as the diagnosis is entertained,** have the surgeons immediately <u>compress the open vein</u> or <u>flood the surgical field with saline solution</u> to stop the entry of air. Simultaneously, limit air entry by positioning the patient so that the heart is higher than the open vein. If much air has already entered, turn the patient to the <u>left lateral decubitus position</u> with the <u>head downward</u> to keep air in the right atrium from moving into the right ventricle. <u>Withdraw air</u> (and blood) through a CVP line (if placed in the right atrium prior to surgery) while giving blood or other fluids through a second IV line. Discontinue anesthetics and administer 100% oxygen while treating arrhythmias and maintaining cardiovascular stability pharmacologically.

D. **Arterial air emboli** may be seen during cardiopulmonary bypass and whenever venous air emboli occur in the presence of a right-to-left intracardiac shunt. Assiduous avoidance of air bubbles in the intravenous infusion is essential when any intracardiac communication exists. Air entering the coronary arteries can rapidly produce ventricular fibrillation and cardiac arrest. Heroic treatment—clamping the aorta, aspirating the ventricle, and performing manual cardiac compression—may avert catastrophe. Arterial air emboli entering the cerebral circulation can cause brain infarction and severe neurologic dysfunction.

VII. Malignant hyperthermia

A. Malignant hyperthermia, a life-threatening disorder of skeletal muscle, should be suspected in patients with a suggestive family or personal history of anesthetic mishap. <u>Malignant hyperthermia is believed due to the decrease in calcium (Ca^{2+}) reuptake by the sarcoplasmic reticulum, resulting in increased resting intracellular Ca^{2+} levels</u>. Rapid rises in intracellular Ca^{2+} levels can occur in susceptible individuals with exposure to triggering agents. The consequent acceleration of both aerobic and anaerobic cellular metabolic processes results in excessive heat, carbon dioxide, and lactic acid production. Malignant hyperthermia can be triggered by all volatile anesthetics, particularly in association with succinylcholine. Cases of malignant hyperthermia have been reported in which, as part of their anesthesia, patients have received IV ketamine, narcotics, barbiturates, and nondepolarizing muscle relaxants. (<u>Notwithstanding concerns expressed in the literature, there have been no reports of amino-amide local anesthetic–triggered episodes.</u>) The specific contribution of these drugs toward triggering malignant hyperthermia is not as clear as is the case for volatile anesthetics and suc-

[margin note: not reuptake but release.]

cinylcholine. It usually appears during anesthesia but may occur postoperatively. The lack of triggering an episode of malignant hyperthermia during a previous (or several previous) anesthetic(s) does not guarantee successful passage through the anesthetic at hand.

B. The anesthesiologist should entertain the diagnosis if any of the following occurs:
1. Unexplained tachycardia.
2. Unexplained cyanosis and tachypnea.
3. Rigidity after succinylcholine administration, or failure of the masseters to relax for intubation. However, the rigidity may present at any time or may never occur.
4. **Fever.** The normal anesthetized patient does not become hyperthermic if the room temperature is below 25.5°C. Regard any rise in temperature of more than 0.5°C in 15 minutes as possible malignant hyperthermia. Fever is a late sign and carries a poor prognosis if therapy has not yet been started.

C. To confirm the diagnosis, the anesthesiologist should
1. Obtain an arterial sample for blood gases and electrolytes. Malignant hyperthermia produces hypoxemia, severe respiratory and metabolic acidosis, and hyperkalemia. A simultaneously obtained peripheral venous sample showing elevated PCO_2 is diagnostic even earlier in the course of the episode. Oximetry or end-tidal carbon dioxide measurements, if available, are valuable diagnostic tools.
2. Double-check the temperature with another thermometer, and exclude other causes, such as a malfunctioning warming blanket.
3. Look for sources of septicemia as an alternative diagnosis.

D. Specific treatment. Dantrolene (Dantrium) specifically attenuates Ca^{2+} release from the sarcoplasmic reticulum to lower intracellular Ca^{2+} levels. The starting dose is 1–2 mg/kg IV, which may be repeated every 5–10 minutes toward a total dose of 10 mg/kg (but more as needed) if symptoms persist. This is the most important treatment, and if quickly employed, need for symptomatic therapy will be minimized. Dantrolene should be continued for 3 days after the episode, to prevent recurrence. The oral dosage is 1–2 mg/kg/day in divided doses.

E. Symptomatic treatment
1. Hyperventilate the patient with 100% oxygen.
2. Stop all anesthetics (and procure another anesthesia machine—with brand-new breathing tubes when convenient). No further anesthesia is needed.
3. Stop surgery as soon as possible.
4. Give sodium bicarbonate ($NaHCO_3$) IV (2–4 mEq/kg) as soon as the first arterial blood gas sample is sent. Once the results of blood gas analysis are

available, administer $NaHCO_3$ according to the following calculations:

$$mEq\ HCO_3 = \frac{\text{Base deficit} \times \text{body weight (kg)}}{3}$$

Since the acidosis is usually severe, it will be hard to overcompensate, and repeated doses may be required. Place an arterial line to follow acid-base balance and blood gases.

5. If **hyperkalemia** is severe and cardiac arrhythmias appear, give regular insulin, 20 units IV, with 50 ml of 50% glucose. As the attack is controlled, transient hypokalemia may be seen, but it should not be treated with potassium replacement unless cardiac arrhythmias occur.

6. **Cooling the patient**

   a. **Children** have a relatively large surface area compared with body weight and can be effectively cooled with surface methods. Apply a cooling blanket, and place ice bags around the neck, axillae, and groin—points where major vessels are close to the surface. Refrigerated saline solution may be given IV. If all these measures fail, immerse the child in a tub of ice water.

   b. **Adults** can be packed in ice, particularly covering the neck, axillae, and groin. Lavage any surgically opened cavities with iced solutions, administer refrigerated saline solution IV, and perform gastric, rectal, and bladder irrigations with iced solutions. Where available, cardiopulmonary bypass can be lifesaving; extracorporeal cooling is the most effective method of heat exchange.

   c. Stop the cooling when the temperature reaches 38°C; restart if and when the temperature begins to rise again.

7. Maintain a high urine output (2 ml/kg/hr) to protect the renal tubules from being damaged by myoglobin and hemoglobin. The combination of tubular myoglobin or hemoglobin inspissation and uncontrolled acidosis, hypovolemia, and hypotension is likely to produce acute tubular necrosis. Start mannitol (25 gm IV), furosemide (20 mg IV), and copious intravenous fluids, and repeat until diuresis occurs; insert an indwelling urinary catheter.

F. **Anesthesia for susceptible patients.** Stress and anxiety should be avoided in the preoperative period. Dantrolene (6 mg/kg) should be given orally in divided doses the day before surgery or 1 mg/kg IV prior to anesthesia. The patient should be well premedicated with fentanyl or droperidol, or both. Local or regional anesthesia is preferred. In the absence of incontrovertible evidence indicating specific narcotics, barbiturates, or relaxants, consensus holds that if general anesthesia is necessary, the safest agents include nitrous oxide, thiopental, fentanyl, droperidol, and pancuronium.

VIII. Transfusion reactions

A. The transfusion of blood products in any form carries certain risks: the transmission of hepatitis, acquired immunodeficiency syndrome (AIDS), malaria, and infectious bacteria; the dilution of the recipient's own platelets and clotting factors; and the administration of mismatched blood, because of either a blood-banking error or anesthetist error in giving properly matched blood to the wrong patient.

B. Leukocyte reactions (found especially in patients who have had multiple transfusions) may not be detected in vitro by standard techniques. The first sign of incompatibility may be an in vivo reaction. For this reason, washed frozen red cells (buffy-coat–poor packed red cells) are the transfusion form of choice for these patients.

C. Mild transfusion reactions may present with stinging or burning along the vein of administration, itching, flushing, urticaria, headache, myalgias and arthralgias (particularly in the flank and low back), chills and fever, and malaise. Along the spectrum toward more severe reactions are hypotension and tachycardia, bronchospasm and respiratory distress, hemolysis, and a generalized clotting deficit. A full-fledged anaphylactic reaction with cardiovascular collapse may occur in the extreme case. Hemoglobinuria may accompany hemolysis; when combined with decreased renal blood flow, acute tubular necrosis may result.

D. For the anesthetized patient, transfusion reactions provide added risk in that they may not be detected until hypotension, bronchospasm, high fever, oliguria, or diffuse oozing in the surgical field becomes severe enough to demand explanation. For this reason, transfusion after surgery is safer, unless cardiovascular stability requires intraoperative blood replacement.

E. As soon as a transfusion reaction is suspected, any blood being given at that time should be taken down immediately. About 10 ml of venous blood should be drawn and sent to the blood bank for tests of hemolysis and for repeat cross-matching. A urine sample should be analyzed for the presence of hemoglobin. The circulation must be maintained, with pressors if necessary, and the renal tubules should be kept open with mannitol-induced diuresis and IV fluid administration. Epinephrine (1 mg in 250 ml of saline as an infusion) may be titrated to counter anaphylaxis, and antihistamines, such as diphenhydramine (25–50 mg IV or IM), may offer symptomatic relief.

IX. High spinal anesthesia

A. The factors that affect the level of spinal cord function interruption after subarachnoid introduction of anesthetic agents include

1. Baricity or specific gravity of the anesthetic solution relative to that of the cerebrospinal fluid.

2. The position of the patient during and after the injection, until the spinal is "fixed."
3. The volume of the anesthetic solution.
4. The total dose of anesthetic agent.
5. The speed and force of injection; the use of barbotage (the repeated aspiration and injection of solution to increase turbulence and flow).

Any number of these factors may combine to give a level much higher than intended. In addition, the inadvertent subarachnoid injection of local anesthetic solution during epidural anesthesia can also produce a total spinal.

B. After completing the injection, the anesthesiologist must frequently check both blood pressure and anesthetic level. As the spinal ascends, blood pressure may fall secondary to preganglionic sympathetic block, causing arteriolar dilatation and decreased venous tone, which in turn will cause decreased cardiac output. Hypotension may progress into a shock state unless volume and pressor administration is instituted. Ephedrine (in 5-mg IV increments) or phenylephrine (10 mg in a 250-ml IV infusion) is commonly titrated to restore sympathetic tone and support blood pressure. Because of its indirect beta-sympathomimetic effect, ephedrine is susceptible to tachyphylaxis on repeated dosings. In large single doses, ventricular irritability and hypertension commonly occur.

Nausea and vomiting, caused by vagal stimulation unopposed by sympathetic nervous system activity, often accompany a rising spinal level and may be treated with atropine. Since nausea and vomiting may be the first sign of a high spinal, blood pressure and breathing ability must be checked immediately.

C. The progressive failure of intercostal muscle movement during inspiration and increased diaphragm activity, along with dyspnea and even loss of consciousness, indicate a high thoracic motor block. Loss of diaphragm (C3, 4, 5) activity, the appearance of nasal flaring, and the use of the sternocleidomastoid and other accessory muscles of respiration indicate that a cervical level has been attained. Although mask ventilation may be adequate, it is prudent to intubate the patient for better airway control and to provide ventilatory assistance until the spinal effect recedes over the next 20–30 minutes. Muscle relaxants may not be required to perform the intubation, and sedation at this point is often not necessary.

29

Recovery Room

David J. Stone

While the recovery room (RR) phase of most anesthetics is uncomplicated, a recent survey at the Massachusetts General Hospital indicates that one or more untoward RR "events" occur after approximately 4% of anesthetics (see Chap. 9). In conjunction with an alert and experienced nursing staff, the RR physician should be able to prevent or treat such problems. It is important to recognize that the most skillful anesthesia and surgery can be undone, or even converted to frank disaster, if RR care is inadequate.

I. **Report.** After the patient arrives in the RR, the admitting nurse should be given a complete but succinct report. The RR physician should also receive a report on cases that have been complicated in any way. Reports should include
   A. Brief synopsis of **prior medical problems** including medications and allergies.
   B. All **medications** administered, including usual medications that have been continued in the perioperative period; premedications; anesthetic agents, including the concentration of inhaled and precise dose of IV anesthetics, relaxants, narcotics, sedatives, vasopressors, inotropes, antiarrhythmics, vasodilators, antihypertensives, and antibiotics.
   C. Course of anesthesia with specific description of problems.
   D. Exact nature of the surgical procedure and the names of the responsible surgeons, who should inform the nurses separately regarding placement and care of drains, patient positioning, and so on.
   E. Descriptions of intravascular cannulas and endotracheal tube, if present; reason for continued intubation and status of patient's mask airway, ease of intubation; status of ventilation and oxygenation.
   F. Extent of residual neuromuscular blockade and/or reversal.
   G. Intraoperative fluids and blood administered, estimated blood loss, and urine output; laboratory values.
   H. Any special features of the patient should be noted, such as blindness, deafness, non–English speaking (and the language the patient speaks); psychiatric, drug, or alcohol problems.
   I. If a patient is unstable in any way, the operating room (OR) anesthesiologist must remain in the RR, until the RR nurses and physician feel that they are ready to assume responsibility for management.

II. **Airway difficulties in the recovery room**
   A. **Inability to "maintain an airway"** may occur in patients who arrive extubated or in those extubated in the RR. The most common cause is obstruction due to the tongue and pharyngeal soft tissues falling backward and occluding the airway. Cardinal signs are lack of air

movement, intercostal and suprasternal retractions, and abdominal wall motion unaccompanied by chest wall elevation. While oxygen is administered, the following maneuvers are used to establish a patent airway:

1. **Neck extension accompanied by chin-lift or jaw-thrust.** If cervical spine surgery has been done, neck extension may be contraindicated.

2. **Repositioning into the lateral decubitus or fully prone position.** The lateral and prone positions may relieve tongue obstruction of the airway, but ventilation may be harder to monitor.

3. **Insertion of an oral or nasal airway.** Nasal airways may be better tolerated in the semiconscious patient and less likely to provoke laryngospasm, salivation, vomiting, or bronchospasm. Before any nasal instrumentation (airway, endotracheal tube, nasogastric tube), the administration of a few drops of 0.25% phenylephrine will vasoconstrict the nasal mucosa to enlarge the area for passage and reduce bleeding. The nasal airway can be lubricated with 5% lidocaine ointment for analgesia. If a nasal airway is not available, an endotracheal tube (6.0–7.5-mm internal diameter [ID]) can be inserted through the nose as far as the posterior pharynx. Occasionally, nasal and oral airways used together are required to relieve obstruction.

4. **Examine the oropharynx** for copious secretions, blood clots, or even forgotten surgical packing and other unexpected foreign bodies.

5. If obstruction cannot be relieved by the measures outlined above, the patient should be gently ventilated with 100% O_2 mask and bag. Endotracheal intubation may be required.

6. If intubation cannot be accomplished, a **cricothyroidotomy** should be performed by the most skillful person available. An uncuffed 5-mm ID endotracheal tube may be used to provide the initial resuscitative ventilation. Alternatively, a 14-gauge cannula can be placed through the cricothyroid membrane and ventilation accomplished by high-pressure wall O_2. However, this provides an extremely small airway and depends on some patency in the upper airway to pop off the high intratracheal pressures that are generated.

7. If surgery has been performed in the area of the airway (thyroid, parathyroid, carotid artery, neck dissection), a **hematoma** may form that can compress the airway. Dressings should be removed and the wound examined. If airway obstruction from hematoma is present, endotracheal intubation may be attempted, despite airway distortion. However, if life-threatening obstruction continues and ventilation is impossible, the wound should be opened to relieve the airway compression and intubation reattempted.

B. **Intubated patients.** Often, patients are brought to the RR while still intubated. Common reasons include

1. **Inability to reverse neuromuscular blockade.** If maximal pharmacologic reversal has been given (neostigmine, 0.07 mg/kg, or edrophonium, 1 mg/kg) and there are no treatable causes of respiratory inefficiency, ventilation should continue while the patient is monitored for adequate recovery . Reversal of neuromuscular blockade should be monitored by peripheral nerve stimulation, bedside pulmonary function, and inspiratory pressure testing, and observing grip strength and ability to elevate the head for 5 seconds (see Chap. 11). While the latter maneuver may be painful in certain patients, it may be the best clinical indicator of recovered muscle strength and ability to maintain an airway.

2. **Difficult airway.** If a patient had a known or unexpectedly difficult mask airway or intubation, the endotracheal tube should be left in place until the patient is fully conscious, that is, easily arousable to verbal stimuli. In semiconscious patients who are "bucking" on the tube, light sedation is appropriate until volatile or narcotic anesthetic agents can wear off more completely. Do not be misled into extubation solely because patients appear to be uncomfortable; "bucking" may be exchanged for laryngospasm when the tube is removed. When in doubt, it is probably best to maintain intubation by means of sedation.

3. **Full stomach.** Scrupulous prevention of aspiration must be continued in the RR; laryngeal reflexes must return before extubating patients with "full stomachs."

4. **Poor gas exchange.** Inadequate oxygenation and CO_2 elimination are often resolved in the RR as the effects of anesthesia, positioning, and surgical retraction fade. If they do not, as a result of intrinsic pulmonary dysfunction, the responsible surgeon and anesthesiologist should be consulted regarding transfer to an intensive care unit.

5. **Hemodynamic instability.** If hemodynamic instability is present from unexpected bleeding, low cardiac output, or sepsis, it is usually wisest to postpone extubation. Bleeding may require reexploration, low cardiac output may adversely affect oxygenation, and sepsis may precede an episode of noncardiogenic pulmonary edema.

6. **"Slow to awaken" patient.** Intubation may continue because patients are too deeply anesthetized to extubate.

7. **Mandibular wiring or banding.** These patients should not be extubated until fully awake. Scissors or wire cutters must be available at the bedside for emergency oral reintubation.

8. Patients who are hypothermic, because shivering

may increase total body and myocardial O_2 consumption by several-fold.

9. Neurosurgical patients in whom central nervous system depression interferes with their ability to maintain and protect their airways.

10. Patients with cervical spine procedures or injury.

11. In contrast, in individuals with myocardial ischemia or increased intracranial pressure (ICP), an endotracheal tube may be detrimental when hypertension and tachycardia result. Provided these patients meet extubation criteria, they should be extubated as soon as is reasonable.

C. **Laryngospasm.** The larynx may close during emergence from anesthesia or just after extubation. Frequently, laryngospasm is associated with mechanical irritation of the glottis by secretions, blood, airway manipulation, and so on.

1. Initial treatment includes the administration of 100% O_2 with anterior mandibular displacement. Gentle continuous positive airway pressure (CPAP) may be applied by mask. If complete obstruction continues, a small dose of succinylcholine (10–20 mg) will open the vocal cords sufficiently to allow ventilation; ventilation must be continued until the relaxant has worn off.

2. Children appear to be more susceptible to laryngospasm, and if extubation has not been accomplished while the patient is deeply anesthetized, intubation should continue until the child is awake.

3. The anesthesiologist should be prepared to treat laryngospasm (tonsil-tip suction, O_2, mask and positive-pressure bag, relaxants, intubation equipment always available) following all extubations.

D. **Laryngotracheal problems after short-term intubation**

1. **Airway swelling**

a. **Glottic edema** may follow traumatic intubations, head and neck surgical manipulation, excessive coughing and "bucking," toxic or allergic reactions to the tube material or an applied lubricant, or irritation by gastric contents. Definitive diagnosis may require fiberoptic laryngoscopy. Obstruction may initially be diagnosed by listening over the trachea for inspiratory stridor. Obstruction is exacerbated during inspiration when the extrathoracic tracheal wall is pulled inward by negative pressure in the airway. Note that a diminution in stridor may not indicate improvement but instead that less air is being exchanged, indicating deterioration. The issue is easily resolved by observing and feeling for air movement.

b. **Subglottic edema** is extremely uncommon in adults but occurs fairly often in small children because the rigid cricoid cartilage is the narrowest part of the pediatric airway and cannot expand. Other predisposing factors include the use of an oversized or inappropriately cuffed endotracheal tube and a recent upper respiratory infection.

  c. Treatment of glottic and/or subglottic edema includes

    (1) Administration of warmed, humidified O_2 by mask.

    (2) Inhalation of racemic epinephrine 2.25% (0.5–1 ml in 2 ml of normal saline); repeat in 20 minutes as needed, then continue every 4 hours as needed.

    (3) Administration of dexamethasone IV (0.5 mg/kg, to a total of 10 mg in patients > 20 kg) before extubation to patients who may be at high risk for developing subglottic edema. Though the effectiveness of steroids (and epinephrine) has not been conclusively demonstrated, clinical experience favors their use. Dexamethasone may also be administered by Medihaler (2 puffs every 4 hours).

    (4) If these measures fail, reintubation with a smaller tube to relieve the obstruction.

  2. Vocal cord paralysis must be considered when surgery has been performed in the area of the recurrent laryngeal nerves. It is a very rare complication of endotracheal intubation alone and is thought to be due to compression of the nerve by the cuff in those cases. Unilateral paralysis should not cause airway obstruction unless the other vocal cord is edematous. Then the situation may be managed as glottic edema. Sometimes, direct or fiberoptic laryngoscopy is performed in the OR after thyroid surgery to document vocal cord movement. Reintubation is indicated if airway obstruction occurs due to bilateral cord paralysis.

  3. Hoarseness and sore throat are commonly encountered in the RR; however, a sore throat rarely indicates laryngotracheal damage and almost always resolves without treatment. Occasionally, these symptoms may even occur in patients who have not been intubated.

  4. Laryngeal incompetence. There may be some residual inability to protect the airway from aspiration, even after short periods of intubation. However, this issue is not clinically significant for patients intubated less than 8 hours.

E. Bronchospasm. In intubated patients, nonbronchospastic wheezing may be caused by obstruction of the endotracheal tube (by clot, mucous plug, foreign body, overinflated cuff, bevel against the tracheal wall, kinked tube, patient biting down on oral tube), tension pneumothorax, congestive heart failure (CHF), endobronchial intubation, or nasogastric tube misplacement.

If suprabronchiolar causes of wheezing have been excluded, treatment of bronchospasm may be entertained. In general, clinical status (dyspnea, respiratory rate and pattern, observed effort to breathe, airway pressures if ventilated, and, most importantly, gas exchange) determines the need for and extent of treatment. Medications and other treatments for bronchospasm are discussed in Chap. 32.

III. **Cardiovascular difficulties in the recovery room**

A. **Hypotension.** First, rule out artifacts; due to technical difficulties, discrepancies may exist between arterial catheter or automated oscillometer measurements and those determined by palpation of the pulse and cuff pressure by Korotkoff sounds or Doppler. In patients with extensive peripheral vascular disease, pressures may differ between extremities or may be difficult to obtain in a given extremity. If still unresolved, a central arterial pressure may be obtained by means of a 6-inch, 18-gauge axillary arterial catheter.

1. Once it is established that hypotension is not an artifact, **possible causes** are then considered. In the RR, hypotension is most commonly caused by intravascular hypovolemia. Other possibilities include residual myocardial depression from the administered anesthetic (especially with underlying CHF), perioperative myocardial ischemia or infarct, pericardial tamponade due to ventricular puncture by a central catheter, and tension pneumothorax related to central catheter placement, regional anesthesia, or inadvertent surgical entrance into the pleura. In addition, bradycardia, hypoxemia, anaphylaxis or anaphylactoid reaction, sepsis precipitated by intraoperative instrumentation or manipulation, vasodilatation due to rewarming or drugs, unsuspected adrenal insufficiency, or hypothyroidism can each cause hypotension in the RR.

2. The anesthetic record is quickly reviewed for an overview of intraoperative fluid balance.

   a. It must be judged whether crystalloid and blood product administration was adequate to replace the estimated blood loss, maintenance fluid requirement, and insensible losses. (Postoperative bleeding must also be included in the accounting.) The hematocrit and appropriate coagulation studies should be checked and samples sent for typing and cross-matching, if necessary.

   b. Treatment often begins with elevation of the patient's legs; if the mean arterial blood pressure is reduced by more than 20% from preoperative levels, it may be wise to administer a small fluid bolus (about 250 ml of Ringer's lactate of normal saline in the adult) during evaluation. A small dose of vasopressor (e.g., 5–15 mg IV ephedrine) may be necessary if the hypotension is severe.

    c. As patients warm and vasodilate in the RR, as much as 500–1000 ml of additional crystalloid may be required to avoid hypotension. Administration of additional crystalloid or blood will correct the majority of hypotensive episodes following general anesthesia. Following epidural or spinal anesthesia, phenylephrine IV (start at 20 µg/min and titrate) or boluses of ephedrine may be necessary to limit the amount of crystalloid administered.

3. It is difficult to be absolutely certain of intravascular volume postoperatively.

    a. Patients may appear edematous from tissue trauma, gravitational effects of positioning, and excess extracellular volume but actually are intravascularly depleted. In the absence of diuretic administration, hyperglycemia, or urinary concentrating defect, a urine output of greater than 1 ml/kg/hr argues strongly against hypovolemia. In patients remaining unacceptably hypotensive after a prudent fluid challenge, **invasive monitoring** is indicated to distinguish between hypovolemia and pump failure.

    b. A central venous pressure (CVP) catheter is probably adequate to monitor patients with normal left ventricular function, but a pulmonary artery catheter is preferable for patients with left ventricular dysfunction or suspected myocardial ischemia. Pulmonary artery catheters also allow rapid and repeated determinations of cardiac output, stroke volume, and calculation of systemic vascular resistance, which are critical guides to therapy. Cardiac outputs can be obtained with a CVP (and arterial cannula) by the dye dilution technique, but it is expensive, cumbersome, and requires a trained technician.

    c. If stroke volume is normal (60–80 ml/beat), then hypovolemia is excluded. A low stroke volume does not distinguish between hypovolemia and cardiac dysfunction, but in conjunction with information regarding filling pressures (pulmonary capillary wedge pressure or CVP) following fluid infusion, stroke volume can be used to guide therapy. Elucidating the role of cardiac output versus systemic vascular resistance in the hypotension will indicate whether inotropes, vasopressors, or vasodilators should be chosen if support becomes necessary.

4. The choice of fluid used to restore intravascular volume is controversial. Large amounts of crystalloid (6–10 liters) may be administered to patients with normal capillary integrity, but septic or severely traumatized patients may develop "leaky capillar-

ies" and require careful fluid resuscitation. In addition, patients who have difficulty handling large amounts of resorbed fluid over 2–4 days postoperatively (elderly, CHF, renal dysfunction) may benefit from 250–1000 ml of 5% albumin instead of additional crystalloids. Hydroxyethyl starch (Hetastarch) 6% is a less expensive alternative. If blood and fresh-frozen plasma are indicated, other colloids become unnecessary.

B. **Hypertension.** Pain, inadequately treated preexisting hypertension, hypercarbia, and bladder distention are common reasons for hypertension in the RR.

1. Treatment is not always necessary. In healthy individuals moderate hypertension (30% elevation of mean arterial blood pressure) is not harmful in itself. If CHF, coronary disease, cerebrovascular disease, or increased intracranial pressure is present, treatment should begin before physiologic consequences occur.

2. Adequate oxygenation and ventilation should be maintained.

3. As a rule, postoperative hypertension is transient, requiring drug treatment for only a few hours. Choices include the following:

   a. **Hydralazine** (5–20 mg IV). Disadvantages include delayed onset of action (about 15 minutes) and reflex tachycardia (which may be blunted by simultaneous administration of a beta blocker).

   b. **Beta blockers** such as propranolol (in 0.5-mg IV increments for adults) and metoprolol (in 5-mg IV increments) are quite useful because high catecholamine levels are likely to be present. They do not increase intracranial pressure and may improve cardiac ischemia. They should be used with caution if there is a history of CHF or chronic obstructive pulmonary disease and avoided if bronchospasm is active. Labetalol (in 5-mg IV increments), a combined alpha and beta blocker, acts more rapidly and predictably than the combination of propranolol and hydralazine.

   c. If myocardial ischemia is a concern, dermal **nitroglycerin** (1–4 inches every 8 hours) or IV nitroglycerin (start at 10–20 µg/min) is useful. **Nifedipine** (10–20 mg sublingually) may also be used.

   d. **Methyldopa (Aldomet)** IV does not take effect for several hours, so it is not useful in treatment of acute hypertension. It is used perioperatively to prevent rebound hypertension after discontinuing clonidine.

   e. Refractory hypertension can be treated with **sodium nitroprusside** (SNP) but is seldom indicated in the RR. A very labile blood pressure during SNP use may represent underlying hypovolemia unmasked by vasodilatation. Blood pressure should be monitored by intraarterial catheter if SNP is used.

C. **Dysrhythmias.** Staff in the RR may be confronted by the following:

1. **Premature atrial contractions** seldom require treatment as long as blood pressure is stable. Work up as per premature ventricular contractions if judged necessary.

2. **Premature ventricular contractions** (PVCs) are very common postoperatively and do not necessarily indicate underlying heart disease. If present preoperatively, work up should proceed, but treatment threshold should be higher. Hypokalemia, hypoxia, and hypercarbia should be ruled out. If pain is stimulating sympathetic output, then morphine may be the drug of choice. A central catheter may cause ectopy by mechanical irritation of the right ventricle. A more grave possibility is myocardial ischemia, necessitating review of a 12-lead ECG. PVCs occur in the setting of myocardial ischemia, produce hypotension, and may be coupled or multifocal; lidocaine (1.5 mg/kg IV bolus, then 1–4 mg/min) should be administered.

3. **Atrial fibrillation** may appear following thoracic surgery in the settings of high catecholamine output, or accompanying abrupt fluctuations in volume status. Beta blockers, verapamil (2.5- to 5.0-mg increments), or digoxin (0.25-mg increments with additional 0.25-mg doses at 2- to 4-hour intervals up to 1.0–1.5 mg) may be used. When used in combination, however, bradycardia, heart block, or severe hypotension may result.

D. **Myocardial ischemia or infarction**

1. **Definite ischemia.** Unambiguous ECG evidence of myocardial ischemia (> 1 mm S–T elevation or depression, hyperacute or deeply inverted T waves) is a medical emergency. **Treatment** consists in immediate O_2 administration, analgesia if necessary, and nitrates, beta blockers, and/or calcium channel antagonists. Treatment should begin with IV nitroglycerin until mean arterial blood pressure has been reduced by about 10%. (Nitroglycerin may be given without intraarterial monitoring, but an arterial cannula should be inserted if blood pressure is low or labile.)

2. Perioperative myocardial infarctions have a higher mortality rate than those occurring in other settings.

3. **Possible ischemia.** Electrocardiograms obtained in the RR may show T-wave flattening or minimal inversion, sometimes associated with slight (< 1 mm) S–T depression. Comparison with a previous ECG is essential, if one is available, as such "changes" may actually represent baseline abnormalities (or normal variants). In fact, T-wave

changes found in the RR setting are unlikely to represent ischemia, even in patients with coronary disease. Cold, stress, invasive surgery, electrolyte abnormalities, various drug effects, and extracardiac disease are factors that may nonspecifically alter the ECG. A repeat ECG in a normothermic patient who is no longer in severe pain may reveal improvement or even complete resolution of the changes. In short, these patients do not seem to suffer adverse outcomes or require invasive monitoring. Nevertheless, it is advisable to continue close surveillance (daily ECGs) into the postoperative period.

E. Oliguria

1. Oliguria (< 0.5 ml/kg/hr of urine) is usually a result of some hemodynamic derangement. However, mechanical causes must be eliminated, that is, obstructed Foley catheter or need for bladder catheterization. If the bladder is empty, hypovolemia is likely. Postrenal causes include ureter ligation or renal vein compression from very high intraabdominal pressures. Other etiologies of oliguria are discussed in Chap. 4.

2. Diuretics should not be administered routinely, as they may both confound diagnostic studies and worsen hypovolemia. Once intravascular volume and cardiac output have been optimized, mannitol, loop diuretics, or low-dose dopamine (1–3 μg/kg/min) may be used to increase urine volume.

IV. Pain

A. Pain control (see Chap. 33) is an essential part of RR care. It is advisable to wait 15–20 minutes between doses of IV narcotics to observe the patient for respiratory depression because many of the drugs used in anesthesia (inhaled anesthetics, preoperative or intraoperative narcotics, barbiturates, relaxants, benzodiazepines) may combine with postoperative narcotics to produce hypoventilation. Anesthetic records should be studied carefully for the amounts and times of administration of such drugs.

B. Postoperative agitation may be due to pain but may result from hypoxia or other causes. Oxygenation, ventilation, and hemodynamic performance should be reviewed before patients are medicated. Sedation of the hypoxic patient is an all too common reason for cardiopulmonary arrest in the RR and elsewhere.

C. In adults not taking monoamine oxidase inhibitors, meperidine (25–50 mg IV) can be used in place of morphine although it may increase heart rate. Some outpatient centers prefer fentanyl (25 μg IV doses in adults) or agonists/antagonists like butorphanol (Stadol) for analgesia in order to avoid late respiratory depression. Children may receive morphine in 0.02 mg/kg IV doses, although it must be used with great care in infants under 6 months of age, who may be more susceptible to respiratory depression.

D. After regional anesthesia, narcotics may be required as the block recedes. Epidural narcotics are often useful in this setting; regimens may be found in Chap. 33.

E. Administration of a local nerve block diminishes the need for analgesia in the RR. Intercostal blocks provide analgesia and improve chest wall expansion after thoracotomy or upper abdominal surgery. Their use is most safely limited to patients with chest tubes already in place because of the risk of pneumothorax. The block can be performed with a 23-gauge needle and 3–4 ml of 0.5% bupivacaine (with or without epinephrine) per segment, up to a total bupivacaine dose of 3 mg/kg.

F. Transcutaneous nerve stimulators have also been used to treat postoperative pain. They involve little risk and may be started in the RR.

G. Administration of methadone (2.5–10.0 mg IV in increments) to patients in intensive care unit settings has also been described and seems to provide excellent analgesia for up to 24 hours.

H. Naloxone (Narcan) is the only pure narcotic antagonist presently available. To reverse narcotic-induced respiratory depression, naloxone should be administered in small IV increments (40–100 μg), as sudden large boluses can precipitate nausea and vomiting, dysrhythmias, hypertension, and pulmonary edema. Large doses will also eliminate all analgesia and produce a very uncomfortable patient. Naloxone, with a duration of about 45 minutes after IV administration, is generally shorter acting than the narcotics. The reversal dose may be doubled when given IM to last 2–4 hours. Nevertheless, patients who receive naloxone must be monitored for a period sufficient to assure that renarcotization does not occur.

V. **Hypoxemia.** Although arterial blood gases are required to quantify arterial oxygenation, pulse oximeters provide a rapid and noninvasive measure of hemoglobin saturation. Almost instantaneously, this value will indicate whether to withhold or begin evaluation or therapy. Cyanosis is an extremely late sign and may not appear as soon as oxygenation becomes inadequate.

A. In the RR, **diminished FIO_2** is a rare cause of hypoxemia (i.e., wall O_2 malfunction).

B. Hypoxemia may be due to hypoventilation with low tidal volumes leading to atelectasis and $\dot{V}A/\dot{Q}$ abnormalities. Functional residual capacity may also be reduced by abdominal distention (pregnancy, obesity, ascites, postoperative distention), surgical dressings, and abdominal pain.

C. Other causes of $\dot{V}A/\dot{Q}$ mismatch include intrapulmonary shunts, increased O_2 consumption, or reduction in cardiac output. Postoperative $\dot{V}A/\dot{Q}$ abnormalities may persist from intraoperative effects of position, positive-pressure ventilation, and anesthetics themselves.

1. **Increased O_2 consumption** or **decreased cardiac output** may decrease $P\bar{v}O_2$ (mixed venous ox-

ygen tension) and PaO_2. Increased O_2 consumption may be due to shivering, hyperthermia, emergence excitement, hyperthyroidism, or malignant hyperthermia.

2. Continued gas exchange abnormalities are more likely to occur in patients who have undergone a procedure that affects their ability to breathe deeply. Age and obesity are important underlying factors that exaggerate these effects. Patients who cannot breathe deeply will have difficulty expanding established areas of **atelectasis** and will tend to develop new ones; they may not be able to cough effectively and clear secretions.

D. **Diffusion hypoxia** should not be a significant problem by the time a patient reaches the RR but can be obviated by administering O_2 as N_2O is discontinued.

E. **Upper airway obstruction** and **bronchospasm** should be treated, if present.

F. Evaluation of preoperative pulmonary function should be reviewed since underlying **pulmonary disease** may be worsened by the effects of anesthesia and surgery.

G. **Pneumothorax** may occur as a complication of surgery, central line placement, or regional anesthesia. If the patient is stable, treatment may await the results of a chest x-ray. If tension pneumothorax is suspected (hypotension, deviated trachea, tympanitic hemithorax), a 14-gauge cannula should be inserted through the second intercostal space in the midclavicular line as an emergency measure, preferably with surgical consultation. In general, a thoracostomy tube should be inserted for tension pneumothorax, for a greater than 20% pneumothorax on an anteroposterior chest x-ray, or for even a small pneumothorax if mechanical ventilation is planned.

H. **Pulmonary edema** may result from cardiogenic or pulmonary capillary etiology. Fluid overload in the absence of myocardial dysfunction is rare. However, noncardiogenic pulmonary edema in the RR may follow pulmonary aspiration, reaction to white blood cell components of blood transfusion, allergic drug reaction, upper airway obstruction, and sepsis.

1. Physical examination is not always diagnostic, since rales are heard in many RR patients; a chest x-ray is required for diagnosis.

2. If fluid overload seems likely, diuresis should be attempted. When fluid balance is uncertain, a pulmonary artery catheter will distinguish between left ventricular failure and increased permeability. In any case, gas exchange must be maintained, possibly with positive-pressure ventilation.

I. **Pulmonary embolus** is frequently considered, but rarely encountered, in the RR. Emboli may be thrombotic, air, tumor, or fat. Treatment is often a dilemma, as anticoagulation may be contraindicated postoperatively. In cases where the diagnosis has been established by pulmonary angiography, a mechanical filter in the inferior vena cava may be needed.

J. **Hypoxemia not due to a specific cause** is likely due to a combination of factors: anesthesia, age, obesity, underlying pulmonary disease, and hypoventilation from pain. Pain relief is required, but narcotics suppress the normal occurrence of intermittent "sighing." Thus, deep breaths must be actively encouraged by inducing coughing and other chest physical therapy techniques. Pain relief per se does not reverse the abnormalities in postoperative lung volumes. Mask CPAP and incentive spirometry can also be used to increase lung volumes. Mask CPAP (5–15 cm H_2O) may be applied for 15 minutes every 2 hours and is the quickest and least painful method to increase FRC; however, gastric distention and pulmonary aspiration are possible. Consequently, CPAP technique should not be employed unless patients are awake. Incentive spirometry is another option but requires cooperation and is not clearly better than conservative therapy. Intermittent positive-pressure breathing is not necessary in routine postoperative care but is useful in patients with neuromuscular diseases and/or chest wall deformities (such as kyphoscoliosis).

VI. **Hypercarbia** may be due to decreased central drive (residual anesthesia), impairment of the bellows mechanism of the lung (disorders of neuromuscular transmission with respiratory muscle weakness), intrinsic pulmonary disease or $\dot{V}_A/\dot{Q}$ mismatching, or increased carbon dioxide production.

A. **Decreased central drive** may result from a central neurologic deficit following neurosurgery in the area of the respiratory center. Much more commonly, anesthetics reversibly depress central drive. Administered oxygen may diminish central drive in patients with chronic obstructive pulmonary disease but mainly causes hypercarbia by reducing hypoxic pulmonary vasoconstriction and increasing dead space in less perfused lung areas. Hypoventilation due to narcotics may be treated specifically with naloxone, while physostigmine (1–4 mg IV in 1-mg increments) may produce a general arousal reaction reversing the effects of other central depressants. Cholinergic side effects are uncommon, but if bronchospasm and bradycardia occur, glycopyrrolate (0.2 mg IV) may be administered.

B. **Muscle weakness** is most often caused by residual neuromuscular blockade (criteria for reversal are discussed in Chap. 11). If relaxants have been fully reversed but the train-of-four is not normalized, ventilation should be continued until the relaxant has worn off. Excessive administration of anticholinesterases may actually worsen weakness. Abdominal distention, pain, and surgical dressings may all contribute to a net decrease in effective respiratory muscle activity.

C. Patients with chronic hypercarbia due to **intrinsic lung dysfunction** are expected to be hypercarbic postoperatively. Such patients will be more sensitive to the effects of anesthesia and have relatively large increases in $PaCO_2$ compared to normals.

D. Increased carbon dioxide production may be produced by shivering, hyperthermia, or emergence excitement. This CO_2 challenge will not become a problem unless ventilation cannot be increased.

VII. Nausea and vomiting

A. Nausea and vomiting are common sequelae of general anesthesia and generally do not require any treatment. The possibility of pulmonary aspiration must be considered in patients who vomit before airway reflexes have returned.

B. Treatment to prevent vomiting may be indicated in patients undergoing eye surgery, considering the theoretical risk of suture disruption. Also, patients with a history of severe postoperative nausea and vomiting may benefit from prophylaxis before their next anesthetic. Droperidol (1.25 mg IV) given during the anesthetic may be useful in adults but may contribute to postoperative somnolence.

C. Antiemetic treatment alternatives include haloperidol (Haldol, 0.5–2.0 mg IV), prochlorperazine (Compazine, 5–10 mg IM or IV), or promethazine (Phenergan, 12.5–25.0 mg IM or IV). Suppository administration (e.g., prochlorperazine 25 mg) may be used as well. All of these compounds are dopamine receptor antagonists and thus have the potential for causing extrapyramidal side effects. Benzaquinamide (Emeticon) does not have this effect and is thus an alternative in parkinsonism. A single dose of dexamethasone (10 mg IV) may provide relief in refractory cases if there are no contraindications. Nausea due to narcotics may be treated with small doses of naloxone.

D. Dystonia caused by phenothiazines or butyrophenones results from blockade of basal ganglion dopaminergic transmission. Patients may become quite rigid and unable to open their mouths or breathe deeply. Treatment consists of either diphenhydramine (Benadryl, 25–50 mg IV or IM), an antihistamine with central anticholinergic actions, or benztropine (Cogentin, 1–2 mg IV), an anticholinergic drug.

VIII. Hypothermia

A. Hypothermia is common, due to the many causes of heat loss during surgery. The most important of these is an ambient OR temperature of less than 21°C. Other factors include direct hypothalamic effects of anesthetics, evaporative heat loss through thoracic and abdominal exposures, and latent heat loss through inhalation of dry, unheated anesthetic gases.

B. Vasoconstriction is an undesirable effect of hypothermia; it may impair peripheral perfusion and cause metabolic acidosis. Hypovolemia may be masked by vasoconstriction, only to become apparent on rewarming. Vasodilators may be needed but should be used judiciously.

C. Shivering may result from hypothermia or from direct

effects of anesthetics on the central nervous system. Shivering increases O_2 consumption and carbon dioxide production, which are poorly compensated because of residual anesthetic effects on the heart and lungs. If cardiac output does increase, so does myocardial O_2 demand, which may produce myocardial ischemia in susceptible patients. If a patient with coronary disease is even moderately hypothermic, ventilation should be controlled and shivering prevented with sedation, narcotics, and/or relaxants to allow a controlled emergence and rewarming without increasing $M\dot{V}O_2$. Low-dose vasodilators (e.g., nitroglycerin, 0.25–2.0 μg/kg/min IV) may be used to "smooth out" the inevitable vasodilatation and accelerate rewarming. Arterial blood gases should be checked to monitor the effects of shivering on gas exchange and tissue perfusion.

D. Every effort should be made to prevent hypothermia in newborns and infants since neonatal hypothermia leads to acidosis, hypoglycemia, and hypoxemia. Keeping infants heads (and bodies) covered will prevent a substantial portion of heat loss, as will maintaining a high room temperature.

IX. Hyperthermia

A. Hyperthermia is less common than hypothermia in the RR.

B. Exacerbation of preoperative infections, exposure to contaminated substances, or manipulation of infected tissue during surgery may produce fever and septicemia. Antibiotics are the key to therapy but should be administered only after obtaining appropriate blood cultures.

C. Pulmonary aspiration is a cause of early fever. Atelectasis, on the other hand, classically causes fever on the first postoperative day, but not usually in the RR.

D. Thyroid storm is rare but should be considered. Treatment is discussed in Chap. 6. Salicylates should be avoided in thyroid storm, as they may increase the amount of unbound hormone. Adrenal insufficiency and pheochromocytoma can also cause fever.

E. Anticholinergic toxicity may be produced by anticholinergics like atropine, scopolamine, or benztropine (Cogentin). Delirium, erythematous rash, and the absence of sweating are observed. Physostigmine IV is therapeutic.

F. Malignant hyperthermia may first appear in the RR and should be evaluated and treated as described in Chap. 28.

G. The onset of the malignant neuroleptic syndrome due to antinausea medication is unlikely in the RR, as it typically develops over 24–72 hours. Unlike malignant hyperthermia, which is a disorder of muscle, malignant neuroleptic syndrome is due to a central, probably presynaptic, abnormality. Dantrolene may eventually prove to be an effective treatment.

H. The combination of monoamine oxidase (MAO) inhibitors and meperidine (or dextromethorphan) can produce hyperpyrexia and death. It is still uncertain whether all synthetic narcotics can trigger this reaction, but it is probably wise to use morphine or codeine in patients who have been taking MAO inhibitors. A partial list includes tranylcypromine (Parnate), phenelzine (Nardil), isocarboxazid (Marplan), pargyline (Eutonyl), and procarbazine (Matulane).

I. Once investigated, fever should be symptomatically treated, particularly in patients less able to cope with hypermetabolic demands (e.g., patients at the extremes of age, as well as those with coronary insufficiency, CHF, and anemia). Rectal acetaminophen (650–1300 mg or 10 mg/kg in children) is usually effective. External cooling with ice packs or a cooling blanket may be necessary.

X. **Recovery from regional anesthesia**

A. **Epidural/spinal/caudal.** While exact standards for adequate recovery vary between institutions, all patients should have some degree of motor and autonomic recovery. Ability to flex the hip reveals motor recovery to the L3 level and, combined with the return of sensation at about L1, should be adequate criteria for discharge of inpatients. By definition, these criteria imply a low level of sympathetic blockade. Outpatients should have complete neurologic recovery, although it may occasionally be quite delayed. For example, in the elderly, a tetracaine spinal prolonged by epinephrine or phenylephrine may last 6–8 hours. However, if recovery seems unduly delayed, neurosurgical consultation should be obtained regarding the possibility of cord compression from hematoma.

Hemodynamically, patients should have a stable, acceptable blood pressure in the absence of vasopressors. Continuing hypotension in the absence of continued sympathetic block mandates investigation for other causes of hypotension.

B. **Other regional anesthetic methods**

1. Monitoring in the RR is probably not indicated after cervical, brachial, or lumbosacral plexus blocks as long as the procedure was sufficiently long that any complications would have been detected in the OR. However, if heavy sedation has been given, or other medical problems exist, a period of monitoring in the RR is warranted.

2. Also, patients may require monitoring as a result of specific surgery, for example, after regional anesthesia for carotid surgery or insertion of ICP monitor under standby or "monitored anesthesia care."

3. Both patients and their nurses should be aware of the estimated time for complete recovery. Similarly, outpatients should be discharged with careful, written instructions. Finally, patients should be protected from self-harm due to lack of strength or sensation.

XI. **Emergence problems**

A. In the absence of severe hypotension or hypoxia, delayed recovery usually reflects the extremes of individual responses to anesthetics. Metabolic causes include profound hypoglycemia, sepsis, and acid-base or electrolyte derangements.

B. If emergence is delayed in a neurosurgical patient, the surgeon should be notified immediately. Residual subdural hematoma, intracerebral bleeding, or edema may produce persistent obtundation. Most neuroanesthetics are planned to allow patients to recover relatively quickly, so that early postoperative assessment of their level of consciousness can be performed.

C. The anesthetic record may contain clues to delayed recovery. Scopolamine premedication may be responsible, as can administration of benzodiazepines, ketamine, and droperidol. Large doses of barbiturates (e.g., > 30 mg/kg of thiopental) will overwhelm redistribution mechanisms and delay recovery until metabolism progresses. Concurrent administration of cimetidine may decrease the metabolism of many drugs, including benzodiazepines, amide local anesthetics, and morphine. The record may also reveal that inhalation anesthesia was quite "deep" and not "lightened" toward the end of the case. Administration of narcotics with potent inhaled agents will slow the ventilatory clearance of the volatile anesthetics. If patients are stable (from respiratory and cardiovascular standpoints) and the neurologic examination is otherwise unremarkable, there is no need to accelerate recovery. If necessary, physostigmine or naloxone may be administered.

D. It is important to establish that **emergence excitement** is not due to hypoxia, hypercarbia, acidosis, sepsis, or cerebral ischemia before causes of lesser import are considered or sedation begun. Discomfort from incisional pain, bladder or gastric distention, or dressings and casts may cause agitation and can be treated specifically. Young patients undergoing procedures with emotional overtones, such as genital or rectal surgery, seem particularly prone to agitation postoperatively. In other patients, emergence delirium may simply represent prolonged excitement during recovery from general anesthesia. Small doses of narcotics or benzodiazepines will provide sedation and smooth emergence.

E. Excitement is more common in patients who have received scopolamine, barbiturate, phenothiazine, or droperidol premedications. Physostigmine may be administered specifically to reverse anticholinergic agitation or nonspecifically to improve delirium in other cases. In adults, emergence from ketamine may be associated with unpleasant dreams and hallucinations. Pretreatment with a benzodiazepine or removal to a quiet recovery area seems to prevent ketamine delirium. The RR staff should be informed of the reasons for choosing ketamine (e.g., hypotension, IM induction in agitated or retarded patient, difficult airway in a child) as part of the RR report.

XII. Criteria for discharge. After general anesthesia, patients should be easily arousable with verbal stimuli and as oriented to person, place, and time as before. Patients should be able to maintain and protect their airways and have stable respiratory and cardiovascular function. Pain should be under reasonable control; however, it is unlikely that it will be completely eliminated in all patients before discharge. Nausea and vomiting should be minimal or absent. For inpatients, IVs should be maintained until oral intake is sufficient, and body temperature should be near normal.

Suggested Reading

Breslow, M. J., et al. Changes in T-wave morphology following anesthesia and surgery: A common recovery room phenomenon. *Anesthesiology* 64:398, 1986.

Craig, D. B. Postoperative recovery of pulmonary function. *Anesth. Analg.* 60:46, 1981.

Cullen, D. J. Acute Renal Failure: Pathophysiology and Prevention. In R. D. Miller (ed.), *Anesthesia.* New York: Churchill Livingstone, 1986.

Fairley, H. B. Oxygen therapy for surgical patients. *Am. Rev. Respir. Dis.* 122s:37, 1980.

Guze, B. H., and Baxter, L. R. Neuroleptic malignant syndrome. *N. Engl. J. Med.* 313:163, 1985.

Herling, I. M. Intravenous nitroglycerin: Clinical pharmacology and therapeutic consideration. *Am. Heart J.* 108:141, 1984.

Schecter, W. P., and Wilson, R. S. Management of upper airway obstruction in the ICU. *Crit. Care Med.* 9:577, 1981.

Stock, M. C., et al. Prevention of postoperative pulmonary complications with CPAP, incentive spirometry and conservative therapy. *Chest* 87:151, 1985.

III

Patient Care
in Other Settings

30

Adult, Pediatric, and Newborn Resuscitation

James K. Alifimoff

Successful resuscitation from cardiac arrest depends on rapid diagnosis and prompt initiation of basic life support (BLS) measures. Because external cardiac massage does not reliably generate more than 6–30% of normal blood flow, restoration of spontaneous circulation by advanced life support (ALS) must be accomplished as soon as possible to achieve optimal recovery of vital organ system function, particularly the central nervous system (CNS).

When cardiac arrest occurs in the operating room (OR), where equipment and drugs necessary for ALS should be readily available, it is still essential that BLS be performed optimally and with minimal interruption. Adequate personnel are usually available, but their efficient deployment should be the responsibility of a single leader. Anesthesiologists qualify for this role because of their expertise in airway management, as well as in cardiopulmonary physiology and pharmacology.

This chapter will focus on management of intrahospital cardiac arrest. Pertinent discussions of airway management may be found in Chaps. 10 and 27. However, neonatal airway management is considered here in detail, owing to the special equipment and skills that are necessary. Pharmacologic agents used to support the circulation once resuscitation has been achieved are discussed in Chap. 16.

I. **Pathophysiology of cardiac arrest.** With cardiac arrest, blood flow ceases, preventing oxygen delivery to vital tissues, and anaerobic metabolism begins. Lactic acid is generated through anaerobiosis in excess of the buffering capacity of the blood. Acidosis produces vasodilatation and depression of catecholamine action.

II. **Causes of cardiac arrest**
   A. **Primary cardiac arrest**
      1. Myocardial ischemia with irritability in the ischemic region, leading to ventricular fibrillation (VF).
      2. Asystole secondary to intrinsic heart disease.
   B. **Secondary cardiac arrest** is commonly associated with asphyxia, blood or fluid loss, electrical shock, or drug effect.
      1. **Hypoxemia** may result from inhalation of hypoxic gas mixtures, airway obstruction, pulmonary parenchymal disease, low cardiac output, or apnea/hypoventilation from a CNS insult or drugs.
      2. **Hypovolemia** from any cause, producing inadequate cardiac preload, leading to poor or inadequate perfusion.
      3. **Hypotension** caused by cardiac tamponade, tension pneumothorax, vena caval obstruction, anaphylaxis, sepsis, or vasodilating drugs.
      4. **Myocardial depression** secondary to drug over-

dose, including inhalation anesthetics, hypokalemia, antiarrhythmics, and negative inotropes (calcium channel antagonists, beta blockers).

III. **Diagnosis of cardiac arrest.** While all expedience in treatment is necessary to assure optimal outcome, it must be absolutely certain that technical problems, for example, a disconnected ECG lead, do not lead to an erroneous diagnosis. While **absence of a pulse in a major vessel** (e.g., carotid or femoral artery) **is diagnostic of cardiac arrest** (and should be employed to confirm diagnosis prior to starting cardiopulmonary resuscitation [CPR]), the following may be highly suggestive as well:

A. Absent blood pressure by sphygmomanometer or direct intraarterial pressure monitoring.

B. Asystole, VF, or ventricular tachycardia (VT) on ECG.

C. Lack of bleeding in the surgical field or "dark blood."

D. Inaudible heart sounds.

E. Cyanosis and/or agonal respirations.

F. Sudden loss of consciousness.

G. Profound desaturation on pulse oximeter.

IV. **Treatment of cardiac arrest.** The diagnosis of cardiac arrest during anesthesia mandates immediate initiation of basic and advanced life support measures. All anesthetic agents should be discontinued, 100% O_2 administered, and the adequacy of ventilation and intravascular volume assured. In addition, possible reflex or mechanical causes must be sought and corrected, including traction on the peritoneum, manipulation of the carotid sinus or heart, or compression of the inferior vena cava.

A. **Basic life support.** The following highlights pertinent sections of the **1986 American Heart Association guidelines.**

1. **Airway.** Securing the airway is discussed in Chap. 10.

2. **Breathing.**

3. **Circulation.** Artificial circulation is provided by external cardiac compressions. The heel of one hand is placed two fingerbreadths above the xiphoid process, and the other is placed on top of the first with the fingers interlocking. Patients should be placed on a firm, stable surface, with the head on the same level as the heart. Compressions are performed with pressure exerted from the shoulders through arms locked at the elbows. In adults, the sternum is depressed 1.5–2.0 inches, and compression should account for 50% of each compression-relaxation cycle.

a. **Single resuscitator.** External compressions are performed at a rate of 80–100/min, with two breaths interposed between groups of 15 compressions.

b. **Two resuscitators.** The compression rate is 80–100/min, with one breath interposed after every 5 compressions.

4. **Precordial thump.** The small epicardial potential produced by a precordial thump can terminate VF.

While a precordial thump can convert VT or complete heart block into sinus rhythm, it can also precipitate VF. Therefore, when this technique is used for a patient in VT with a pulse, a defibrillator should be immediately available because of the danger of inducing VF.

B. **Advanced life support** treats cardiac arrest definitively with drugs, fluids, DC countershock, or artificial pacemaker when appropriate. However, continuation of effective BLS remains important, to maintain vital organ perfusion and assure circulation of lifesaving drugs to their sites of action.

1. **Administration of drugs** may be done through a peripheral IV, central venous pressure catheter (CVP), endotracheal tube, or by intracardiac injection.

   a. **A peripheral IV** should be established in an antecubital vein as soon as possible by a team member who is not performing CPR. However, drugs injected by this route may take minutes to reach their sites of action.

   b. If restoration of spontaneous circulation is not accomplished after administration of drugs through a peripheral IV, a **central venous catheter** should be started by the internal jugular, subclavian, or femoral approach with only minimal interruption of CPR. Cannulation of the internal jugular or femoral vein requires less interruption of CPR and is also less likely to cause a pneumothorax. (See Chap. 8.)

   c. If venous access cannot be rapidly established, certain essential drugs may be given through the **endotracheal tube;** there is sufficient pulmonary arterial/venous uptake of atropine, epinephrine, and lidocaine to achieve therapeutic concentrations. Since optimal doses for this route of administration have not been established, it is currently suggested that the same doses be used as for IV administration. Dilution of these drugs in up to 10 ml of sterile saline will assure a volume sufficient to reach the alveolar level. **Sodium bicarbonate ($NaHCO_3$) and calcium chloride ($CaCl_2$) should never be given by this route!** Endotracheal administration of drugs should replace the older method of intracardiac injection.

   d. **Intracardiac administration** is not recommended during closed-chest CPR; endotracheal administration avoids the risks of pneumothorax or intramyocardial injections.

2. **Drugs for ALS**

   a. **Oxygen (100%)** should be used to ventilate all cardiac arrest victims. In hemodynamically stable patients with VT, supplemental O_2 should be supplied by face mask. (See Chap. 32.)

   b. **Epinephrine's** alpha- and beta-agonist effects

are beneficial; the alpha effect (vasoconstriction) increases perfusion pressures during external cardiac compressions, while the beta effects enhance myocardial contractility or, at least, coarsen fine VF.

    (1) Initial dose of 0.5–1.0 mg IV (5–10 ml of 1 : 10,000 solution).

    (2) Repeat every 5 minutes.

c. Following the administration of epinephrine, **NaHCO₃** is typically given when there has been prolonged cardiac arrest or when metabolic acidosis has been documented by arterial blood gases (ABGs). However, recent evidence indicates that NaHCO₃ administration does not seem to improve defibrillation or survival in laboratory animals, shifts the oxyhemoglobin-dissociation curve (decreasing O_2 availability to tissues), and might paradoxically produce acidosis by promoting carbon dioxide production.

    (1) Initial dose of 1 mEq/kg IV.

    (2) Subsequent dose of 0.5 mEq/kg every 10 minutes.

    (3) If ABGs are available, the dosage can be calculated as follows:

$$NaHCO_3 \text{ (mEq)} = 0.3 \times \text{body weight (kg)} \times \text{base deficit (mEq/L)}$$

d. Lidocaine is used for the treatment of ventricular arrhythmias, including recurrent or refractory VF. Lidocaine must be used cautiously in patients with atrial fibrillation or flutter, as it can cause dangerous acceleration in the ventricular response.

    (1) Initial dose of 1 mg/kg IV.

    (2) Repeated doses of 0.5 mg/kg may be given every 8 minutes to a total dose of 3 mg/kg.

    (3) Dosage should be decreased in the presence of low cardiac output and with hepatic dysfunction.

e. Procainamide should be used to treat ventricular arrhythmias, either when lidocaine has failed or is contraindicated.

    (1) A dose of 50 mg IV every 5 minutes up to a total of 1 gm may be given until ventricular ectopy is abolished, hypotension occurs, or the QRS complex is widened by 50%.

    (2) Emergently, 20 mg/min IV may be given, up to 1 gm.

    (3) Maintenance infusion rate is 1–4 mg/min.

    (4) Dosage should be decreased in renal failure.

f. Bretylium is used in the treatment of refractory ventricular arrhythmias and VF. It may initially cause release of catecholamines. Since it is also a postganglionic adrenergic blocking agent, hypotension often follows approximately 5 minutes after administration. Its use is indicated when lidocaine and DC cardioversion have failed to resolve VF, or when lidocaine and procainamide have not suppressed VT without hemodynamic compromise.

    (1) For VF, a 5 mg/kg IV initial bolus is given; a subsequent dose of 10 mg/kg may be repeated every 15 minutes to a total dose of 30 mg/kg.

    (2) For recurrent VT, 5–10 mg/kg of bretylium in 50 ml of 5% D/W is given IV over 10 minutes; a continuous infusion of 1–2 mg/min may then be started.

g. Atropine decreases vagal tone, increases atrioventricular node conduction, and stimulates sinus node discharge. It is useful for the treatment of sinus bradycardia with hypotension or ventricular escape beats, as well as asystole.

    (1) Initial dose of 0.4–1.0 mg IV for symptomatic bradycardia.

    (2) For asystole, the initial dose is 1 mg IV, which may be repeated to a total of 3 mg.

    (3) Doses of less than 0.4 mg may be parasympathomimetic, that is, cause bradycardia.

h. Calcium (Ca^{2+}) has previously been recommended for the treatment of asystole and electromechanical dissociation. However, there is little support for the efficacy of this therapy, and recent evidence associates Ca^{2+} accumulation with cellular death. In fact, Ca^{2+} channel blocking agents may provide cerebral protective effects during cerebral ischemic-anoxic insults. For these reasons, the use of Ca^{2+} during ALS is no longer recommended, unless hypocalcemia is documented or suspected. The use of Ca^{2+} may also be considered in the treatment of hyperkalemia, hypermagnesemia, and Ca^{2+} antagonist overdose.

    (1) Dose of 2–4 mg/kg IV of $CaCl_2$ (1.5–3.0 ml of 10% $CaCl_2$ solution).

    (2) Alternatively, calcium gluconate (10%) may be used at a dose of 5–8 ml IV for a full-sized adult.

i. Isoproterenol is a beta-sympathomimetic agent that had previously been recommended for use in asystolic cardiac arrest. Currently, however, its only use is in the patient with atropine-resistant bradycardia. Its infusion rate is 2–10 µg/min.

C. Specific cardiac arrest scenarios. To some extent, resuscitations must be individualized. The following scenarios are those most pertinent to OR care, but the steps that are specified do not preclude alternative or additional therapies as deemed appropriate by the anesthesiologist.

1. **Monitored VF,** that is, less than 1 minute in duration.
   a. Precordial thump.
   b. Start BLS CPR until defibrillator is charged.
   c. Confirm rhythm with defibrillator oscilloscope or ECG.
   d. Defibrillate with 200 joules.
   e. If VF is not terminated, continue BLS CPR while recharging the defibrillator, and defibrillate with 200–300 joules.
   f. Repeat (**e**) with a third countershock below 360 joules.
   g. If third countershock is unsuccessful, administer epinephrine, 1 mg IV or by endotracheal tube, during CPR.
   h. Defibrillate with 360 joules.
   i. Continue CPR, and administer lidocaine, 1 mg/kg IV or by endotracheal tube.
   j. Defibrillate with 360 joules.
   k. Administer bretylium, 5 mg/kg IV. Alternatively, use additional lidocaine and consider NaHCO$_3$ as discussed in section **IV.B.2.c.**

2. **Ventricular tachycardia without hemodynamic compromise** or change in mental status.
   a. Lidocaine, 1 mg/kg IV.
   b. Repeat lidocaine, 0.5 mg/kg, every 8 minutes up to a total dose of 3 mg/kg, or start a lidocaine infusion at 2 mg/min after the first bolus, and increase by 1 mg/min to a maximum of 4 mg/min after each additional bolus.
   c. Procainamide, 20 mg/min IV, up to 1 gm.
   d. **Synchronized cardioversion** starting at 50 joules. Consider sedation during cardioversion.

3. **Ventricular tachycardia with hemodynamic compromise** or change in mental status, indicating poor cerebral perfusion.
   a. **Synchronized cardioversion** at 50 joules.
   b. Repeat at 100 joules, then 200 joules, and if necessary, 360 joules.
   c. If VT recurs or persists, administer lidocaine, and cardiovert at an energy level that was previously successful.
   d. If unsuccessful, procainamide as in **2.c** or bretylium, 5 mg/kg IV.

4. **Asystole** may follow VF or may be due to excessive parasympathetic tone. Causes for bradycardia are reviewed in Chap. 15. Very fine VF may appear to be asystole; therefore, countershock at 200 joules may be justified initially. Two different ECG lead readings are necessary to make the diagnosis for this reason.

       a. Immediate BLS CPR.

       b. Epinephrine, 1 mg IV or by endotracheal tube.

       c. Atropine, 1 mg IV or by endotracheal tube, and repeat every 5 minutes to a total dose of 3 mg.

       d. Consider NaHCO$_3$ IV.

       e. Insertion of a transvenous or transthoracic pacemaker may result in a ventricular rhythm in rare instances and should be considered following failure of pharmacologic therapy.

    5. Electromechanical dissociation is characterized by organized electrical activity without effective mechanical myocardial function and carries a grave prognosis. Treatment consists of

       a. Immediate BLS CPR.

       b. Epinephrine, 1 mg IV or by endotracheal tube.

       c. Consider correctable causes, which include cardiac tamponade, tension pneumothorax, profound hypovolemia, pulmonary embolism, and profound hypoxemia or acidosis.

       d. Consider NaHCO$_3$.

D. Open-chest CPR currently is indicated for

    1. A patient whose chest is already open.

    2. Penetrating thoracic trauma.

    3. Profound hypothermia.

    4. Suspected massive pulmonary embolism.

    5. Tension pneumothorax.

    6. Cardiac tamponade.

    7. Severe chest deformity, as in advanced emphysema, which precludes adequate performance of external cardiac compression.

    8. Failure of adequately performed external cardiac compression and refractory VF (rare).

E. When to terminate CPR. The decision to suspend CPR in the OR is a difficult one for medical, ethical, and legal reasons.

    1. Unambiguous determination that a patient has suffered irreversible brain damage is the **main criterion** for such a decision. However, this is impossible *during* CPR efforts. Fixed and dilated pupils may be the result of drug therapy and/or anesthesia and are thus not a definitive index of cerebral function or ultimate neurologic outcome. Since we lack sound neurologic criteria for termination of ALS measures, the decision must be based on the cardiovascular status. As discussed in the American Heart Association's "Standards and Guidelines for Cardiopulmonary Resuscitation and Emergency Cardiac Care" (see **Suggested Reading**), it must be possible to state that both "BLS and ALS were employed in a manner and for a time adequate to test the responsiveness of the victim's cardiovascular system." In this context, cardiovascular unresponsiveness indicates that the heart is no longer viable and thus eliminates the need to establish irreversible loss of neurologic function.

   2. Meticulous documentation of the resuscitation should
   establish that efforts were pursued to the appropriate end-point.

   3. However, if doubts about when to terminate CPR
   exist, resuscitative efforts should be continued.

F. Do not resuscitate (DNR) orders. A perplexing situation for the anesthesiologist arises when patients with
DNR orders are scheduled for a surgical procedure.
While the operation is usually only palliative, the patient may still suffer cardiac arrest in the OR or recovery room. Under such conditions, resuscitation should
still be performed with the understanding that reversi-
bility is possible when the arrest has been caused or
precipitated by a therapeutic maneuver rather than the
underlying disease process. However, in these circumstances, it is absolutely essential that this be discussed
openly, and in detail, with the patient (if competent),
the family, the primary physician, and the surgeon, and
documented in the consent form and medical record.

Pediatric Resuscitation

Differences in the anatomy and physiology of infants and
children necessitate additional skills in both BLS and ALS
on the part of the anesthesiologist. Cardiac arrest in the pediatric population is rarely a primary event, but rather is
**usually secondary to hypoxemia from respiratory
compromise.** For this reason, securing a clear airway and
providing adequate ventilation are the fundamental concerns. Airway management and ventilation in pediatric patients are discussed in Chap. 23.

I. Basic life support
   A. Airway control.
   B. Breathing.
   C. Circulation. In determining pulselessness in **infants**
   (< 1 year), the brachial or femoral pulse is sought,
   rather than the carotid because the infant's short neck
   makes palpation of this artery difficult. In **children** (>
   1 year), either the carotid or femoral artery may be palpated.

      1. The heart is lower in the mediastinum of infants
      than previously thought. To locate the appropriate
      position for external cardiac compressions, an im-
      aginary line is drawn between the nipples, and
      compressions are performed one fingerbreadth be-
      low this line. In children, the correct position for
      external cardiac compression is determined as in
      the adult.

      2. In infants, the tips of two fingers are used for
      compressions. Alternatively, and probably more ef-
      fectively, the infant's chest may be encircled with
      both hands, and the sternum compressed with the
      thumbs. For children, the heel of one hand is used
      for performing cardiac compressions. In all cases,
      patients should be placed on a firm surface.

3. For respective rates, depths of compression, and compression-ventilation ratios, see Table 30-1. An important difference between adult and pediatric CPR is the need to interrupt compressions systematically to allow for ventilations. The use of this **programmed breath** avoids hypoventilation, which may occur when ventilations compete with chest compressions.

II. Advanced life support

A. The majority of cardiac arrests in pediatric patients occur in infants. While respiratory obstruction with secondary cardiac arrest is the most common etiology, the principles of resuscitation are the same as those applied to the adult, and all arrests should be approached with a similar systematic therapeutic scheme. Rapid initiation of BLS CPR is the first step. Then IV catheters are established and drugs administered. However, drug dosages (in mg/kg) must be recalculated according to regimens established for pediatrics.

B. **Administration of drugs and fluids**

1. In infants and children, drugs and fluids may be administered through a peripheral IV, CVP catheter, or by intraosseous, endotracheal, or intracardiac injections.

2. In children, peripheral IVs may be started in the median basilic, antecubital, or cephalic veins in the upper extremity, although these may be difficult to cannulate in an obese child. Scalp veins are the least desirable because attempts at cannulation may impede CPR efforts, and they are easily dislodged. As an alternative, the femoral vein allows access to the central circulation when a catheter of suitable length is used. In skilled hands, saphenous vein cutdowns can also be quickly performed. Sites of central venous access in children are the same as those in adults.

3. **Intraosseous injection** is another mode of vascular access that may be preferable to endotracheal or intracardiac injection. A spinal or bone marrow needle with stylet is inserted into the anterior tibial bone marrow to gain access to the circulation.

4. Recommendations for **endotracheal instillation** are the same as in adults with respect to the drugs that may be administered by this route.

5. The complications of intracardiac injections are the same as discussed previously in sec. **IV.B.1.d.**

C. **Drugs for pediatric ALS**

1. **Epinephrine**
   a. Initial dose of 0.01 mg/kg by IV bolus (0.1 ml/ kg of 1 : 10,000 solution).

   10 µg/kg

   b. Repeat every 5 minutes.

2. Considerations for the use of **calcium** are similar to those in sec. **IV.B.2.h.** The initial dose is 2 mg/kg of 10% $CaCl_2$ by IV bolus.

3. In infants, cardiac output is rate dependent. Thus **atropine** is indicated in the treatment of bradycar-

Table 30-1. Pediatric cardipulmonary resuscitation

Age	Ventilations/min	Compressions/min	Ventilation-Compression Ratio	Depth (inches)
Infant	20–24	100–120	1 : 5	0.5–1.0
Young child (> 1–4 years)	20	100	1 : 5	1.0–1.5
Older child (> 4 years)	16	80	1 : 5	1.5–2.0

dia (heart rates < 80), even without accompanying hypotension, and in asystolic cardiac arrest. The initial dose is 0.02 mg/kg IV or IM with a minimum dose of 0.1 mg.

4. **Isoproterenol** infusion may also be used to treat bradyarrhythmias. The initial rate is 0.1 µg/kg/min followed by titration to effect.

5. **Sodium bicarbonate.** Following adequate ventilation and administration of epinephrine, $NaHCO_3$ may be administered when there has been prolonged cardiac arrest or when there is documented metabolic acidosis with ABGs. (See sec. **IV.B.2.c.**)

   a. Initial dose of 1 mEq/kg for both IV and intraosseous administration, followed by 0.5 mEq/kg every 10 minutes.

   b. If ABGs are available, subsequent doses are based on the base deficit (see sec. **IV.B.2.c.(3)**).

D. **Ventricular fibrillation** is an uncommon event in infants and children. Bradyarrhythmias and heart block are the usual precursors of cardiac arrest. Therefore, defibrillation should be attempted only if ECG monitoring shows VF.

1. **Size of electrode paddles.** Electrodes should be well separated; since the propagated current is directly proportional to the size of the paddle, the largest diameter that still allows separation should be employed. A 4.5-cm electrode is adequate for infants; the 8-cm paddle is for older children.

2. **Electrode interface.** Because of the small size of these patients, a bridge of electrode cream or saline can form between the two defibrillating electrodes. This must be avoided, since it will lead to insufficient energy traversing the myocardium. **Alcohol pads must never be used,** since doing so may cause serious burns.

3. The initial dose is 2 joules/kg; thereafter, doses should be doubled and repeated twice. If defibrillation does not result from the higher doses, more aggressive correction of acid-base abnormalities is indicated. As in adults, defibrillation of children receiving digoxin can result in irreversible cardiac arrest. In such patients, defibrillation should begin with the lowest energy setting that the defibrillator will deliver, then cautiously increased.

Newborn Resuscitation

Optimal newborn resuscitation requires an individual to ventilate, one to perform cardiac compressions, and a third to administer drugs and fluids. Modern fetal monitoring techniques have facilitated early identification of neonates who are at highest risk for cardiopulmonary depression after birth (see Chap. 25 for a discussion of fetal monitoring). Thus preparedness and coordination of the team is more possible than ever and are the keys to successful resuscitations. Stabilization of resuscitated newborns then continues in the intensive care unit setting and is discussed in Chap. 31.

I. Temperature regulation

A. Although all neonates have difficulty tolerating cold environments, asphyxiated newborns have particularly unstable thermoregulatory systems, and hypothermia exacerbates acidosis.

B. To minimize heat loss, all neonates should be
  1. Completely dried of amniotic fluid (especially their heads, since its relatively large surface area predisposes to heat loss).
  2. Maintained in a prewarmed environment, that is, the delivery suite should be warm and the infant placed under a radiant warming device.

II. Newborn assessment. Initial preparation and evaluation of all newborns should be systematic.

A. The oropharynx is suctioned with a bulb-type suction at the time of delivery by the obstetrician.

B. The baby is placed under a radiant heating device.

C. Oropharyngeal suctioning is repeated. If the amniotic fluid is meconium-stained, manage as described in sec. **V.A.5.**

D. Dry the head, torso, and extremities.

E. Determine APGAR score.

III. The APGAR score

A. Newborns are assessed at 1 and 5 minutes after delivery using an objective scoring system that includes five categories: **A**ppearance, **P**ulse, **G**rimace, **A**ctivity, and **R**espiration. A score from 0–2 is possible in each category; thus a perfect score would be a 10. However, few newborns achieve a score of 10, since almost all have some acrocyanosis. In general, the 1-minute score correlates well with umbilical vein pH and is indicative of intrapartum asphyxia, while the 5-minute score appears to correlate with eventual neurologic outcome. The APGAR score is summarized in Table 30-2.

B. **Neonatal depression** is usually due to one of three causes:
  1. Uteroplacental insufficiency.
  2. Maternal medication (e.g., opiates).
  3. Neonatal disease.

IV. Intervention based on APGAR score

A. **APGAR score 8–10.** These infants require no further specific treatment. Monitoring must be performed for at least another 5 minutes to be certain that hypoventilation does not occur, and care must be taken to maintain normothermia.

B. **APGAR score 5–7.** These infants have had minor asphyxia during birth and require stimulation and an O_2-enriched atmosphere. Stimulation is accomplished by vigorous rubbing of the baby's back or by gentle slaps on the soles of the feet. Oxygen can be supplied from a Ma-

Table 30-2. The APGAR score

Clinical sign	Points assigned		
	0	1	2
Appearance	Cyanotic	Acrocyanotic	Pink
Pulse (determined either by auscultation of the precordium or by palpation of the umbilical artery)	< 60	60–100	> 100
Grimace or reflex irritability to oropharyngeal suctioning	No response	Weak cry	Vigorous cry
Activity or muscle tone	Flaccid	Weak	Good
Respiratory effort	Apnea	Irregular	Regular

pleson-type resuscitation bag; Hope-type ventilation bags deliver O_2 only during positive-pressure ventilation and thus are ineffective for this purpose.

C. **APGAR score 3–4.** Bag and mask ventilation should be started when stimulation does not establish adequate respiration or if the heart rate decreases to less than 100/min.

D. **APGAR score 0–2.** These infants require immediate initiation of CPR (BLS and ALS).

V. **Specific resuscitative measures**

   A. **Airway**

   1. Suctioning is important, as blood, mucus, or meconium can obstruct the airway. A bulb and syringe suction device is most appropriate, as it is not dependent on external power. In addition, its descent into the hypopharynx is limited. Each nasal opening should be suctioned after the mouth to assure patency of the nasal passages, as neonates are obligate nose-breathers.

   2. Suctioning should be limited to 10 seconds, and ventilation with 100% O_2 (either spontaneously or with assistance) should be done between attempts.

   3. Monitoring during suctioning is necessary because suctioning can cause bradycardia by either a vagal reflex or be secondary to hypoxemia.

   4. If obstruction is below the level of the vocal cords, endotracheal intubation and suctioning are indicated. Suction only as the catheter is being withdrawn to minimize damage to the tracheal mucosa.

5. The presence of watery or thin meconium does not mandate routine endotracheal intubation, although thin meconium, if aspirated, can cause lung injury. However, **meconium aspiration** has probably occurred if there is thick, particulate, meconium-stained fluid. In such cases, patients should be treated as follows:

   a. Immediate suctioning should be performed after delivery of the head, using a DeLee trap.

   b. Laryngoscopy and endotracheal intubation should be accomplished prior to applying positive-pressure ventilation; after intubation, suction is applied by mouth or directly from wall suction as the endotracheal tube is withdrawn.

   c. Repeat **b** until meconium is no longer obtained from the endotracheal tube.

B. **Breathing**

   1. **Bag and mask ventilation.** A ventilatory rate of 30–40 breaths/min at an airway pressure of 20–30 cm H_2O should provide an adequate minute ventilation. However, higher inflation pressures may be required in asphyxiated infants. Adequacy of ventilation is assessed by symmetric chest expansion and the presence of equal breath sounds in the mid-axillary line. A variety of face mask sizes should be available: size 0 for the premature infant ($<$ 2500 g) to size 1 for the full-term neonate.

   2. **Endotracheal intubation.** Types and sizes of endotracheal tubes are summarized in Table 30-3. Cole tubes, which have tapered ends, are to be avoided, since the distal ends are readily occluded with secretions. The technique of endotracheal intubation is as follows:

      a. Place the infant in the **"sniffing" position,** and perform laryngoscopy with a Miller blade (size 0 or 1). The tip of the blade is placed in the vallecula, although occasionally it is necessary to elevate the epiglottis directly to expose the glottic opening.

      b. A **stylet** will provide rigidity to the endotracheal tube and facilitate intubation; however, extreme care must be taken to keep the stylet tip within the endotracheal tube to avoid damage to the trachea.

      c. **Endotracheal tube position.** In full-term neonates, the distance from glottis to carina is 5 cm. The tube should be 2.5 cm below the level of the cords. Most tubes are marked for this purpose.

      d. In premature infants, the distance from glottis to carina is less than 5 cm. In these patients, limit the endotracheal tube length below the cords to 1.0–1.5 cm. Note that these small distances make neonates particularly vulnerable to inadvertent extubation or endobron-

Table 30-3. Endotracheal tube sizes

Infant weight (gm)	Endotracheal tube* (internal diameter, mm)	Suction catheter size (French gauge)
< 1250	2.5	5 Fr
1250–3000	3.0	6 Fr
> 3000	3.5	8 Fr

*Endotracheal tube internal diameter most commonly used for respective weights. However, a range of tube sizes, from one size smaller to one size larger than anticipated, should be available to accommodate exceptional patients.

chial intubation during resuscitation, mandating added vigilance.

C. **Cardiac compressions.** If the heart rate decreases to less than 80 beats/min and does not respond to ventilation with 100% O_2, external cardiac compressions should be started. The preferred approach in neonates is the **chest encircling technique** with overlapping thumbs compressing in the midline just below the nipple line. With larger infants, adequate compressions may require three fingers with the opposite hand supporting the back. The sternum is depressed ½–¾ inch at 120 compressions/min. The lungs are inflated at a rate of 40/min, to produce a ventilation-compression ratio of 1 : 3. As in pediatric CPR, it is important to allow a pause for an effective **programmed breath.** If no response occurs, appropriate drug therapy should be started.

D. **Drugs and fluids** can be administered either through an umbilical vein catheter, endotracheal tube, or intracardiac route.

　1. **Technique of umbilical vein cannulation**

　　a. The umbilical cord stump and surrounding skin are prepped and draped in a strictly aseptic fashion (i.e., sterile gown and gloves).

　　b. A sterile umbilical tape is placed at the base of the cord, but not tightened.

　　c. The cord is trimmed with a scalpel blade 1 cm above the skin attachment, while holding firmly to prevent bleeding.

　　d. The umbilical vein is identified. (There are two arteries, which have thick muscular walls, while the vein is the thin-walled, largest vessel.)

　　e. An umbilical vein catheter (size 5 Fr for full-terms and 3.5 Fr for prematures), previously flushed with heparinized saline and connected to a three-way stopcock to eliminate any air, is inserted to a distance sufficient to gain access to the central circulation. If resistance is encountered or if there is no free flow of blood, insert the catheter 2.5–5.0 cm beyond the end of the cord. Free blood flow is reconfirmed.

f. Obtain a blood sample for pH determination, and attach a syringe to the stopcock for the administration of drugs.

g. Air embolism must be prevented, as this may be fatal in neonates with a patent foramen ovale.

h. If bleeding occurs, the tie at the base of the cord stump is tightened.

i. Hypertonic solutions such as 25–50% D/W, undiluted $NaHCO_3$, or $CaCl_2$ should not be administered by this route, as they may cause parenchymal damage to the liver.

j. Considering the dangers of infection and portal vein thrombosis, the catheter is usually removed following resuscitation if the infant is stable.

2. As in the adult, epinephrine, atropine, and lidocaine may be administered through the endotracheal tube in the same doses as described below.

3. Dextrose. Hypoglycemia from diminished glycogen stores is common in asphyxiated infants. Rapid infusion of dextrose will correct unrecognized hypoglycemia; however, determination of blood glucose levels should not delay administration of glucose.

a. Initial dose of 0.5 gm/kg IV (2 ml/kg of 25% D/W).

b. Then a continuous infusion of 10% D/W at a rate of 4 ml/kg/hr or less.

4. The use of $NaHCO_3$ following brief arrests or episodes of bradycardia is discouraged. However, administration will decrease hydrogen ion load, improve myocardial contractility, and optimize catecholamine action in prolonged resuscitations. Since there is an association between $NaHCO_3$ infusion and **intraventricular hemorrhage** in premature infants related to the high osmolar load, the neonatal preparation (0.5 mEq/ml) should be administered slowly and with adequate ventilation.

a. Initial dose of 1 mEq/kg given IV over 2 minutes.

b. Subsequent dose of 0.5 mEq/kg IV every 10 minutes during resuscitation.

c. When ABGs are available, subsequent doses are based on the base deficit (see the first part of this chapter, sec. **IV.B.2.c.(3)**).

5. Epinephrine is indicated when there is profound bradycardia or asystole. The initial dose is 0.1–0.3 ml/kg of 1 : 10,000 solution IV and repeated every 5 minutes.

6. Calcium and **atropine** are no longer recommended during the acute phase of neonatal resuscitation.

7. Naloxone is a specific competitive antagonist of

narcotics at opiate receptors. It is indicated in neonates with respiratory depression following maternal administration of narcotics. The duration of action of naloxone (15–30 minutes) is shorter than
that of most narcotics, and so continued apnea
monitoring is required. In the newborn child of a
narcotics addict, naloxone may precipitate an acute
narcotic withdrawal syndrome. The initial dose is
0.01 mg/kg IV, repeated every 2–3 minutes. Administration may also be endotracheal or, if perfusion
is adequate, SQ or IM.

(handwritten margin note: 10 µg/kg)

E. Hypovolemia
  1. Hypovolemia should be considered as an etiology of
  arrest in any neonate who requires resuscitation.
  2. Symptoms and signs
    a. Pre- or intrapartum hemorrhage.
    b. Faint pulses with normal heart rate, tachycar-
    dia, or bradycardia.
    c. Severe asphyxia.
    d. Hypotension.
    e. Persistent pallor, after adequate oxygenation
    and circulatory support are provided.
  **3. Correction of suspected intravascular volume
  deficit** can be accomplished with the following initial amounts and repeated as necessary:
    a. Albumin (5%), 10 ml/kg.
    b. Lactated Ringer's solution, 10 ml/kg.
    c. O-negative whole blood, 10 ml/kg, cross-matched
    with maternal blood.

Suggested Reading

American Heart Association. Standards and guidelines for cardiopulmonary resuscitation (CPR) and emergency cardiac
care (ECC). *J.A.M.A.* 255:2095, 1986.

Geller, S. A., Elliot, P. L., and Rogers, M. C. Update on cardiopulmonary resuscitation. *Adv. Anesth.* 3:323, 1986.

Gregory, G. A. Resuscitation of the newborn. *Anesthesiology*
43:225, 1975.

Orlowski, J. P. Cardiopulmonary resuscitation in children. *Pediatr. Clin. North Am.* 27(3):495, 1980.

Safar, P. *Cardio-Pulmonary-Cerebral-Resuscitation.* Philadelphia: Saunders, 1981.

Todres, I. D., and Rogers, M. C. Methods of external cardiac
massage in the newborn infant. *J. Pediatr.* 86:781, 1975.

31

Newborn Intensive Care

Randall S. Glidden

Anesthesiologists may care for sick neonates in the delivery room, neonatal intensive care unit (NICU), or operating room. Optimal care for these small patients requires an understanding of perinatal physiology, the NICU environment, basic care needs, and the spectrum of disorders that are unique to the newborn. Since many disorders arise from an abnormal transition from fetal to neonatal life, pertinent aspects of normal fetal growth and development and transition of extrauterine life will be reviewed. Next, the initial evaluation of a newborn in distress and principles of basic care are outlined, and finally, specific neonatal problems will be discussed. Care of the neonate in the delivery room (including resuscitation) may be found in Chap. 30, and surgical management of the neonate is discussed in Chap. 23.

I. Physiology
A. Fetal growth and development
1. Organogenesis is virtually complete after the 12th gestational week. Further cellular growth occurs until delivery.
2. **Lung development** is usually insufficient for survival until the 23rd or 24th week, while secretion of surfactant is marginal until the last few weeks gestation. Fetal lung maturation can be augmented by maternal steroid administration.
3. The **circulatory system,** in its final form by the 12th week, is a system of parallel circuits supplying oxygen to fetal organs through the umbilical vessels, intraorgan shunts (ductus venosus, foramen ovale), and the ductus arteriosus.
4. The **kidneys** excrete urine in the second half of pregnancy. Full ability to regulate fluid and electrolytes is incomplete until several months after birth.
5. Body stores of calcium, iron, and phosphate are acquired in the last trimester, with half accumulating in the last 4 weeks.

B. Transition to extrauterine life
1. With the first breath, lung compliance increases and pulmonary vascular resistance acutely falls. Both ventilation and lung perfusion then rapidly increase.
2. **Circulatory readjustments** at birth arise from changes in pulmonary mechanics. The fall in right atrial pressure causes functional closure of the foramen ovale. Right-to-left flow through the ductus arteriosus decreases and then reverses, becoming left-to-right (aorta to pulmonary artery). With increasing PaO_2, constriction of the ductus occurs within several hours, leading to functional closure.

II. Initial evaluation
A. History
1. **Prenatal.** This should include preexisting or acquired maternal disorders (e.g., hypertension, diabetes), specific pregnancy-related problems (e.g., preeclampsia, premature labor, sepsis), maternal drug use (prescribed and recreational), smoking, and alcohol use, all of which could have an effect on the fetus.
2. **Perinatal**
   a. The immediate perinatal course should be reviewed. This should include all relevant data, including number of weeks gestation, time of onset of labor and rupture of membranes, use of tocolytics and fetal monitors, signs of fetal distress, anesthesia, type of delivery (spontaneous, forceps, cesarean), condition of infant at delivery, APGAR scores, and immediate resuscitation steps required. Check to see if vitamin K and antibacterial eye care were given at birth; these important prophylactic measures are easily overlooked.
   b. If the infant was transferred to the NICU from an outside hospital, a summary of the events during transport should be included.
3. **Family history.** Relevant family history includes other abnormal labors/deliveries, preterm births, or siblings with congenital malformations.

B. Physical examination
1. **General inspection.** Although the thorough organ-system approach is as appropriate for neonates as it is for adults, a careful inspection of the naked infant (front and back) will often yield more useful information regarding the infant's immediate needs. Focus on color (especially the oral mucosa, since it is normal to have acrocyanosis; note any jaundice), respiratory effort (comfortable breathing versus grunting, nasal flaring, intercostal retractions, periods of apnea), degree of activity (floppy versus irritable; seizure activity), and any obvious malformations/deformities. **Note:** The presence of one malformation should lead to a thorough search for others.
2. **Vital signs**
   a. **Pulse.** 110–120/min at term (140–180 preterm).
   b. **Respiratory rate.** 35–40 breaths/min at term (50–70 preterm). Note pattern and depth.
   c. **Blood pressure.** 60–90/40–60 at term (40–60/20–40 preterm).
   d. **Temperature.** Normal is 37.5°C (rectally).
3. **Systems examination**
   a. **Head, eyes, ears, nose, and throat.** Record head circumference and presence of any scalp swellings (hematoma versus caput). The fonta-

nelles should be flat and the eyes checked for possible cataracts (i.e., abnormal red reflex). Assure patency of nares by alternately occluding each side and assessing any effect on respirations (newborns are obligate nose-breathers).

  b. **Chest.** Note retractions, rales, rhonchi, or asymmetry of breath sounds.

  c. **Cardiac.** Assess rate, rhythm, and murmurs (may be absent initially but appear after 24–48 hours as intracardiac pressure gradients change). Note peripheral pulses, degree of capillary refill in nail beds, and cyanosis.

  d. **Abdomen.** Note contour (protruding versus scaphoid); number of vessels in umbilical cord (two arteries, one vein); size of liver, spleen, right and left kidneys, and other masses; and bowel sounds. Note the patency of the anus.

  e. **Extremities.** Note any limb deformities, unusual posturing or asymmetric movement of limbs. Examine hips for possible dislocation. Check feet for forefoot adduction and clavicles for possible fracture (especially if delivery was difficult). Note any cyanosis or edema. Examine back for presence of sinus tracts or midline swellings.

  f. **Genitalia.** Is there any ambiguity? Both testes should be palpable; note the presence of hernias.

  g. **Skin.** In addition to color, examine for any unusual pigmented/depigmented areas.

  h. **Neurologic.** Note motor activity, strength, symmetry, and tone and the presence of such newborn reflexes as Moro, tonic neck, grasp, and step/place. Newborns usually have an upgoing Babinski reflex and brisk deep tendon reflexes. The standardized Dubowitz examination may be performed as an aid in estimating gestational age.

C. Laboratory studies

  1. Typical blood tests for sick neonates include arterial blood gases (ABGs), hemoglobin/hematocrit, platelet count, prothrombin time, partial thromboplastin time, WBC with differential, electrolytes, glucose, BUN, creatinine, calcium, phosphate, and bilirubin (total and direct). Urinalysis is done routinely, and more elaborate liver function tests or cardiac enzymes may sometimes be indicated. Similarly, chest x-ray and ECG are obtained if specifically indicated.

  2. If history or physical examination suggests the presence or risk of infection, appropriate cultures should be obtained (see sec. **IV.E**). A gastric aspirate can be gram-stained for evidence of amni-

onitis. "TORCH" group (**T**oxoplasmosis, **O**thers, **R**ubella, **C**ytomegalovirus, **H**erpes simplex virus) acute and convalescent titers and serum IgM may be obtained if a prenatal viral infection is suggested.

D. Assessment. After integrating the history, physical examination, and laboratory evaluation, a problem-oriented assessment should be made. Remember to include a description of the gestational age and size appropriateness. Neonates may be classified in the following manner:

1. **Gestational age**
   a. **Term** (38–42 weeks).
   b. **Preterm** (< 38 weeks). Preterms have a higher incidence of pulmonary immaturity, hemodynamic lability, poor feeding tolerance, and decreased ability to excrete water and solute loads. They are also at increased risk for developing hypoglycemia (glucose < 30 mg/dl) and hypocalcemia (total calcium < 7 mg/dl) and have poor temperature regulating ability.
   c. **Post-term** (> 42 weeks). Post-term infants often suffer from placental insufficiency and may be meconium stained or asphyxiated at birth. They may also exhibit hypoglycemia and polycythemia (hematocrit > 65%).

2. **Weight,** as a function of gestational age, may be plotted on standardized graphs to categorize an infant as "appropriate," "large," or "small" for apparent gestational age (AGA, LGA, SGA).
   a. **Small for gestational age** (SGA) implies "intrauterine growth retardation." The size of these infants may be the result of chromosomal defects, maternal hypertension or smoking, chronic placental insufficiency, or congenital infection; thus an attempt should be made to determine the etiology. These infants have a high incidence of hypoglycemia, hypocalcemia, and polycythemia.
   b. **Large for gestational age** (LGA) infants are associated with maternal diabetes and should be followed for hypoglycemia resulting from high circulating insulin levels.
   c. Infants with birth weights less than 1.5 kg are termed **very low birth weight** (VLBW).

III. Basic care

A. Environment. The physical environment in the NICU has evolved in response to the special needs of neonates.

1. **Infection**
   a. Sick neonates are particularly vulnerable to infection, and there is an increased risk of nosocomial infection and colonization in NICUs.
   b. Infectious transmission may be reduced by using separate equipment and isolettes (or warming tables) for each infant, by scrupulous hand-

washing before and after each handling, and by having all personnel and visitors wear cover gowns or scrub clothes.

2. Hypothermia

a. Neonates are inherently prone to large heat losses because of a large surface area–body weight ratio. They also have less subcutaneous fat and minimal brown fat stores to fuel non-shivering thermogenesis. These conditions are most pronounced in preterm and SGA infants. Heat loss leads to detrimental increases in oxygen and caloric consumption.

b. Management

   (1) Warmed isolette walls help prevent radiant and convective heat loss. Isolette temperature should be set to maintain "neutral thermal environment."

   (2) Warming table with skin temperature probe (used for sicker infants) also prevents radiant heat loss.

   (3) Use warmed, humidified oxygen in ventilator circuits.

   (4) Use warming lights for procedures outside isolettes.

   (5) Heat loss must be prevented by using warmed isolettes and prewarmed procedure rooms when infants travel outside the NICU for procedures.

B. Fluids and electrolytes

1. Physiology

a. A **"physiologic diuresis"** normally occurs after birth. With decreasing gestational age, extracellular fluid (ECF) accounts for a larger fraction of total body water (85% in 36-week, 75% in term infant). It is normal to lose 5–10% of the ECF in the first few days, so initial fluid therapy should allow for a 5–10% weight loss while supplying adequate water, electrolytes, and calories. Renal function differs from that of the older child in that the neonate is less able to concentrate urine and to handle solute loads.

b. Maintenance fluids are based on

   (1) Normal expected ECF loss (first week only).

   (2) Insensible water loss. This is normally 60–120 ml/kg/day and is increased with lower birth weight, phototherapy, radiant warmer use, and fever.

   (3) Ongoing abnormal losses.

   (4) Caloric needs may be partially met with 10% D/W.

   (5) Electrolyte administration is aimed at maintenance of normal serum concentrations and normal osmolarity. Usual requirement is 1–3 mEq/kg/day for sodium and potassium. With physiologic diuresis, there is usually no need for added electrolytes in the first 24 hours.

2. Management
a. First 24 hours
(1) If body weight is greater than 1.0 kg: 60–100 ml/kg/day 10% D/W (no added electrolytes).

(2) If body weight is less than 1.0 kg: 100–120 ml/kg/day 10% D/W.

(3) If under radiant warmer, may need to adjust upward.

b. After 24 hours
(1) Increase or decrease total fluids to maintain approximately 1% loss in body weight/day (for the first week only) and a urine output of at least 0.5 ml/kg/hr.

(2) Can usually add 1–2 mEq/kg/day of sodium and potassium (as chloride salts), based on serum concentrations and osmolality.

(3) Infants who are VLBW may require less dextrose; they often become hyperglycemic on 10% solutions.

(4) Infants on ventilators will gain a large amount of free water from the humidified gases.

(5) Follow weights (daily or twice daily), skin turgor, color, capillary refill, and urine output to assess adequacy of therapy.

C. Nutrition
1. Physiology
a. Nutritional requirements (in addition to fluids/electrolytes) may be met by enteral (ideally) and/or parenteral means.

(1) **Calories.** 60–80 kcal/kg/day for maintenance of weight, 100–130 kcal/kg/day for growth.

(2) **Protein.** 2–4 gm/kg/day.

(3) **Essential fatty acids.**

(4) **Vitamins.** Folate; vitamins E, D, and K.

(5) **Minerals.** Calcium (180–220 mEq/kg/day), phosphate, magnesium, zinc, copper, manganese, and iron.

b. The gastrointestinal tract is functional at 28–30 weeks' gestation but is of limited capacity.

2. Management
a. Enteral route
(1) **Formulas.** If the mother's breast milk is not available, a variety of products exist designed especially for the premature infant. The ideal infant formula is an imitation of human breast milk, with a high whey to casein ratio (60 : 40). Fat should provide 40–50% of the calories. Although lactose is the usual source of carbohydrate, the preterm infant may have lac-

tose intolerance; other formulas are available that use glucose, glucose polymers, or corn syrup.

(2) Feeding. Infants over 32 weeks' gestation without other problems may have adequate suck reflex to feed from breast or bottle, with occasional gavage supplementation if necessary. Under 32 weeks, infants often have poor suck and gag reflexes and should be fed by gavage by a small feeding catheter. Usually begin with 1–5 ml every 2–4 hours (depending on size), starting with sterile water and advancing to dextrose-water and then dilute formula as tolerated.

(3) If unable to supply adequate calories for growth by enteral means alone within 72 hours, consider parenteral supplementation.

(4) Very ill neonates and those with high respiratory rates should be fed by gavage or parenterally.

b. Parenteral route

(1) A peripheral route (small IV catheter) or central route (subclavian cannula) must be established. Up to 12.5% dextrose can be safely administered by peripheral vein.

(2) After calculating fluid requirements, estimated calories are supplied as follows: dextrose, 5–15% (4 kcal/gm) based on infant's ability to tolerate glucose load; protein, 2–3 gm/kg/day (4 kcal/gm); and fat to supply remainder of caloric needs (but not to exceed 40–50% of total calories). Fat is supplied as 10% fat emulsion (e.g., Intralipid, 1.1 kcal/ml). Most hospitals have protocols for adding vitamin and mineral supplements to the nutrition solution.

(3) Monitoring. Besides serum glucose, electrolytes, osmolality, and urine output, liver function tests, BUN, and creatinine should be monitored, since these may be adversely affected by protein infusions. Fat emulsions have been associated with hyperlipemia, rare acute reactions, decreased platelet adhesiveness, eosinophilia, and fat deposition in the lungs. Fat emulsion infusion may be contraindicated in infants with thrombocytopenia.

IV. Common neonatal problems

A. Respiratory system

1. Initial considerations

a. Physical examination may reveal tachypnea, grunting, retractions, nasal flaring, cyanosis.

b. Initial laboratory studies should include an arterial (or arterialized capillary) blood gas, hematocrit, and chest x-ray. Additional studies will be necessary to confirm or rule out potential etiologies, as suggested by the differential diagnoses.

c. **Differential diagnosis**

(1) **Airway obstruction.** Consider choanal atresia, vocal cord palsy, laryngomalacia, hemangioma, tracheal stenosis, obstruction of trachea by external masses (e.g., cystic hygroma, vascular ring anomalies).

(2) **Developmental anomalies.** Tracheoesophageal fistula, diaphragmatic hernia, congenital emphysema, lung cysts.

(3) **Lung parenchyma.** Hyaline membrane disease, pneumonia, meconium aspiration, transient tachypnea, pneumothorax.

(4) **Nonpulmonary.** Cyanotic congenital heart disease, persistent pulmonary hypertension, congestive heart failure (CHF), metabolic disturbances (e.g., acidosis).

2. **Specific respiratory disorders**

a. **Respiratory distress syndrome** (RDS)

(1) Respiratory distress syndrome (also known as hyaline membrane disease) is a major cause of morbidity and mortality in premature infants. The lungs of some preterm infants lack surfactant, which leads to either the failure of alveoli to expand or collapse of those already expanded. The persistence of significant atelectasis alters lung mechanics, greatly increases the work of breathing, and promotes $\dot{V}_A/\dot{Q}$ mismatch. This in turn leads to increased pulmonary vascular resistance and right-to-left shunting across the foramen ovale and the ductus arteriosus. These events may ultimately produce life-threatening hypoxemia and respiratory failure. Differential inflation of some areas of the lung can predispose to pneumothorax and pneumomediastinum.

(2) Infants at risk for RDS include premature infants, infants of diabetic mothers, infants born by cesarean delivery, asphyxiated infants, and those with previously affected sibling(s). Infants at risk may be identified prenatally by amniocentesis and evaluation of amniotic fluid for lecithin-sphingomyelin (L/S) ratio less than 2 : 1 or saturated phosphatidylcholine (SPC) less than 500 µg/dl. Glucocorticoids given prior to delivery may prevent or attenuate the severity of the illness.

(3) Infants with RDS demonstrate tachypnea, grunting, nasal flaring, retractions, and hypoxemia within several hours af-

ter birth. The chest x-ray will show a "ground-glass" pattern and air bronchograms. A **"shake test"** for surfactant in swallowed amniotic fluid confirms the diagnosis (bubbles will not appear if insufficient surfactant is present). Besides respiratory involvement, infants may also demonstrate signs of cardiovascular and metabolic abnormalities (e.g., patent ductus and acidosis).

  (4) Management

    (a) Initial treatment consists of providing warmed, humidified oxygen by hood and following PaO_2 and $PaCO_2$. The PaO_2 should be maintained between 50 and 80 mm Hg (or $< 95\%$ SaO_2 if using a pulse oximeter) to obviate the possible risk of retinopathy associated with hyperoxia. Samples can be obtained through a radial or umbilical artery catheter or arterialized capillary sample ("cap gas"). Saturation may be followed with a pulse oximeter. A transcutaneous Clark electrode may be used to display $PtcO_2$ continuously.

    (b) If deterioration occurs (> 0.60 FiO_2 is needed or increasing tachypnea), continuous positive airway pressure (CPAP) can be provided either by nasal prongs, nasopharyngeal tube, or by endotracheal tube. Usually start CPAP at 5 cm H_2O.

    (c) If carbon dioxide retention, hypoxemia on greater than 0.60 FiO_2, or apnea develops, mechanical ventilation is indicated (see sec. **IV.A.3**).

  (5) Since RDS is indistinguishable from sepsis/pneumonia caused by group B beta-hemolytic streptococcus, broad-spectrum antibiotics (usually ampicillin and gentamicin) are begun after obtaining appropriate culture (see sec. **IV.E**).

  (6) Continued monitoring of cardiovascular, renal, and metabolic function is extremely important, especially with severe RDS. Positive-pressure ventilation may adversely affect cardiac preload (and hence cardiac output), leading to poor perfusion to other organ systems.

  (7) As the child improves, respiratory support should be slowly weaned. Weaning steps should always be done gradually, changing one parameter at a time (see sec. **IV.A.3.i**).

(a) Generally, peak inspiratory pressure is slowly lowered to less than 30 cm H_2O.

(b) Then FIO_2 is lowered in increments of 0.05 until less than 0.50.

(c) Intermittent mandatory ventilation can then be reduced ($PaCO_2$ permitting), ultimately leading to CPAP alone.

(d) Extubation can usually be accomplished when ABGs are in an acceptable range, the FIO_2 is less than 0.40, and CPAP is reduced to 2–3 cm H_2O ("physiologic CPAP").

(e) After extubation, infants are placed in oxygen hoods at the same FIO_2 and are observed closely for any sign of respiratory distress.

(8) Various **complications** may occur during recovery from RDS. For instance, a tension pneumothorax may develop when, as compliance improves, relative hyperinflation during positive-pressure ventilation leads to air leak. Other frequent short-term complications include superimposed infections, intraventricular hemorrhages, and the reopening of a ductus arteriosus. Sicker victims of RDS may suffer from longer term effects, such as bronchopulmonary dysplasia and retinopathy of prematurity.

b. Pneumothorax

(1) Pneumothorax is a frequent complication seen in mechanically ventilated infants and occasionally in otherwise normal term infants. Uneven ventilation with overdistention of airways and alveoli is the probable etiology.

(2) The diagnosis should be considered in any neonate with respiratory distress or in the ventilated infant with an acute change in condition (e.g., sudden cyanosis, hypotension, agitation). Often one hears asymmetric breath sounds, but this is not a constant finding. Transillumination of the chest with a strong light usually will show a hyperlucent hemithorax; a chest x-ray will confirm the diagnosis.

(3) Treatment consists in aspiration with an IV needle and should be performed before obtaining a chest x-ray if the infant becomes unstable. Reaccumulation of air after aspiration warrants immediate placement of a chest tube.

(4) Other air leak syndromes include pneumo-

mediastinum and pneumopericardium. Although occasionally asymptomatic, drainage is required if symptoms occur.

c. Meconium aspiration

  (1) The passage of meconium in utero is often seen during the stresses of the perinatal period, with an incidence of about 1% of all live births. Often these infants are postmature or have shown signs of distress on fetal monitoring.

  (2) Infants delivered through thick meconium-stained fluid should be intubated and suctioned, preferably before they have taken the first breath. Absence of meconium in the oropharynx does not exclude its presence in the trachea.

  (3) Disruption of pulmonary physiology may be due to complete large airway obstruction by large particles of meconium, obstruction of terminal airways (with subsequent atelectasis and right-to-left shunt), incomplete (ball-valve) obstructions (with overinflation and pneumothorax), or pneumonia (either chemical or by superimposed bacterial infection).

  (4) Treatment includes respiratory support as needed and usually broad-spectrum antibiotics. Such infants often demonstrate persistent pulmonary hypertension.

d. Apnea

  (1) Periods of apnea longer than 20 seconds are usually considered "true apnea" as opposed to the normal brief pauses ("periodic breathing") often demonstrated by the premature infant. True apnea is often accompanied by bradycardia.

  (2) True apnea stems from immaturity of the premature infant's respiratory control center. Other causes include airway obstruction, sepsis, hypoxemia, hypo- or hyperthermia, gastroesophageal reflux, hypocalcemia, hypoglycemia, anemia, other central nervous system (CNS) disease (hemorrhage or seizures), and maternal drug use; such causes should always be considered before labeling apneic episodes "physiologic" or "apnea of immaturity."

  (3) Individual episodes usually require only tactile stimulation and continued monitoring for any new episodes. Further treatment includes the correction of any underlying problems, the use of oscillating water mattresses to provide stimulation, decreasing the temperature to the lower end of the neutral thermal zone, and/or the use of respiratory stimulants.

Theophylline PO or IV (loading dose of 5–7 mg/kg, then 1.5–2.0 mg/kg/6hr) has often been beneficial. The therapeutic serum level is 5–15 μg/ml.

(4) Severe recurrent episodes may require intubation and CPAP or mechanical ventilation.

3. **Mechanical ventilation**

   a. **Indications** for mechanical ventilation include an FIO_2 requirement greater than 0.60, $PaCO_2$ over 50, and/or obvious indications of respiratory fatigue. The goal of mechanical ventilation is to provide for gaseous exchange without producing any sequellae.

   b. Although volume-preset neonatal ventilators exist, **pressure-limited time-cycled ventilators** are used most often. In essence, these devices consist of a source for a warmed, humidified mixture of air and oxygen, connected by a T to the infant's endotracheal tube and the outside environment. By intermittently occluding the exhaust end of the T, a quantity of gas is diverted to the infant, producing a tidal volume breath. The timing of the occluding valve determines the inspiratory and expiratory times, and a "pop-off" valve limits the peak inspiratory pressure (PIP) generated. Placing a resistance at the exhaust valve generates positive end-expiratory pressure (PEEP).

   c. **Oxygenation** can be improved by increases in FIO_2, mean airway pressure, and PEEP. Carbon dioxide elimination is dependent on minute ventilation ($\dot{V}m$), which can be increased by increasing rate or tidal volume (V_T) (e.g., increase PIP or inspiratory time) and by decreasing PEEP.

   d. Babies with **RDS** usually have high airway resistance and low lung compliance. The usual starting rate is in the 30s with an inspiratory time of 0.5–1.0 seconds and an expiratory time of 1.0–1.5 seconds. A maximum inspiratory time of 1.0–1.5 seconds and a minimum expiratory time of 0.3 seconds may be required to provide adequate ventilation in sicker neonates. Other initial settings can be estimated after hand ventilating with a Mapleson circuit and manometer and observing for adequacy of chest movement and PIP required. Positive end-expiratory pressure may be added in increments, usually starting with 5 cm H_2O, but rarely exceeding 10. FIO_2 should be kept at an appropriate minimum to prevent lung toxicity.

   e. If the infant "fights" the ventilator, sedation with morphine (0.1 mg/kg), and possibly muscle relaxation, may be required. Such behavior may actually represent hypoventilation, hypoxemia, or hypoperfusion; these must be ruled out before proceeding with sedation or paralysis.

f. Close monitoring of ABGs is essential, particularly after changing ventilator settings or deterioration in the infant's condition.

g. A **sudden worsening** in condition mandates immediate checking of the apparatus (from wall connections to endotracheal tube). When in doubt, disconnect from the mechanical ventilator and ventilate the infant by hand. Besides mechanical problems, check for blocked or kinked endotracheal tube, endobronchial intubation, and pneumothorax.

h. As RDS improves, lung compliance increases; overinflation at the previously preset PIP can lead to pneumothorax unless it is carefully adjusted downward during this time.

i. **Weaning** should proceed by discontinuing the elements with the most potential for harm. For example, PIP should be less than 30 cm H_2O and FIO_2 less than 0.6 before changing rate or PEEP. FIO_2 should be decreased gradually, usually 0.05–0.10 at a time; PIP is lowered 2–3 cm H_2O at a time. Then rate can also be reduced, ultimately allowing the infant to breathe spontaneously. Extubation is considered once the infant is on 2–3 cm H_2O CPAP and FIO_2 not more than 0.4 and is not tachypneic when breathing spontaneously.

B. **Cardiovascular system**

1. **Congenital heart disease.** Neonates with cardiac disease may demonstrate cyanosis, CHF, arrhythmias, and murmurs. Physical examinations should include four-extremity blood pressure measurements and, in the presence of cardiac signs and symptoms, chest x-ray, arterial blood gases, hematocrit, and often two-dimensional echocardiography.

a. **Cyanosis**

(1) Arterial desaturation is characteristic of cardiac lesions that produce right-to-left shunting. Blood entering the right heart may be shunted to the left (usually through the foramen ovale) because of structural obstruction at the tricuspid and/or pulmonic valve level or because of rearrangements in the outflow tracts (as with transposition of the great arteries). Most of these lesions depend on the patency of the ductus arteriosus to provide flow through the lungs. Examples of "ductus-dependent" lesions include transposition of the great arteries, pulmonic stenosis/atresia, tricuspid atresia, tetralogy of Fallot, and Ebstein's anomaly.

(2) The diagnosis of cardiac shunt as the cause of cyanosis can usually be confirmed by the failure of the infant to raise PaO_2 above 150 mm Hg on an FiO_2 of 1.0. With positive-pressure ventilation and PEEP, a PaO_2 of greater than 150 mm Hg is usually achieved at this FiO_2 in the presence of pulmonary disease or persistent pulmonary hypertension. Other noncardiac causes of cyanosis include polycythemia and methemoglobinemia.

(3) Initial management consists in optimizing hemoglobin saturation and stabilizing any accompanying problems, in anticipation of surgical correction or palliation. Infants should be placed in an atmosphere of 50% oxygen; higher FiO_2 adds risk of direct pulmonary toxicity and will not raise PaO_2 if a fixed shunt exists. Hematocrit should be 40 or more. If a ductus-dependent lesion exists, ductal closure may be prevented by placing the infant in room air and by infusing prostaglandin E_1 [Prostin VR], 0.1–0.5 µg/kg/min). Prostaglandin side effects include apnea, hypotension, and seizure activity.

b. **Congestive heart failure**

(1) Congestive heart failure usually presents with tachypnea, tachycardia, diaphoresis, excessive weight gain, signs of decreased perfusion (e.g., poor capillary refill, oliguria), and decreased growth.

(2) Lesions responsible for CHF usually do so because of increased flow (patent ductus arteriosus, ventricular septal defect) or obstruction of outflow (aortic stenosis, coarctation of the aorta). Left-to-right shunt, with greatly augmented pulmonic blood flow, is a frequent finding.

(3) Treatment consists in fluid and sodium restriction, maintenance of normal hematocrit and PaO_2, diuresis as indicated, and digitalization. Infusion of PGE_1 may be used to improve CHF in preductal aortic coarctation, by providing ductal flow to the postductal aorta.

(4) Congestive heart failure refractory to the above, or with signs of hypoperfusion, may be treated with inotropes (e.g., dopamine, dobutamine, or isoproterenol).

c. **Patent ductus arteriosus**

(1) Patent ductus arteriosus is often found in the premature infant and is characterized by a murmur at the left sternal border, bounding peripheral pulses, excessive

weight gain, and evidence of increased pulmonary blood flow (e.g., failure to wean from mechanical ventilation).

(2) Treatment includes the same measures as for CHF; however, digoxin is of questionable effectiveness. Pharmacologic closure with indomethacin (0.2 mg/kg PO every 12 hours for 3 doses) may be tried if other medical management fails to close the ductus within 24–48 hours. Surgical closure may be indicated if pharmacotherapy fails.

d. Arrhythmias

(1) The most frequent arrhythmia seen in neonates is paroxysmal atrial tachycardia (PAT).

(2) Vagal maneuvers (such as nasopharyngeal stimulation or immersing the face in ice water) may be tried with caution.

(3) Digitalization will usually convert the PAT to sinus rhythm; maintenance for 1 year is subsequently indicated. Propranolol or quinidine is a reasonable alternative medication, but DC conversions may be necessary.

2. Persistent pulmonary hypertension (PPH)

a. Persistent pulmonary hypertension, also referred to as persistent fetal circulation (PFC), is a disorder of varied etiologies seen most often in infants near term. It is manifested by an increase in pulmonary vascular resistance (PVR) with resulting pulmonary arterial hypertension, right-to-left shunting across the ductus and foramen ovale, and profound cyanosis.

b. A predisposing condition (e.g., asphyxia, meconium aspiration, bacterial pneumonia/sepsis) may cause alveolar hypoxia, which triggers a reflex increase in PVR. Initially infants may seem to have normal lungs, but once initiated, the manifestations of PPH may become life-threatening. In some cases, infants may have underlying pathology of their pulmonary vasculature and exhibit even more exaggerated responses. Babies with diaphragmatic hernia often have PPH, probably secondary to pulmonary hypoplasia.

c. Markedly cyanotic infants may present after a stormy delivery, with decreased pulmonary vascular markings on chest x-ray and no evidence of lung pathology. Usually there is also marked hypoxemia ($PaO_2 < 60$ mm Hg) even on 100% oxygen (which excludes most lung parenchymal causes, where a marked positive response in SaO_2 is seen). A dramatic improvement may follow active positive-pressure hyperventilation, as PVR normalizes secondary to decreased

$PaCO_2$. This hyperventilation maneuver excludes true right-to-left shunt (as seen in cyanotic congenital heart disease), but cardiac echocardiography will still be needed to rule out congenital heart disease. (One added complication to ABG interpretation is that a gradient may be present between well-oxygenated preductal arterial blood [by right radial] and desaturated postductal blood [by umbilical artery line] that will vary with changes in PVR.)

d. Management consists in intubation and mechanical ventilation, often with high rates (maintaining a $PaCO_2$ in the 20–30 mm Hg range) and high FIO_2 (which also serves to diminish PVR). Lung mechanics are usually normal, so short inspiratory times and little (if any) PEEP will suffice. Paralysis may aid in ventilation. Profound analgesia induced with fentanyl infusion (1–3 μg/kg/hr) may help ablate PVR elevations from noxious stimuli. Systemic acidosis may require sodium bicarbonate infusion.

(1) If needed, support can be given with dopamine, isoproterenol, or crystalloid or colloid to maintain preload.

(2) Elevated PVR may respond to tolazoline (1 mg/kg IV over 10 minutes; continue if a response is seen). However, this is a nonselective vasodilator that may lower systemic blood pressure as well. Prostaglandins have been used with qualified success.

(3) If improvement occurs, gradual reduction of FIO_2 can be tried. These infants may demonstrate exquisite sensitivity to minute changes in FIO_2 (the so-called flip-flop phenomenon), leading to a sudden increase in PVR and a fall in PaO_2, so extreme vigilance is warranted during weaning.

e. Despite best efforts, many patients show a progressive deterioration of respiratory function, often succumbing to the combined effects of PPH and the morbidity of prolonged mechanical ventilation.

C. Gastrointestinal system
   1. Surgical diseases
      a. Esophageal atresia
         (1) Esophageal atresia should be suspected when a nasogastric tube cannot be passed into the stomach. The majority of esophageal atresias are of the blind pouch variety with a distal tracheoesophageal fistula (TEF). This distal TEF may produce respiratory distress, another frequent find-

ing in this disorder. Other variations, such as the H-type TEF, are relatively rare.

(2) X-ray verification of a nasogastric tube held up in an esophageal pouch will usually confirm the diagnosis.

(3) Treatment consists in surgical decompression with a gastrostomy tube, followed later by definitive repair. Initially, however, the nasogastric tube should be placed on continuous suction. Endotracheal intubation and ventilation are indicated if respiratory compromise occurs. The tip of the endotracheal tube should be positioned distal to the fistula (usually close to the carina) to avoid gastric distention during positive-pressure ventilation; this will necessitate close observation for possible endobronchial migration of the tip.

b. Diaphragmatic hernia

(1) Diaphragmatic hernia should be suspected in the neonate with respiratory distress and a scaphoid abdomen. Although diaphragmatic hernia usually presents within 24 hours after birth, the diagnosis may be delayed in infants with less severe pulmonary involvement. Often profound cyanosis and unilaterally decreased breath sounds are present. A chest x-ray will reveal abdominal contents (e.g., gas shadows) in the thorax (usually the left side).

(2) Most of the morbidity and high mortality rate are due to varying degrees of pulmonary hypoplasia with resultant pulmonary hypertension, $\dot{V}A/\dot{Q}$ mismatch, and right-to-left shunting across the ductus arteriosus and foramen ovale.

(3) Initial management includes nasogastric decompression of the stomach and, usually, endotracheal intubation and ventilation utilizing a rapid rate with high FIO_2, low PIP, and no PEEP. Anesthesia with a continuous fentanyl infusion (3 µg/kg/hr) and paralysis may reduce sympathetic responsiveness and facilitate ventilation. Inotropes and volume support may be required.

(4) Surgical repair should be performed as soon as possible after the initial stabilization.

(5) Management after surgery is similar to that discussed for PPH (sec. **IV.B.2**).

c. Duodenal atresia. This condition usually presents with bile-stained emesis, upper abdominal distention, and increased volume of gastric aspirates. Abdominal x-ray often reveals the "double bubble," representing air in the stomach and upper duodenum. Seen more frequently in infants with Down's syndrome, duodenal atresia may coexist with other intestinal malformations. Treatment consists in nasogastric decompression and surgical correction.

d. **Pyloric stenosis.** Although usually seen in the second or third week of life, pyloric stenosis may present in the immediate newborn period with persistent nonbilious vomiting and (often) a metabolic alkalosis from loss of gastric hydrochloric acid. An abdominal mass consisting of the hypertrophic pylorus ("olive") may be palpable. The diagnosis is confirmed by abdominal x-ray (gastric dilatation) and by barium swallow. After metabolic abnormalities are corrected, nasogastric drainage and surgical repair are indicated.

e. **Volvulus**
   (1) Volvulus may occur as a primary lesion or as the result of intestinal malrotation. If present in utero, intestinal necrosis may be present at birth, and emergency resection is indicated.
   (2) Usual manifestations include abdominal distention, bilious vomiting, and occasionally, signs of shock and sepsis. The diagnosis of malrotation is made by barium enema, which demonstrates an abnormally positioned ligament of Treitz.

f. **Gastroschisis and omphalocele**
   (1) These disorders are caused by failure of the abdominal wall to close completely, allowing the viscera to remain outside the abdominal cavity. The abdominal contents may be covered with intact or ruptured peritoneum (omphalocele), or they may be entirely open to the external environment (gastroschisis).
   (2) Medical stabilization includes nasogastric drainage and protection of the viscera prior to repair of the abdominal defect. If the peritoneal sac is intact, the omphalocele should be covered with sterile, warm petrolatum gauze to decrease heat and water loss and the risk of infection. If the sac has ruptured (or if the infant has a gastroschisis), saline-soaked gauze should be used to wrap the exposed viscera; the infant should then be wrapped in warmed sterile towels. The infant should be carefully positioned to avoid kinking the blood supply from the mesentery.

2. **Necrotizing enterocolitis**
   a. Necrotizing enterocolitis is a syndrome of acute intestinal necrosis occurring predominantly in premature infants (80% are < 1000 gm). It usually develops after the first week of life and almost always after the institution of enteral feedings. Mortality may be as high as 40%.
   b. Pathogenesis is unclear but probably involves overgrowth of intestinal microflora and invasion of ischemic enteric mucosa, with subsequent development of coagulative necrosis, which may lead to intestinal perforation.
   c. Presenting signs include an increase in gastric aspirates, abdominal distention, emesis, abdominal wall erythema, and ileus. The infant may show such systemic signs as temperature instability, lethargy, respiratory and circulatory instability, oliguria, and bleeding diathesis.
   d. Laboratory evaluation should include abdominal x-ray (may show fixed loops of bowel, pneumatosis intestinalis, or portal air), CBC (thrombocytopenia), ABGs (acidosis), stool guaiac, and stool Clinitest (evidence of bleeding and/or carbohydrate malabsorption). Since the differential diagnosis includes sepsis, cultures of blood, urine, CSF, and stool should also be obtained.
   e. When necrotizing enterocolitis is suspected, enteral feedings are discontinued, and the stomach is decompressed with a nasogastric tube. The child is then kept NPO for at least 2 weeks and supported with parenteral feedings. Broad-spectrum antibiotics are begun (ampicillin, gentamicin, and if perforation is suspected, clindamycin). Serial platelet counts may help predict exacerbation or resolution of the illness. Surgical consultation is usually warranted.
3. **Hyperbilirubinemia**
   a. **Pathophysiology**
      (1) After hemoglobin degradation, unconjugated bilirubin is bound to albumin, conjugated in the liver, and then excreted through the gastrointestinal tract. Unconjugated ("indirect acting") bilirubin is lipid-soluble and is capable of entering the central nervous system if serum levels exceed the binding capacity of circulating albumin. Toxic buildup of bilirubin in the CNS stains the basal ganglia and hippocampus (kernicterus). This can produce a variety of neurologic sequelae, ranging from severe cerebral palsy to a syndrome of minimal brain dysfunction appearing later in childhood.
      (2) In general, hyperbilirubinemia may result from overproduction (e.g., hemolysis),

underconjugation (e.g., immature liver), underexcretion (e.g., biliary atresia), or a combination of the above.

b. Specific causes

   (1) Physiologic jaundice is common in most neonates because of increased red cell turnover and decreased conjugating ability of the liver. Although rarely of significance in the term infant, the premature infant may reach potentially toxic levels by this mechanism alone.

   (2) Hemolytic disease (especially Rh induced) was once the major cause of severe hyperbilirubinemia; the routine use of Rh immune globulin (RhoGAM) has now made Rh disease uncommon. However maternal sensitization to ABO blood group antigens (and others such as Kell) can produce a milder hemolysis in the neonate leading to jaundice. Hemolysis may also accompany primary red cell abnormalities such as spherocytosis.

   (3) Increased bilirubin load may result from absorption of sequestered blood (e.g., bruised infant, cephalhematomas) and polycythemia.

   (4) Hyperbilirubinemia may occur with sepsis, asphyxia, peripheral alimentation, breast milk feeding, and such metabolic disorders as hypothyroidism, hypoglycemia, and galactosemia.

c. Evaluation. Laboratory studies include total and direct bilirubin, Coombs' test, and blood smear for red blood cell morphology. If bacterial infection is suspected, appropriate cultures are indicated.

d. Treatment

   (1) Physiologic and mild hemolytic jaundice are simply monitored with serial bilirubin levels. If tolerated, early feeding is usually indicated to reduce enterohepatic reuptake of bilirubin.

   (2) Charts are readily available that relate birth weight and age to acceptable bilirubin concentrations. The more immature the infant, the lower the maximum allowable bilirubin concentration.

   (3) Phototherapy (irradiation with 420–460 nm light) is usually begun for moderate bilirubin elevations, especially in preterm infants. Exchange transfusion is reserved for those infants with bilirubin levels close to the potentially toxic range, when there is a rapid rate of rise, or when there is evidence of massive hemolysis at birth. Exchange transfusion is indicated if indirect bilirubins from cord blood are greater than 5 mg/dl; preterm infant, greater than 10–15 mg/dl; or term infant, greater than 25 mg/dl.

D. Neurologic system

1. Seizures

a. Seizures are a common neonatal problem and may be generalized, focal, or subtle. Jitteriness alone, however, may also be a manifestation of a seizure disorder.

b. **Etiologies** include birth trauma (with or without intracranial hemorrhage), postasphyxia encephalopathy, metabolic disturbances (hypoglycemia or hypocalcemia), drug withdrawal, and infections (including viral). Pyridoxine dependency is a rare cause of neonatal seizures.

c. **Workup** includes
   (1) Electrolytes, glucose, calcium, magnesium; possibly serum/urine amino acids.
   (2) Appropriate cultures, including cerebrospinal fluid.
   (3) Cranial ultrasound and/or CT scan.
   (4) Electroencephalogram before and during pyridoxine administration.

d. **Treatment.** Underlying problems are corrected, a test dose of pyridoxine (50 mg IV) is administered, anticonvulsants are started, and any respiratory/cardiovascular compromise is supported.

e. **Anticonvulsants**
   (1) **Phenobarbital.** 10 mg/kg IV load, two times over several minutes; maintenance dosage of 5 mg/kg/day (divide every 12 hours) to maintain a serum level of 20–40 μg/ml.
   (2) **Phenytoin** (Dilantin). 10 mg/kg IV load, two times (no faster than 1 mg/kg/min); maintenance 5 mg/kg/day (divide every 12 hours), to a therapeutic level of 15–30 μg/ml.
   (3) **Diazepam.** 0.1–0.3 mg/kg IV (may cause apnea).
   (4) **Paraldehyde** (rectal). 0.1–0.3 ml/kg.

2. Intracranial hemorrhage

a. Intracranial bleeding sites can include the subdural, subarachnoid, and (most commonly) intraventricular spaces. Intraventricular hemorrhage probably occurs in over 40% of infants below 1500 gm.

b. Although intracranial hemorrhage of all types may present with seizures or other CNS signs, intraventricular hemorrhage is often silent and is diagnosed by cranial ultrasound. Grading of intraventricular hemorrhage is based on the amount of blood seen and whether or not intracerebral extension of blood is present.

    c. Surgical decompression of subdural hematomata is usually indicated. Intraventricular hemorrhage is usually treated supportively.

    d. The major complication of intraventricular hemorrhage is hydrocephalus due to intraventricular cerebrospinal fluid obstruction (which often requires shunting). Daily measurement of head circumference and frequent repeat ultrasound examinations are therefore mandatory.

    e. Since hypertonic agents (e.g., sodium bicarbonate and 50% D/W) have been implicated as an etiology of intraventricular hemorrhage, judicious use of the more dilute solutions manufactured specifically for neonates is probably safest.

E. Infectious diseases

  1. Prolonged rupture of membranes

    a. Leakage of amniotic fluid for over 24 hours is associated with a high incidence of amnionitis and subsequent bacterial infection in the neonate.

    b. Workup of the infant includes Gram's stain and culture of gastric aspirate, CBC with differential, and sedimentation rate.

    c. If frank amnionitis or neonatal infection seems likely, cultures of blood, urine, and possibly cerebrospinal fluid are obtained, and antibiotic coverage with ampicillin and an aminoglycoside is begun.

  2. Neonatal sepsis

    a. Early neonatal bacterial infections can include generalized sepsis, pneumonia, urinary tract infection, and meningitis. Organisms responsible for infections soon after birth are usually acquired in utero or from passage through the birth canal, and can include group B beta-hemolytic streptococcus, *Escherichia coli,* and *Listeria.* Later onset infections may be caused by *Staphylococcus aureus* and *S. epidermidis.*

    b. The clinical presentation of sepsis can be protean and include RDS, shock, temperature instability, CNS signs (seizures, apnea, irritability), and poor feeding. Therefore a high index of suspicion is warranted.

    c. Laboratory evaluation should include appropriate cultures, CBC with platelet count, urinalysis, and chest x-ray. Counterimmunoelectrophoresis or latex fixation tests may be useful in identifying specific pathogens before cultures are available.

    d. Broad-spectrum antibiotics are usually begun (ampicillin or oxacillin plus an aminoglycoside) and continued for 48–72 hours pending culture results. If cultures are positive, treatment should continue as indicated by the severity and location of the infection. Aminoglycoside serum levels should be monitored and dosages adjusted to prevent side effects.

Suggested Reading

Avery, M. E., and Taeusch, H. W. *Schaffer's Diseases of the Newborn* (5th ed.). Philadelphia: Saunders, 1984.

Cloherty, J. P., and Stark, A. R. (eds.). *Manual of Neonatal Care* (2nd ed.). Boston: Little, Brown, 1985.

Klaus, M. H., and Fanaroff, A. A. *Care of the High-Risk Neonate* (3rd ed.). Philadelphia: Saunders, 1986.

Todres, I. D., and Firestone, S. Neonatal Emergencies. In J. F. Ryan, et al. (eds.), *A Practice of Anesthesia for Infants and Children*. Orlando, Fla.: Grune & Stratton, 1986.

32

Respiratory Intensive Care

Thomas A. Mickler and Vincent L. Hoellerich

I. **Respiratory failure**
   A. **Definition.** Respiratory failure is a state of inefficiency in gas exchange such that overall metabolic demands are not met. **Respiration** refers to gas exchange at a cellular level, while **ventilation** is the movement of gas in and out of the lungs. Respiratory failure will always occur with inadequate ventilation but may also occur even when ventilation is adequate if pulmonary, hemodynamic, or metabolic derangements are present.
   B. **Diagnosis.** The arterial PaO_2, $PaCO_2$, and pH obtained by arterial blood gas (ABG) analysis are the key to diagnosing respiratory failure. Specifically, a **PaO_2 below the predicted normal range for the patient's age at the prevalent barometric pressure (in the absence of intracardiac right-to-left shunting) or a $PaCO_2$ greater than 50 mm Hg** (not due to respiratory compensation for metabolic alkalemia) **is respiratory failure.** The age dependence of the PaO_2 can be estimated from $PaO_2 = 109 - (0.43 \times age)$, or by using Table 32-1 (note that the normal $PaCO_2$ for any age is 40). In acute situations, respiratory failure must be assessed by clinical signs, since appropriate measures must be undertaken before ABG results are available. Impending respiratory failure is indicated by a respiratory rate less than 6/min or greater than 30/min, "rocking" motions of the thorax and abdomen during labored breathing, circumoral pallor or cyanosis, or acrocyanosis.
II. **Causes of respiratory failure**
   A. **Ventilatory failure.** Mild or moderate hypoventilation affects carbon dioxide (CO_2) excretion more than it affects oxygenation and will increase the CO_2 content (and the $PaCO_2$) in both arterial and venous blood. However, oxygenation ultimately declines for two reasons: (1) elevation of the alveolar CO_2 tension ($PACO_2$) will cause a concomitant decrease in the alveolar oxygen tension (PAO_2), resulting in a fall in arterial oxygen (O_2) tension (PaO₂) (see sec. **XII.B**), and (2) atelectasis will cause shunting through the pulmonary vasculature and results in further declines in oxygenation. Hypoventilation may result from the following:
      1. **Decreased responsiveness to CO_2.** The $PaCO_2$ is the most important mediator controlling ventilation. The regulatory mechanism is located near the medulla in the brainstem, and metabolic or mechanical depression of the brainstem will interfere with the ventilatory response to increasing $PaCO_2$. Normally, minute ventilation ($\dot{V}E$) rises about 2 L/min/mm Hg rise in $PaCO_2$.
         a. **Drug administration** may attenuate the nor-

Table 32-1. Age-dependence of arterial oxygen tension

Age (yr)	Average PaO_2 (mm Hg)
< 30	94
31–40	87
41–50	84
51–60	81
> 60	< 75

mal ventilatory response to CO_2. Narcotics, inhalation agents, and some sedatives shift the CO_2 response curve (i.e., $\dot{V}E$ versus $PaCO_2$) to the right, either in a parallel fashion or by decreasing the slope.

b. Patients with **chronic obstructive pulmonary disease (COPD) all have decreased responses to CO_2**. A severely affected patient ("CO_2 retainer") will have an elevated $PaCO_2$, but this does not always imply that ventilation is stimulated solely by "hypoxic drive."

c. **Intracranial pathology** from head trauma, subdural or epidural intracranial bleeding, or metabolic imbalance can cause central nervous system (CNS) depression and hypoventilation.

2. **Mechanical failure.** Inadequate ventilatory function may be due to the loss of the integrity of the neuromuscular junction, the diaphragm, the thoracic cage, or obstruction of the airways.

a. **Neuromuscular diseases** may lead to severe diaphragmatic weakness or paralysis; examples include myasthenia gravis, poliomyelitis, Guillain-Barré syndrome, and phrenic nerve palsy. Ventilation may be adequate while at rest, but decompensation can occur from inability to clear secretions or increase ventilation when metabolic demands are increased.

b. **Skeletal injury.** Chest trauma causing fractures of three or more ribs (in two or more places) in the anterior or posterolateral chest may result in a **flail chest.** The flail area is functionally detached from the rib cage; thus this portion of the chest wall is displaced inward when the rib cage moves outward during inspiration. If the flail is large, rebreathing can occur by exchange of air between the flail segment and other portions of the lungs; this may lead to hypercarbia, hypoxemia, and ultimately, ventilatory failure.

c. **Restrictive lung disease.** Parenchymal, chest wall, or pleural processes that impair expansion of the lungs may cause hypoventilation. With severe restrictive disease, hypoxemia may be present at rest, but classically the PaO_2 falls dramatically during periods of exercise or stress. Acute causes of restriction include pleural effusion, burns, and hemothorax; chronic causes include sarcoidosis, pulmonary fibrosis, and chest wall resection, scarring, or reconstruction.

d. **Upper airway obstruction.** Although occasionally due to foreign bodies in the pharynx or larynx, this problem occurs most often in obtunded patients when the tongue falls backward and blocks the hypopharynx. Other causes include epiglottic edema or epiglottitis, vocal cord paralysis from surgical trauma to the recurrent laryngeal nerve, and vocal cord edema after trauma or inhalational injury.

e. **Regional anesthesia.** Spinal and epidural blocks that reach the high thoracic or cervical dermatomes may inhibit intercostal muscle function and, if sufficiently high, the diaphragm.

B. **Pulmonary failure.** Parenchymal abnormalities that interfere with gas exchange may ultimately lead to respiratory failure.

1. **Ventilation/perfusion ($\dot{V}/\dot{Q}$) mismatch.** Gas exchange is most efficient when the best perfused alveolar-capillary units receive the most ventilation and, similarly, when alveoli with minimal ventilation receive little perfusion. A "mismatch" of ventilation and perfusion in multiple alveolar-capillary units will result in less efficient gas exchange and, if severe, may cause both hypoxemia and hypercarbia. Arterial desaturation caused by $\dot{V}/\dot{Q}$ mismatching is usually improved with O_2 therapy and can thereby be distinguished from desaturation caused by pure shunt (see sec. **2**). Pulmonary edema, COPD, and diffuse interstitial pulmonary fibrosis are common causes of $\dot{V}/\dot{Q}$ mismatch.

2. Pure intrapulmonary **shunt** occurs when mixed venous blood enters the systemic arterial circulation without exposure to alveolar gas. In essence, "shunted" alveolar-capillary units are those in which the $\dot{V}/\dot{Q}$ ratio is zero, that is, units that are perfused but not ventilated. Acquired conditions that may result in pulmonary shunts include atelectasis, aspiration or lobar pneumonia, acute respiratory distress syndrome, pneumothorax, and one-lung ventilation. The resulting hypoxemia is generally refractory to O_2 administration alone, and therapy must be directed toward the underlying cause (see sec. **XII.E**).

3. **Increased dead space.** Physiologic dead space (V_D) refers to areas of the lung that are ventilated but not perfused. The normal physiologic dead space is about 2 cc/kg body weight, or in the average adult, about 150 cc; this value is often represented as a fraction of the tidal volume (V_D/V_T) and is nor-

mally about 0.3 (see sec. **XII.F**). Increases in dead space may cause a relative state of hypoventilation and subsequent hypercarbia. Possible causes of increased V_D/V_T in the intensive care unit include air or pulmonary embolism, severe parenchymal lung disease, and excessive V_T or positive end-expiratory pressure (PEEP) in ventilated patients.

4. **Diffusion abnormalities.** The transit of blood through the alveolar capillary takes about 0.75 seconds, and the equilibration of O_2 normally occurs within one-third of that time. In principle, a thickened, diseased alveolar-capillary membrane should impair diffusion of O_2. However, thickening would have to be greater than eightfold to develop an increased A-aDO_2 (alveolar-to-arterial O_2 gradient). Thus, diffusion abnormalities do not usually contribute significantly to hypoxemia.

C. **Hemodynamic instability**

1. **Decreased cardiac output** may contribute to hypoxemia by decreasing O_2 delivery (cardiac output $\times$ O_2 content of blood) to tissues. Acutely, certain tissues adjust to this low flow state not only by slightly decreasing O_2 consumption but also by increasing the extraction of O_2 from the arterial blood, resulting in a decreased mixed venous O_2 content ($C\bar{v}O_2$). Unless additional O_2 is given, this decrease in $C\bar{v}O_2$ will cause a direct decrease in arterial O_2 content and exacerbate hypoxemia.

2. **Hypovolemia** causes respiratory compromise by decreasing cardiac output and pulmonary perfusion, potentially resulting in a relative increase in V_D/V_T.

D. **Metabolic disturbances**

1. **Increased O_2 consumption**

a. **Fever** increases metabolism: for each 1°C increase in temperature, O_2 consumption increases by about 10%. Reducing temperature in febrile patients may reduce hypoxemia.

b. **Sepsis** increases metabolic rate and O_2 consumption, even in the absence of fever.

c. **Muscle activity,** including shivering, increases O_2 consumption.

2. **Increased CO_2 production**

a. Carbon dioxide production follows O_2 consumption as temperature is increased or decreased.

b. The **respiratory quotient** (RQ) is the ratio of the amount of CO_2 produced to the amount of O_2 consumed. This ratio depends, in part, on the substrates that are metabolized; if only carbohydrate is used, the RQ will be 1.0; if only fat is metabolized, the RQ will be 0.7. The average RQ for healthy adults on an average American diet is 0.8. The RQ can exceed 1.0 if metabolism is anaerobic or if fat is synthesized from carbohydrate (values as high as 1.3 have been reported in patients receiving total parenteral nutrition). Such an increase in the RQ may lead to respiratory failure in patients who are unable to compensate for a relative increase in CO_2 production.

3. **Shifts in the O_2-hemoglobin dissociation curve.** If shifted to the **right,** O_2 binding will be inhibited and unloading of O_2 to tissues will be facilitated. This occurs when these factors are increased: temperature, hydrogen ion concentration, CO_2 tension, and 2, 3-diphosphoglycerate. Conversely, a **left** shift facilitates uptake of O_2 but inhibits unloading; this may occur when those same factors are diminished.

III. Therapeutic measures for respiratory failure in non-intubated patients

A. **Oxygen** administration is a logical first treatment step. Except when used for routine postoperative care, the need for and the efficacy of O_2 therapy should be documented by clinical signs (e.g., cyanosis, diaphoresis, tachycardia, tachypnea, hypertension), pulse oximetry, or ABG analysis.

1. **Guidelines.** Oxygen is most helpful when treating hypoxia from $\dot{V}/\dot{Q}$ abnormalities and hypoventilation. In postoperative patients, supplemental O_2 will alleviate diffusion hypoxemia resulting from the washout of anesthetic gases (see Chap. 10). Patients with COPD who are CO_2 retainers may respond to O_2 therapy by decreasing alveolar ventilation ($\dot{V}A$); although such a response may require 100% O_2, it is prudent to use the lowest FIO_2 that relieves hypoxia. If hypoventilation occurs without relief of hypoxia, intubation and ventilation are indicated.

2. The major considerations in selecting the best **device for supplying supplemental O_2** are patient comfort and compliance, the level of FIO_2 that is needed, how narrow the range of FIO_2 must be maintained, and the level of humidification desired. In general, the FIO_2 delivered by these devices varies because they may allow entrainment of room air. Room air may be entrained if the patient's peak inspiratory flow rate (about 40 L/min at normal tidal breathing) exceeds the limits of the device or if the devices are not worn properly by the patient (e.g., noncompliance). Table 32-2 shows the relationship between FIO_2 and flow rates for these devices.

a. **Nasal cannulas** are well tolerated and allow for continuous O_2 delivery, even during eating and coughing. The final concentration of O_2 reaching the trachea is a function of both the O_2 flow rate from the cannulas and the total $\dot{V}E$ of ambient air. The final FIO_2 will be high if the $\dot{V}E$ is low (hypoventilation) and low if the $\dot{V}E$ is high (hyperventilation). Thus if a narrow range of FIO_2 must be maintained, this device should

Table 32-2. Oxygen delivery devices for nonintubated patients

Equipment	O_2 Flow (L/min)	FIO_2
Nasal cannulas	1–6	0.25–0.55
Open face mask	6–12	0.35–0.65
Face mask/nasal cannula combination	6–12 (mask) 6 (cannulas)	0.44–0.85
Face tent	8–10	0.21–0.55
Nonrebreathing mask (mask with reservoir)	Any rate that prevents the reservoir from collapsing	0.60–0.80
Venturi mask	4–12	0.24, 0.28, 0.31, 0.35, 0.40

not be selected. At flow rates above 6 L/min, the nasal mucosa can become very dry because little humidification is supplied with this device.

b. Venturi masks provide delivery of O_2 over a narrow range of FIO_2. With this system, air is entrained into a low flow of O_2 (4–12 L/min), and the FIO_2 is independent of both $\dot{V}E$ and inspiratory flow rate (provided the latter does not exceed the limiting flow-rate capability of the mask, which is usually about 40 L/min). Venturi masks guarantee that the FIO_2 will not exceed a prescribed level, so they are a good choice for patients with both hypoxemia and hypercarbia. However, this device has a limited ability to deliver humidification and is not appropriate for patients who require highly humidified O_2.

c. Open mask O_2 is limited by the inability to deliver supplemental O_2 within a narrow range of FIO_2. However, it can deliver higher levels of humidity because of the wider bore of its tubing; an FIO_2 as high as 0.5 can be delivered without causing drying of the nasal mucosa. These masks are most efficient when tight-fitting; however, discomfort or inconvenience often results in improper positioning on the face, which markedly alters the O_2 concentration delivered.

d. Masks with reservoir bags ("nonrebreathing" masks) can deliver a high FIO_2 to a nonintubated patient.

e. Combining nasal cannulas and O_2 masks will enhance the delivered O_2 concentrations; however, high flows through the nasopharynx (6–15 L/min) are required and are seldom tolerated well by patients for prolonged periods.

3. The pulmonary **toxicity of O_2** is a function of **dose** (FIO_2) and the **duration** of administration. It results in thickening and edema of the pulmonary interstitium and can result in decrease in lung compliance and PaO_2. Supplemental O_2 at an FIO_2 below 0.5 can usually be administered indefinitely without sequelae; consequently, it is a major objective of O_2 therapy that the FIO_2 be kept below 0.5 while maintaining the PaO_2.

B. **Mobilization and removal of secretions**

1. **Humidification of gases** decreases the viscosity of mucus and supports ciliary function and mucous clearance, all of which are needed to prevent respiratory tract infection. Normally, alveolar gas is 100% humidified at 37°C and contains 44 ml H_2O/L. Typically, inspired room air is 50% humidified at 21°C and contains 9 ml H_2O/L. Thus, the nasopharynx and tracheal mucosa both increase the temperature of inspired air and supply 35 ml H_2O for each liter inspired. Hospital and tank O_2 gas is completely dry and must be humidified to prevent drying of secretions.
   Unheated humidifiers bring gases up to a relative humidity of 90% at room temperature, while **heated humidifiers** completely humidify gases at 37°C. **Hydrosphere units** use ultrasonic nebulization to produce a dense fog containing particulate water and complete humidification. The water content can be from 50–100 ml H_2O/L; 30 minutes of therapy every 1–2 hours can help mobilize dried or thickened secretions. This technique has not been shown to be any more efficacious than other methods of humidification.

2. Although the small "insensible" losses of water that occur from breathing dry gases will rarely contribute to the overall fluid status of patients, **intravascular hydration** must be maintained for "topical" humidification in the airway to be effective.

3. **Mucolytic agents** make secretions less viscous and therefore easier to clear. N-Acetylcysteine (Mucomyst) has been shown to decrease the viscosity of secretions, improve the forced expiratory volume at 1 second (FEV_1) and the forced vital capacity (FVC), and produce positive subjective responses from patients. Because N-acetylcysteine may cause bronchospasm, a bronchodilator such as isoetharine (Bronkosol) should be administered to minimize airway reactivity.

4. **Blind nasal endotracheal suctioning** can be a very effective means to generate coughing and to remove thick secretions. A soft catheter is passed through the nose and pharynx blindly into the trachea and 1–5 ml of sterile saline injected (O_2 may be connected to the catheter to avoid hypoxia). Suction is applied for no longer than 15 seconds; then

O_2 by mask is resumed. Electrocardiographic monitoring should be done during and after suctioning, since arrhythmias (especially bradycardias) during this procedure are common. Relative contraindications include coagulopathies, recent laryngeal or tracheal surgery with fresh anastomoses, and severe bradyarrhythmias.

5. **Bronchoscopy** is used for both diagnosis and therapy. Specimens for culture uncontaminated by upper airway flora can be obtained, and bronchial plugs of thick inspissated mucus can also be removed through the bronchoscope. Collapsed lung segments may be expanded by bronchoscopy when other maneuvers have failed. Flexible bronchoscopy may be performed without an endotracheal tube in place, although it is technically easier to accomplish in intubated patients (a tube size of at least 8.0 mm internal diameter [ID] is required for passage of adult-sized units).

C. **Reversal of bronchospasm or stridor**

1. **Bronchospasm** should be treated initially by removing precipitating inhaled irritants or drugs (e.g., beta blockers). Inhaled bronchodilators cause fewer cardiovascular side effects than systemically administered drugs and are the first line of therapy; they may be given to intubated and nonintubated patients.

   a. **Inhaled agents**

      (1) **Isoetharine** (Bronkosol), 0.5 ml in 2.5 ml saline, can be given every 2–4 hours.

      (2) **Metaproterenol** (Alupent or Metaprel) has less beta-1 activity than isoetharine and may cause less tachycardia; either 0.3 ml in 2.5 ml saline is given every 6–8 hours, or a metered-dose inhaler is used (two "puffs" [0.65 mg/puff] every 3–4 hours).

      (3) **Albuterol** (Proventil or Ventolin) has the least beta-1 activity and is packaged in a metered-dose inhaler. A special fitting mask must be used for effective administration to nonintubated patients; two puffs (90 µg/puff) are given every 4–6 hours. A nebulizer solution (5 mg/ml) is expected to be commercially available in 1987.

      (4) **Beclomethasone** (Vanceril) is a steroid that may potentiate the effects of inhaled bronchodilators; supplied in a metered-dose inhaler, two puffs (50 µg/puff) are given every 4–6 hours.

   b. **Intravenous agents**

      (1) **Aminophylline** acts synergistically with inhaled bronchodilators. A loading dose of 5 mg/kg (IV over 30 minutes) is administered, followed by continuous infusion

(0.5–1.0 mg/kg/min). Maintenance doses should be reduced by half in the presence of liver disease or reduced hepatic perfusion. The infusion rate is increased until either wheezing subsides, tachycardia occurs, or a dose of 1 mg/kg/min has been infusing for more than 3 hours. Serum levels of theophylline may be followed, but clinical response (and/or side effects) usually dictates the dosage. Intravascular volume must be monitored closely, since aminophylline has diuretic properties, especially in younger patients.

    (2) Epinephrine (0.25–1.0 μg/min) or **isoproterenol** (0.5–10 μg/min) by continuous infusion is occasionally needed to control refractory bronchospasm.

    (3) Methylprednisolone (Solu-Medrol), 30–60 mg every 6 hours, may also be beneficial in refractory cases.

  2. Stridor may result from laryngeal edema, vocal cord paralysis, or epiglottic edema. Restriction of air movement may be severe enough to cause ventilatory failure, so equipment and personnel for intubation and tracheostomy should be readily available. Therapy should be instituted with the following:

    a. Racemic epinephrine (Vaponefrin, 0.5 ml of 2.25% solution in 2.5 ml of normal saline) should be given by nebulizer with humidified O_2 to reduce laryngeal edema. Treatments may be repeated every 1–2 hours as tolerated (side effects are rare but include tachycardia, hypertension, arrhythmias, and agitation).

    b. Steroids may also be administered either IV (dexamethasone [Decadron], 4–8 mg as a single dose) or by aerosol (beclomethasone, 2 puffs every 4 hours as needed).

D. Reversal of drug effects

  1. Central nervous system depressants may diminish the normal respiratory drive, shifting the CO_2 response curve to the right, and thus contribute to respiratory failure. Such drugs include, but are not limited to, the narcotics, inhalation anesthetics, barbiturates, and benzodiazepines.

Narcotic-induced respiratory depression may be reversed by administering the pure opiate antagonist naloxone (Narcan). The clinical use of naloxone is discussed in Chap. 10. Mixed agonist-antagonists such as nalbuphine (Nubain) may produce "smoother" reversals.

Physostigmine (Antilirium) has broad CNS-stimulating properties and has been used (1–2 mg IV) to treat confusion from benzodiazepines and other drugs (e.g., scopolamine and droperidol) that produce "central cholinergic syndrome." However, physostigmine has not been shown to be effective in reversing benzodiazepine-induced respiratory depression. With severe CNS depression from tricyclic antidepressants or multiple sedatives, intubation and mechanical ventilation should be instituted.

2. **Muscle relaxants.** The partially curarized patient may appear to ventilate adequately during quiet breathing, but the ability to protect the airway, clear secretions, or breathe deeply may be markedly impaired. Hypocalcemia, hypermagnesemia, hypothermia, respiratory acidosis, and antibiotics (e.g., aminoglycosides) can all potentiate neuromuscular blockade; monitoring the reversal of relaxants is considered in Chap. 11.

E. **Chest physical therapy** includes percussion and vibration, postural drainage, and enhancement of coughing. Chest **percussion and vibration** are used to loosen inspissated secretions and stimulate coughing. Special caution should be exercised in patients who may develop hemoptysis from carcinoma, tuberculosis, lung abscess, or bronchiectasis. Percussion and vibration may be modified for the elderly or osteoporotic patient and after recent thoracic surgery. **Postural drainage** is applied when there is hypersecretion and retention of sputum, such as in cystic fibrosis, bronchiectasis, and lung abscess.

F. **Analgesia.** Patients recovering from thoracic or abdominal procedures may "splint" from pain at the surgical site. This can result in hypoventilation and atelectasis.

1. **Intravenous and intramuscular narcotics** are still the mainstays of postoperative analgesia (see Chap. 33). However, all narcotics, even the new mixed agonist-antagonist types, cause central respiratory depression; this effect may be potentiated by residual anesthetics following surgery.

2. **Intercostal nerve blocks** are useful for post-thoracotomy patients and are discussed in detail in Chap. 19.

3. **Epidural analgesia** is particularly convenient after procedures that have employed epidural anesthesia, but a catheter can also be placed postoperatively for pain relief. Either local anesthetics or narcotics may be used effectively in this setting. Lumbar epidural catheters, especially when used to administer narcotics, provide excellent analgesia for patients with painful thoracic incisions and may obviate the need for thoracic epidurals or intercostal nerve blocks. Epidural analgesia is discussed in Chap. 33.

G. **Incentive spirometry.** Atelectasis can be treated and possibly prevented by certain voluntary maneuvers. Specifically, a maximal deep inspiration that is held for a period of time with the glottis open (i.e., a yawn) is the best way to open collapsed alveoli. During incentive spirometry, patients perform precisely this maneuver and are given positive feedback as their ability improves. Lessons should be given preoperatively, and the use of this device encouraged frequently (every 2 hours while awake) after surgery. Other devices promote deep breathing without an inspiratory pause; this will not reverse atelectasis, and some that promote the expiratory maneuvers may even exacerbate collapse.

H. **Mask continuous positive airway pressure** (CPAP) provides positive pressure against which patients must exhale. With a tight-fitting mask, pressures of 5–20 cm H_2O may be provided. Continuous positive airway pressure prevents closure of unstable airways and increases FRC and thus may help to prevent and treat atelectasis. When using mask CPAP, patients must be awake and cooperative, spontaneously breathing, and hemodynamically stable. The major complication of mask CPAP is gastric distention from swallowed air and aspiration of gastric contents; it can be safely administered to patients with nasogastric tubes, but it is contraindicated soon after esophageal surgery. Mask CPAP is usually administered every 1–2 hours for 10- to 15-minute intervals; initially, a pressure of 5 cm H_2O is used, but this may be increased in 2.5–5.0 cm H_2O increments to a maximum of 15–20 cm H_2O as needed and as tolerated.

IV. **Respiratory failure requiring intubation and mechanical ventilation**

A. **Intubation**

1. **Indications**

a. Respiratory arrest.

b. Prevention of aspiration in comatose or obtunded patients.

c. Pulmonary toilet.

d. Mechanical ventilation.

2. **Techniques**

a. **Tube size and type.** Polyvinylchloride endotracheal tubes with high-volume, low-pressure cuffs are least likely to cause tracheal damage. Usually, a 7.0 mm ID tube is appropriate for women, while an 8.0 mm ID tube is best suited for men. In emergencies, a styleted 7.0 mm ID tube should be used. Tubes should not be cut until a postintubation chest x-ray is reviewed (see sec. **XI**).

b. **Oral intubation** is the most expedient and surest approach in urgent situations. In cases in which cervical spine injury is suspected, blind nasal intubation or nasal intubation guided by flexible bronchoscopy may be indicated.

c. In elective situations, the **nasal approach** is used when intubation will be required for more than 24 hours. Nonsedated patients may be more comfortable with nasal tubes because it is easier to close the mouth, which prevents drying of the oral mucosa.

(1) The nasal turbinates limit the size of tube that may be used. When tube diameters are less than 6.5 mm, airway resistance and the work of breathing are increased, and clearance of secretions may be more difficult.

(2) Nasal hemorrhage, sinusitis, and necrosis of the nares are occasional **complications.** Relative contraindications include neutropenia, basilar skull fracture, Le-Forte type 3 facial fracture, and coagulopathies.

d. **Awake intubation** should be considered for patients in respiratory failure who are spontaneously breathing, may be difficult to intubate, or are at increased risk for aspirating. Intravenous sedation is used sparingly during emergency intubation to avoid respiratory or cardiovascular depression; however, in patients with coronary artery disease or valvular heart disease who require intubation, fentanyl (1–2 μg/kg) and/or lidocaine (1 mg/kg) given 2–3 minutes prior to intubation may attenuate unwanted cardiovascular responses to airway manipulation.

e. **Rapid sequence intubations** (see Chap. 10) should be considered for patients who may aspirate or are uncooperative or combative. Contingency arrangements for ventilation (e.g., mask ventilation, cricothyroidotomy) are made prior to administering muscle relaxants, should attempts at intubation be unsuccessful.

f. **Endotracheal tube cuffs** must be inflated with the minimum volume to achieve a seal at 20–30 cm H_2O positive pressure, usually 5–10 cc of air. Cuff pressures should be kept below 40 cm H_2O, since this approximates the tracheal mucosal capillary perfusion pressure, and greater pressure may cause mucosal ischemia.

3. **Complications of intubation.** The most serious complications involve misplacement of the endotracheal tube, so a systematic evaluation of tube position is mandatory after every intubation:

a. Manually ventilate patient.

b. Observe the chest for bilateral expansion, especially at the apex of each hemithorax.

c. Auscultate over the stomach for inflation; if none, listen for breath sounds bilaterally.

d. Note the endotracheal tube markings at the lips or nares.

e. Obtain and evaluate a chest x-ray for the position of the tip of the tube.

(1) **Esophageal intubation** requires immediate reintubation. If vomiting occurs while the tube is in the esophagus, it

should be left in place until endotracheal intubation is accomplished. Diagnosing esophageal intubations may be difficult because there are other reasons for diminished breath sounds and poor compliance, including severe bronchospasm, pleural effusions, or pulmonary consolidation. When in doubt, laryngoscopy should be repeated immediately with the tube in place.

(2) **Endobronchial intubation** is almost always into the right mainstem bronchus. The diagnosis is made by asymmetric breath sounds or perhaps by postintubation chest x-ray; breath sounds may be transmitted and thus not completely absent over the nonventilated lung. The tube markings at the incisors should be between 18 and 24 cm in an average-size adult; if inserted further, endobronchial intubation is likely.

(3) **False passage** into the retropharynx may complicate nasal intubation. Gentle, steady pressure rather than abrupt brute force is the safest way to pass by the nasal turbinates. The diagnosis is confirmed by laryngoscopy and is usually followed by consultation with an otolaryngologist.

(4) The majority of patients with tracheal stenosis following intubation have had prolonged intubations; stenosis rarely occurs following brief periods of intubation (24 hours). In this context, tracheal stenosis may occur at three sites: the subglottic area, the cuff site, or rarely, the tip site. In patients who require prolonged intubation (> 2 weeks), tracheostomy should be performed—both to reduce patient discomfort and to minimize the risks of laryngotracheal injury.

B. **Continuous positive airway pressure** of 5 cm H_2O is commonly applied when patients are intubated but breathing spontaneously. It helps to maintain FRC and may prevent atelectasis, since the normal mechanism for maintaining airway and alveolar patency—mild resistance to air flow by the epiglottis and upper airway structures—is bypassed by the endotracheal tube. Since CPAP raises intracranial pressure, it should be avoided in the presence of intracranial pathology. Continuous positive airway pressure usually hinders complete exhalation and therefore promotes air trapping and hyperinflation in patients with COPD. Rarely, it may serve to "stent" the airways and facilitate exhalation in COPD patients; however, unless accurate flow-pressure measurements are made to document the stenting effect, CPAP should not be used in these patients.

C. Mechanical ventilation and PEEP

   1. **Indications.** Mechanical ventilation is necessary whenever spontaneous ventilation is inadequate to maintain gas exchange. Table 32-3 indicates the level of compromise of various respiratory parameters associated with the need for mechanical ventilation.

   2. A detailed description of **ventilator modes** can be found in sec. **V.**

   3. **Ventilator settings** (for intermittent mandatory ventilation [IMV] mode).

      a. **Tidal volume** (V_T) is initially set at 10–15 ml/kg. If the peak inspiratory pressure (PIP) is greater than 60 cm H_2O, V_T is decreased in 50- to 100-ml increments until the PIP is less than 60 cm H_2O. If this results in $\dot{V}_E$ insufficient to maintain an appropriate $PaCO_2$, the IMV rate is increased. A PIP greater than 60 cm H_2O may occasionally be needed to ventilate patients with severely reduced compliance.

      b. **Respiratory rate** (IMV) is initially set at 8–10 breaths/minute; $\dot{V}_E$ is then adjusted to maintain $PaCO_2$ in the 35–40 mm Hg range (or near a chronically compensated value).

      c. **F_{IO_2}** is initially set at 1.0 to assure the best possible O_2 saturation; the F_{IO_2} can then be titrated to keep either the PaO_2 in the 80–100 range or the O_2 saturation at 95–100%. Whenever possible, the F_{IO_2} should be reduced to at least 0.50 to minimize O_2 toxicity.

      d. **Positive end-expiratory pressure** is set at 3–5 cm H_2O to prevent atelectasis and maintain FRC. It should not be used in patients with elevated intracranial pressure unless intracranial pressure monitoring is available (see Chap. 22) and should be administered with caution in patients with COPD (see sec. **IV.B**). Positive end-expiratory pressure improves oxygenation by reexpanding ("recruiting") closed alveolar units. However, PEEP may have hemodynamic consequences, including reduced venous return from increased intrathoracic pressure and/or a direct effect on cardiac output depending on the compliance of the lungs, chest wall, and left ventricle. (In general, the more compliant the lungs, the greater the hemodynamic consequences of PEEP; IV fluid and inotropic support may be needed to maintain adequate cardiac output and blood pressure.) It is usually increased in 2.0–2.5 cm H_2O increments until arterial O_2 saturation can be maintained with an F_{IO_2} less than 0.6.

      e. **Inspiratory to expiratory (I/E) time** is usually started at 1 : 2. This means that at a respiratory rate of 10/min, 2 seconds are allowed for inspiration, 4 seconds for expiration. An I/E ra-

Table 32-3. Clinical parameters associated with respiratory failure

Respiratory parameter	Usual range	Intubation/ventilation may be indicated
Respiratory rate (per min)	12–25	> 35
Vital capacity (ml/kg)	30–70	< 15
Inspiratory force (cm H_2O)	50–100	< 25
Oxygenation		
PaO_2 (mm Hg)	75–100	< 60
A-aDO_2 (mm Hg)[a]	10–200	> 350
Ventilation		
V_D/V_T	0.3–0.4	> 0.6
$PaCO_2$ (mm Hg)	35–45	> 55[b]

[a]After 10 minutes on 100% O_2.
[b]Except for patients with chronic CO_2 retention.

tio of 1 : 2.5 or 1 : 3 may be used when there is a prolonged expiratory phase, as in patients with COPD. Ratios approaching 1 : 1 are needed with high respiratory rates, since peak inspiratory flow rates are limited and time is required to deliver the preset V_T.

4. **Endotracheal suctioning** is necessary to remove secretions from intubated patients who cannot effectively cough. It is usually part of chest physiotherapy, but it may be needed more frequently when secretions are copious. For patients on ventilators, the consistency, color, and volume of secretions should always be noted, and sterile suction catheters and gloves should also always be used. Before and during endotracheal suctioning, patients should breathe 100% O_2 to prevent transient hypoxemia from lowered FRC. Critically ill patients may become bradycardic when disconnected from ventilators, and atropine should be available; new "in-line" suction catheters may obviate this problem.

D. **Paralysis and deliberate hypothermia**

1. **Paralysis** improves compliance by relaxing the chest wall musculature and preventing "bucking" or straining or against inflations. Patients who breathe against an inspiratory cycle will ventilate ineffectively because the elevated airway pressures cause the "pop-off" valve to open, and a portion of the preset V_T will be lost. Paralysis potentially reduces total body O_2 consumption by preventing excessive O_2 utilization from muscle activity, especially during shivering.

a. **Indications.** Severe respiratory acidosis (pH < 7.30) in patients ineffectively ventilated with PIP above 60 cm H_2O should be paralyzed.

   b. **Method.** Heavy sedation is required before paralysis; a narcotic may be used either alone or combined with a benzodiazepine or barbiturate. (Ventilatory compliance may be vastly improved with this step alone.) A nondepolarizing muscle relaxant, such as curare (0.5 mg/kg IV), is given over a period of several minutes, followed by a continuous infusion (6–15 mg/hr).

2. **Deliberate hypothermia.** Oxygen consumption is the only parameter that can be altered to improve persistent hypoxemia despite high FIO_2, PEEP, and adequate cardiac output. Oxygen consumption is reduced in parallel with metabolic rate, leading to an increased $C\bar{v}O_2$ and SaO_2.

   a. **Indications.** If PEEP is greater than 20 cm H_2O in a paralyzed patient and increasing the cardiac output fails to alleviate arterial hypoxemia (despite an $FIO_2 > 0.6$), deliberate hypothermia may be appropriate.

   b. **Method.** Patients are placed on cooling blankets with thermostatic control. Core temperature is measured with a pulmonary artery catheter or other thermistor and is allowed to fall to about 32°C. (Hypothermia can precipitate atrial or ventricular fibrillation, so core temperatures below 32°C are dangerous and must be avoided.)

V. Mechanical ventilators

A. Conventional ventilators

1. **Ventilation modes**

   a. **Control.** The ventilator is responsible for initiation and delivery of each VT; patients' respiratory efforts will not trigger delivery of the preset VT.

   b. **Assist.** Patient is totally responsible for initiation of the inspiratory phase; the ventilator then delivers a preset VT when triggered. The VE delivered is thus entirely dependent on the number of patient-initiated inspirations.

   c. **Assist/control.** The ventilator functions in the assist mode unless the patient's respiratory rate falls below a preset level, at which time the machine converts to the control mode.

   d. **Intermittent mandatory ventilation.** The ventilator delivers a preset VT at a preset rate, but patients can breathe spontaneously between cycles and thus assume a portion of their ventilatory needs. A demand valve is present on most IMV ventilators that must be opened by an inspiratory effort before fresh gas can be inhaled. The work required to open this valve is generally minimal, but it may still inhibit spontaneous ventilation and thus hinder weaning in patients with marginal reserve. The Emerson-IMV unit supplies a continuous fresh gas flow of 60 L/min between cycles without a demand valve.

   e. **Synchronized IMV (SIMV).** Patients breathe spontaneously from ventilator-supplied gases through a demand valve, and at preset intervals, preset VT is delivered. Whenever possible, ventilator cycles are not initiated during the expiratory phase of patients' breathing.

   f. **Continuous positive airway pressure.** Patients breathe spontaneously through a demand valve or high-flow system; no positive-pressure breaths are delivered.

   g. **Positive end-expiratory pressure.** Positive airway pressure is maintained at end expiration, that is, between machine-assisted breaths.

   h. **Pressure support.** During spontaneous breathing, the ventilator functions as a constant pressure generator. When triggered by an inspiratory effort, a preset level of pressure (e.g., 10–30 cm H_2O) rapidly develops in the system and remains until spontaneous flow rates decrease to 25% of peak inspiratory flow. This mode may be used either independently, in conjunction with CPAP, or in conjunction with SIMV +/− PEEP). Pressure support may decrease the work of breathing, which is helpful in patients with neuromuscular disease.

   i. **Extended mandatory minute ventilation** (EMMV). Minute volume is preset; patients then receive this volume while breathing spontaneously, during mechanical ventilation, or a combination of both. If the spontaneous V̇E falls below the preset minimum, mechanical ventilation makes up the difference.

2. **Other ventilator controls**

   a. **Sigh.** Periodic delivery of a VT that is greater (commonly by 50%) than the preset VT.

   b. **Inflation hold** (also called **inspiratory hold** or **inspiratory pause**) is incorporation of a static phase at the end of inspiration.

   c. **Flow taper** allows for the gradual reduction of flow rate during inspiration; modification of the rate may begin at any time during inspiration. Adjustments in this setting may improve the distribution of inspired gas.

   d. **Negative end-expiratory pressure** (NEEP) is defined as the maintenance of airway pressure below atmospheric at end exhalation. Theoretically, NEEP could prevent a significant increase in mean intrathoracic pressure, but it is rarely used because it promotes air trapping and pulmonary edema and actually has little effect on intrathoracic pressure.

   e. **Expiratory retard.** Resistance to exhalation decreases expired gas flow and hence lengthens the time it takes peak airway pressure to return to baseline. This maneuver is used to prevent premature closure of small airways during exhalation and may be helpful when used in patients with COPD.

   3. Specifications of some commercial mechanical ventilators (Table 32-4).
 B. High-frequency jet ventilation (HFJV) is produced by injecting gas into the trachea through an 18- or 16-gauge catheter, usually at rates of 75–150/min. It is commonly instituted with a "background" of controlled ventilation of 4–6 breaths/min and is thus different than either conventional ventilatory modes used at rapid rates or high-frequency oscillatory ventilation (600–1200/min). High-frequency jet ventilation maintains gas exchange with lower airway pressures than would otherwise be needed, so it may be specifically indicated in the presence of a large bronchopleural fistula. Survival seems to be prolonged in fistula patients when HFJV is used, but improvement in overall mortality rate has yet to be established.

VI. Complications from mechanical ventilation
 A. Barotrauma results in pneumothorax, pneumomediastinum, or subcutaneous emphysema. It occurs during positive-pressure ventilation with a reported incidence of 0.5–18%. The risk of barotrauma appears to be more a function of underlying parenchymal pathology rather than the level of PIP. Patients with COPD and infectious processes seem predisposed to barotrauma, regardless of ventilatory mode or airway pressure.
 B. Effects on hemodynamic measurements. During mechanical ventilation with PEEP, intrapleural pressure increases, and intracardiac pressures (as measured by the pulmonary artery catheter) are falsely elevated (above the actual transmural pressure, i.e., intracardiac minus intrapleural pressure). How much PEEP is "transmitted" depends on the compliance of the lungs and chest wall; with high compliances, pressure values may be falsely elevated by up to one-third of the applied PEEP. With low compliances, fewer artifacts are introduced (see sec. **XII.A** for calculation of compliances). However, as a rule, critically ill patients are not disconnected from ventilators to measure pulmonary artery pressures because (1) O_2 desaturation may occur, (2) several minutes may be needed for the values to reach a steady state, and (3) monitoring trends, rather than absolute values, obtained during mechanical ventilation are usually sufficient.

VII. Weaning from mechanical ventilation. Consideration for weaning begins when the acute phase of pulmonary illness subsides. In general, the time needed to wean is directly related to the length of the period of mechanical ventilation.
 A. Method. When IMV is used, patients will begin "weaning" spontaneously (i.e., gradually assuming a greater portion of their $\dot{V}_E$ requirements), and the need for me-

Table 32-4. Mechanical ventilators

Ventilator	Modes	Driving mechanism	Features
Bear I, II	C, A/C, SIMV, CPAP	Pneumatic with solenoids and regulators	1, 2, 3, 4
Bennett MA-1	C, A/C, A, IMV, CPAP, SIMV (opt.)	Bellows system by gas from electronic compressor	1 (opt.), 2, 5, 6 (opt.)
Bennett MA-2	C, A/C, A, SIMV, CPAP, IMV (opt.)	Bellows system by gas from electronic compressor	1, 2, 3
Bird Mark 7 & 8	A, A/C, C	Pneumatic by Venturi device with pneumatic clutch and needle valve	6 (Mark 8)
Emerson 3-MV (IMV Ventilator)	C, IMV	Rotary piston, electronic motor	1, 2
Engstrom ERICA	C, A/C, SIMV, CPAP, EMMV, Pressure Assist	Modified bellows by electronically regulated compressed gases	1, 2, 3, 4
Puritan-Bennett 7200	C, A/C, SIMV, CPAP, EMMV (opt.), PS (opt.)	Pneumatic by microprocessors operating solenoid valves	1, 2, 3, 9
Servo 900B, 900C	C, A/C, SIMV, CPAP, PS (900 C)	Pneumatic with servo mechanisms	1, 2, 3, 6 (opt.), 7, 8

Features:
1. PEEP
2. Sigh
3. Inflation hold
4. Flow taper
5. Expiratory retard
6. NEEP
7. Pressure control: functions as a time-cycled pressure-limited unit
8. Accelerating flow pattern
9. Selectable flow wave forms

chanical ventilation will diminish. During an **"IMV wean,"** the IMV rate is progressively decreased in parallel with the patient's ability to increase spontaneous respiration and to maintain satisfactory ABGs. Intermittent mandatory ventilation progresses to CPAP, then patients are evaluated for possible extubation. During a **"CPAP wean,"** patients are removed intermittently from ventilator-assisted breathing. Progressively longer intervals without IMV are allowed and performance during spontaneous breathing assessed (see Table 32-3).

B. **Weaning marginal patients** may take several days or even weeks; to prevent needless patient fatigue and frustration, their metabolic and nutritional status (see sec. **IX**) must be optimized. When ventilators with demand valves are used (see sec. **V.A.1.d**), the extra work required to open the valve may fatigue respiratory muscles and delay weaning. Inspiratory muscles may be strengthened by short (initially 5 minutes) sessions off the ventilator with a T piece or CPAP every 2–4 hours during waking hours. Alternatively, the IMV rate may be decreased by 10–20% for 10–60 minutes every 2–4 hours while awake.

VIII. Extubation

A. **Criteria.** Successful extubations are associated with

1. A maximum inspiratory pressure after airway occlusion for 10 seconds of greater negative magnitude than -30 cm H_2O.

2. A vital capacity of less than 15 cc/kg.

3. A PaO_2 greater than 80 mm Hg with an FIO_2 less than 0.4 (since the maximum FIO_2 that can dependably be delivered to nonintubated patients is 0.5 [see sec. **III.A**]).

4. Ability to protect the airway (i.e., intact gag and cough reflexes) and clear secretions.

5. Cardiovascular and metabolic stability and no residual neuromuscular blockade.

B. **Method.** Oxygen (100%) is administered for 5 minutes; the endotracheal tube lumen, mouth, and pharynx are then suctioned thoroughly. When the cuff is deflated, positive pressure is applied to assess whether a leak is present. (The absence of a leak may indicate that subglottic edema is present, and it may be prudent to postpone extubation to allow the edema to resolve.) The tube is withdrawn with a single, steady motion during positive-pressure ventilation; an O_2 mask is then applied. The SaO_2 may be continuously monitored, but ABGs are still checked 10–20 minutes later.

IX. Nutritional support. Inadequate nutrition may delay recovery of critically ill patients by compromising immune function, promoting muscle atrophy, and delaying wound healing.

A. **Enteral nutrition.** The alimentary tract is the first choice for administering nutrition (Table 32-5). Alimentary feeding obviates the need for dedicated central lines, avoids the risk of line sepsis, reduces the fluid

Table 32-5. Commercial solutions for enteral nutrition

Solution	Kcal/ml	CHO (gm/ml)	Protein (gm/ml)	Fat (gm/ml)	Osm (mOsm/L)	Sodium (mEq/L)
Amin Aid	1.90	0.370	0.0020	0.0450	1050	15.0
Enrich	1.10	0.162	0.0397	0.0372	480	36.8
Ensure	1.06	0.145	0.0372	0.0372	470	36.8
Isocal	1.06	0.133	0.0342	0.0444	300	23.0
Osmolite	1.06	0.145	0.0372	0.0385	300	27.6
Pulmocare	1.50	0.106	0.0626	0.0921	490	57.0
Vital (high N_2)	1.00	0.185	0.0417	0.0108	500	20.3
Vivonex (high N_2)	1.00	0.204	0.0443	0.0010	810	23.0

necessary to deliver a caloric load, and buffers gastric acids. Enteral feeding is contraindicated in patients with a bowel fistula or ileus or in those unable to protect their airway unless a cuffed endotracheal or tracheostomy tube is in place.

B. Parenteral nutrition. When enteral feeding is not possible, nutritional supplements may be administered through a peripheral vein, or total parenteral nutrition (TPN) given through a central vein. The osmolality of the solution administered determines which route is appropriate (Table 32-6); for example, solutions containing more than 10% D/W will cause sclerosis of peripheral veins and must be given centrally. **Complications of parenteral nutrition** include

1. **Hyperglycemia,** which is initially managed with a "sliding scale" of regular insulin (IV or SQ, every 4–6 hours) titrated to blood sugars. Subsequently, the total daily dose of insulin can be added directly to the solution.

2. **Hypoglycemia,** which may occur as a rebound effect after sudden discontinuation of a TPN infusion. Another concentrated glucose infusion (e.g., 10% D/W) should be substituted if TPN is abruptly stopped.

3. **Electrolyte disturbances** may occur and can be treated by adding appropriate replacements to the TPN solutions. Serum electrolytes should be monitored at least twice weekly.

4. **Hypercarbia,** which may result from increased CO_2 production ($\dot{V}CO_2$) in patients who are unable to increase alveolar ventilation ($\dot{V}A$) enough to maintain $PaCO_2$. $PaCO_2$ is proportional to $\dot{V}CO_2/\dot{V}A$. Substitution of fat (Liposyn 10%, 500 ml three times weekly) for some of the carbohydrate calories will decrease CO_2 production. However, if hypercarbia persists, the total caloric intake may have to be adjusted.

X. Monitoring

A. Cardiovascular system

1. **Arterial catheters** are placed if there is hemodynamic instability or if multiple ABGs or other blood tests are anticipated.

2. **Central venous pressure (CVP) catheters** are useful to reflect right heart response to fluid administration or changes in ventilatory regimens, or for central drug administration.

3. **Pulmonary artery catheters** are indicated in patients with respiratory failure when right or left ventricular dysfunction is suspected or if intermittent cardiac output determinations are required. Hemodynamically unstable patients who require ventilation with PEEP greater than 15 cm H_2O or $\dot{V}E$ greater than 20 L/min will also need pulmonary artery monitoring. The method and risks of inserting pulmonary artery catheters are discussed in Chap. 8.

Table 32-6. Solutions for parenteral nutrition

Solution	Calories (kcal/L)	Dextrose (gm/L)	Amino acids (gm/L)	Osm (mOsm/L)
Peripheral	300	50	30	650
Regular TPN	1000	250	42.5	1900
Fluid-restricted TPN	1320	350	30.6	2500
Renal TPN	1250*	350*	12.8*	2510*

*Values for 750-ml volume.

B. Respiratory system

  1. **Pulse oximeters** are noninvasive means to assess SaO_2 and are particularly useful in critically ill patients, in whom sudden declines in SaO_2 may occur. The efficacy of all ventilatory regimens is still assessed by ABG analysis, although FIO_2 may be titrated to the SaO_2.

  2. **Arterial blood gases** establish the PaO_2, $PaCO_2$, and pH, provided the samples are handled and analyzed properly.

     a. **Arterial blood gas syringes** contain either lyophilized or liquid heparin; with the latter, only the amount needed to wet the syringe walls should be used. If excessive liquid heparin is used, values will be spurious, since liquid heparin has a pH of 6.90 and PCO_2 and PO_2 of room air (0 and 150, respectively). The sample should be placed on ice immediately and analyzed within 15 minutes. If left at room temperature, a falsely low PaO_2 may be reported. This is especially true in patients with very high white blood cell counts, since white blood cells actively metabolize O_2.

     b. The use of the **Siggaard-Andersen nomogram** for ABG interpretation (reprinted on the inside back cover of this book) is discussed in sec. **XII.J.**

  3. **End-tidal CO_2 analyzers** reflect values that correlate well with $PaCO_2$. Although the accuracy of readings is reduced in patients with a high VD/VT or rapid respiratory rate, these devices do reduce the need for ABG determinations.

  4. **Pulmonary mechanics** include measurement of the average resting VT, vital capacity, and inspiratory force. These last two parameters are obtainable only when patients can cooperate and respond to commands. Patients on ventilators should have daily determinations to monitor clinical progress and assess the ability to wean.

  5. **Sputum Gram stains** should be obtained daily from patients intubated for more than 24 hours, since there is a substantial risk of acquiring a pulmonary infection. Colonization of the respiratory tract with potential pathogens is common in the intensive care unit; the use of antibiotics is therefore indicated only if other signs of infection are present (e.g., fever, leukocytosis, infiltrate on chest x-ray, white blood cells with intracellular organisms on Gram stain).

  6. **Chest tube function** should continuously be assessed; Fig. 32-1 illustrates the most common system for drainage of the pleural space, the Pleur-Evac.

     a. The Pleur-Evac is a derivative of the traditional "three-bottle" system, where the proximal bot-

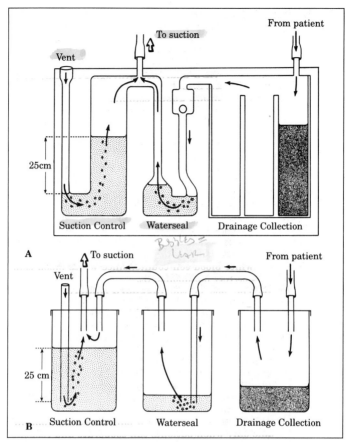

Fig. 32-1. Chest tube drainage apparatus. The Pleur-Evac system (A), a derivative of the traditional "three-bottle" collection system (B).

tle traps the drainage, the middle bottle prevents air or fluid from being drawn into the thorax (i.e., the "waterseal"), and the distal bottle regulates the level of suction that reaches the pleural cavity. Application of constant vacuum to the suction-control chamber produces a steady stream of bubbles and subatmospheric pressures in all three chambers. The negative pressure is independent of strength of the wall suction and depends only on the height of the water column in the suction-control chamber.

   b. **To examine a Pleur-Evac,** confirm
     (1) That the water level in the middle chamber varies with respirations, especially

> when disconnected from suction (absence of respiratory variation suggests mechanical obstruction of the chest tube).
>
> **(2)** Whether the volume and nature of any pleural drainage has changed.
>
> **(3)** Whether bubbling is occurring in the waterseal chamber (this is evidence of a bronchopleural leak). A qualitative assessment of the size of a bronchopleural leak can be made from the magnitude of the bubbling in the waterseal chamber.

XI. Radiology in the intensive care unit. In general, portable anteroposterior chest x-rays are obtained whenever there is a sudden deterioration in vital signs or ABGs; pneumothorax, aspiration, pulmonary edema, and endobronchial intubation are reversible causes of respiratory failure that may first be appreciated by this technique. Daily chest x-rays are useful for following the effects of chest physiotherapy, antibiotics, and diuretic therapy. Besides acute emergencies, other specific indications for chest x-ray include

A. Central venous catheter placement. Catheter tips should be in the superior vena cava, not the right atrium, since transmural erosion can occur, leading to cardiac tamponade. Pneumothorax, particularly after subclavian catheter placements, should be ruled out by examining the chest x-rays with a spot light.

B. Feeding tube placement. Soft feeding tubes placed with the aid of a stylet can enter the trachea, even when cuffed endotracheal or tracheostomy tubes are in place. In contrast, larger-diameter nasogastric tubes (14 Fr or larger) are much less likely to pass into the trachea, and chest x-rays are not routinely needed after these are placed.

C. Postintubation. In adults, the tip of the endotracheal tube should be 5–8 cm beyond the vocal cords and overlie the T2–T3 vertebral body. The neck should be in a neutral position when chest x-rays are taken; neck flexion will cause both nasal and oral endotracheal tubes to advance further into the trachea, while neck extension causes the movement to be outward. If the tip is close to the carina when the neck is in a neutral position, an endobronchial intubation may occur with flexion.

XII. Tests of respiratory function and equations

A. Compliance is the change in volume for a given change in pressure. The compliance of healthy lungs during spontaneous ventilation is 150–200 ml/cm H_2O (a change of 2–4 cm H_2O in intrapleural pressure allows the lung to accommodate a V_T of about 500 ml). With positive-pressure mechanical ventilation, compliance is quite different; here, normal compliance is 40–60 ml/cm H_2O.

Compliance = change in volume (V)/change in pressure (P)

where V = tidal volume
P = (PIP − PEEP)

The dynamic compliance is determined clinically using the PIP obtained about 0.5 second after a V_T has been given (the plateau pressure). The calculated compliance may be falsely low due to the artifacts produced by high flow rates, as well as the resistances in the connecting tubing and endotracheal tube.

B. The alveolar gas equation is used to calculate the alveolar-to-arterial O_2 gradient (A-aDO_2).

$$PaO_2 = (P_B - P_{H_2O}) (FiO_2) - (PaCO_2/RQ)$$
$$+ (PaCO_2) (FiO_2) [(1 - RQ)/RQ]$$

where PaO_2 = alveolar O_2 tension

P_B = barometric pressure

P_{H_2O} = water vapor pressure at 37°C (47 mm Hg)

FiO_2 = the fractional concentration of inspired O_2

$PaCO_2$ = the arterial CO_2 tension obtained from an ABG

RQ = the respiratory quotient (usually about 0.8)

Since the last term is a small correction factor, the equation may be simplified for clinical use:

$$PaO_2 = (P_B - P_{H_2O}) (FiO_2) - PaCO_2/RQ$$

The PaO_2 calculated above is equivalent to the ideal alveolar capillary blood PO_2. In the absence of lung disease, there is normally a 0–10 mm Hg difference between the calculated alveolar and actual arterial PO_2 when $FiO_2 = 0.21$. The alveolar-arterial PO_2 gradient increases with increasing FiO_2 (up to 25–50 mm Hg) even when lung function is normal (for reasons that are unclear).

C. Oxygen content of blood. It is difficult to measure O_2 content of blood directly; however, the O_2 content of the alveolar capillary, arterial, or venous blood can be calculated from the respective PO_2 and the hemoglobin concentration by

$$CaO_2 = (1.39 \text{ cc } O_2/\text{gm Hgb}) (\text{gm Hgb/dl blood}) (SO_2)$$
$$+ \text{dissolved } O_2$$

where dissolved $O_2 = (PO_2) (0.003 \text{ ml } O_2/\text{mm Hg/dl blood})$

Estimates of the constant for O_2-carrying capacity of hemoglobin vary between 1.34 and 1.39. SO_2 can be measured with an oximeter or calculated from the PO_2. Although some ABG analyzers have algorithms for calculating O_2 content of partially saturated blood, this is inaccurate because algorithms do not include compensations for shifts in the O_2-hemoglobin dissociation curve.

D. Fick equation relates cardiac output, $\dot{V}O_2$, and the O_2

content difference between arterial and mixed venous blood:

$$CO = \dot{V}O_2/(CaO_2 - C\bar{v}O_2)$$

where CO = cardiac output in dl/min
$\dot{V}O_2$ = oxygen consumption in ml/min
CaO_2 and $C\bar{v}O_2$ are the O_2 contents of arterial and mixed venous blood in ml O_2/dl blood, respectively

The Fick equation is commonly rearranged to calculate O_2 consumption as follows:

$$\dot{V}O_2 = [CO] [CaO_2 - C\bar{v}O_2)]$$

This only approximates O_2 consumption because of inaccuracies in both thermodilution cardiac output measurement and the calculation of O_2 content.

E. **The shunt equation.** The alveolar-arterial O_2 gradient calculation is an indicator of oxygenating efficiency, but its value depends on a number of factors other than the efficiency of the lung (e.g., cardiac output and tissue O_2 consumption). The shunt equation is useful only to quantitate lung inefficiency in oxygenation:

$$\dot{Q}s/\dot{Q}_T = (CcO_2 - CaO_2)/(CcO_2 - C\bar{v}O_2)$$

where $\dot{Q}s/\dot{Q}t$ = shunt flow as a proportion of total lung blood flow
CcO_2 = alveolar capillary O_2 content
CaO_2 = arterial O_2 content
$C\bar{v}O_2$ = mixed venous O_2 content

Alveolar capillary PO_2 is assumed to be equal to PaO_2 (from the alveolar gas equation), and SaO_2 is usually calculated from this PO_2. PaO_2 and $P\bar{v}O_2$ are measured by ABG analysis. For arterial and alveolar capillary blood, if the PO_2 is greater than 100 mm Hg, 100% O_2 saturation is assumed. $S\bar{v}O_2$ saturation must be estimated from an O_2-hemoglobin dissociation curve (based on the $P\bar{v}O_2$).

F. V_D/V_T represents the **physiologic dead space as a fraction of the tidal volume** and is a useful measure of lung dysfunction. Values greater than 0.6 are usually incompatible with weaning from mechanical ventilation.

$$V_D/V_T = (PaCO_2 - P\bar{e}CO_2)/PaCO_2$$

where $PaCO_2$ = arterial PCO_2
$P\bar{e}CO_2$ = average PCO_2 in expired gas collected over time (usually 3–5 minutes)

G. **Oxygen consumption** ($\dot{V}O_2$) is usually calculated using the Fick equation (see sec. **XII.D**) and is normally 3–4 ml/min/kg. It may also be calculated by measuring the difference between the amount of O_2 that enters the lung and the amount that is exhaled. This calculation requires collection of expired gas over a known period of ventilation and measurement of the concentrations of expired O_2 ($F\dot{E}O_2$), CO_2 ($F\dot{E}CO_2$), and N_2 ($F\dot{E}N_2$):

$$\dot{V}O_2 \text{ (ml/min)} = \{ [(FN_2) (FIO_2/FIN_2)] $$
$$- [FO_2] \} \times (\dot{V}E) \text{ (at STPD)}$$

where $FN_2 = 1.0 - (FO_2 + FCO_2)$
FIN_2 = fractional concentration of inspired N_2
FIO_2 = fractional concentration of inspired O_2
$\dot{V}E$ = measured minute ventilation (expired)

H. **Carbon dioxide production** ($\dot{V}CO_2$) is usually 2.4–3.2 cc/min/kg and is measured by collecting expired gas in an impermeable ("Douglas") bag over a known period of steady-state ventilation. The concentration of the mixed expired CO_2 ($F\dot{E}CO_2$) is measured and the $\dot{V}E$ is calculated:

$$\dot{V}CO_2 \text{ (cc/min)} = (F\dot{E}CO_2) \times (\dot{V}E) \text{ (at STPD)}$$

Correction factors to convert expired gas volumes to dry volumes at standard temperature and pressure are available in most physiology texts.

I. **Respiratory quotient** (RQ) is the ratio of CO_2 production to O_2 consumption:

$$RQ = CO_2 \text{ production (ml/min)}/O_2 \text{ consumption (ml/min)}$$

The normal value for RQ is 0.8 but depends on the patient's source of calories at the time RQ is calculated (see sec. **IX**).

J. **Practical use of the Siggaard-Andersen nomogram for ABG interpretation** (see inside back cover). This nomogram is used to diagnose, quantitate, and treat acid-base abnormalities by determining the base excess (principally HCO_3^-) in a given sample of arterial blood. Regardless of the absolute pH, a positive base excess indicates metabolic alkalosis, while a negative value (base deficit) reveals an underlying metabolic acidosis. To use the nomogram, a straight line drawn through the measured values for the patient's $PaCO_2$, pH, and hemoglobin will intersect the scales at the appropriate value for the base excess.

Suggested Reading

Chernow, B. (ed.). *The Pharmacologic Approach to the Critically Ill Patient*. Baltimore: Williams & Wilkins, 1983.

Dantzker, D. R. (ed.). *Cardiopulmonary Critical Care*. Orlando, Fla.: Grune & Stratton, 1986.

Kacmarek, R. M., Mack, C. W., and Dimas, S. *The Essentials of Respiratory Therapy*. Chicago: Year Book, 1985.

Pontoppidan, H., et al. Respiratory intensive care. *Anesthesiology* 47:96, 1977.

Rie, M. A., and Wilson, R. S. Acute Respiratory Failure. In J. Tinker and M. Rapin (eds.), *Care of the Critically Ill Patient.* New York: Springer, 1983.

Suter, P. M., Fairley, H. B., and Isenberg, M. D. Optimum end-expiratory airway pressure in patients with acute pulmonary failure. *N. Engl. J. Med.* 292:284, 1975.

33

Pain

Daniel B. Carr

I. Pain and the anesthesiologist

A. **Acute pain.** Anesthesiologists play a unique role in the treatment of acute pain. Intraoperative blockade of afferent stimuli, or the central response to such, is the hallmark of successful anesthetic management. Once the patient leaves the recovery room, responsibility for further analgesic management ordinarily lies with the surgeon. Departures from this routine may occur when conventional analgesics prove ineffective postoperatively (or are avoided from fear of, e.g., respiratory depression), when pain is expected to persist (e.g., after a noncurative cancer operation), or when pain patterns do not fit the objective findings. In such cases, an inpatient "pain consult" is often sought for adjustment of pharmacotherapy, for diagnostic and therapeutic nerve blocks, or other interventions ranging from (permanent) neurolysis to placement of catheters for prolonged drug delivery.

B. **Chronic pain.** Patients with long-standing symptoms are referred to anesthesiologist consultants for diagnosis as well as therapy. Few other specialists are prepared to perform selective nerve blocks to judge the importance of an individual facet joint, nerve root, or sympathetic chain within a symptom complex. Such referrals often originate with orthopedic surgeons or neurosurgeons. Prognostic importance also attaches to local anesthetic blockade performed to simulate neurolysis, for example, of intercostal nerves in a patient with malignant involvement of the chest wall or of celiac plexus in a patient with inoperable pancreatic cancer. Thoracic or general surgeons or oncologists might refer such cases. Therapeutic trials of local anesthetics and corticosteroids instilled epidurally, or into suspected "trigger points," are undertaken in patients referred by internists, orthopedists, or rheumatologists.

Apart from technical facility with neural blockade, anesthesiologists are consulted to help manage patients whose pain has a more obscure anatomic basis. Chronic neuropathic, myofascial, or idiopathic pain is often managed medically, the regimen for which is a consensus between specialists in anesthesia, psychiatry, and neurology. Familiarity with analgesic, anxiolytic, anti-inflammatory, anticonvulsant, and antidepressant drugs has led anesthesiologists to serve as valuable members—even leaders—of comprehensive pain management teams.

II. Pathways and mediators

A. **Neural.** Afferent pathways have been best studied in animals subject to nociceptive stimuli such as heat, irritant chemicals, local pressure, or tooth pulp stimulation. Accordingly, their participation in clinical pain (e.g., visceral pain) is often extrapolation, albeit useful.

1. **Nociceptors** are of two major types: **high-threshold mechanoceptors** and **polymodal nociceptors.** High-threshold mechanoceptors do not respond to heat or chemical irritation but do respond to strong pressure provided this is applied to a wide area of skin (often over 1 cm^2). High-threshold mechanoceptor axons are myelinated and of **A delta** caliber, that is, they conduct rapidly (5–25 m/sec). Polymodal nociceptors respond not only to pressure but also to heat and algesic substances; their axons are unmyelinated and conduct in the **C fiber** range (< 2 m/sec). Other classes of nociceptor, such as polymodal nociceptors with axons in the A delta range, are recognized. All nociceptors increase in sensitivity after mild injury.

2. **Primary afferents** with cell bodies in dorsal root ganglia lead from nociceptors to the spinal cord. Afferent impulses in either fast, myelinated A delta or slow, unmyelinated C fibers are perceived as pain. A delta stimulation yields "first" pain: sharp, pricking, localized, and rapid in onset. C fibers underly "second" pain: dull, aching, poorly localized, and prolonged. **Visceral afferents** are also of A and C caliber but—in contrast to **somatic afferents**—reach the spinal cord through sympathetic, parasympathetic, and splanchnic nerves, or even through ventral roots. Dorsal root afferents project rostrocaudally across several segments.

3. **Dorsal horn** processing of afferent input takes place in a cascade system arrayed in six laminae described by Rexed. **Substantia gelatinosa** (SG), corresponding to laminae I (Wall) and/or II (Duggan) and/or III (Bonica), contains neurons responding essentially only to pain, that is, **nociceptive-specific.** In contrast, **wide dynamic range** cells, particularly in lamina V, respond to different modes of input (e.g., mechanical, chemical, thermal) even at levels below the pain threshold. Dorsal horn neurons are inhibited by small SG interneurons (**"gate theory"**); selective triggering of the latter by large myelinated peripheral afferents mediates analgesia due to **transcutaneous electrical nerve stimulation** (TENS). Reflex activation of **sympathetic efferent** outflow at the segmental level may perpetuate a vicious cycle of pain.

4. **Ascending pain pathways** originate largely as crossed projections of dorsal horn cell axons at the segmental level. The **spinothalamic tract** ascends in anterolateral cord to ventroposterior and medial thalamic nuclei, which project to associative and somatosensory areas of cerebral cortex. Classically it is identified with localization and discrimination of pain. **Spinoreticular** neurons underly arousal, affective sensations, and autonomic responses. Persistence or recurrence of pain sensa-

tions after severing of both these major pathways argues for the clinical function of other tracts (e.g., **spinomesencephalic** or multisynaptic, **propriospinal** paths). In actuality, collateral fibers often link theoretically "distinct" tracts.

5. **Psychological factors** presumably take place at cortical and subcortical levels, although electrical stimulation of the cortex itself rarely produces pain. Emotional and cognitive aspects assume great importance in chronic pain states and underlie individual variability in pain perception or analgesic requirements; their neurobiologic bases are at present poorly understood.

B. **Chemical mediators** of pain offer opportunities for drug therapy at multiple sites.

1. **Peripheral algesic substances** activate nociceptors during acute injury or inflammation. Acetylcholine, histamine, serotonin, bradykinin, prostaglandins, adenosine triphosphate, and hydrogen and potassium ions can act alone, or synergistically, to do so. Many of these and others under investigation (e.g., lymphokines, monokines, interleukins) are white blood cell products.

2. **Neuropeptides** function in primary sensory as well as inhibitory ("modulatory") roles. They are always produced as fragments of larger precursors, which often yield several active daughter compounds, each with the primary structure of a chain of amino acids. Twisting of these chains in vivo results in three-dimensional structures that fit specific receptors. **Substance P,** an 11–amino acid peptide, is a major sensory transmitter of primary pain afferents; other peptides with possible sensory roles include cholecystokinin, angiotensin II, and vasoactive intestinal peptide. Analgesic peptides include somatostatin, calcitonin gene-related peptide, and **endorphins.** The last include several families of opioid peptides, each with part of their structure resembling morphine, but with other regions having actions distinct from narcotics (e.g., immune modulation). Endorphins and their receptors are found in the dorsal horn (where they inhibit substance P release), periaqueductal grey, raphe nucleus, and limbic structures. Beta endorphin is derived from the same precursor as adrenocorticotropic hormone, and both are cosecreted during stress.

3. **Monoamines** include dietary amino acids (glycine) or their enzymatically produced derivatives (e.g., catecholamines from tyrosine, or serotonin from tryptophan). Catecholamines function as excitatory sympathetic transmitters and also are released systemically as hormones that sensitize nociceptors. Yet norepinephrine and serotonin not only transmit key inhibitory brainstem signals to dorsal horns but also contribute to the analgesia produced by

morphine or by certain forms of environmental stress. Indeed, opiate-monoamine interactions are well recognized: profound, synergistic analgesia results from co-administering intrathecal morphine and serotonin or norepinephrine.

III. **Acute pain.** Postoperative or posttraumatic pain responds to interference with anatomic pathways using drugs that block nerve conduction or act selectively on one or another mediator. A stepwise approach that balances the strength of analgesic to severity of pain, adjusting doses in the presence of regional anesthesia, is appropriate. Preoperative patient education is recognized to decrease postoperative analgesic requirements.

A. **Nonsteroidal anti-inflammatory drugs** (NSAIDs) diminish nociceptor activation by inhibiting prostaglandin biosynthesis, thereby reducing tissue injury and inflammation. Prostaglandins also amplify peripheral nociceptor responses to algesic mediators (e.g., bradykinin or histamine). Nonsteroidal anti-inflammatory drugs are bound to peripheral proteins, which leak into the damaged site, and are locally concentrated in the acidic environs of damaged tissue. Although NSAIDs have central effects (e.g., antipyresis), their analgesic effects in acute pain essentially reflect peripheral actions. Individual responses to different NSAIDs are variable. Optimizing therapy, therefore, by serial trials of different NSAIDs is feasible and rational (Table 33-1). Most NSAIDs share side effects of gastrointestinal intolerance, tinnitus, fluid retention, platelet dysfunction, and hepatic or renal dysfunction, and appropriate laboratory studies should be obtained every 4–6 months if usage becomes chronic. In the short term (e.g., postoperatively), NSAIDs may be as effective as morphine.

B. **Regional anesthetic techniques** impede nociceptive afferent and/or spinal cord pain transmission. Local anesthetics are used at both sites; their pharmacology and clinical use are discussed in Chaps. 12 and 13. Opioids overlap with local anesthetics in pharmacodynamics, physicochemical properties (pK, molecular weight, and oil-water solubility), and in some cases (e.g., meperidine) even structure. Yet opioids and local anesthetics contrast in that true toxicity (convulsions or cardiovascular collapse) is very rare with the former. Also, opioids act on specific spinal and supraspinal receptors, while local anesthetics block axonal sodium channels. Opiates selectively impair pain transmission, but local anesthetics block sensory, motor, and sympathetic fibers; the former are incomplete blockers of acute surgical or obstetric pain, yet with the latter complete block is possible. Thus in lower limb surgery for which complete anesthesia plus vasodilatation is desired, local anesthetics would be best, but for postoperative analgesia, and long-term relief of cancer pain without sensorimotor impairment, opioids would be preferable.

Epidural narcotics (Table 33-2) are more commonly used than intrathecal narcotics, because the epidural route has less risk of headache or meningitis and thus is safer if prolonged drug delivery becomes desirable. Nonetheless **"one-shot" intrathecal narcotics** cannot be disregarded, as several studies have found persistent postoperative analgesia after co-administration of 1 mg or less of morphine along with local anesthetic. Epidural and intrathecal opioids act at the same sites— the former after diffusion across dura and cerebrospinal fluid (CSF)—and either may lead to **tolerance** and **narcotic side effects** (urinary retention, pruritus, nausea, and vomiting). Epidural opioids diffusing through CSF may be carried rostrally to ventilatory centers to produce **central respiratory depression** that is late in onset (6–12 hours) and unheralded by patient panic. At therapeutic doses, morphine, which is water-soluble and persistent in CSF, is much more likely to cause this than fentanyl, which is lipid-soluble and segmentally concentrated, or meperidine, which has intermediate solubility. Respiratory depression is potentiated by other central nervous system depressants (including parenteral narcotics), old age, respiratory disease, raised intrathoracic or intraabdominal pressure, morphine doses in excess of 5 mg, or inadvertent dural puncture. These and all other side effects of narcotics are reversible with naloxone, 0.2–0.4 mg IV, repeated as necessary.

C. **Systemic narcotics** are the traditional mainstay for acute pain (see Table 33-1). Codeine, which is metabolized to morphine, or morphine itself is a **narcotic agonist** that binds to prototypical **mu** (for morphine) **receptors.** Other drugs such as butorphanol or metkephamid are selective agonists at other types of opiate receptors (i.e., **kappa** and **delta,** respectively) and are chosen because of their apparent "ceiling" effects on respiratory depression. However, such drugs often block mu receptors and hence may precipitate withdrawal symptoms in patients chronically treated with mu agonists; for this reason, they are termed **mixed agonist-antagonist** drugs. **Partial agonists** such as buprenorphine act on only one class of receptor (e.g., mu) but have a response plateau below that of a full agonist and so may also precipitate withdrawal in tolerant patients. Narcotics given to normal patients with acute pain rarely produce euphoria; instead depersonalization or frank **dysphoria** are common, more so with selective or partial agonists.

D. **Adjuvant medications** are useful to treat narcotic side effects such as sedation (dextroamphetamine), nausea (droperidol), or constipation (stool softeners). Nonsteroidal anti-inflammatory drugs, hydroxyzine, and dextroamphetamine are valuable to potentiate narcotic analgesia, each by distinct mechanisms. Individualization of adjuvants suggests adding antibiotics where superinfection contributes to pain (e.g., ulcer debridement), muscle relaxants such as diazepam or baclofen if spasm is present, or anxiolytics.

Table 33-1. Analgesics and related drugs

Generic name	Proprietary name	Oral dosage (mg)[a]	Parenteral dosage (mg)
Nonsteroidal anti-inflammatory agents			
Aspirin		650 q3–4h	
Ibuprofen	Motrin, Advil	200–800 q6h	
Naproxen	Naprosyn	250–500 q12h	
Indomethacin	Indocin	25–50 q8h	
Acetaminophen[b]	Tylenol	650 q3–4h	
Narcotics			
Propoxyphene	Darvon	65 q3–4h	
Codeine		15–60 q4–6h	30–60 q4–6h
Butorphanol	Stadol		2–4 q3–4h
Buprenorphine	Buprenex		0.3–0.6 q4–6h
Oxycodone	In Tylox, Percocet, Percodan	5–10 q4–6h	
Morphine			5–20 q3–4h
Meperidine	MS-Contin, Roxanol	10–30 q12h	
Meperidine	Demerol	50–200 q2–3h	50–100 q3–4h
Hydromorphone	Dilaudid	2–4 q4–6h	2–4 q4–6h
Methadone	Dolophine	10–20 q6–8h	2.5–10 q6h
Antidepressants			
Amitriptyline	Elavil	50–150 hs	
Imipramine	Tofranil	50–150 hs	

Desipramine	Norpramin	50–150 hs	5–10 q4h
Phenelzine	Nardil	15 tid	
Doxepin	Adapin	25–50 tid	
Anxiolytics, muscle relaxants			
Diazepam	Valium	5 qid	
Clonazepam	Klonopin	0.5–1.0 tid	
Alprazolam	Xanax	0.5–1.0 tid	
Cyclobenzaprine	Flexeril	10–20 tid	
Baclofen	Lioresal	5–15 tid	
Methocarbamol	Robaxin	500 tid	
Hydroxyzine	Vistaril	50–100 qid	50–100 q6h
Anticonvulsants (non-benzodiazepine)			
Carbamazepine	Tegretol	100–200 tid	
Phenytoin	Dilantin	50–100 tid	
Valproate	Depakene	100–400 tid	
Antinauseants, major tranquilizers			
Prochlorperazine	Compazine	5–10 tid	5–10 q3–4h
Chlorpromazine	Thorazine	10–25 q6h	25–50 q3–4h
Haloperidol	Haldol	0.5 q8h	1–2 q6h
Droperidol	Inapsine	5–15 q8h	1.25 q6h

[a]Dosages are for an average 70-kg adult.
[b]Not anti-inflammatory, but efficacious in acute pain.

Table 33-2. Single-dose intraspinal narcotics in the adult

Drug	Dose (mg)	Latency (min)	Duration (hr)
Epidural			
Morphine	2–4	20–30	6–24
Fentanyl	0.1	4–10	3–6
Meperidine	100	5	4–20
Intrathecal			
Morphine	0.5–1.0	10	18–48
Meperidine	10–30	5	?–48

NOTE: Only morphine has FDA approval for epidural or intrathecal use, but extensive clinical experience has been gained with the other drugs as well. To control clinical response for volume of drug given, we dilute epidural drugs to a volume of 3 ml and intrathecal drugs to 1 ml in saline. Preservative-free drugs and saline diluent are employed.

    E. Patient-controlled analgesia (PCA, or demand analgesia) allows standard drugs such as morphine to be given from bedside or portable devices operated directly by the patient, whenever the patient desires. These devices typically employ an electrically powered pump with safety limits on IV or SQ infusion rates. Patient-controlled analgesia is feasible for selected patients; its wider adoption awaits comparative analyses of costs, risks, and impact on postoperative course (e.g., duration of stay, pain scores, morbidity, and mortality).

IV. Chronic pain syndromes. Chronic pain syndromes are both varied and complex in their manifestations. Significant **behavioral changes** often are present when pain of any etiology has persisted more than a few months. Irritability, insomnia, dependency on family members and/or drugs, and lack of motivation are common. **Depression** is frequent enough to warrant empiric therapy. Tricyclics and monoamine oxidase inhibitors both act on analgesic pathways directly and through effects on neuromodulators such as endorphins; side effects include drowsiness, which is helpful if after a bedtime dose.

    Prior to starting any palliative therapy, the referring physician's diagnosis must first be confirmed; for example, "facet pain" may actually be due to a symptomatic bony metastasis. Careful review of the history and physical findings will ordinarily suffice, although at times the opinion of another consultant is necessary and leads to further workup. A few of the most prevalent pain syndromes are discussed in the sections that follow.

    A. Myofascial pain (formerly **fibrositis**) is extremely common yet often undiagnosed. Hyperirritable sites in muscle and nearby connective tissue, termed **trigger points,** result from minor trauma, fatigue, or tension, which then produce reflex muscle spasm, ischemia, and pain. Trigger points are tender nodules or sometimes ropelike and have been described in virtually every muscle group. **Treatment** consists in either cooling the site with chlorofluoromethane and then passively stretching the involved muscles or local injection. "Dry needling" of the trigger point, saline injection, local anesthetic alone, or local anesthetic with corticosteroid each has advocates. We employ 2–3 ml of xylocaine 1% or bupivacaine 0.5% injected through a 22-gauge needle to assess the initial response and, at subsequent visits, 2–3 ml of a 1 : 9 solution of triamcinolone (2.5% as Aristocort or 1% as Kenalog) in xylocaine 1% or bupivacaine 0.5%. Injections are repeated at least a week apart.

B. **Low back pain** occurs in at least half of all adults through multiple, often coexistent mechanisms. Organic disease (e.g., retroperitoneal tumor) must be excluded, anatomic derangements (e.g., bony fragments) characterized thoroughly, and surgical options (e.g, foraminotomy) considered with orthopedists or neurosurgeons prior to selecting nonsurgical management. Sensorimotor function, including tenderness and pain on flexion or extension of the spine and extremities, should be documented at each stage of treatment. Bowel or bladder dysfunction argue for aggressive surgical intervention, as does persistent decrease in motor power or sensation.

1. **Radicular pain** may arise from a **ruptured** or **herniated intervertebral disk** with intraspinal bulging or lateral compression of the exiting nerve root between the disk (anterior) and facet joint (posterior). Pain on the affected side produced by passive straight leg raising of the opposite leg (**crossed straight leg raising**) is seen with lateral disk herniation. Facet joint hypertrophy, nerve root scarring, or dorsal root ganglion compression likewise causes radicular pain. **Spinal stenosis** may produce a neurogenic pattern of claudication, often relieved by rest.

2. **Epidural steroid** injection is offered when symptoms persist despite 2 or more weeks of strict bed rest. Benefits of this procedure may result from decreased inflammation and shrinkage of scar tissue. It also appears promising in treatment of spinal stenosis. Midline injections are technically simplest and therefore tried first; **paravertebral** or **caudal** approaches are reserved for nonresponders, if local root scarring is present, or if anatomic barriers exist (e.g., after posterior fusion). Patients may be placed in the prone position, with blankets under the stomach of slender patients, to decrease lumbar lordosis. With arms dangling over the sides of the table, which is radiolucent to permit intermittent C-arm fluoroscopy, needle hubs are used to mark appropriate vertebrae and pressed into the skin leaving indentations. After preparing the skin,

draping, and infiltrating the skin, a styletted 22-gauge spinal needle is inserted to the ligamentum flavum, the stylet removed, and a 10-cc syringe attached. With air under continuous pressure as the barrel is moved piston-style, the needle and syringe are slowly advanced until the epidural space is identified by loss of resistance to air. At L4–L5, this depth usually is 4–6 cm. After negative aspiration, 2 ml of 1% xylocaine containing epinephrine 1 : 200,000 is instilled and the patient observed for tachycardia or spinal anesthesia for 5 minutes. During this time, a permanent x-ray is obtained. Then, 3 ml of triamcinolone (2.5% as Aristocort or 1% as Kenalog) is instilled. Other steroids have been advocated but may cause arachnoiditis after (inadvertent) intrathecal injection. The patient is warned that soreness or increased symptoms may occur for the next several days. Telephone follow-up is at 2 weeks, and repeat injections are no more frequent than monthly for a total of three at the same site.

3. **Lumbar paravertebral** injections are useful not only for steroid administration but also for gauging contributions of specific root afferents to a patient's pain syndrome. For the latter purpose, local anesthetics are used without steroid. The patient is positioned as for midline epidural injection, and the skin is marked above the root foramen, that is, the lateral margin of the vertebral body just caudad to the pedicle. The needle entry site is marked 5–8 cm lateral to the midline, just caudad to the level of the transverse process (or slightly differently when necessary if the iliac crest or ribs lie in the needle path). Under local anesthesia (1.5% xylocaine containing epinephrine 1 : 200,000), a 22-gauge, 10-cm "finder" needle is advanced to the transverse process. The finder is removed and replaced with a 22-gauge, 3.5-inch (9 cm) spinal needle directed caudal to the transverse process, advanced until the root is identified by a paresthesia. Infiltration of local anesthesia around the root is avoided, since it will prevent a paresthesia. Needle tip position adjacent to the foramen is confirmed by lateral x-ray. Xylocaine 1.5% with epinephrine, or a 1 : 9 mixture of 1% tetracaine in 1.5% xylocaine with epinephrine, is given 1–2 ml at a time to produce dermatomal anesthesia; total volumes more than 2 or 3 ml will readily spread to anesthetize nearby roots and blur the diagnostic benefit. Some clinicians mix sodium bicarbonate with local anesthetics to enhance their action by raising pH. For therapeutic trials, up to 75 mg of triamcinolone may be given with the local anesthetic. Adequate muscular recovery from the anesthetic must occur before discharge.

4. **Facet joint** irritation is perceived as an ache in the lower back, sometimes referred to the buttocks or

thighs; sensorimotor compromise is rare. Classically, there is local tenderness over the involved joint(s) and worsening of pain on twisting or bending forward, sideways, or (especially) backward. Facet and disk degeneration may coexist, for example, as narrowing of the disk space alters facet anatomy. Selective injection of a facet joint is accomplished by positioning the patient prone or turned slightly laterally to provide a clear fluoroscopic view of the articular surfaces. Blankets folded beneath the patient will open the joint maximally. After preparing and infiltrating the skin, the tip of a styletted 22-gauge spinal needle is advanced into the joint and its position confirmed by rolling the patient laterally and seeing the needle tip remain within the joint. The stylet is removed and reinserted after injecting 1–2 ml of local anesthetic; the needle remains in place while a permanent x-ray is taken. If by this point the pain is gone, 1 ml of Aristocort or Kenalog is instilled prior to removing the needle.

C. **Reflex sympathetic dystrophy** presents with burning pain, hyperesthesia, blanched and cool skin, and edema following trauma as trivial as a blister or sprain, or as invasive as lumbar surgery. When present with nerve injury, it is termed **causalgia.** Local osteoporosis occurs in advanced cases.

1. **Treatment** by sympathetic blockade employs local anesthetics without epinephrine. For **stellate block,** the patient is supine with the neck hyperextended and a C-arm fluoroscope in place. A 22-gauge 5-cm needle is advanced between the trachea and carotid artery to touch the lateral portion of the anterior surface of C7 or T1, a negative aspiration is obtained, and 10 ml of 1% xylocaine or 0.25% bupivacaine is slowly injected. This produces **Horner's syndrome** (ptosis, anhidrosis, enophthalmos, and miosis) and also scleral injection, hoarseness, or bradycardia. **Lumbar sympathetic block** uses a technique akin to paravertebral block (see sec. **B.3**) except the needle enters the skin just cephalad to the L2 transverse process and, after touching the transverse process, is redirected cephalad to touch the L2 vertebral body without hitting a somatic nerve root. The needle bevel is then turned toward the vertebral body to allow the needle tip to slide inward along its lateral surface. The needle tip is advanced until its bevel is half on the vertebral body and half deep to it on lateral x-ray. A total of 30 ml of 1% xylocaine or 0.1% tetracaine in 1% xylocaine is given in three doses.

2. Loss of **galvanic skin response** confirms interruption of sympathetic outflow to the limb. Warming of finger or toe by 20°F (starting at nearly room temperature in a room at 68°F) also indicates an effective block. Blocks may be repeated weekly, four

to five times, without harm, or three times a day by catheter for a week. A currently available alternate or supplemental treatment employs **intravenous regional injection** of guanethidine (15–20 mg) in 25–50 ml saline for an arm or twice the drug in twice the volume for a leg. Results with oral alpha or beta blockers, calcium channel antagonists, transcutaneous electrical nerve stimulation, or calcitonin are less consistent.

D. **Neuropathic pain** may result from diffuse insults such as diabetes or local trauma including limb ischemia or amputation. Injured nerves, regardless of their particular pathology (e.g., demyelination, neuroma formation, sprouting), may fire spontaneously or after stimuli other than normal nociceptor activation. Accordingly, anticonvulsants may produce relief (see Table 33-1); an antidepressant is often added empirically. Ordinary analgesics or surgical excision usually help little, except when painful nerve compression or entrapment (e.g., ilioinguinal nerve after herniorrhaphy) may be relieved. Peripheral neurolytic blocks are inadvisable in pain of nonmalignant origin because of the eventual high incidence of ethanol- or phenol-induced neuritis and the likelihood of slow spontaneous improvement in neuropathy resulting from acute trauma. **Postherpetic neuralgia** (PHN) is more common after acute varicella zoster in patients who are older and/or immunocompromised. No method has been proved to prevent PHN after acute zoster, although favorable anecdotal outcomes have followed treatment of the acute phase with subcutaneous injection of triamcinolone in xylocaine (see sec. **IV.A**) or sympathetic block; the latter is especially effective in zoster ophthalmicus. These measures occasionally help in established PHN, but drug treatment with antidepressants such as amitriptyline and/or anticonvulsants (see Table 33-1) is more often effective and thus used first. Associated myofascial pain should be treated and, when possible, averted by early physical therapy.

E. **Chronic or learned pain behavior** may complicate any of the above syndromes or occur as a form of conversion reaction without evident pathology (**"psychogenic pain"**). Even after the pain of a known illness or operation should have abated, pain may persist due to **"centralization"** (i.e., autonomous central neuronal firing no longer dependent on peripheral nociceptors). Spinal or epidural blocks with increasing concentrations of local anesthetics might, in theory, isolate contributions of distinct afferents to a complex pain syndrome; in practice, such **"differential blocks"** do not separate sympathetic and somatic sensation and offer little diagnostic or prognostic benefit.

Insofar as exploring the meaning of the illness with the patient may strengthen therapeutic rapport and unearth treatable symptoms such as anxiety or depression, this is valuable. However, options for specific behavioral therapies are numerous and often best accomplished through referral to the appropriate psychiatrist, psychologist, or other specialist. Such options encompass relaxation techniques (e.g., biofeedback), hypnosis, psychotherapy, and conditioning. Rehabilitation and physical therapy are useful to improve mobility and functional level. These varied approaches share key goals of removing drug dependency and restoring disrupted family, social, and employment spheres.

V. **Cancer pain.** Nearly half of all patients with cancer, and three-quarters of advanced cases, experience pain. Palliation of cancer pain draws on all skills already outlined as well as expertise in chemotherapy, radiotherapy, surgery, and pastoral care. Patient discomfort—a mix of acute and chronic pain—will fluctuate spontaneously and during such therapies, as will analgesic goals and needs. The mechanism of pain should be sought, particularly with changes in quality or intensity, and therapy tailored appropriately (e.g., fixation or radiotherapy for pathologic fracture, rather than automatic increase in analgesics; antibiotics for ulcer infection).

A. **Pharmacotherapy** proceeds stepwise, starting with NSAIDs, then adding mild opiates such as codeine or strong opioids such as methadone (see Table 33-1). The goal is to keep the patient pain-free for the greatest number of hours per day, rather than waiting for pain to appear every few hours before treating it. Nonsteroidal anti-inflammatory drugs alone may surpass narcotics for certain types of pain, such as bone metastasis, and suffice for a patient's entire course. When pain is severe, we use round-the-clock methadone, plus hydromorphone if needed briefly; consistent need for the latter prompts us to raise the methadone dose. Narcotics should not be deemed a failure until their dosage is increased to the point of drowsiness; even then it is possible to raise the dosage more, decrease sedation, and enhance analgesia by adding dextroamphetamine (Dexedrine), 5 mg every 6 hours.

1. **Adjuvant medicines** (see sec. **III.D** and Table 33-1) include stool softeners or cholinomimetics to avert severe constipation or urinary retention during narcotic therapy; anxiolytics; antidepressants; major tranquilizers; and glucocorticoids for tumor-related or perineural edema. Nitrous oxide (e.g., 50–60% in oxygen) has been used for brief bedside anesthesia during temporary, painful procedures such as dressing changes.

2. **Drug delivery** systems permit targeting of agents at the best site (e.g., intraspinal) and/or at the best time (e.g., PCA). Numerous reports document the effectiveness of epidural (or, less frequently, intrathecal) opiates for long-term pain relief of cancer pain (see Table 33-2). We prefer epidural to intrathecal routes because infection and CSF leak appear less likely with the former, and we proceed to a permanent catheter only after a successful tem-

porary catheter trial. Tolerance invariably develops with long-term use, forcing higher and higher doses. Low doses of an epidural local anesthetic may produce analgesia with preserved motor function. Certain pains (e.g., nerve compression) seem opiate-resistant from onset; epidural nonopioid analgesics such as clonidine or somatostatin are now being evaluated in this setting.

B. Nerve blocks aid in diagnosis (e.g., assessing one nerve's or root's contribution to a complex pain syndrome) and therapy. **Neurolytic blocks** employ either alcohol (100% ethanol) or phenol (6–10% in glycerine or Renografin) to destroy nerves. Both agents have been administered into the subarachnoid or epidural spaces to palliate cancer pain, but if this is contemplated, it should be done only after repeated trials of local anesthetics to ensure reproducibility and efficacy. Even then, paraparesis and sphincter dysfunction are possible. Alcohol blocks are transiently painful and so should be preceded by a local anesthetic. Compared to phenol, they are more likely to be permanent and also to eventuate in a painful neuritis.

Techniques of nerve blocks have been described in sec. **IV.C.1** and in Chap. 13, except for **celiac plexus block** for abdominal visceral pain. The patient and C-arm fluoroscope are positioned as for lumbar sympathetic block (see sec. **IV.C.1**). Under local anesthesia, 15-cm, 20-gauge needles are inserted bilaterally just below the twelfth rib at the level of L1, then advanced cephalad and deep until they touch the anterolateral surface of the L1 vertebral body. The C-arm is turned to the lateral view, and then the needles are advanced anteriorly (i.e., down toward the table) until their tips lie 2 cm anterior to the vertebral body or aortic pulsations are felt (on the left). After a negative aspiration, 10 ml of 50% Renografin is injected to confirm position by demonstrating a periaortic shadow. Initial test dosage employs 25 ml/needle of 0.25% bupivacaine with epinephrine 1 : 200,000. Subsequent neurolysis can be accomplished with 25 ml/needle of 6% phenol or 50% alcohol. Complications include temporary postural hypotension and, if x-ray localization is not used, paresis or sphincter dysfunction from subarachnoid, epidural, or intrapsoas injection. Less likely are pneumothorax, bowel perforation, kidney trauma, and retroperitoneal hematoma.

C. Neurosurgical techniques range from implantation of permanent intraspinal or intraventricular catheters, to insertion of stimulating electrodes, to interference with a variety of pathways inaccessible to the anesthesiologist. Dorsal rhizotomy, dorsal root entry zone lesions, spinal tractotomy or cordotomy, and more cephalad lesions all have their supporters. Lesions or interruptions of still more cephalad tracts (e.g., cingulotomy) fall into the realm of psychosurgery, which may nonetheless be helpful in carefully selected cases. **Pi-**

tuitary destruction by any of several techniques (alcohol injection, radiofrequency probe, or transsphenoidal resection) results in prompt pain relief for several months to a year. Such pain relief is independent of the hormonal responsiveness of the tumor, although hormone-dependent tumors (e.g., breast or prostate) may indeed regress after this procedure. Mechanisms of this central analgesic effect are obscure, possibly involving endorphins.

Suggested Reading

Aronoff, G. M. (ed.) *Evaluation and Treatment of Pain.* Baltimore: Urban and Schwarzenberg, 1985.

Brena, S. V., and Chapman, S. L. (eds.). Chronic Pain: Management Principles. *Clinics in Anaesthesiology,* Vol. 3. Philadelphia: Saunders, 1985.

Cousins, M. J., and Bridenbaugh, P. O. (eds.). *Neural Blockade in Clinical Anesthesia and Management of Pain.* Philadelphia: Lippincott, 1980.

Cousins, M. J., and Mather, L. E. Intrathecal and epidural administration of opioids. *Anesthesiology* 61:276, 1984.

Foley, K. M., and Inturrisi, C. E. (eds.). Opioid analgesics in the management of clinical pain. In J. J. Bonica (ed.), *Advances in Pain Research and Therapy,* Vol. 8. New York: Raven, 1986.

Linson, M. A., Leffert, R., and Todd, D. P. The treatment of upper extremity reflex sympathetic dystrophy with prolonged continuous stellate ganglion blockade. *J. Hand Surg.* 8:153, 1983.

Simon, L. S., and Mills, J. A. Nonsteroidal antiinflammatory drugs. *N. Eng. J. Med.* 302:1179, 1980.

Stanton-Hicks, M., and Boas, R. A. (eds.). *Chronic Low Back Pain.* New York: Raven, 1982.

Sternbach, R. A. (ed.). *The Psychology of Pain.* New York: Raven, 1978.

Stoll, B. A., and Parbhoo, S. (eds.). *Bone Metastasis: Monitoring and Treatment.* New York: Raven, 1983.

Swerdlow, M. Anticonvulsants in the therapy of neuralgic pain. *The Pain Clin.* 1:9, 1986.

Wall, P. D., and Melzack, R. (eds.). *Textbook of Pain.* New York: Churchill Livingstone, 1984.

Willis, W. D. *The Pain System: The Neural Basis of Nociceptive Transmission in the Mammalian Nervous System.* New York: Karger, 1985.

Yaksh, T. L., and Hammond, D. L. Peripheral and central substances involved in the rostrad transmission of nociceptive information. *Pain* 13:1, 1982.

Drug Appendix

Glossary of Equivalent Drug Names

United States	United Kingdom
Acetaminophen	Paracetamol
Dibucaine	Cinchocaine
Echothiophate	Ecothiopate
Epinephrine	Adrenaline
Ergonovine	Ergometrine
Furosemide	Frusemide
Hydralazine	Hydrallazine
Isoproterenol	Isoprenaline
Lidocaine	Lignocaine
Meperidine	Pethidine
Methohexital	Methohexitone
Nitroglycerin	Nitroglycerine
Norepinephrine	Noradrenaline
Penicillin G	Benzyl penicillin
Pentobarbital	Pentobarbitone
Phenobarbital	Phenobarbitone
Scopolamine	Hyoscine
Secobarbital	Quinalbarbitone
Succinylcholine	Suxamethonium
Tetracaine	Amethocaine
Thiopental	Thiopentone
Trimethaphan	Trimetaphan

Table A-1. Commonly Used Drugs

W. Andrew Kofke and Leonard L. Firestone

Generic and trade names[a]	Uses	Dose[b]	Onset[c,d]	Duration[d]
Acetylcysteine (Mucomyst)	Viscous respiratory secretions	Inhaled via nebulizer: 2–5 ml of 5–20% solution q6–8h. Directly instilled into endotracheal tube or tracheostomy: 1–2 ml 10–20% solution q1–4h	Inhaled: 1 min	Inhaled: 4–8 hr
Aminophylline (theophylline ethylene diamine)	Bronchospasm CHF	IV: LD: 6.0 mg/kg at < 25 mg/min. MD: Young, healthy: 0.7 mg/kg/hr × 12h, then 0.5 mg/kg/hr. Old, healthy: 0.6 mg/kg/hr × 12h, then 0.3 mg/kg/hr. CHF, liver disease: 0.5 mg/kg/hr × 12 hr, then 0.1–0.2 mg/kg/hr. PR: 250–500 mg q8–24h (suppository or enema). PO: 100–250 mg q6–8h	IV: Rapid IM: 30–60 min PR: Suppository 2–4 hr; Enema 30–60 min PO: 1–4 hr	6–12 hr

Key to abbreviations:
@—at the rate of; μg—microgram; ACT—activated clotting time; AV—atrioventricular; BBB—blood-brain barrier; CHF—congestive heart failure; CNS—central nervous system; CO—cardiac output; D—day(s); U—units; VT—ventricular tachycardia; SL—sublingual; Dx—diagnosis; E—major excretion route of metabolites and unchanged drug; epi—epinephrine; ETT—endotracheal tube; GI—gastrointestinal; Hb—hemoglobin; h(hr)—hour(s); HR—heart rate; IM—intramuscular; IV—intravenous; K—thousand; kg—kilogram; LD—loading dose; LFT—liver function test; M—major sites of metabolism; M²—meter squared; MAOI—Monoamine oxidase inhibitor; MAP—mean arterial pressure; max—maximum; MD—maintenance dose; metHb—methemoglobin; mg—milligram; min—minute; ml—milliliter; mo—months old; ng—nanogram; NSS—normal saline solution; AH—atrial-His; PO—per os; PR—per rectum; prn—as needed or indicated; PT—prothrombin time; PTT—partial thromboplastin time; q—every; RBF—renal blood flow; s—second; SQ—subcutaneous; SVR—systemic vascular resistance; SVT—supraventricular tachycardia; $t_{1/2\alpha}$—redistribution half-life; tE—elimination half-life; TL—therapeutic level; VA—ventricular arrhythmia; VF—ventricular fibrillation; wo—weeks old; yo—years old; ~—approximately; ≅—approximately equivalent; >—greater than;

Half-Life[e]	Pharmacologic effects[f]	Comments[g]	Fate
tE 1.35 hr	Disruption of disulfide bonds with reduction of viscosity of pulmonary secretions and increase in mucociliary clearance	May cause bronchospasm, bronchial bleeding, nausea, or vomiting Inactivates some aerosolized antibiotics May damage rubber endotracheal tubes	M: Liver E: Liver, kidney
tE 3–10 hr	Inhibition of phosphodiesterase, resulting in bronchodilatation with positive inotropic and chronotropic effects	May cause tachyarrhythmias, CNS stimulation, GI upset, or diuresis IM injection painful Follow serum levels closely TL = 10–20 mg/L	M: Liver E: Kidney (10% unchanged)

≥—greater than or equal to; <—less than; ≤—less than or equal to.
[a]Does not include all brands of a given drug.
[b]Unless otherwise specified, dosages are those usually given to a 70-kg adult. Clinical situations may indicate higher or lower doses than those noted.
[c]Onset of clinically notable effect; not time to peak effect.
[d]May be altered with conditions that alter renal or hepatic metabolism or perfusion, or by conditions that affect metabolism or perfusion of the target organ(s).
[e]Depending on the mechanism of action of a drug and its solubility in the target organ(s), the distribution or elimination half-life may not coincide with the half-life for the biological effect.
[f]Includes only pharmacologic effects needed for a given clinical indication.
[g]Major side effects and noteworthy points only; i.e., some adverse effects and contraindications may not be mentioned.
[h]Duration of narcotics is affected by degree of pain, tolerance to the drug, other drugs concomitantly administered, and the patient's physical condition.
[i]Doses of CNS-depressant drugs are those usually given to healthy 70-kg patients and may vary with the patient's condition or concomitant drug intake. Older or debilitated patients may require smaller doses.

Table A-1 (continued)

Generic and trade names[a]	Uses	Dose[b]	Onset[c,d]	Duration[d]
Amiodarone (Cordarone)	Refractory or recurrent VT or VF	PO: 400 mg/day (maintenance)	2–21 days	> 24 hr
Amrinone (Inocor)	Management of acute ventricular failure	IV: 0.75 mg/kg bolus over several minutes, then infuse at 5–10 μg/kg/min to a maximum dose of 10 mg/kg/day. Infusion mixtures (100 mg in 250 ml) must not contain dextrose	10 min	Bolus: 0.5–2 hr Infusion: 3–4 hr
Atenolol (Tenormin)	Hypertension β_1-adrenergic receptor blockade	PO: 50–100 mg/day		> 24 hr
Atracurium (Tracrium)	Neuromuscular blockade	IV (intubation): 0.4–0.5 mg/kg Continuous IV infusion: 50 or 100 mg in 500 ml 5% D/W or NSS; 5–10 μg/kg/min titrated vs. train-of-four response	IV: 3–5 min	IV: 20–45 min
Atropine	Bradycardia Antisialagogue Decreasing GI motility	As adjunct to neostigmine and pyridostigmine reversal of neuromuscular	IV: Rapid IM/SQ/PO: 1–2 hr	IM/SQ/PO: 4 hr

Half-Life[e]	Pharmacologic effects[f]	Comments[g]	Fate
tE 20–100 days	Depresses the SA node and prolongs the PR, QRS, and QT intervals and produces α- and β-adrenergic blockade	May cause severe sinus bradycardia and AV block, liver and thyroid function test abnormalities, hepatitis, and cirrhosis Pulmonary fibrosis may follow long-term use Increases serum levels of digoxin, oral anticoagulants, diltiazem, quinidine, procainamide, and phenytoin	M: Liver E: Intestine
tE 3.5–6 hr	Increase in cardiac output from both inotropic and vasodilating effects	May cause thrombocytopenia	M: Liver E: Kidney, intestine
tE 6–7 hr	β_1-selective adrenergic receptor blockade	Relatively cardioselective High doses block β_2-adrenergic receptors; therefore contraindicated in CHF, asthma, and heart block	M: None E: Kidney, intestine
tE 20 min	Nondepolarizing competitive blockade of neuromuscular junction	No significant cardiovascular effects May cause histamine release with bolus dosage of > 0.6 mg/kg Duration is not prolonged in the presence of renal failure	M: Blood (Hofmann elimination and ester hydrolysis)
$t_{1/2\alpha}$ 1 min tE 2 hr	Competitive blockade of acetylcholine at muscarinic receptors	May cause tachyarrhythmias, AV dissociation, premature ventricular contractions, bradycardia (low dose),	M: Minimal E: Kidney (77–94%), liver

Table A-1 (continued)

Generic and trade names[a]	Uses	Dose[b]	Onset[c,d]	Duration[d]
		blockade: IV: 0.02–0.03 mg/kg As adjunct to edrophonium reversal of neuromuscular blockade: IV: 0.015 mg/kg For drying secretions: IV/IM/SQ/PO: 0.4–0.8 mg For bradycardia: IV: 0.4–1.0 mg *Pediatric* For preop. control of secretions: IV/IM/SQ/PO: 0.01 mg/kg/dose (< 0.4 mg) For bradycardia: IV: 0.01 mg/kg/dose (< 0.4 mg)		
Bicarbonate, sodium (NaHCO$_3$)	Metabolic acidosis Alkalinization of urine Hyperkalemia	For metabolic acidosis: IV: mEq NaHCO$_3$ = [base deficit × wt (kg) × 0.2–0.3] (subsequent doses titrated vs. patient's pH) Neonatal solution is 4.2% (~ 0.5 mEq/ml); adult solution is 8.4% (~ 1.0 mEq/ml) For alkalinization of urine: PO: LD: 4g MD: 1–2g q4h	IV: Rapid	IV: Variable
Butorphanol (Stadol)[h,i]	Pain Sedation	For perioperative analgesia (dosage individualized)[j]: IV: 0.5–2.0	IV: Rapid IM: 10–30 min	Variable

Half-Life[e]	Pharmacologic effects[f]	Comments[g]	Fate
		dry mouth, or urinary retention; crosses BBB and placenta	
	H^+ neutralization	May cause metabolic alkalosis, hypercarbia, or hyperosmolality Administration of hyperosmolar solution to neonates may cause intraventricular hemorrhage Central hypertonic bolus can cause transiently decreased CO, SVR, and myocardial contractility with hypotension and increased intracranial pressure Crosses placenta	M: Blood E: Lung (as CO_2), kidney
tE 2.5–3.5 hr	Analgesia CNS depression Narcotic antagonism	May cause hypotension, nausea, vomiting, dizziness, depression of respiration, increase in	M: Liver E: Kidney

Table A-1 (continued)

Generic and trade names[a]	Uses	Dose[b]	Onset[c,d]	Duration[d]
		mg (in increments) prn IM: 1.0–4.0 mg prn (2 mg ≅ 10 mg morphine)		
Bretylium (Bretylol)	VF VT	For immediately life-threatening VA: IV: 5–10 mg/kg q15–30 min prn to max 30 mg/kg (undiluted) For other VAs: LD: IV: 5–10 mg/kg in 50–100 ml 5% D/W over 10–20 min repeated once after 1–2 hr prn MD: IV: 5–10 mg/kg in 50–100 ml 5% D/W over 10–20 min q6h, or, preferably, as constant infusion, 1–2 mg/min IM: 5–10 mg/kg q6–8h (undiluted)	IV:minutes (VF) 2 min–2 hr (VT) IM: 15 min	IV: 6–24 hr IM: 10–24 hr
Calcium chloride ($CaCl_2$)	Hypocalcemia Hyperkalemia Hypermagnesemia Hypotension	(10% $CaCl_2$ = 1.36 mEq Ca^{2+}/ml = 27.2 mg Ca^{2+}/ml) For life-threatening hypocalcemia, hyperkalemia: IV: 5–10 mg/kg prn	Rapid	Variable
Calcium gluconate (Kalcinate)	Hypocalcemia Hyperkalemia	(10% calcium gluconate = 0.45 mEq Ca^{2+}/ml =	Rapid	Variable

Half-Life[e]	Pharmacologic effects[f]	Comments[g]	Fate
		biliary pressure, or narcotic withdrawal syndrome (in addicts) Higher incidence of sedation than with agonist narcotics Crosses placenta	
tE 5.5–10 hr	Initially, release of norepinephrine into circulation, followed by prevention of synaptic release of norepinephrine Supression of VF and VAs Increase in myocardial contractility (direct effect)	May cause initial hypertension and ectopy followed by decrease in SVR with hypotension (potentiated by quinidine or procainamide), aggravation of digoxin-induced arrhythmias, or drowsiness Muscle atrophy or necrosis with repeated IM injections (no more than 5 ml/IM site) Not a first-line drug for VAs	M: Minimal E: Kidney (mostly), liver (very small amount)
	Essential for maintenance of cell membrane integrity, muscular excitation-contraction coupling, glandular stimulation-secretion coupling, and enzyme function	May cause bradycardia or arrhythmia (esp. with digitalis) Irritating to veins	Protein bound Incorporated into muscle, bone, and other tissues
	See Calcium chloride	Ca^{2+} less available than with $CaCl_2$, due to binding to gluconate	See Calcium chloride

Table A-1 (continued)

Generic and trade names[a]	Uses	Dose[b]	Onset[c,d]	Duration[d]
	Hypermagnesemia Hypotension	9.0 mg Ca^{2+}/ml) For life-threatening hypocalcemia, hyperkalemia: IV: 15–30 mg/kg IV prn		
Captopril (Capoten)	Hypertension CHF	PO: 25–150 mg q8–12h	1 hr	8–12 hr
Chloral hydrate (Noctec, Somnos, Aquachloral)[i]	Insomnia Sedation	For sedation: PO/PR: 500–2000 mg	PO/PR: 15–60 min	PO/PR: 4–8 hr
Chlordiazepoxide (Librium)[i]	Sedation Ethanol withdrawal syndrome	(Dosage individualized) IM/IV: 5–100 mg q4–6h prn PO: 5–25 mg q6–12h	IV: 3–30 min IM: 15 min–several hr PO: 15 min–2 hr	IV: 0.5–4 hr IM: Variable PO: 4 hr
Chlorothiazide (Diuril)	Edema Hypertension	IV: 500–2000 mg/day in divided doses PO: 500–2000 mg/day in divided doses	IV: 15 min PO: 1–2 hr	IV: 2–4 hr PO: 6–12 hr
Chlorpromazine (Thorazine)[i]	Psychosis Agitation Nausea and vomiting Hiccoughs Sedation Prevention of shivering	(Dosage individualized) IV: 25–50 mg in 500–1000 ml NSS infused slowly (< 1 mg/min), or dilute to 1 mg/ml and give at 1 mg/min	IV: Rapid IM: 30 min PO: 30–60 min	IM: 3–4 hr PO: 4–6 hr

Half-Life[e]	Pharmacologic effects[f]	Comments[g]	Fate
		May cause bradycardia or arrhythmia (esp. with digitalis)	
Apparent tE: < 3 hr	Angiotensin I-converting enzyme inhibition decreases angiotensin II and aldosterone levels Reduces both preload and afterload in patients with CHF	May cause neutropenia and agranulocytosis	M: Liver E: Renal (50% unchanged)
tE (of trichloroethanol) 8–11 hr	CNS depression	May cause skin and mucous membrane irritation or GI upset Minimal respiratory or hemodynamic effect May potentiate oral anticoagulants Crosses placenta	M: Liver and RBC to trichloroethanol (active) E: Kidney (mostly), liver
$t_{1/2\alpha}$ 15–45 min tE 5–30 hr	CNS depression Anticonvulsant effect	May cause paradoxical CNS excitement, respiratory depression at high doses IM injection painful, with erratic absorption Frequent dosing may result in accumulation of active metabolites Crosses placenta	M: Liver (to several active metabolites) E: Kidney, liver
tE 1–2 hr Anephric: tE 2–5 hr	Increase in renal excretion of Na^+, Cl^-, K^+, Mg^{2+}, Br^-, I^-, H_2O, with decrease in excretion of Ca^{2+}	May cause electrolyte imbalance, dehydration, or glucose intolerance IM or SQ injection irritating Crosses placenta	M: Minimal E: Kidney, liver
tE 16–30 hr	Control of psychoses CNS depression Suppression of nausea and vomiting	May cause hypotension from α-adrenergic blockade and myocardial depression Weak anticholinergic effects, extrapyramidal reactions, cholestatic jaundice, or alteration of thermoregulation	M: Liver E: Liver, kidney

Table A-1 (continued)

Generic and trade names[a]	Uses	Dose[b]	Onset[c,d]	Duration[d]
		until desired effect, or 25 mg injected PO/IM: 10.0–50 mg q6–8 prn		
Cimetidine (Tagamet)	Reduction of gastric volume and raising of pH (pulmonary aspiration prophylaxis) Hiatus hernia Gastric acid hypersecretion Anaphylaxis	IV/IM/PO: 300 mg q6h (q12h in renal failure)	PO: 45–90 min	IV/IM: 4–5 hr PO: 4–5 hr
Clonidine (Catapres)	Hypertension	PO: 0.2–1.2 mg/day in divided doses (2.4 mg/day max dose)	PO: 30–60 min	PO: 8 hr
Dantrolene (Dantrium)	Malignant hyperthermia	Prophylactic preoperative or intraoperative treatment is generally not recommended If signs of the syndrome develop: 3 mg/kg IV bolus; if syndrome persists after 30 min, repeat dose, up to 10 mg/kg	IV: 30 min	
Dexamethasone (Hexadrol, Decadron)	See Hydrocortisone	(Significant variation in indications and doses among clinicians) For most non-life-threatening conditions:		

Half-Life[e]	Pharmacologic effects[f]	Comments[g]	Fate
		Crosses placenta	
tE 2 hr	Antagonism of histamine action on H_2 receptors, with inhibition of gastric acid secretion	May cause small increase in creatinine, increase in blood levels of concurrently administered propranolol or benzodiazepines, reduction in activity of some liver microsomal enzymes, potentiation of oral anticoagulants or somnolence	M: Liver E: Kidney (75%)
tE 12–20 hr Anephric: tE 25–37 hr	Central α-adrenergic stimulation, resulting in decrease in SVR and heart rate	Abrupt withdrawal may cause rebound hypertension May cause drowsiness, nightmares, restlessness, anxiety, or depression IV injection may cause transient peripheral α-adrenergic stimulation	M: Liver E: Kidney (80%), liver (20%)
tE 5 hr	Reduction of Ca^{2+} release from sarcoplasmic reticulum	May cause muscle weakness, GI upset, drowsiness, sedation, or abnormal liver function (chronically) Additive effect with neuromuscular blocking agents Tissue irritant	M: Liver E: Kidney
tE 4–5 hr	See Hydrocortisone Has 25 times the glucocorticoid potency of hydrocortisone Minimal mineralocorticoid effect	See Hydrocortisone	M: Liver (microsomes) E: Kidney, liver (15%)

Table A-1 (continued)

Generic and trade names[a]	Uses	Dose[b]	Onset[c,d]	Duration[d]

		IV/IM: 0.50–24 mg/day
		For cerebral edema:
		IV:
		  LD: 10 mg
		  MD: 4 mg q6h (tapered over 6 days)
		IM:
		  MD: 4 mg q6h (tapered over 6 days)
		For life-threatening conditions:
		IV: 1–6 mg/kg q2–6h prn *or*
		IV:
		  LD: 20 mg
		  MD: Infusion: 3 mg/kg/day		

Dextran 40 (Rheomacrodex)	Inhibition of platelet aggregation
	Volume expansion (controversial)
	Low flow states
		IV (10% solution):
		  LD: 100 ml over 30 min
		  MD: 10–15 ml/kg/day
			IV: Rapid	

Diazepam[i] (Valium)	Anxiety
	Agitation
	Convulsions
	Spasticity
	Sedation
	Barbiturate or ethanol withdrawal
		(Dosage individualized)
		Sedation:
		  IV: 0.03–0.10 mg/kg q4h or prn
		  PO: 0.05–0.15 mg/kg q6–12h prn
		Induction of general anesthesia:
		  IV: 0.1–0.5 mg/kg
		Seizures:
		  IV: 0.1 mg/kg, and titrate vs. response
			IV: Rapid
			IM: 15–30 min
			PO: 30–60 min
				IV: 15 min–3 hr

Half-Life[e]	Pharmacologic effects[f]	Comments[g]	Fate
By molecular wt: 14–18 K: 15 min 44–55 K: 7.5 hr > 55 K: several days	Immediate, short-lived plasma volume expansion Adsorption to RBC surface, resulting in prevention of RBC aggregation and decrease in blood viscosity Decrease in platelet adhesiveness	May cause volume overload, anaphylaxis, bleeding tendency, interference with blood matching, or false elevation of blood sugar Can cause renal failure, but this can be limited by keeping urine specific gravity < 1.030 Use in hypovolemia controversial	M: Minimal E: Kidney (unchanged)
tE 7–10 hr tE (active metabolites) 2–8 days	CNS depression Amnesia Increase in seizure threshold	May cause hypotension, idiosyncratic increase in anxiety, psychosis, mild respiratory depression (apnea occasionally), or thrombophlebitis Tissue irritant: IV injection painful; IM injection painful Frequent dosing may result in accumulation of active metabolites	M: Liver (to active metabolites—⅓ oxazepam) E: Kidney (70%)

Table A-1 (continued)

Generic and trade names[a]	Uses	Dose[b]	Onset[c,d]	Duration[d]

Digoxin (Lanoxin)	Heart failure
	Supraventricular tachyarrythmias
		IV/IM:
		  LD: 0.5–1.0 mg/day in divided doses
		  MD: 0.125–0.5 mg qd
		PO:
		  LD: 1–1.5 mg/day in divided doses
		  MD: 0.125–0.5 mg qd
		Pediatric
		  IV/IM: (divided doses)
		  LD: (2–10 yo) 15–35 µg/kg/day
		  LD: (2 wo–2 yo) 30–50 µg/kg/day
		  LD: (neonates) 15–30 µg/kg/day
		  MD: 20–30% of LD qd
		  PO:
		  LD: (2–10 yo) 20–40 µg/kg/day
		  LD: (1 mo–2 yo) 35–60 µg/kg/day
		  LD: (neonates) 20–35 µg/kg/day
		  MD: 20–30% of LD qd
			IV: 15–30 min
			IM: 30 min
			PO: 1–2 hr
				IV/IM/PO: 2–6 days

Diltiazem (Cardizem)	Chronic angina pectoris Variant angina from coronary artery spasm	PO: 30–60 mg q6h	1–3 hr	
Diphenhydramine (Benadryl)[i]	Allergic reactions Drug-induced extrapyramidal reactions Sedation	IV/IM: 10–50 mg q6–8h PO: 25–50 mg q6–8h *Pediatric* IV/IM/PO: 5.0 mg/kg/day in 4 divided doses (max 300 mg)	IV: Rapid PO: 15–30 min	IV: 4–6 hr PO: 3–6 hr

Half-Life[e]	Pharmacologic effects[f]	Comments[g]	Fate
tE 42 hr Anephric: tE 108 hr	Increase in myocardial contractility Decrease in conduction in AV node and Purkinje fibers	May cause arrythmias, ECG changes, GI upset, or blurred vision Toxicity potentiated by hypokalemia, hypomagnesemia, hypercalcemia Cautious use in Wolff-Parkinson-White syndrome IM injection painful Concurrent quinidine use increases tE TL = 1–2 ng/ml	M: Minimal E: Kidney (60–90%); dosage lower with renal failure
tE 4 hr	Calcium channel blocker which slows conduction through SA and AV nodes, dilates coronary and peripheral arterioles, and reduces myocardial contractility	Bradycardia and heart block May interact with β-blockers to seriously impair contractility	M: Liver E: Kidney
tE 3–7 hr	Antagonism of histamine action on H_1 receptors Anticholinergic effect CNS depression	May cause hypotension (IV), tachycardia, dizziness, or seizures	M: Liver E: Kidney

Table A-1 (continued)

Generic and trade names[a]	Uses	Dose[b]	Onset[c,d]	Duration[d]
Dobutamine (Dobutrex)	Heart failure	Infusion mix: 250 mg in 250–1000 ml 5% D/W IV: Infusion at 2.5–15 µg/kg/min titrated vs. patient response	IV: 2 min	IV: 10 min
Dopamine (Intropin)	Hypotension Oliguria	Infusion mix: 200–800 mg in 250 ml 5% D/W For hypotension: IV: Infusion at 2–30 µg/kg/min titrated vs. patient response For oliguria: IV: Infusion at 1–2 µg/kg/min	IV: 5 min	IV: 10 min
Droperidol (Inapsine)[i]	Nausea, vomiting Agitation Sedation Adjunct to neurolept-anesthesia	(Dosage individualized) IV: 1.25–10 mg prn IM: 2.5–10 mg prn	IV/IM: 5–8 min	IV/IM: 3–6 hr
Edrophonium (Tensilon)	Supraventricular tachycardia Diagnosis of myasthenia gravis Reversal of neuromuscular blockade	For reversal of neuromuscular blockade: IV: 0.5–1.0 mg/kg (cautiously with atropine) For supraventricular tachycardia: IV: 10 mg	Neuromuscular block reversal: IV: 1–5 min Other uses: IV: 30–60 sec IM: 2–10 min	Neuromuscular block reversal: IV: 1.1 hr Other uses: IV: 5–10 min IM: 5–30 min
Ephedrine	Hypotension	IV/SQ/IM: 5–50 mg q3–4h prn	IV: Rapid	IV: 1 hr

Half-Life[e]	Pharmacologic effects[f]	Comments[g]	Fate
tE 2 min	β-adrenergic stimulation	May cause hypertension, arrhythmias, or myocardial ischemia Can increase ventricular rate in atrial fibrillation	M: Liver, nerve endings E: Kidney, liver
tE 2 min	Dopaminergic, β-, and α-adrenergic stimulation	May cause hypertension, arrhythmias, or myocardial ischemia Primarily dopaminergic effects (increased RBF) at 1–5 μg/kg/min Primarily α- and β-adrenergic effects at ≥ 15 μg/kg/min	M: Kidney, liver, nerve endings (partly to norepinephrine) E: Kidney
	Psychic indifference to environment Antipsychotic effect Antiemetic effect	May cause inner anxiety, extrapyramidal reactions, or hypotension (from moderate α-adrenergic and dopaminergic antagonism) Residual effects may persist ≥ 24 hr	M: Liver E: Kidney, liver (10% unchanged)
$t_{1/2\alpha}$ 7.2 min tE 1.8 hr	Cholinesterase inhibition	See Neostigmine	
tE 3–6 hr	α- and β-adrenergic stimulation Induction of norepinephrine release at nerve endings	May cause hypertension, arrhythmias, myocardial ischemia, CNS stimulation, decrease in uterine activity or mild bronchodilatation Minimal effect on uterine blood flow	M: Liver E: Kidney (60–75% unchanged)

Table A-1 (continued)

Generic and trade names[a]	Uses	Dose[b]	Onset[c,d]	Duration[d]
Ephinephrine (Adrenalin)	Heart failure Hypotension Broncho-spasm Anaphylaxis Cardiac arrest Topically and by infiltration for hemostasis	Infusion mix: 1 mg in 250 ml 5% D/W IV: Infusion initially at 0.5 μg/min, then titrated vs. patient response SQ/IM: 1 : 1000 soln (1.0 mg/ml), 0.1–0.5 ml q10–15 min × 3 prn For cardiac arrest: IV or intracardiac: 1–10 ml of 1 : 10,000 solution (0.1 mg/ml) *Pediatric* IV (for cardiac arrest): 1 : 10,000 solution, 0.1 ml/kg SQ/IM: 1 : 1000 solution, 0.01 ml/kg/dose q15 min × 3 prn	IV: Rapid SQ: 3–5 min	IV: 10 min
Epinephrine, racemic (Vaponefrin)	Broncho-spasm Airway edema	Inhaled via nebulizer: 0.5 ml of 2.25% solution in 2.5–3.5 ml NSS q 1–4h prn *Pediatric* Inhaled via nebulizer: 0.5 ml of 2.25% solution in 2.5–3.5 ml NSS q4h prn	Inhaled: 1–5 min	Inhaled: 2–3 hr
Ergonovine (Ergotrate)	Postpartum hemorrhage	For postpartum hemorrhage: IV: 0.2 mg in 5 ml NSS over ≥ 1 min (emergency) IM: 0.2 mg q2–4h prn for ≤ 5 doses, then PO: 0.2–0.4 mg q6–12h × 2 days or prn	IV: Rapid IM: 2–5 min PO: 5–15 min	IM: 3 hr PO: 3 hr

Half-Life[e]	Pharmacologic effects[f]	Comments[g]	Fate
	α- and β-adrenergic stimulation	May cause hypertension, arrhythmias, or myocardial ischemia With local anesthesia, causes vasoconstriction Crosses placenta	M: Liver, nerve endings E: Kidney, liver (10%)
	See Epinephrine Mucosal vasoconstriction	See Epinephrine	See Epinephrine
	Constriction of uterine and vascular smooth muscle	May cause hypertension from systemic vasoconstriction (especially in eclampsia and hypertension), arrhythmias, coronary spasm, uterine tetany, or GI upset	M: Probably liver

Table A-1 (continued)

Generic and trade names[a]	Uses	Dose[b]	Onset[c,d]	Duration[d]
Ethacrynic acid (Edecrin)	Edema Hypercalcemia Hypertension	(Dosage individualized) IV: 0.5–1.0 mg/kg dose PO: 50–100 mg q12–24h	IV: 15 min PO: 30 min	IV: 2–3 hr PO: 6–8 hr
Etomidate (Amidate, Hypnomidate)	Induction of general anesthesia	IV: 0.3–0.4 mg/kg	30–60 sec	3–5 min (redistribution)
Fentanyl (Sublimaze)[h,i]	Pain Induction of general anesthesia	For perioperative analgesia (dose individualized): IV: 10–100 µg (in increments) prn IM: 50–100 µg prn For cardiac anesthesia: IV: up to 50–100 µg/kg (in increments) titrated vs. patient response (100 µg ≅ 10 mg morphine)	IV: 2 min IM: 7–15 min	IV: variable IM: variable
Fluorescein (Fluorescite)	Assess tissue perfusion	IV: 10 mg/kg rapidly	IV: Rapid	IV: several hours
Flurazepam (Dalmane)[i]	Insomnia Sedation	PO: 15–30 mg at bedtime	PO: 15–45 min	PO: 7–8 hr
Furosemide (Lasix)	Edema Hypercalcemia Hypertension Intracranial hypertension	(Dosage individualized) IV/IM: 10–40 mg (initial dose) PO: 20–200 mg/day	IV: 2–10 min IM: 5–30 min PO: 30–60 min	IV: 2 hr PO: 6–8 hr

Half-Life[e]	Pharmacologic effects[f]	Comments[g]	Fate
tE 30–70 min	See Furosemide	See Furosemide Tissue irritant May potentiate oral anticoagulants	M: Liver E: Liver (30–40%), kidney (30–65%)
tE: 1–5 hr	Hypnosis without analgesia	Minimal cardiovascular effects and histamine release Significant myoclonic muscle movements and pain on IV injection	M: Liver, plasma esterases
$t_{1/2\alpha}$ 1–2 min tE 4 hr	Similar to those of morphine	Similar to those of morphine Chest wall rigidity more frequent than with morphine Accumulation with frequent dosing	M: Liver E: Kidney (10–20% unchanged)
tE 28 min (rabbits)	Uptake by viable cells only	May cause nausea, vomiting, false hemoglobin elevation, or hypersensitivity reactions (with slow infusion) Minimal cardiovascular effect	M: Minimal E: Kidney, liver
Two active metabolites with tE 2–4 hr and 47–100 hr	CNS depression	May cause idiosyncratic excitement, abnormal liver function, nausea, vomiting	M: Liver E: Kidney
tE 1 hr Anephric: 3 hr	Increase in excretion of Na^+, Cl^-, K^+, PO_4^{-3}, Ca^{+2}, and H_2O	May cause electrolyte imbalance, dehydration, deafness, hyperglycemia, or hyperuricemia	M: Minimal E: Liver, kidney (mostly)

Table A-1 (continued)

Generic and trade names[a]	Uses	Dose[b]	Onset[c,d]	Duration[d]
Gallamine (Flaxedil)	Neuromuscular blockade Bradycardia	For neuromuscular blockade (intubation) IV: 3–4 mg/kg For bradycardia (with preexisting blockade): IV: 10–20 mg	IV: 1–2 min	IV: 15–20 min
Glucagon	Duodenal or choledochal relaxation	IV/IM/SQ: 0.5–1.0 U/dose; repeat in 20 min prn	IV: 5–20 min	IV: 10–30 min
Glycopyrrolate (Robinul)	Bradycardia Decreasing GI motility Antisialagogue	As adjunct to neostigmine and pyridostigmine reversal of neuromuscular blockade: IV: 0.01–0.02 mg/kg For drying secretions: IV/IM/SQ: 0.1–0.2 mg PO: 1–2 mg For bradycardia: IV: 0.1–0.2 mg/dose	IV: 1–4 min IM/SQ: 20–40 min PO: 1 hr	IV: 2–4 hr IM/SQ: 4–6 hr PO: 6 hr
Haloperidol (Haldol)[i]	Psychosis Agitation	(Dosage individualized) IV: 1–2 mg prn IM: 2–5 mg q1–8h prn PO: 0.5–5.0 mg q8h prn	IV: 10–15 min IM: 10 min PO: 1–2 hr	≤ 3 days
Heparin (Lipo-Hepin, Liquaemin Sodium, Panheprin)	Anticoagulation	For thromboembolism: IV: LD: 5000 U MD: 1000 U/hr or 5000–10,000 U q4–6h SQ: MD: 8000–10,000 U q8h (preferably), or 15,000–20,000 U q12h Titrate vs. PTT or ACT	IV: immediate SQ: 1–4 hr	IV: 2–6 hr SQ: 12–16 hr

Half-Life[e]	Pharmacologic effects[f]	Comments[g]	Fate
$t_{1/2\alpha}$ 5 min tE 2.5 hr	Nondepolarizing competitive blockade of neuromuscular junction	May cause tachycardia and hypertension from indirect sympathomimetic and positive inotropic effects Dialyzable Crosses placenta	M: Minimal E: Kidney
tE 5 min	GI tract relaxation	May cause anaphylaxis, nausea, vomiting, hyperglycemia, or positive inotropic and chonotropic effects High doses potentiate oral anticoagulants	M: Liver
	See Atropine	See Atropine Does not cross BBB or placenta	M: Probably minimal E: Probably kidney
tE 13–36 hr	Blockade of central effects of dopamine with antipsychotic effects CNS depression	May cause extrapyramidal reactions or very mild α-adrenergic antagonism Antiemetic effect	M: Liver E: Liver, kidney
tE 1–2 hr	Blockade of conversion of prothrombin and activation of other coagulation factors Decrease in platelet agglutination	May cause bleeding, acute reversible thrombocytopenia, allergic reactions, or diuresis (36–48 hr after a large dose) Half-life increased in renal failure and decreased in thromboembolism and liver disease Does not cross placenta	M: Liver E: Kidney

Table A-1 (continued)

Generic and trade names[a]	Uses	Dose[b]	Onset[c,d]	Duration[d]
		For cardiopulmonary bypass: IV: LD: 300 U/kg MD: 100 U/kg/hr Titrate MD vs. ACT or heparin level		
Hydralazine (Apresoline)	Hypertension	(Dosage individualized) IV: 2.5–20 mg q4–6h or prn IM: 20–40 mg q4–6h or prn PO: 10–50 mg q6h prn	IV: 2.5–20 min IM: 10–30 min PO: 20–30 min	IV: 2–6 hr IM: 2–6 hr PO: 2–6 hr
Hydrocortisone (Solu-Cortef)	Adrenal insufficiency Inflammation and allergy Septic shock CNS trauma	(Significant variation in doses and indications among clinicians) For non-life-threatening conditions: IV/IM: 100–500 mg q2–10h prn For life-threatening conditions: IV: 50 mg/kg over several minutes q4–24h not longer than 2–3 days)		
Hydroxyzine (Vistaril, Atarax)[i]	Anxiety Nausea and vomiting Allergies Sedation	IM: 25–100 mg q4–6h PO: 25–100 mg q6–8h	PO: 15–20 min	PO: 4–6 hr
Indigo carmine	Evaluation of urine output Localization of ureteral orifices during cystoscopy	IV: 40 mg slowly IM: 50–100 mg	IV/IM: 10–30 min	IV/IM: Several hours

Half-Life[e]	Pharmacologic effects[f]	Comments[g]	Fate
tE 2–4 hr	Relaxation of vascular smooth muscle (arteriole > venule)	May cause hypotension, reflex tachycardia, SLE syndrome, or Coombs'-positive hemolytic anemia Increases coronary, splanchnic, cerebral, and renal blood flows	M: Liver E: Kidney
tE 1–1.5 hr	Stimulation of gluconeogenesis Inhibition of peripheral protein synthesis Membrane stabilizing effect Anti-inflammatory and antiallergic effect Mineralocorticoid effect	May cause adrenocortical atrophy (Addison's crisis with abrupt withdrawal), delayed wound healing, CNS disturbances, osteoporosis, or electrolyte disturbances	M: Liver (reductase) E: Kidney
tE 3 hr	Antagonism of histamine action on H_1 receptors CNS depression Antiemetic effect	May cause dry mouth Minimal cardiorespiratory depression IV injection may cause thrombosis Arterial injection may cause gangrene Crosses placenta	M: Liver E: Liver, kidney
tE 5 hr		Hypertension from adrenergic stimulation (for about 15–30 min after IV dose)	M: Minimal E: Kidney

Table A-1 (continued)

Generic and trade names[a]	Uses	Dose[b]	Onset[c,d]	Duration[d]
Indocyanine green (Cardio-Green)	Cardiac output measurement by indicator dilution	IV (diluted in 1 ml): 5 mg rapidly injected into central circulation		
Insulin	Hyperglycemia Hyperkalemia	For hyperglycemia (dosage highly individualized): SQ: Usually 5–10 U prn (regular insulin) For uncontrolled diabetes: IV: LD: 10–20 U (regular insulin) MD: 0.1–0.2 U/kg/hr (regular insulin)	SQ: Regular: 15 min Semilente: 30 min Globin: 2–3 hr NPH: 3 hr Lente: 3 hr PZI: 3–4 hr Ultralente: 3–4 hr	SQ: Regular: 6–8hr Semilente: 12–16 hr Globin: 12–18 hr NPH: 18–24 hr Lente: 18–28 hr PZI: 24–36 hr Ultralente: 30–36 hr
Isoetharine (Bronkosol, Bronkometer)	Bronchospasm	Inhaled (aerosol or IPPB): 0.25–0.5 ml of 0.5–1.0% solution diluted in 1.5–2.5 ml NSS given over 15–30 min q4h prn Inhaled (metered nebulizer [Bronkometer]): 1–2 puffs (0.34 mg/puff) with 1 min between puffs q4h prn	Inhaled: 5 min	Inhaled: 1–4 hr
Isoproterenol (Isuprel)	Heart failure Heart block Bronchospasm Pulmonary hypertension	Infusion mix: 1 mg in 250 ml 5% D/W IV: Infusion initially at 1 µg/min, then titrated vs.	IV: rapid Inhaled: 2–5 min	IV: 1–2 min Inhaled: 1–3 hr

Half-Life[e]	Pharmacologic effects[f]	Comments[g]	Fate
tE 3–4 min (increased in liver disease)	Almost complete binding to plasma protein, with distribution within plasma volume	May cause allergic reactions or transient increase in bilirubin Absorption spectra changed by heparin Cautious use with iodine allergy (contains 5% NaI)	M: Minimal E: Liver
IV: (Regular) 5–15 min (increased in renal failure)	Facilitation of glucose transport into cells Shift of K^+ and Mg^{2+} into cells	May cause hypoglycemia, allergic reactions, or synthesis of insulin antibodies	M: Liver E: Kidney ($< 10\%$)
	β-adrenergic stimulation (β_2, β_1), resulting in bronchodilatation	May cause tachycardia, hypertension, peripheral vascular vasodilatation, CNS stimulation, or bronchial irritation Tachyphylaxis and paradoxic bronchospasm can occur with excessive use	M: Lung, liver E: Kidney (10% unchanged)
$t_{1/2\alpha}$ 2.5–5 min	β-adrenergic stimulation	May cause arrhythmias, myocardial ischemia, hypertension, or CNS excitement Tachyphylaxis after repeated inhaled doses	M: Liver, nerve endings E: Kidney, liver

Table A-1 (continued)

Generic and trade names[a]	Uses	Dose[b]	Onset[c,d]	Duration[d]
	β-Blocker overdose	patient response Inhaled (aerosol or IPPB): 0.5 ml of 0.5% solution in 1.5–2.5 ml NSS over 15–20 min q5h prn Inhaled (metered nebulizer): 1–2 puffs (0.13 mg/puff) with 2–5 min between puffs q4h prn		
Ketamine (Ketalar, Ketaject)[i]	Induction of general anesthesia	IV: LD: 1–3 mg/kg as 1% solution MD: ⅓–½ LD prn (usually q5–30 min) IM: LD: 5–10 mg/kg as 5%–10% solution	IV: rapid IM: 3–5 min	IV: 5–10 min IM: 10–20 min
Labetalol (Normodyne, Trandate)	Hypertension (including hypertensive crisis) Combined α- and β-adrenergic blockade during induced hypotension	IV: 5–10 mg increments at 10-min intervals, to a dose of 40–80 mg Infusion at 2 mg/min, up to 300 mg (hypertensive crisis) PO: 200–400 mg q12h	IV: 5 min PO: 1–2 hr	IV: 2–12 hr PO: 6–8 hr

Half-Life[e]	Pharmacologic effects[f]	Comments[g]	Fate
$t_{1/2\alpha}$ 10–18 min tE 2.5 hr	Somatic analgesia with poor visceral analgesia Block of cerebral association pathways	Usually preserves and exaggerates airway reflexes May cause transient, modest hypertension and tachycardia (possibly potentiated by atropine), regurgitation (rarely, aspiration can occur), salivation (needs an antisialagogue), lacrimation, diaphoresis, increase in intraocular pressure, bronchodilatation, or dreams and hallucinations on emergence (treat with a benzodiazepine) Can increase cerebral blood flow, cerebral metabolic rate, intracranial pressure Crosses placenta	M: Liver E: Kidney, liver
IV: tE 2–4 hr PO: $t_{1/2\alpha}$ 3–8 hr	Selective α_1-adrenergic blockade with nonselective β-adrenergic blockade	May cause bradycardia, AV conduction delays, bronchospasm in asthmatics, and postural hypotension	M: Liver E: Kidney, liver

Table A-1 (continued)

Generic and trade names[a]	Uses	Dose[b]	Onset[c,d]	Duration[d]

Lidocaine (Xylocaine)	VAs
	Local anesthesia
	Adjunct to general anesthesia
	Intracranial hypertension
	Cough suppression
		For arrhythmias:
		IV:
		  LD: 1 mg/kg × 2 (2nd dose 20–30 min after 1st dose)
		  MD: 15–50 μg/kg/min
		IM: 4 mg/kg
			IV: 10–90 sec
			IM: 5–30 min
				IV: 5–20 min
				1–2 hr

Lorazepam (Ativan)[i]	Anxiety Sedation	(Dosage individualized) IV/IM: 1–4 mg (0.05 mg/kg) prn PO: 1–10 mg/day in divided doses	IV: 5–20 min IM: 0.5–2 hr PO: 1–2 hr	IV: 4–6 hr IM: 8 hr PO: 8 hr
Mannitol (Osmitrol)	Intracranial hypertension Neurosurgery Prophylaxis of renal failure Glaucoma Diuresis	IV: 0.25–1.0 g/kg as 20% solution over 30–60 min (in acute situation can give bolus of 12.5–25.0 gm over 5–10 min)	IV: 15 min	IV: 2–3 hr
Meperidine (Pethidine, Demerol)[h,i]	Pain Sedation	For perioperative analgesia (dose individualized): IV: 0.5–1.0 mg/kg (in increments) prn IM/SQ: 0.5–1.0 mg/kg prn PO: 1 mg/kg prn (usually q2–4h) (100 mg ≅ 10 mg morphine)	IV: 5 min IM/SQ: 10 min PO: 15 min	Variable
Metaproterenol (Alupent, Orciprenaline)	Bronchospasm	Inhaled (metered aerosol): 2–3 puffs (0.65 mg/puff) q3–4h prn (max 12 puffs/day) Inhaled (IPPB): 0.2–0.3 ml of 5% solution	Inhaled: 2–10 min PO: 15–30 min	Inhaled: 1–5 hr PO: 4 hr

Half-Life[e]	Pharmacologic effects[f]	Comments[g]	Fate
$t_{1/2\alpha}$ 1 min tE 1.5 hr	Antiarrhythmic effect Sedation Neural blockade	May cause dizziness, seizures, disorientation, heart block (with myocardial conduction defect), or hypotension Crosses placenta TL = 1–5 mg/L	M: Liver E: Kidney (10% unchanged)
tE 14 hr	CNS depression Amnesia (dose dependent)	May cause paradoxical CNS excitement or very mild respiratory depression Minimal cardiovascular depression Crosses placenta	M: Liver E: Kidney
tE 1.7 hr	Increase in serum osmolality, resulting in decrease in brain size and amount of intraocular fluid, osmotic diuresis, and transient expansion of intravascular volume	Rapid administration may cause vasodilation and hypotension May worsen or cause pulmonary edema, intracranial hemorrhage, systemic hypertension, or rebound intracranial hypertension	M: Minimal E: Kidney (80% unchanged)
tE 1.5–4 hr	Similar to those of morphine Mild vagolytic effect	Similar to those of morphine May cause tachycardia Mild negative inotropic effect Metabolic products can cause CNS excitement in high doses Avoid concurrent (within 2 wk) use of monoamine oxidase inhibitors Crosses placenta	M: Liver E: Kidney
tE 6 hr	β-adrenergic stimulation (mostly β_2), resulting in bronchodilatation	May cause arrhythmias, hypertension, CNS stimulation, nausea, vomiting, or inhibition of uterine contractions Tachyphylaxis can occur	M: Liver E: Liver (13%), kidney (79%)

Table A-1 (continued)

Generic and trade names[a]	Uses	Dose[b]	Onset[c,d]	Duration[d]
		in 2.5 ml NSS q4h PO: 20 mg q6–8h		
Methadone (Dolophine, Westa-done)[h,i]	Pain	For perioperative analgesia (dose individ-ualized): IV: 2.5–10 mg (in incre-ments) prn IM/SQ: 2.5–10 mg prn PO: 2.5–10 mg prn (usually q3–4 h) (10 mg ≅ 10 mg mor-phine)	PO: 30–60 min	Variable
Methohexital (Brevital)[i]	Induction of general anesthesia	IV: 1–2 mg/kg (1% solution) *Pediatric* PR: 20–30 mg/kg (10% solu-tion)	IV: Rapid PR: 7 min	IV: 5–10 min PR: 45 min
Methyldopa (Aldomet)	Hyperten-sion	IV: 250–1000 mg in 100 ml 5% D/W over 30–60 min q6h prn (max 1 gm q6h) PO: 250 mg q6–12h × 48 hr, then titrated vs. patient response (max 3 gm/day)	IV: 1–2 hr PO: 4–6 hr	IV: 10–16 hr PO: 24 hr
Methylene blue (me-thylthio-nine chlo-ride, Urolene Blue)	Urinary tract diag-nostic aid Methemo-globinemia	For methemoglo-binemia: IV: 1–2 mg/kg as 1% solu-tion over 10 min, and re-peat in 1 hr prn For diagnostic aid: PO: 65–130 mg q8–12h		
Methylergo-novine (Mether-gine)	Postpartum hemor-rhage	IV: 0.2 mg in 5 ml NSS/dose over ≥ 1 min (emergency) IM: 0.2 mg q2–4h	IV: 1 min IM: 2–5 min PO: 5–10 min	IV/IM: Several hours

Half-Life[e]	Pharmacologic effects[f]	Comments[g]	Fate
tE 15–30 hr	Similar to those of morphine Low incidence of sedation at lower doses	Similar to those of morphine Cumulative effects with frequently repeated doses	M: Liver E: Liver, kidney
tE 1–2 hr	CNS depression	May cause hiccoughs, respiratory depression, mild cardiovascular depression, muscle tremors, or pain along injection site	M: Liver E: Liver, kidney
tE 2 hr Anephric: tE > 4 hr	May be a false neurotransmitter, resulting in decrease in mean arterial pressure without increase in heart rate or change in CO	May cause sedation, psychosis, depression, hypotension, liver damage, or Coombs'-positive hemolytic anemia	M: Liver E: Kidney
	Low dose promotes $MetHb \rightarrow Hb$ High dose promotes $Hb \rightarrow MetHb$	May cause RBC destruction (prolonged use), hypertension, bladder irritation, nausea, diaphoresis May inhibit nitrate-induced coronary artery relaxation	M: Tissues E: Liver, kidney (75% unchanged)
$t_{1/2\alpha}$ 1.5–2 min tE 20–44 min	See Ergonovine	See Ergonovine Hypertensive response less marked than with ergonovine	M: Probably liver

Table A-1 (continued)

Generic and trade names[a]	Uses	Dose[b]	Onset[c,d]	Duration[d]
		prn (≤ 5 doses) PO (after IM or IV doses): 0.2–0.4 mg q6–12h × 2–7 days		
Methyl-predniso-lone (Solu-Medrol)	See Hydro-cortisone	(Significant variation in doses and indications among clinicians) For non-life-threatening conditions: IV/IM: 10–250 mg q4–24h (IV given over 1 min) For life-threatening conditions: IV: 100–250 mg q2–6h *or* 30 mg/kg q4–6h for 24–48 hr (given over 15 min) prn		
Metoclo-pramide (Reglan)	Gastro-esophageal reflux Premedica-tion for patients with a hiatus hernia (pulmo-nary aspiration prophylaxis) Antiemetic	IV/IM: 10 mg PO: 10–15 mg q6h	IV: 1–3 min IM: 10–15 min PO: 30–60 min	PO/IV/IM: 1–2 hr
Metocurine (Metubine)	Neuromus-cular blockade	IV (intubation): 0.3–0.4 mg/kg	IV: 2–4 min	IV: 25–90 min
Metoprolol (Lopressor)	Hyperten-sion Angina pectoris	PO: 50–100 mg q6–12h	PO: 15 min	PO: 6 hr

Half-Life[e]	Pharmacologic effects[f]	Comments[g]	Fate
tE 3–4 hr	See Hydrocortisone; 5 times glucocorticoid and 0.5 times mineralocorticoid potency of hydrocortisone	See Hydrocortisone	M: Liver (microsomes) E: Kidney
PO: tE 2–6 hr	Increases gastric and small intestinal motility (which improves emptying) and lower esophageal sphincter tone	Rarely may produce extrapyramidal reactions	M: Liver E: Kidney
tE 6 hr Anephric: 11.4 hr	Nondepolarizing competitive blockade of the neuromuscular junction	Large bolus can cause hypotension Small amount of histamine liberation	M: Minimal E: Kidney, liver (slight)
tE 3–4 hr	β_1-Adrenergic antagonism (β_2-adrenergic antagonism in high doses)	May cause bradycardia, clinically significant bronchoconstriction (when doses > 100 mg/day), dizziness, fatigue, insomnia Crosses placenta and BBB	M: Liver E: Kidney

Table A-1 (continued)

Generic and trade names[a]	Uses	Dose[b]	Onset[c,d]	Duration[d]
Midazolam (Versed[i])	Sedation Hypnotic adjunct to balanced anesthesia Induction of general anesthesia	IV (sedation): 0.07–0.08 mg/kg in 1–2-mg increments (induction): 0.25–0.35 mg/kg IM (sedation): 0.07–0.08 mg/kg	IV: 1–3 min IM: 15–30 min	IV: 2–6 hr (induction dose) IM: 1–2 hr
Morphine[h,i]	Pain Sedation	For perioperative analgesia (dose individualized): IV: 0.1 mg/kg (in increments) prn IM: 0.1 mg/kg prn For cardiac anesthesia: IV: up to 1 mg/kg (in increments) titrated vs. patient response Epidural: 2–5 mg (preservative-free solution only) Intrathecal: 0.2–1 mg (preservative-free solution only)	IV: 5–10 min IM: 30–60 min SQ: 30–90 min Epidural: 20–30 min Intrathecal: 10 min	Variable
Nadolol (Corgard)	Angina pectoris Hypertension	PO: 40–320 mg/day		> 24 hr
Nalbuphine (Nubain)[h,i]	Pain Sedation	For perioperative analgesia (dose individualized): IV: 0.14 mg/kg (in increments) prn IM/SQ: 0.14 mg/kg prn (10 mg ≅ 10 mg morphine)	IV: 2–3 min IM/SQ: 15 min	Variable

Half-Life[e]	Pharmacologic effects[f]	Comments[g]	Fate
tE 1–4 hr	CNS depression Amnesia Increases seizure threshold	Water-soluble, so uptake is predictable and IV injection is painless when administered IM Doses should be reduced by 25% in the elderly, and when used in combination with narcotics Cimetidine increases plasma levels	M: Liver E: Kidney
tE 2–4 hr	Analgesia CNS depression Euphoria	May cause respiratory depression, bronchospasm (rare), chest wall rigidity, bradycardia, hypotension, nausea, vomiting, dysphoria, diaphoresis, allergic reactions, histamine release, increase in biliary pressure or decrease in GI and GU motility With epidural use, pruritus is common and delayed respiratory depression may occur Crosses placenta	M: Liver E: Kidney
tE 20–24 hr	Nonselective β-adrenergic blockade	May cause severe bronchospasm	E: Kidney (unchanged)
tE 5 hr	Similar to those of butorphanol	Similar to those for butorphanol	M: Liver E: Kidney

Table A-1 (continued)

Generic and trade names[a]	Uses	Dose[b]	Onset[c,d]	Duration[d]
Naloxone (Narcan)	Reversal of narcotic effects	For postoperative narcosis: IV: 0.1–0.4 mg doses titrated vs. patient response q2–3 min *Pediatric* For postoperative narcosis: IV: 1–10 µg/kg (in increments) q2–3 min (up to 0.4 mg) titrated vs. patient response	IV: 1–2 min IM/SQ: 2–5 min	IV: 1 hr IM/SQ: 1–4 hr
Neostigmine (Prostigmin)	Reversal of neuromuscular blockade Myasthenia gravis	For reversal of neuromuscular blockade: IV: 0.06–0.07 mg/kg (cautiously with an anticholinergic agent)	IV: 1–5 min IM/SQ: 10–30 min	IV: 2.5–4 hr
Nifedipine (Procardia)	Coronary artery spasm Myocardial ischemia	PO: 10–30 mg TID	PO: 15–20 min	
Nitrite, sodium	Cyanide poisoning	IV: 300 mg (10 ml of 3% solution) at 2.5–5 ml/min *Pediatric* IV: 6 mg/kg (0.2 ml/kg) (≤ 300 mg) slowly (Adult and pediatric administration: repeat ½ dose 2–48 hr later prn); Give with sodium thiosulfate		

Half-Life[e]	Pharmacologic effects[f]	Comments[g]	Fate
tE 1–1.5 hr	Antagonism of narcotic effects	May cause reversal of analgesia, hypertension, arrhythmias, pulmonary edema, delirium, or withdrawal syndrome (in addicts)	M: Liver E: Kidney
$t_{1/2\alpha}$ 3–4 min tE 1.3 hr Anephric: tE 3 hr	Cholinesterase inhibition	May cause bradycardia, hypotension, CNS stimulation or depression, GI cramps, or cholinergic crisis Cautious use with fragile bowel or bowel anastomoses	M: Liver E: Kidney
$t_{1/2\alpha}$ 2.5–3 hr tE 4–5 hr	Blockade of slow calcium channels in heart Systemic and coronary vasodilatation and increase in myocardial perfusion	May cause reflex tachycardia, GI upset, or mild negative inotropic effects Little effect on automaticity and atrial conduction May be useful in asymmetrical septal hypertrophy Drug solution is light sensitive	M: Liver E: Liver, kidney
	Formation of metHb, which can then bind with cyanide	May cause hypotension May decrease O_2-carrying capacity of Hb by formation of metHb	

Table A-1 (continued)

Generic and trade names[a]	Uses	Dose[b]	Onset[c,d]	Duration[d]
Nitroglycerin (glycerol trinitrate, Nitrostat, Nitrol)	Myocardial ischemia Esophageal spasm Biliary colic CHF Hypertension Pulmonary hypertension	Infusion mix: 30–50 mg in 250 ml 5% D/W IV: Infusion initially at 10 μg/min, then titrated vs. patient response Sublingual: 0.15–0.6 mg/dose Topical: 2% ointment 0.5–5 inches q4–8h	IV: 1–2 min SL: 1–3 min PO: 1 hr Topical: 30–60 min	IV: 10 min SL: 30 min PO: 8–12 hr Topical: 3 hr
Nitroprusside (Nipride)	Hypertension Induction of deliberate hypotension CHF Pulmonary hypertension	Infusion mix: 30–50 mg in 250–1000 ml 5% D/W IV: Infusion initially at 0.1 μg/kg/min, then titrated vs. patient response to max. 10 μg/kg/min (total dose < 1–1.5 mg/kg over 2–3 hr)	IV: Rapid	IV: 1–10 min
Norepinephrine (Levarterenol, Levophed)	Hypotension	Infusion mix: 4 mg in 250 ml 5% D/W IV: Infusion initially at 1–8 μg/min, then titrated vs. patient response	IV: Rapid	IV: 1–2 min
Oxytocin (Pitocin, Syntocinon)	Postpartum hemorrhage Induction of labor Oxytocin challenge	Infusion mix: 10–40 U in 1000 ml crystalloid For postpartum hemorrhage: IV: Infusion at	IV: < 1 min IM: 3–7 min	IV: < 60 min IM: 30–60 min

Half-Life[e]	Pharmacologic effects[f]	Comments[g]	Fate
tE 1.9 min	Smooth muscle relaxation, resulting in favorable redistribution of coronary blood flow, coronary vasodilatation, bronchodilatation, and biliary, GI, and GU tract relaxation	May cause reflex tachycardia, hypotension, headache Tolerance and dependence with chronic use May be absorbed by plastic in IV tubing	M: Smooth muscle, liver
	Smooth muscle relaxation	May cause excessive hypotension, reflex tachycardia, or decrease in the thyroid iodine uptake Can accumulate cyanide in the presence of liver dysfunction and can accumulate thiocyanate in the presence of renal dysfunction Prolonged therapy can be associated with hypothyroidism, increase in plasma cyanide, and thiocyanate Avoid with Leber's hereditary optic atrophy, tobacco amblyopia, severe liver or renal disease, hypothyroidism, or vitamin B_{12} deficiency	M: RBC and tissues → HCN, then to liver → thiocyanate (half-life 1 wk) (0.44 mg cyanide/mg nitroprusside) E: Kidneys
	α- and β-adrenergic stimulation (mostly α)	May cause hypertension, arrhythmias, myocardial ischemia, increased uterine contractility, constricted microcirculation, or CNS stimulation	M: Liver, nerve endings E: Kidney
tE 1–5 min	Oxytocic effects, e.g., uterine contraction, milk release Renal, coronary, and cerebral vasodilatation Reduction of postpar-	May cause uterine tetany and rupture, fetal distress, or anaphylaxis IV bolus can cause hypotension, tachycardia, arrhythmias	M: Liver, kidney, mammary glands E: Kidney (small

Table A-1 (continued)

Generic and trade names[a]	Uses	Dose[b]	Onset[c,d]	Duration[d]
	test	rate necessary to control atony IM: 10 U after delivery of placenta		
Pancuronium (Pavulon)	Neuromuscular blockade	IV (intubation): 0.08–0.1 mg/kg	IV: 1–3 min	IV: 35–55 min
Pentobarbital (Nembutal)[i]	Sedation	IV: 1 mg/kg slowly; wait 1 min, and titrate slowly up to 500 mg or desired effect IM: 100–200 mg PO: 100–200 mg	IV: 1 min IM: 10–30 min PO: 30–60 min	IV: 15 min IM: 2–3 hr PO: 3–4 hr
Phenoxybenzamine (Dibenzyline)	Hypertension from catecholamine excess Vasospasm Malignant hyperreflexia	PO: 10–200 mg/day (start at 10 mg/day and increase dosage by 10 mg/day every 4 days prn)	PO: 2 hr	
Phentolamine (Regitine)	Hypertension from catecholamine excess Vasospasm Pulmonary hypertension Extravasation of α-agonist	For catecholamine excess states: IV: 2–5 mg prn BP rise IV/IM: 2–5 mg 1–2h preop PO: 50 mg q6–8h For extravasation of α-agonist: Into affected area: 5–10 mg in 10 ml NSS within 12 hr For pulmonary hypertension: LD: 0.1 mg/kg at < 0.5 mg/min MD: Infusion: 1–2 μg/kg/min	IV: 1–2 min IM: 15–20 min	IV: 10–13 min IM: 3–4 hr

Half-Life[e]	Pharmacologic effects[f]	Comments[g]	Fate
	tum blood loss		amount)
$t_{1/2\alpha}$ 5 min tE 1–2 hr	Nondepolarizing competitive blockade of the neuromuscular junction	May cause tachyarrhythmias or hypertension from mild indirect sympathomimetic effects	M: Liver (partial) E: Kidney (mostly), liver
tE 20–50 hr	CNS depression	May cause hypotension, hiccoughs, laryngospasm, or respiratory depression May antagonize oral anticoagulants Exacerbates porphyria Crosses placenta	M: Liver E: Kidney (mostly), liver
tE 24 hr	Noncompetitive α-adrenergic antagonism	May cause hypotension (which may be refractory to norepinephrine) or tachycardia Accumulates in fat	E: Liver, kidney
tE 19 min (1 subject)	Competitive α-adrenergic antagonism, resulting in vasodilatation	May cause hypotension, reflex tachycardia, arrhythmias, stimulation of GI tract, or hypoglycemia	

Table A-1 (continued)

Generic and trade names[a]	Uses	Dose[b]	Onset[c,d]	Duration[d]
Phenyleph-rine (Neo-Syn-ephrine)	Hypotension Systemic va-sodilata-tion Supraven-tricular tachycar-dia Nasal congestion	Infusion mix: 10–30 mg in 250 ml 5% D/W IV: Infusion initially at 10 μg/min, then titrated vs. patient response IV bolus: 100–500 μg/dose Topical nasal: 0.125%–1% solution	IV: Rapid	IV: 5–20 min
Phenytoin (di-phenylhy-dantoin, Di-lantin)	Seizures Digoxin-in-duced ar-rhythmias Refractory VT Tic doulou-reux	For seizures: IV: LD 2–5 mg/kg at < 50 mg/min (up to 1000 mg, cautiously, with ECG monitoring) PO: MD: 300–600 mg/day in 3 divided doses For neurosurgical prophylaxis: IV/IM: 100–200 mg q4h (IV < 50 mg/min) For arrhythmias: IV: 100 mg at < 50 mg/min q10–15 min until ar-rhythmia is abolished, side effects occur, or 10–15 mg/kg is given	IV: 3–5 min IM: Vari-able	IV/IM/PO: Variable
Physostig-mine (eser-ine, Antili-rium)	Postop delir-ium Tricyclic an-tidepres-sant over-dose Reversal of CNS ef-fects of an-ticholi-nergic drugs	For postop delir-ium IV: 0.5–2 mg q15min prn	IV/IM: 3–8 min	IV/IM: 30 min–5 hr

Half-Life[e]	Pharmacologic effects[f]	Comments[g]	Fate
	α-Adrenergic stimulation with small degree of induced release of norepinephrine	May cause hypertension, bradycardia, constricted microcirculation, uterine contraction, or uterine vasoconstriction	M: Liver, intestine
$t_{1/2\alpha}$ 38 min tE 7–42 hr	Anticonvulsant effect Antiarrhythmic effects similar to those of quinidine or procainamide	May cause nystagmus, diplopia, ataxia, drowsiness, gingival hyperplasia, GI upset, hyperglycemia, or hepatic microsomal enzyme induction IV bolus may cause bradycardia, hypotension, respiratory arrest, cardiac arrest, CNS depression Tissue irritant Erratic IM absorption Crosses placenta Significant interpatient variation in dose needed to achieve TL tE increases as plasma level increases TL = 7.5–20 µg/ml	M: Liver E: Kidney (< 2% unchanged)
tE 30–60 min	Inhibition of cholinesterase, resulting in central and peripheral cholinergic effects	May cause bradycardia, tremor, hallucinations, psychiatric or CNS depression, mild ganglionic blockade, or cholinergic crisis Crosses BBB	M: Acetylcholinesterase (incompletely understood) E: Kidney

Table A-1 (continued)

Generic and trade names[a]	Uses	Dose[b]	Onset[c,d]	Duration[d]
Phytonadione (Aqua-MEPHY-TON)	Deficiency of vitamin K-dependent clotting factors	IV: 2.5–25 mg at ≤ 1 mg/min IM/SQ/PO: 2.5–25 mg If 8 hr after IV/IM/SQ dose, PT is not improved, repeat dose prn	IV: 15 min IM: 1–2 hr PO: 6–12 hr	IV/IM: Normal PT in 12–14 hr

Procainamide (Pronestyl)	Atrial and ventricular arrhythmias
	Malignant hyperthermia
		For arrhythmias:
		IV:
		  LD: 10–50 mg/min until toxicity or desired effect occurs up to 12 mg/kg. Stop if ≥ 50% QRS widening or PR lengthening
		  MD: Infusion at 2 mg/kg/hr
		IM:
		  LD: 6–12 mg/kg
		  MD: 6 mg/kg q3–8h
		PO:
		  LD: 12 mg/kg
		  MD: 6 mg/kg q3h
		For malignant hyperthermia:
		IV: Up to 10 mg/kg at ≤ 10–50 mg/kg. Stop if ≥ 50% QRS widening or PR prolongation
			IV: < 5 min
			IM: < 15 min
			PO: 15–30 min
				IV/IM/PO: 3 hr

Prochlorperazine (Compazine)	Nausea and vomiting	For nausea and vomiting: IV: 5–10 mg/dose (≤ 40 mg/day) IM: 5–10 mg q2–4h prn (<	IV: Rapid IM: 10–20 min PR: 60 min PO: 30–40 hr	IM/PR/PO: 3–4 hr

Half-Life[e]	Pharmacologic effects[f]	Comments[g]	Fate
$t_{1/2\alpha}$ 20 min tE 2–2.5 hr	Promotion of synthesis of clotting factors II, VII, IX, X	Excessive dose can make patient refractory to further oral anticoagulation May fail with hepatocellular disease IV administration occasionally causes hypotension, fever, diaphoresis, bronchospasm, anaphylaxis, or pain at injection site Crosses placenta	
$t_{1/2\alpha}$ 5 min tE 2–4 hr (active metabolites: tE 6 hr) Anephric: tE 6–10 hr	Antiarrhythmic effect	May cause increased ventricular response in atrial tachyarrhythmias, asystole (with AV block), CNS excitement, SLE syndrome, or liver damage IV administration can cause QRS widening and PR prolongation on the ECG or hypotension from vasodilatation Decrease LD by ⅓ in CHF or shock IM injection painful Hypotensive response may be accentuated with general anesthesia TL = 4–8 mg/L	M: Liver, plasma (to active metabolite) E: Kidney
	Similar to those of chlorpromazine, with more antiemetic and fewer sedative effects	May cause hypotension (especially when given IV), extrapyramidal reactions, or cholestatic jaundice	

Table A-1 (continued)

Generic and trade names[a]	Uses	Dose[b]	Onset[c,d]	Duration[d]
		40 mg/day) PR: 25 mg q12h prn PO: 5–10 mg q6–8h prn		
Promethazine (Phenergan)	Nausea, vomiting Allergies Sedation	IV/IM/PO: 12.5–50 mg q4–6h prn *0.25 mg/kg child*	IV: 3–5 min IM/PO: 20 min	IM/PO: 4–6 hr
Propranolol (Inderal)	Atrial and ventricular arrhythmias Myocardial ischemia Hypertension Hyperthyroidism Migraine headache Hypertrophic cardiomyopathy	IV: Test dose of 0.25–0.5 mg, then 1–5 mg/dose at ≤ 1 mg/min titrated vs. response PO: 10–40 mg q6–8h, increased prn *Pediatric* IV: 0.05–0.1 mg/kg over 10 min	IV: 2 min PO: 30 min	IV: 1–6 hr PO: 6 hr
Protamine	Reversal of effects of heparin	IV: 1 mg/90 U of lung heparin activity *or* 1 mg/115 U of intestinal heparin activity	IV: 5 min	IV: 2 hr
Pyridostigmine (Regonol, Mestinon)	Reversal of neuromuscular blockade Myasthenia gravis	For reversal of neuromuscular blockade: IV: 0.24 mg/kg (cautiously with an anticholinergic agent)	IV: 2–5 min IM: 15 min PO: 30–45 min	IV: 1–3 hr PO: 3–6 hr

Half-Life[e]	Pharmacologic effects[f]	Comments[g]	Fate
tE 4.4–7 hr	Antagonism of histamine action on H_1 receptors CNS depression Amnesia Antiemetic effect	May cause mild hypotension or mild anticholinergic effects May interfere with blood grouping Intraarterial injection can cause gangrene Relatively free of extrapyramidal effects Crosses placenta	M: Liver E: Kidney, liver
$t_{1/2\alpha}$ 10 min tE 2–5 hr	β-adrenergic blockade	May cause congestive heart failure (unusual in low doses), bradycardia, AV dissociation, bronchospasm (unusual in low doses), drowsiness (in high doses), or hypoglycemia Crosses placenta and BBB	M: Liver E: Kidney, liver
	Formation of protamine-heparin complex	May cause myocardial depression and peripheral vasodilatation with sudden hypotension or bradycardia Protamine-heparin complex antigenically active Transient reversal of heparin may be followed by rebound heparinization Can cause anticoagulation if given in excess relative to amount of circulating heparin (controversial)	
$t_{1/2\alpha}$ 7 min tE 1.9 hr Anephric: $t_{1/2\alpha}$ 4 min tE 6.3 hr	Cholinesterase inhibition	See Neostigmine Does not cross BBB significantly in usual doses	M: Tissue and liver cholinesterases E: Liver, kidney (75%)

Table A-1 (continued)

Generic and trade names[a]	Uses	Dose[b]	Onset[c,d]	Duration[d]
		For myasthenia gravis (individualized): PO: 600 mg–1.5 g/day in divided doses IV/IM: ~ $\frac{1}{30}$ PO dose		
Quinidine gluconate (Quinaglute)	Atrial and ventricular arrhythmias	For acute arrhythmias: IV: 800 mg in 50 ml 5% D/W, giving 300–750 mg at ≤ 16 mg/min (≤ 1 ml/min). Stop IV infusion if 25–50% QRS widening, HR < 120, loss of P waves, or arrhythmia ablated IM: 600 mg, then up to 400 mg q2h as needed for arrhythmia control	IV: 4–6 min IM: 15 min PO: 1–3 hr	PO: 6–8 hr
Quinidine sulfate	Atrial and ventricular arrhythmias	For arrhythmias: PO: 200–600 mg q6–8h	PO: 1–3 hr	PO: 6–8 hr
Ranitidine (Zantac)	Duodenal ulcers Reduction of gastric volume and raising of pH (pulmonary aspiration prophylaxis)	IV/IM: 50–100 mg q6–8h PO: 100–300 mg q12h	IV: rapid IM: 15 min PO: 1–3 hr	IV/IM: 6–8 hr PO: 12 hr
Ritodrine (Yutopar)	Premature labor	IV (continuous infusion): Mix 150 mg in 5% D/W, infuse 0.10–0.35 mg/min PO: 10–20 mg q4–6h to a maximum of 120 mg/day	IV: < 10 min PO: 30–60 min	

Half-Life[e]	Pharmacologic effects[f]	Comments[g]	Fate
$t_{1/2\alpha}$ 7 min tE 3–7 hr	Antiarrhythmic effect	May cause hypotension (from vasodilatation and negative inotropic effects), increased ventricular response in atrial tachyarrhythmias, AV block, CHF, mild anticholinergic effects, increase in serum digoxin level, cinchonism, or GI upset May potentiate action of oral anticoagulants IM injection painful, with erratic absorption TL = 3–6 mg/L	M: Liver E: Kidney (15–40% unchanged)
tE 5 hr Anephric: 4–14 hr	See Quinidine gluconate	See Quinidine gluconate	M: Liver E: Kidney
tE: 2–3 hr	Histamine H_2-receptor antagonist Inhibits basal, nocturnal, and stimulated gastric acid secretion	Doses should be reduced by half with renal failure	M: Liver E: Kidney
IV: tE 2–2.5 hr IV/PO: tE 12 hr	β_2-selective adrenergic receptor agonist which inhibits uterine contractility Dose-related increases in maternal and fetal heart rate and blood pressure Crosses the placenta	Pulmonary edema may occur, particularly in patients also given corticosteroids Potentiation of cardiovascular effects by magnesium sulfate, potent volatile general anesthetics, parasympatholytics (e.g., atropine)	E: Kidney (70–90% unchanged)

Table A-1 (continued)

Generic and trade names[a]	Uses	Dose[b]	Onset[c,d]	Duration[d]
Scopolamine (hyoscine[i])	Antisial- agogue Amnesia and sedation	IV/IM/SQ: 0.3– 0.6 mg	IV: 1 min	
Secobarbital (Seconal[i])	Sedation Seizures	For sedation: IV: 50 mg/15 sec until de- sired effect or 250 mg given IM: 100–200 mg PO: 100–200 mg	IV: 1–3 min IM: 7–10 min PO: 15–30 min	IV: 15 min IM: 3–4 hr PO: 3–4 hr
Succinyl- choline (Anectine)	Induction of neuromus- cular blockade	IV: 1–1.5 mg/kg *Pediatric* IV: 1–1.5 mg/ kg IM: 2–4 mg/kg	IV: 30–60 sec IM: 2–3 min	IV: 10–15 min IM: 10–30 min
Sufentanil (Sufenta[h,i])	Pain Induction of general anesthesia	IV (adjunct to balanced anesthesia): 0.2–0.8 μg/kg	< 1 min	IV: vari- able

Half-Life[e]	Pharmacologic effects[f]	Comments[g]	Fate
		Contains sulphur and thus may cause serious allergic reactions, including anaphylaxis	
		Contraindicated in eclampsia, pulmonary hypertension, hyperthyroidism	
	Anticholinergic effect CNS depression	May cause excitement or delirium, tachycardia, hyperthermia, or mild antiemetic effect	E: Kidney (partly unchanged)
		Crosses BBB and placenta	
tE 20–28 hr	CNS depression	See Pentobarbital	M: Liver E: Kidney
	Depolarizing neuromuscular blockade	May cause arrhythmias, myoglobinuria, transient muscarinic and nicotinic stimulation, slight increase in intraocular and intragastric pressures, myotonic response in myotonia congenita and myotonia dystrophica, prolonged blockade with pseudocholinesterase deficiency, phase II block (esp. with infusion), or increase in serum K^+ (0.5–1.0 mEq normally)	M: Blood pseudocholinesterase E: Kidney (2% unchanged)
		Accentuated K^+ release may occur with burns, massive tissue trauma, paralysis, muscular dystrophy, Guillain-Barré syndrome, etc.	
$t_{1/2\alpha}$ 10–13 min tE 2.5–3 hr	Similar to those of morphine, but with minimal cardiovascular depression	Dose-related muscle rigidity and bradycardia	M: Liver, small intestine E: Kidney

Table A-1 (continued)

Generic and trade names[a]	Uses	Dose[b]	Onset[c,d]	Duration[d]
		(induction of general anesthesia): 10–30 μg/kg		
Terbutaline (Brethine, Bricanyl)	Bronchospasm Premature labor	For bronchospasm: SQ: 0.25 mg. Repeat in 15 min prn (use < 0.5 mg/4 hr) PO: 2.5–5.0 mg q6h (< 15 mg/day) *Pediatric* SQ: 3.5–5.0 μg/kg	SQ: < 15 min PO: < 30 min	SQ: 1.5–4 hr PO: 4–8 hr
Thiopental[i] (thiopentone, Pentothal)	Induction of hypnosis or sedation Intracranial hypertension	IV: 1–4 mg/kg (2.5% solution) or infusion, 1000 mg in 250 ml 5% D/W, titrated to desired effect	IV: Rapid	IV: 10–15 min
Thiosulfate, sodium	Cyanide poisoning	IV: 12.5 gm in 50 ml 5% D/W infused over 10 min *Pediatric* 7 g/m² (about 200 mg/kg) (not > 12.5 g)		
Trimethaphan (Arfonad)	Induction of deliberate hypotension Hypertension	Infusion mix: 500 mg in 500 ml 5% D/W IV: 1–4 mg/min × 5–10 min, then titrate vs. patient response (usually about 1 mg/min)	IV: Rapid	IV: 5–20 min
Trimethobenzamide (Tigan)	Nausea and vomiting	IM/PR: 200 mg q6–8h prn PO: 250 mg q6–8h prn	IM: 15 min PO: 20–40 min	IM: 2–3 hr PO: 3–4 hr

Half-Life[e]	Pharmacologic effects[f]	Comments[g]	Fate
tE 7 hr	β-adrenergic stimulation ($\beta_2 > \beta_1$), resulting in bronchodilatation	May cause arrhythmias, hypokalemia, or CNS excitement	M: Liver, intestinal wall E: Kidney
$t_{1/2\alpha}$ 3 min tE 5–10 hr	CNS depression Decrease in cerebral blood flow and intracranial pressure	May cause hypotension (from myocardial depression and peripheral vasodilatation), tachycardia, CHF, respiratory depression, bronchospasm, or anaphylaxis Intraarterial injection can cause gangrene Exacerbates porphyria Crosses placenta	M: Liver E: Kidney
	Combines with CN⁻ to yield thiocyanate	Give with sodium nitrite	E: Kidney
	Ganglionic blockade	May cause prolonged hypotension (especially with high doses), histamine release, bronchospasm, mydriasis, or potentiation of the effects of succinylcholine	M: Blood E: Kidney
	Antiemetic effect	May cause hypotension, sedation, extrapyramidal reactions, or mild antihistamine effect	E: Kidney

Table A-1 (continued)

Generic and trade names[a]	Uses	Dose[b]	Onset[c,d]	Duration[d]
d-Tubocurarine (curare)	Neuromuscular blockade	IV (intubation): 0.6 mg/kg	IV: 3–5 min	IV: 30 min
Vasopressin (antidiuretic hormone, Pitressin)	Diabetes insipidus GI bleeding	For diabetes insipidus: IM/SQ: 5–10 U q8–12 h For GI bleeding: IV: 0.1–0.4 U/min		SQ/IM: 48–96 hr (tannate), 2–8 hr (injection)
Vecuronium (Norcuron)	Neuromuscular blockade	IV (intubation): 0.08–0.10 mg/kg	IV: 3–5 min	IV: 25–40 min
Verapamil (Isoptin, Calan)	Supraventricular tachycardia Atrial fibrillation or flutter Wolff-Parkinson-White syndrome Lown-Ganong-Levine syndrome	IV: 5–10 mg (75–150 µg/kg) over ≥ 2-min period. If no response in 30 min, repeat 10 mg (150 µg/kg) *Pediatric* IV (0–1 yr): 0.1–0.2 mg/kg IV (1–15 yr): 0.1–0.3 mg/kg. Repeat dose once if no response in 30 min	IV: 1–10 min PO: 15–30 min	IV: Hemodynamic effects 10–20 min (AV node effects 6 hr)
Warfarin (Coumadin, Panwarfin, Athrombin-k)	Anticoagulation	IV/IM/PO: LD: 40–60 mg (½ in older or debilitated) > 1–3 days MD: 2–10 mg qd Dosage titrated vs. PT	IV/IM: 1–9 hr PO: 2–12 hr	IV/IM/PO: 2–5 days

Half-Life[e]	Pharmacologic effects[f]	Comments[g]	Fate
tE 3 hr	Nondepolarizing competitive blockade of neuromuscular junction	May cause histamine release and transient moderate ganglionic blockade with hypotension, or (rarely) bronchospasm	M: Minimal E: Liver (40%), kidney (60%)
10–20 min	Increase in urine osmolality and decrease in urine volume Smooth muscle contraction, resulting in splanchnic, coronary, muscular, and skin vasoconstriction	May cause water intoxication, hypertension, bradycardia, myocardial ischemia, abdominal cramps (from increased peristalsis), gallbladder, urinary bladder, and uterine contraction, pulmonary edema, oliguria, vertigo, or nausea	M: Liver, kidney E: Kidney
tE 65–75 min	Nondepolarizing competitive blockade of neuromuscular junction	No significant cardiovascular effects	M: Blood E: Liver, kidney
$t_{1/2\alpha}$ 15–30 min tE 5–7 hr	Blockade of slow calcium channels in heart Prolongation of PR and AH intervals with negative inotropy and chronotropy Systemic and coronary vasodilatation	May cause severe bradycardia, tachycardia, AV block, or worsening of CHF (1% incidence of life-threatening tachycardia, bradycardia, asystole, or hypotension)	M: Liver E: Liver, kidney
tE 48 hr	Interference with utilization of vitamin K by the liver, thereby inhibiting synthesis of factors II, VII, IX, X	May cause bleeding Crosses placenta May be potentiated by ethanol, antibiotics, chloral hydrate, cimetidine, dextran, d-thyroxine, diazoxide, ethacrynic acid, glucagon, methyldopa, monoamine oxidase inhibitors, phenytoin, prolonged use of narcotics, quinidine,	M: Liver E: Kidney, intestine

Table A-1 (continued)

Generic and trade names[a]	Uses	Dose[b]	Onset[c,d]	Duration[d]

Half-Life[e]	Pharmacologic effects[f]	Comments[g]	Fate
		sulfonamides, CHF, hyperthermia, liver disease, malabsorption, etc.	
		May be antagonized by barbiturates, chlordiazepoxide, haloperidol, oral contraceptives, hypothyroidism, hyperlipidemia, etc.	

References

American Hospital Formulary Service. *American Hospital Formulary.* Bethesda, Md.: American Society of Hospital Pharmacists, 1981.

Behrman, R. E., and Vaughan, V. C., III. *Nelson Textbook of Pediatrics* (12th ed.). Philadelphia: Saunders, 1983.

Campbell, J. W., and Frisse, M. (eds.). *Manual of Medical Therapeutics* (25th ed.). Boston: Little, Brown, 1983.

DiPalma, J. R. (ed.). *Drill's Pharmacology in Medicine* (4th ed.). New York: McGraw-Hill, 1971.

Gilman, A., et al. (eds.). *The Pharmacological Basis of Therapeutics* (7th ed.). New York: Macmillan, 1980.

Govoni, L. E., and Hayes, J. E. *Drugs and Nursing Implications* (3rd ed.). New York: Appleton-Century-Crofts, 1978.

Graef, J. W., and Cone, T. E., Jr. (eds.). *Manual of Pediatric Therapeutics* (3rd ed.). Boston: Little, Brown, 1984.

Osol, A., et al. (eds.). *Remington's Pharmaceutical Sciences* (16th ed.). Easton, Pa.: Mack Publishing Co., 1980.

Physicians' Desk Reference (41st ed.). Oradell, N.J.: Medical Economics Company, 1987.

Pribor, H. C., Morrell, G., and Scherr, G. H. *Drug Monitoring and Pharmacokinetic Data.* Park Forest South, Ill.: Pathotex, 1980.

Ritschel, W. A. *Handbook of Basic Pharmacokinetics.* Washington, D.C.: Drug Intelligence Publications, 1976.

Shirkey, H. C. *Pediatric Drug Handbook.* Philadelphia: Saunders, 1977.

Index

Index

J.w.s : www.hourglass2.org /